W9-ALW-314

THE ENCYCLOPEDIA OF

THE HEART AND HEART DISEASE

Second Edition

THE ENCYCLOPEDIA OF

THE HEART AND HEART DISEASE

Second Edition

Otelio S. Randall, M.D.
Director of the Howard University Hospital (HUH)
Preventive Cardiology Program

Nathan M. Segerson, M.D.
Director of Clinical Cardiac Electrophysiology,
Kitsap Cardiology Consultants

Deborah S. Romaine

AN AMARANTH BOOK

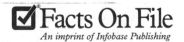
Facts On File
An imprint of Infobase Publishing

The Encyclopedia of the Heart and Heart Disease, Second Edition

Facts On File, Inc.
An imprint of Infobase Publishing, Inc.
132 West 31st Street
New York NY 10001

Library of Congress Cataloging-in-Publication Data
The encyclopedia of the heart and heart disease / Otelio S. Randall, Nathan Segerson,
Deborah S. Romaine. — 2nd ed.
p. ; cm. — (Libnrary of health and living)
"An Amaranth book."
Includes biobliographical references and index.
ISBN-13: 978-0-8160-7751-9 (hardcover : alk. paper)
ISBN-10: 0-8160-7751-7 (hardcover : alk. paper) 1. Heart—Encyclopedias. 2. Heart—Diseases—Encyclopedias. I. Randall,
Otelio Sye, 1937– II. Segerson, Nathan. III. Romaine, Deborah S., 1956– IV. Series: Facts on File library of health and living.
[DNLM: 1. Heart—Encyclopedias—English. 2. Heart Diseases—Encyclopedias—English. WG 13 E557 2010]
QP111.4.R36 2010
612.1'7—dc22   2009053594

Facts On File books are available at special discounts when purchased in bulk quantities for businesses, associations, institutions, or sales promotions. Please call our Special Sales Department in New York at (212) 967-8800 or (800) 322-8755.

You can find Facts On File on the World Wide Web at http://www.factsonfile.com

Text design by Annie O'Donnell
Composition by Hermitage Publishing Services
Cover printed by Art Print, Taylor, Pa.
Book printed and bound by Maple Press, York, Pa.
Date printed: July 2010

Diagrams from Human Body On File™: Physiology, adapted by Sholto Ainslie

Printed in the United States of America

10 9 8 7 6 5 4 3 2 1

This book is printed on acid-free paper.

In memory of
Walter Kwiczola, one strong heart:
Roses are red, violets are blue,
life is beautiful and so are you.

CONTENTS

FOREWORD

Few people are surprised to hear that heart disease is one of the most common serious health conditions affecting our population. And we can all recite the basic tenets of a heart-healthy lifestyle that have been broadcast for years in homes and schools. Nonetheless, the natural reaction patients have when their doctors first diagnose them with a heart condition is one of shock and unfamiliarity. But gradually, as the intimidation of their diagnosis wears off, the reality of being personally affected by heart disease drives people to a want for knowledge and understanding. In my experience, this is exactly the reaction they should have.

In reality, patients need not live in fear of heart disease. Our understanding of this broad science and our therapies for these diseases have evolved greatly in our generation. No longer should cardiac diagnosis mark the end of active lifestyles. No longer should cardiac patients be controlled by limitations of their disease, when they can instead become knowledgeable partners in their own care and take control of their own heart health. Indeed, as is so often the case, fear can be overcome easily by understanding.

The Encyclopedia of the Heart and Heart Disease, Second Edition provides a unique tool to patients and to students of cardiovascular sciences to better their understanding of the commonest heart conditions. At a glance, this work provides a comprehensive go-to resource for readers to efficiently decode the language of cardiology. But the true value in this work is the context and perspective it provides to more invested readers whose interest may go beyond the mere terminology of a subject. Underneath the veil of unfamiliar vocabulary, those readers will be led to simple and often fascinating concepts about the workings of the human heart that will give direction and focus to their further exploration.

Whether you are personally affected by heart disease, are formally studying cardiac sciences, or perhaps are just intrigued by this topic, I hope this resource inspires your curiosity to go to the next level.

—Nathan M. Segerson, M.D.,
Director of Clinical Cardiac Electrophysiology
Kitsap Cardiology Consultants
Bremerton, Washington

PREFACE

This second edition of *The Encyclopedia of the Heart and Heart Disease* features hundreds of updated and new entries covering the gamut from the latest discoveries in cardiovascular technology to the most effective lifestyle approaches for heart health. Research continues to reveal the secrets of the heart's function, resulting in new ways to connect and even reverse cardiovascular dysfunction and disease. Cardiologists are learning more about how lifestyle factors intersect with genetics, which factors matter more on both sides of the equation, and how the use this knowledge to individualize therapies to treat heart disease as well as more effective preventive measures to help keep the heart healthy and strong.

The immune system has stepped to front and center in unraveling the complexities of conditions such as coronary artery disease (CAD). New medications abound, expanding treatment options for managing blood cholesterol levels, arrhythmias, hypertension, and heart failure. In only five years, automated external defibrillators (AEDs) have move from high-tech novelties to become commonplace in community settings, providing the means for ordinary people to save the lives of heart attack victims. And while nutrition remains a significant dimension of cardiovascular health, the conclusion of several major studies throws a questioning light on the role of nutritional supplements such as antioxidants.

This revised edition of *The Encyclopedia of the Heart and Heart Disease* also features editorial enhancements, such as improved cross-referencing and entry formatting, to make it easier to find related entries. Consistent headings within entries help to focus key information. Entries for cardiovascular conditions include risks and emphasize preventive measures when they exist. Recent studies also affirm that much of cardiovascular disease is preventable through lifestyle choices, so across entries the highlight is on heart *health*.

INTRODUCTION

In every family in the United States, someone is receiving treatment for some form of heart disease—nearly 62 million people. Cardiovascular diseases are the leading causes of death in the United States today, claiming more lives each year than all other conditions combined. They also are the leading causes of disability. There is a wide variety of these diseases. Atherosclerosis and its related diseases account for many of them and for the majority of heart attacks. Atherosclerosis also is the most common cause of renal artery stenosis, which leads to kidney failure. Hypertension is the leading cause of stroke. These conditions affect people of all ages and ethnic backgrounds.

Since 1974 I have worked in cardiac intensive care units at the University of Michigan and at Howard University, and I have seen over and over the ways heart disease changes people's lives. Not just the lives of people who have heart disease, but also the lives of their family members and loved ones. As a cardiologist and as a clinical researcher I have been passionately dedicated throughout my career to a practice of preventive cardiology, working especially in the areas of hypertension and obesity.

Some forms of heart disease develop from causes we cannot prevent, such as congenital heart malformations and heart disease that occurs as a result of genetic mutations. But most heart disease is preventable, and most of the causes of heart disease arise from lifestyle. Smoking, high-fat, high-salt, and high-calorie diets, and physical inactivity, are major cardiovascular risk factors. We now know that obesity is itself an independent risk factor for heart disease, beyond the roles of diet and exercise. Further, we see that most cardiovascular diseases, especially those resulting from diabetes, dyslipidemia, and hypertension, develop over an extended time, which gives us opportunity to halt and even reverse damage. It is clear that, as cliché as it sounds, prevention is the best treatment for heart disease. Though this gives us great hope for eventually eliminating preventable forms of heart disease, it is not so simple or easy for individuals to make the required changes.

Necessity calls for a wide spectrum of different kinds of treatment, including surgical, medical, and behavior modification approaches. We are fortunate in the practice of medicine today that we have available a broad spectrum of pharmacological agents and technological procedures at our disposal. The ways we treat and manage many cardiovascular diseases is vastly different than even just 10 years ago, with results that are little short of miraculous. Yet even with such therapeutic interventions, we are continually learning about the heart and cardiovascular functions and the causes and mechanisms of altered functions.

It is essential to have an invaluable encyclopedia such as this to help clarify the many different concepts regarding the heart in health and in disease that have evolved and continue to evolve. There are many people building their foundation of heart knowledge for various personal or professional reasons; for each of them this encyclopedia presents a readily available and accessible source on what we know about the heart, as well as where our knowledge is headed. For students of medical technology, nursing, pharmacy, and even medicine, this encyclopedia presents useful, current, and reliable research. For people who want to reduce their risk of heart disease or who have heart disease, this encyclopedia facilitates further learning and brings much-needed context and understanding. *The Encyclopedia of the Heart and Heart Disease* is a very important volume in the Facts On File Library of Health and Living series, one that will appeal greatly to *all* of its users, prompting successful investigations on all questions of, and yielding authoritative information on all matters of, the heart.

—Otelio S. Randall, M.D.
Professor of Internal Medicine
Director of the Howard University Hospital (HUH)
Preventive Cardiology Program
Howard University Hospital
Washington, D.C.

ENTRIES A–Z

abdominal aortic aneurysm A bulging or ballooning of the aorta in the abdomen, most commonly just below the renal arteries (the arteries that supply BLOOD to the kidneys). The aorta is the body's largest artery and is the primary conduit carrying oxygenated blood from the HEART into the body. The abdominal aorta travels from the heart down through the abdomen to the point below the kidneys where it branches into the two iliac arteries that give rise to the femoral arteries that supply blood to the pelvis and legs. In an adult, the abdominal aorta is about one inch in diameter. An aneurysm exists when any point along the aorta becomes enlarged by 50 percent or more of the normal diameter. This enlargement can take the form of a gradual bulging or a prominent split in the wall of the artery. Once an aneurysm manifests, it will not get better on its own.

Symptoms and Diagnostic Path

Most abdominal aortic aneurysms have no symptoms until their diameter exceeds 4 centimeters (about an inch and a half), when they can be detected during routine physical exams. When symptoms are present, they might include:

- A bulging around the belly button, usually to one side or the other (most often to the left)
- Abdominal pulsations
- Pain in the abdomen
- Pain in the middle of the back (in the region of the kidneys)

Tests such as ULTRASOUND or COMPUTED TOMOGRAPHY (CT) SCAN can confirm a suspected abdominal aortic aneurysm. The larger the aneurysm becomes the faster it enlarges, generally spreading along the length of the aorta as well as expanding in diameter. The greatest risk with aneurysm is that it will rupture, causing life-threatening internal bleeding. Undetected aneurysms that rupture cause 15,000 deaths in the United States every year. A rupturing aneurysm can develop a slow leak, in which it oozes blood, or "blow out" in much the same fashion as a bicycle inner tube. A major rupture is a significant threat to life that requires immediate emergency surgery.

Treatment Options and Outlook

Surgical repair of an abdominal aortic aneurysm involves "patching" the weakened artery wall with an autograft (tissue from the person's body, such as a segment of a less significant artery) or with a synthetic material. Because this repair is major surgery that involves cutting open the abdomen, recovery typically takes six to eight weeks.

Risk Factors and Preventive Measures

Often the cause of abdominal aortic aneurysm remains unknown. Family history of aneurysm, untreated or uncontrolled HYPERTENSION (high BLOOD PRESSURE), ARTERIOSCLEROSIS (accumulation of plaque within the walls of the arteries), and cigarette smoking increase the risk for abdominal aneurysm. Sometimes there is a congenital defect in the aorta that causes weakness or vulnerability in the artery's structure. Lifestyle practices to reduce the risk for CARDIOVASCULAR DISEASE (CVD), appropriate treatment for CVD that does develop, and not smoking are the most effective measures to lower the risk for abdominal aortic aneurysm.

See also BRAIN ANEURYSM; CARDIOVASCULAR SYSTEM; ENDOCARDITIS; MARFAN SYNDROME; MYOCARDITIS; SURGERY TO TREAT CARDIOVASCULAR DISEASE.

ablation A method to permanently destroy small areas of cells to alter the way they conduct electrical impulses. Ablation is usually done as a cardiac catheterization procedure and may use extreme cold (cryoablation), extreme heat (RADIOFREQUENCY ABLATION), or laser. Radiofrequency ablation is the most commonly used. Ablation is an effective treatment for many kinds of ARRHYTHMIAS.

Procedure

Ablation is typically an outpatient procedure performed at a hospital or cardiac catheterization center. It is done with the person under sedation and requires fasting (no food or drink) for eight hours before the scheduled procedure, as well as someone to take the person home after the procedure. The cardiologist first inserts a catheter into a central vein such as the femoral vein in the groin and threads it into the HEART using FLUOROSCOPY to guide the catheter to the desired location. The cardiologist uses the catheter to deliver the ablative energy, which creates a very small wound to the area. When the wound heals, the scar tissue is unable to conduct electricity.

Risks and Complications

Any invasive procedure carries the risk for infection and bleeding. Because ablation involves the insertion of a catheter into the heart, there is also risk for inadvertent damage to BLOOD vessels or the heart itself, as well as a risk for heart attack. However, in ablation these risks are very low. The main complication is that the procedure fails to achieve the desired effect and the arrhythmia persists or returns or new arrhythmias develop.

Outlook and Lifestyle Modifications

When it is successful, ablation fully resolves the arrhythmia and there is no further need for medication, if the person had been taking ANTIARRHYTHMIA MEDICATIONS. Most people fully recover from the ablation procedure within a few days and without any residual effects and can return to their usual activities. Regular monitoring is important, however, to make sure other arrhythmias do not develop.

See also PACE MAPPING; SURGERY TO TREAT CARDIOVASCULAR DISEASE.

accelerated idioventricular rhythm (AIVR) An ARRHYTHMIA in which ECTOPIC BEATS cause a ventricular HEART RATE that is faster than normal but not so fast as to be classified TACHYCARDIA (heart rate at rest does not exceed 100 beats per minute). Accelerated idioventricular rhythm commonly accompanies underlying HEART DISEASE such as MYOCARDIAL INFARCTION (MI), though it also can occur as a consequence of DIGITALIS TOXICITY.

Symptoms and Diagnostic Path

AIVR does not usually cause symptoms, but rather is identified on ELECTROCARDIOGRAM (ECG) during evaluation for possible MI or in the period of recovery following treatment for MI. The ECG provides the necessary information to make the diagnosis. Factors that help to distinguish AIVR from other arrhythmias include present or recent MI, recent treatment with THROMBOLYTIC MEDICATIONS ("clot busters"), recent ANGIOPLASTY or CORONARY ARTERY BYPASS GRAFT (CABG), and treatment with DIGOXIN. Because AIVR is nearly always associated with MI, diagnostic blood tests to measure CARDIAC ENZYMES and ELECTROLYTE levels also help to confirm the diagnosis. When there are questions about whether another arrhythmia might be involved, additional diagnostic procedures might include ELECTROPHYSIOLOGY STUDIES (EPS).

Treatment Options and Outlook

Most often, AIVR itself does not require treatment and typically goes away with recovery from the underlying HEART DISEASE (which doctors call self-terminating). However, treatment for the underlying heart disease may include a combination of surgical and medical therapies. When the cause of the AIVR is digitalis toxicity, treatment is adjustment of the digoxin dose and close monitoring of digoxin levels in the blood to maintain a therapeutic level or switching to a different medication. Occasionally other arrhythmias may develop as a consequence of damage to the heart from the MI; these will require appropriate treatment.

Risk Factors and Preventive Measures

AIVR develops as a response to other heart conditions, so the risk factors and preventive measures that apply are those for cardiovascular disease in general. People who have dilated CARDIOMYOPATHY or CONGENITAL HEART DISEASE may also develop AIVR. Most people with these conditions are already receiving regular cardiology testing and monitoring for arrhythmias and other complications.

See also ACCESSORY PATHWAY; DIGOXIN IMMUNE FAB; LIVING WITH HEART DISEASE.

accessory pathway An abnormal, extraneous route of conductivity in the HEART. An accessory pathway allows direct electrical connectivity between the atria and the ventricles, the heart's upper and lower chambers respectively. Accessory pathways are common causes of ARRHYTHMIAS.

In the normal conduction pathway of the healthy heart, a specialized cluster of cells called the ATRIO-VENTRICULAR (AV) NODE serves as a "breaker" to interrupt the flow of electrical impulses from the atria (the heart's upper chambers) to the ventricles (the heart's lower chambers. This slight delay allows the atria to completely empty and the ventricles to completely fill with BLOOD. Accessory pathways bypass the AV node, allowing electrical impulses to flow directly between the atria and the ventricles. They may also allow areas of cells in the heart other than the heart's natural PACEMAKER, the SINOATRIAL (SA) NODE, to initiate the electrical impulse that sets the contraction of the heart in motion, altering the flow and pattern of electrical impulses in ways that often cause the heart's chambers to contract out of synchronization. These altered patterns cause arrhythmias, notably tachycardias (very rapid HEART RATE). The most common arrhythmia disorder associated with accessory pathways is WOLFF-PARKINSON-WHITE SYNDROME.

Accessory pathways are often present from birth as congenital defects, though they may not be detected until adulthood. Rarely, they are associated with other congenital deformities of the heart's structure such as EBSTEIN'S ANOMALY. Accessory pathways are a frequent cause of supraventricular TACHYCARDIAS (SVT), significant arrhythmias that require treatment. Accessory pathways can be classified by their anatomic locations. Common locations include:

- Left-sided pathways. This location connects the left atrium and the left ventricle and is the most

commonly seen accessory pathway. Because access to this location can sometimes be difficult, ABLATION treatment poses some additional risk.

- Anteroseptal accessory pathway. Because this location is very close to the natural conduction pathway of the heart (the AV node), treatment is very likely to require a pacemaker. This accessory pathway is usually seen in the context of Wolff-Parkinson-White syndrome.

- Atriofascicular pathways, which exist between the conductive tissue of the atrium directly into the His-Purkinje system. Because of their connection to the specialized conduction system, these pathways do not change the electrical activation of the ventricle and cannot be detected on a standard ECG. However, they can facilitate SVT.

- Fasciculoventricular accessory pathways, which exist between the His-Purkinje system and the ventricles and are often multiple. These pathways are usually congenital but rarely cause arrhythmias.

- Posteroseptal accessory pathways usually connect the right atrium and the left ventricle and are usually congenital.

- Subepicardial accessory pathways, which exist within the epicardium (the outer layer of the heart muscle), are often seen in association with coronary sinus aneurysms (abnormal dilation in the main vein of the heart).

The usual remedy for accessory pathways is cardiac ablation, a catheter-based procedure that destroys the aberrant cells and restores the heart's normal electrical activation.

See also AGING, CARDIOVASCULAR CHANGES AS A RESULT OF; CONDUCTION SYSTEM; HEART BLOCK; LOWN-GANONG-LEVINE SYNDROME; RADIOFREQUENCY ABLATION; REENTRY; SURGERY TO TREAT CARDIOVASCULAR DISEASE.

Accupril See QUINAPRIL.

acebutolol A BETA ANTAGONIST MEDICATION taken to treat HYPERTENSION (high BLOOD PRESSURE).

Acebutolol blocks both beta-1 and beta-2 adrenergic receptors to regulate the strength and rhythm of the HEART's contractions and sometimes is prescribed to treat PREMATURE VENTRICULAR CONTRACTIONS (PVCs). Physicians sometimes prescribe acebutolol in combination with other medications, particularly DIURETIC MEDICATIONS (water pills), for mild to moderate hypertension and in combination with other ANTIHYPERTENSIVE MEDICATIONS for moderate to serious hypertension.

Acebutolol, like other beta-blockers, can cause undesired side effects such as FATIGUE and ERECTILE DYSFUNCTION. It can interact with a number of other drugs that alter its effectiveness, most common among them cimetidine (Tagamet), ibuprofen (Advil or Motrin), and penicillin. Because of metabolic changes that take place with aging, older people are more sensitive to the effects of acebutolol and other beta-blockers and generally should start with a lower dose until the response is known. Acebutolol is sold in the United States under the brand name Sectral.

See also ALPHA ANTAGONIST MEDICATIONS; EXERCISE; LIFESTYLE AND HEART HEALTH.

ACE inhibitor medications See ANGIONTENSIN-CONVERTING ENZYME INHIBITOR MEDICATIONS.

acetaminophen An over-the-counter medication taken to relieve pain and reduce fever. There are numerous brand names available; the most recognizable is Tylenol. Research studies conducted in the late 1990s suggest that taking therapeutic doses of acetaminophen helps to lower low-density lipoprotein levels, or "bad" cholesterol, in the BLOOD. In these studies, acetaminophen appeared also to have an ANTIOXIDANT effect, helping to limit damage to the HEART following HEART ATTACK and in conditions such as cardiac ISCHEMIA, in which oxygen supply to the heart becomes restricted. However, a 2006 study determined that acetaminophen does not affect blood flow, heart function, blood pressure, or damage to the heart. It does safely reduce fever, however. Clinical studies continue to explore these effects.

Researchers are also investigating whether using acetaminophen to lower fever in people who have suffered strokes can improve their odds for surviving. Fever following stroke is one measure of the stroke's severity. Research continues to explore whether attempting to prevent fever with medications such as acetaminophen can have a beneficial effect.

See also ASPIRIN; CHOLESTEROL, BLOOD; NSAIDs

activities of daily living (ADLs) An objective assessment of a person's ability to carry out the common functions and tasks of everyday life, and a measure of the extent to which HEART DISEASE limits this ability. Clinicians use ADLs to assess recovery from HEART ATTACK (myocardial infarction), heart surgery, and STROKE, measuring short-term progress (including the effectiveness of treatments such as medication) as well as long-term recovery and independence. ADLs also help determine the level of disability a person has as a result of heart disease, and whether and when a person is capable of returning to work.

There are a number of assessment tools to measure ADLs for cardiac status (including stroke), among them the New York Health Association (NYHA) classification system, Motor Assessment Scale (MAS) for stroke, Sunnaas Index of ADL, and Nottingham Health Profile. Some of these measure general ADL capabilities and others correlate ADLs to the degree of heart disease or residual damage that is present. In general, an ADL assessment evaluates a person's ability in these functions:

- ambulation and mobility
- basic household chores
- cooking and eating
- dressing
- fine motor control
- speech and swallowing
- toileting, bathing, and personal hygiene

Heart disease, particularly chronic conditions such as HEART FAILURE and ANGINA, can limit physical activity, which in turn restricts a person's ability to manage ADLs. When the heart does not pump efficiently, it cannot meet the body's increased demand for oxygen during activity. A person with a chronic heart condition might be able to handle basic ADLs, such as personal hygiene and getting dressed without assistance, but not be able to manage the more extensive physical exertion that household chores such as vacuuming require. Stroke, a form of cardiovascular disease in which damage occurs in the brain instead of the heart, can result in serious and permanent ADL limitations. Stroke can cause paralysis that restricts mobility or interferes with swallowing. It also can damage the brain's speech center, causing various speech problems.

Physical therapy, occupational therapy, and speech pathology can teach methods and techniques to compensate for permanent losses, such as resulting from paralysis following stroke, as well as to preserve existing functions. These supportive therapies can expedite recovery following heart surgery, too, for operations such as CORONARY ARTERY BYPASS GRAFT (CABG) and VALVE REPAIR AND REPLACEMENT, in which most people can expect a prompt and full return to independence as well as for operations such as HEART TRANSPLANT, in which recovery is more extensive and might require some lifestyle modifications. ADAPTIVE EQUIPMENT AND ASSIST DEVICES often can improve a person's level of independence and ability to manage the activities of daily living.

Difficulty with ADLs increases with aging, particularly when other health conditions or impairments related to aging are present, such as osteoarthritis, Parkinson's disease, or Alzheimer's disease. In the elderly, it is essential that the ADL assessment incorporate an overall perspective of the person's well-being as well as the effect of heart disease.

See also AMERICANS WITH DISABILITIES ACT (ADA); APHASIA; DYSPHAGIA.

acupuncture A centuries-old method of treatment in which a trained practitioner inserts very fine needles into specific points on the body. From the Eastern medicine perspective in which acupuncture originated, health is a state of balance, and illness or disease is a state of imbalance of the body's life energy, or chi. Chi flows along invisible energy channels in the body called meridians. These meridians roughly correspond to the body's physical nervous system. Acupuncture points along the meridians correlate to body organs, systems, and functions. These points often are in locations distant from their corresponding organs. For example, acupuncture points in the ear (auricular acupuncture) correlate to various body locations as well as certain areas within the brain related to addiction. Acupuncture is an integral element of traditional Chinese medicine (TCM) and other Eastern systems and is used for both diagnosis and treatment.

Western practitioners have adapted the concepts of acupuncture to Western principles of medicine. From the Western medicine perspective, acupuncture points correlate to locations along the nervous system. Needles inserted in these locations alter nerve impulses and stimulate the release of various chemicals that aid in pain relief and healing. It is likely, although not proven, that acupuncture causes cells to release chemicals called endorphins, the body's natural painkillers. Western practitioners often use mild electrical stimulation, heat, or cold applied to the inserted needles to intensify the acupuncture effect.

The National Institutes of Health (NIH) undertook a review of studies conducted to assess the effectiveness of acupuncture and in 1997 released this consensus statement:

Acupuncture as a therapeutic intervention is widely practiced in the United States. While there have been many studies of its potential usefulness, many of these studies provide equivocal results because of design, sample size, and other factors. The issue is further complicated by inherent difficulties in the use of appropriate controls, such as placebos and sham acupuncture groups. However, promising results have emerged, for example, showing efficacy of acupuncture in adult postoperative and chemotherapy nausea and vomiting and in postoperative dental pain. There are other situations such as addiction, stroke rehabilitation, headache, menstrual cramps, tennis elbow, fibromyalgia, myofascial pain, osteoarthritis, low back pain, carpal tunnel syndrome, and asthma, in which acupuncture may be useful as an adjunct treatment or an acceptable alternative or be included in a comprehensive management program. Further research is likely to uncover additional areas where acupuncture interventions will be useful. (*Acupuncture. NIH Consensus Statement Online 1997 Nov. 3–5; 15 (5): 1–34.*)

Acupuncture and Heart Disease

Studies of acupuncture's effectiveness for heart disease are limited. There are a number of acupuncture points for the heart and for blood pressure. Stimulating these points can improve pain caused by ANGINA (restricted blood flow to the heart) and can lower BLOOD PRESSURE. From the perspective of Western medicine, it does so by stimulating the brain to release ENDORPHINS AND ENKEPHALINS, chemicals that cause blood vessels to relax (dilate) and alter the body's biochemical stress response. This improves blood flow and affects many body functions, including heart rate and breathing rate. For the vast majority of people with heart disease, acupuncture cannot replace the need for medications to regulate blood pressure and other cardiovascular functions and should be an ADJUNCT THERAPY.

Acupuncture and Stroke Recovery

Stroke recovery is among the conditions for which the National Institutes of Health (NIH) has determined acupuncture to be useful as an adjunct therapy (used as part of a comprehensive treatment approach). Acupuncture cannot treat a stroke itself; stroke is a medical emergency that requires immediate conventional medical care. Acupuncture helps to relieve the problems that might follow stroke, such as pain, restricted mobility due to paralysis, and speech impairments. Acupuncture points depend on the nature and location of the problem.

Acupressure and Acumassage

There are two methods of stimulating acupuncture points that can be done without needles—acupressure and acumassage. Generally the effect is not quite as strong, but one advantage is that these methods can be learned for home or self-use. Acupressure uses firm, steady pressure applied with the fingertips over an acupuncture point. Among the most common uses of acupressure are for head-

aches, applying pressure to acupuncture points in the head and neck, and for nausea (particularly motion sickness), applying pressure to an acupuncture point on the inside of the wrist. Acumassage is similar to acupressure but incorporates a gentle massaging motion along with the pressure and generally moves along several acupuncture points rather than staying focused on just one. Acupressure and acumassage are often effective in stimulating heart and chest acupuncture points on the ear, which can help to lower blood pressure, relieve anginal pain, and relieve discomforts during stroke recovery.

Finding a Qualified Acupuncturist

As with any form of therapy or treatment, finding a qualified practitioner is essential. In the United States, most states require some form of training and licensing. In many states only those who are already licensed to practice as some form of healthcare provider—such as physician, chiropractor, dentist, registered nurse, naturopathic physician, TCM practitioner—can obtain a license to practice acupuncture. In a few states, only a physician (medical doctor or doctor of osteopathy) can be so licensed. And in a few states, anyone who completes a minimum training program and passes the licensing test can become an acupuncturist.

Look for an acupuncturist who has both adequate training and experience; who always follows sterile technique (uses sterile, disposable needles, new from the package for each treatment session) to prevent infection from needle-borne pathogens such as hepatitis; and who preferably works frequently with people who have heart disease. Doctors often can recommend qualified acupuncturists within the local community.

See also COMPLEMENTARY THERAPIES; STRESS REDUCTION TECHNIQUES; TAI CHI; YOGA.

acute myocardial infarction   See HEART ATTACK.

Adalat   See NIFEDIPINE.

Adams-Stokes disease   See STOKES-ADAMS DISEASE.

adaptive equipment and assist devices Items and modifications to help people with disabilities to perform common tasks and ACTIVITIES OF DAILY LIVING (ADLS). Adaptive equipment and assist devices are helpful during recovery from a serious health crisis such as HEART ATTACK or STROKE as well as when there is long-term or permanent loss of function. There are many aids and accommodations available to meet a person's specific needs. These include:

- mobility aids such as walkers and wheelchairs
- large button and speaker telephones, voice-activated dialing
- lever-style light switches and sound- or touch-activated lighting and appliances
- lever-style door handles to replace conventional doorknobs
- bed rails and trapeze devices for lifting and turning in bed
- railings in bathrooms, elevated toilet seats, shower chairs, and wide-door showers with no sill for ease in bathing or showering
- clothing that easily slips on and off, slip-on or hook-and-loop closure shoes

Medicare and Medicaid provide limited coverage for certain adaptive equipment such as mobility aids, and private insurance might provide additional coverage. An occupational therapist can evaluate the home environment to make suggestions for improving ease of access and personal safety. Some modifications are easy to make, such as replacing light switches and door handles. Others, such as replacing steps with ramps and installing safety railings, might require professional assistance.

See also AMERICANS WITH DISABILITIES ACT (ADA); CARDIAC REHABILITATION; HEART DISEASE.

adenosine A drug that has several diagnostic and therapeutic applications for CARDIOVASCULAR DISEASE (CVD). Common brand names include Adenocard and Adenoscan. Adenosine is always administered intravenously, with ELECTROCARDIO-GRAM (ECG) monitoring and close medical supervision. It is very short acting in the body and has few side effects.

Diagnostically, adenosine is administered by IV to simulate the changes that take place in the HEART with EXERCISE. It does this by causing the coronary arteries to dilate, which increases BLOOD flow to the heart muscle. An ADENOSINE STRESS TEST is a nuclear imaging study done on an outpatient basis at a hospital. This test is performed to assess CORONARY ARTERY DISEASE (CAD), heart function following heart surgery (including HEART TRANSPLANT), and damage to the heart following MYOCARDIAL INFARCTION (MI).

Therapeutically, adenosine is administered intravenously at a higher dose than when used diagnostically to treat an episode of supraventricular tachycardia (SVT). Adenosine slows the travel of electrical impulses through the ATRIOVENTRICULAR (AV) NODE, a specialized cluster of cells the role of which is to regulate electrical flow between the atria (upper chambers of the heart) and ventricles (lower chambers of the heart). This slows ventricular contractions and may also reestablish the normal CONDUCTION PATHWAY for an extended time. The therapeutic use of adenosine is called pharmacological CARDIOVERSION.

Side effects that may occur during the administration of adenosine include flushing, LIGHT-HEADEDNESS, a sense of pressure in the chest, and, when used therapeutically, anxiety and brief loss of consciousness. Adenosine cannot be administered to a person who takes dipyridamole, a commonly prescribed ANTICOAGULANT MEDICATION. Complications of adenosine cardioversion may include the emergence of other ARRHYTHMIAS. As well, the cardioversion may not last very long, in which case the cardiologist will recommend other treatment options for SVT.

See also ACCESSORY PATHWAY; ANTIARRHYTHMIA MEDICATIONS; DIPYRIDAMOLE STRESS TEST; EXERCISE STRESS TEST; MEDICATIONS TO TREAT HEART DISEASE.

adenosine stress test A diagnostic drug infusion procedure, performed usually for myocardial perfusion imaging, that uses the drug ADENOSINE to simulate the increased flow of BLOOD to the HEART and changes in heart rate and pumping effort as would occur with EXERCISE. Adenosine administered via IV causes the arteries supplying the heart to dilate; a small amount of a radioisotope tracer also injected into the bloodstream allows a gamma camera or magnetic resonance imaging (MRI) to capture images of the changes that take place in the heart. An adenosine stress test requires minimal preparation and recovery and takes four to six hours, although not all of this time is for the test itself. It is a good idea to allow a full day for the test.

Reasons for Doing This Test

An adenosine stress test helps to evaluate CHEST PAIN (ANGINA), occluded (blocked) coronary arteries, damage following MYOCARDIAL INFARCTION (MI), heart function following surgery (including HEART TRANSPLANT), HEART FAILURE, and certain ARRHYTH-MIAS. Most commonly, the cardiologist requests an adenosine stress test for a person who is unable to undergo a traditional EXERCISE STRESS TEST. People who have significant lung disease, such as CHRONIC OBSTRUCTIVE PULMONARY DISEASE (COPD), should discuss the various testing options with their cardiologists, as adenosine can cause worsen breathing problems.

Preparation, Procedure, and Recovery

Preparation for an adenosine stress test requires fasting (no food or drink, including water) for up to eight hours before the scheduled test time, as well as no CAFFEINE or tobacco for 24 and preferably 48 hours before. The caffeine and tobacco restriction is especially important because caffeine and NICOTINE affect the blood vessels and HEART RATE. It might also be necessary to temporarily stop certain medications, notably DIPYRIDAMOLE and theophylline; the cardiologist will make this determination. Upon arriving at the facility for the test, it is necessary to undress from the waist up and put on a hospital gown. A technologist starts one or two IVs for the administration of fluids, the adenosine solution, and the radioisotope injection and also places electrodes on the chest for ELECTROCARDIOGRAM (ECG) monitoring during the test.

Typically, the adenosine stress test begins with administration of the radioisotope solution and imaging of the heart's blood flow at rest. Then the adenosine is administered through the IV over several minutes, followed by another injection of the radioisotope and another session of imaging that shows the heart's blood flow under stress (simulated exercise). The time between the scans varies from one to four hours, during which the person is usually free to walk around and drink fluids (without caffeine) but not eat. After a period of rest to monitor heart activity and make sure ECG, heart rate, and BLOOD PRESSURE are normal, the test is complete and the person may dress and go home. From start to finish the adenosine stress test may take up to six hours.

Risks and Complications

There are very few risks associated with adenosine stress testing. The insertion of the IVs may cause mild discomfort, and the IV sites may be sore or develop bruising after the procedure. Some people become uncomfortable while lying still for the scanning. Some people experience flushing, headache, LIGHT-HEADEDNESS, and a sensation of chest pressure when the adenosine is being administered, and, rarely, cardiac arrhythmias can be induced; these side effects quickly go away after the adenosine solution is finished. Radiation exposure is minimal, about the same as with a chest X-ray. It is important to eat and drink following the procedure to help eliminate the radioisotope from the body.

See also CORONARY ARTERY DISEASE (CAD); DIPYR-IDAMOLE STRESS TEST.

adjunct therapy   Treatment that augments primary treatment for a heart condition, generally focusing on relieving secondary symptoms rather than targeting the cause of the cardiovascular condition. EXERCISE, for example, improves cardiovascular efficiency and general health overall, but it does not directly affect blocked arteries that cause STROKE or ANGINA. Often adjunct therapies accommodate the side effects of primary treatment, as when potassium supplements are taken to offset the potassium depletion that can develop when taking diuretic medications to treat hypertension or HEART FAILURE. Adjunct therapies also can include COMPLEMENTARY THERAPIES such as herbal remedies and ACUPUNCTURE.

See also LIFESTYLE AND HEART HEALTH; MEDICATION MANAGEMENT; MEDICATION SIDE EFFECTS.

adrenaline See EPINEPHRINE.

adrenergic receptor A molecular structure on a cell that can receive, or bind with, the molecular structure of EPINEPHRINE. Adrenergic receptors exist in many types of cells, most predominantly those of smooth muscle such as the walls of the ARTERIES, cardiac myocytes (HEART cells), and walls of other organ structures such as the intestines and the urinary bladder. There also are adrenergic receptors in the lungs and in the brain (central adrenergic receptors). When an adrenergic receptor is activated, it allows certain nerve signals to communicate instructions to other cells. These instructions result in an action on the part of the cell; with smooth muscle cells, the action is to relax or to contract depending on what kind of adrenergic receptor is activated. There are two main types of adrenergic receptors, alpha and beta, each of which has subtypes. Although all adrenergic receptors elicit certain general responses, each subtype regulates specific responses.

Some adrenergic receptors will also bind with NEUROTRANSMITTERS other than epinephrine, such as NOREPINEPHRINE and DOPAMINE. Using drugs to stimulate or block adrenergic receptors generates effects that can treat heart problems, particularly HYPERTENSION.

See also ALPHA ANTAGONIST MEDICATIONS; BETA ANTAGONIST MEDICATIONS.

advance directives Documents providing written instructions regarding treatment decisions should a person become incapacitated and unable to express such desires when care is needed. Advance directives are particularly important with regard to crisis care and end-of-life care decisions. Each state has procedures and processes for completing and implementing advance directives. In most states, two documents comprise advance directives, a living will and a durable power of attorney for health care (DPHC). Local hospitals, medical clinics, physician offices, senior centers and programs, and extended care facilities such as assisted living centers, skilled nursing facilities, and long-term care centers typically have information about advance directives specific to relevant laws, regulations, and procedures to follow to make certain advance directives are valid and are followed if needed.

In most cardiac surgery centers, the admissions process includes a discussion of advance directives. Everyone undergoing heart surgery should have advance directives in place before having surgery. Although heart surgery is safer and more successful than ever, it still involves considerable risk. The best way to make sure treatment for emergencies is consistent with personal preferences is to have those preferences documented in writing and part of the medical record.

Adrenergic Receptor	Tissues	Action/Result
Alpha 1	blood vessels; urinary bladder; penis	contracts muscle fibers; increases blood pressure
Alpha 2	blood vessels; nerve endings in all cells; intestinal walls; liver; platelets	contracts smooth muscle fibers; increases blood pressure; inhibits norepi nephrine release in nerve endings; increases platelet clumping (aggregation)
Beta 1	heart muscle; kidneys	increases force and rate of heart contraction; increases blood pressure
Beta 2	small blood vessels (arterioles) that supply the heart and lungs; bronchial tissues; uterus; skeletal muscle	relaxes muscle fibers; dilates blood vessels; dilates bronchial structures
Beta 3	fat	lipid breakdown

It is important for family members or close friends to know about advance directives and the desires these documents specify. The person most responsible for assisting with care, or who would be most likely to make health-care decisions on the incapacitated person's behalf, should receive copies of advance directive documents. Copies also should go to the physician responsible for care for inclusion in the medical record. A person may always modify or withdraw advance directives. Some states have laws requiring hospitals and other health-care providers to locate free or low-cost legal services to assist patients in understanding and structuring advance directives. It is a Joint Commission on Accreditation of Healthcare Organizations (JCAHO) accreditation standard for hospitals in the United States that the admissions process includes discussion of advance directives.

Living Will

A living will stipulates a person's preferences for medical treatment at the end of life, including whether to initiate or continue CPR (cardiopulmonary resuscitation), lifesaving measures such as mechanical ventilation; and other considerations. The easiest way to prepare a living will is to fill out and sign standardized forms available through many health-care providers, bookstores, and stationery stores. It is important to use forms or documents that follow relevant state laws and procedures. Some states require the signatures of witnesses for a living will to be valid, while others require only the signature of the person completing the living will. The person who signs a living will can change or revoke it at any time, even during a medical crisis when death seems imminent if the person is capable of communicating his or her wishes.

Durable Power of Attorney for Health Care (DPHC)

Durable power of attorney for health-care (DPHC), called health-care proxy in some states, is a legal document that gives one person the right to make medical treatment decisions on behalf of another person. This can be a trusted family member or friend. In most states, it cannot be a doctor, nurse, or other health-care professional unless there is a relationship by blood, adoption, or marriage.

Because DPHC is a legal document, it is more formal than a living will and requires the signatures of two witnesses (in most states). The witnesses typically cannot be the person to whom the DPHC is assigned (sometimes called the health-care agent), although health-care professionals and employees can. It is a good idea to designate a primary and an alternate health-care agent; some DPHC forms require this. A DPHC can be changed simply by replacing it with a revised document. Make sure all copies, including those provided for inclusion with health-care records at the doctor's office and at the hospital, are replaced.

A DPHC assignee, or health-care agent, is authorized to make decisions regarding the person's medical treatment including end-of-life decisions. It is important that this assignee understands the person's desires and is willing to make sure they are followed. These desires might include those expressed in a living will as well as other preferences related to matters such as surgery and emergency medical care. A DPHC covers any circumstance in which the person becomes unable to make his or her own health-care decisions, not just at the end of life. Because it is not possible to anticipate when or how such an inability might occur, it is a good idea to have a DPHC in place in advance.

Do Not Resuscitate (DNR) Orders

Do not resuscitate (DNR) orders are written instructions to health-care personnel saying that no means of life support should be initiated if the person goes into cardiac arrest or other life-threatening state. DNR orders may be freestanding from a living will and typically become a consideration when a person has a serious health circumstance from which recovery is unlikely and in which the person's health situation will not improve as a result of life-sustaining measures.

See also HOSPICE; INFORMED CONSENT.

aerobic capacity The maximum amount of oxygen the body can consume during exercise. The higher the aerobic capacity, the higher the level of aerobic fitness and, in general, the better the state of overall health. Aerobic capacity represents a blend of HEART function and lung function, and is related to overall PHYSICAL FITNESS. Clinicians measure aerobic capacity through various methods; the most common is respirometry, in which a person breathes in and out of a tube connected to a machine that measures the amounts of oxygen and CARBON MONOXIDE in the breath while the person exercises on a treadmill. Respirometry also measures the volume of air that the lungs can take in. Clinicians typically present aerobic capacity in units called METs, or METABOLIC EQUIVALENTS, that derive from a series of mathematical calculations. People with heart disease typically have moderate to pronounced reductions in aerobic capacity, indicating the extent to which there is damage to the heart.

Following a program of regular exercise that is designed to accommodate specific and individual needs can improve cardiac capacity and overall cardiovascular health for most people, even those with HEART DISEASE or those who have had heart attacks (under supervision and guidance of a physician). People who are simply out of shape because they do not get regular physical activity also have reduced aerobic capacity, which they can improve by engaging in a progressive program of regular aerobic exercise. Athletes use strenuous aerobic EXERCISE to extend aerobic capacity for improved athletic performance.

See also FITNESS LEVEL; HEART RATE; LIFESTYLE AND HEART HEALTH; LUNG CAPACITY; NUTRITION AND DIET.

aerobic exercise   See EXERCISE.

African Americans and cardiovascular disease
CARDIOVASCULAR DISEASE, including HEART DISEASE, is a significant health concern among Americans of all ethnicities. For reasons that researchers do not fully understand, however, cardiovascular disease affects some ethnicities disproportionately. While heart disease affects 30 percent of adults of all ethnicities, it affects 40 percent of African Americans. African Americans are at particular risk for HYPERTENSION (high BLOOD PRESSURE) and in fact have one of the highest rates of hypertension in the world. African Americans also are more likely than people of other ethnicities to die from cardiovascular disease.

Hypertension
One in three African Americans has hypertension; health experts estimate that half of those who have hypertension do not know it. Hypertension develops at earlier ages among African Americans than among people of other ethnicities and tends to be more severe at onset as well as to have a more significant progression after diagnosis. African Americans are three times more likely than white Americans to die from hypertension. Hypertension is now second only to diabetes mellitus as the leading cause of kidney disease and kidney failure in African Americans. Hypertension is the leading complication of diabetes, which also disproportionately affects African Americans.

Hypertension can exist independently, but more often it coexists with other forms of heart disease. Most notable are HYPERLIPIDEMIA (elevated blood levels of cholesterol and triglycerides), ATHEROSCLEROSIS (a buildup of PLAQUE, or fatty deposits, along the inside walls of the arteries that narrows and stiffens the arteries), and CORONARY ARTERY DISEASE (CAD; blockage of the arteries that supply the heart). Because hypertension is more prevalent in African Americans, people of African-American heritage should have regular blood pressure checks beginning in early adulthood. Factors such as family history of hypertension and the presence of other risk factors for high blood pressure such as OBESITY and DIABETES determine how frequently blood pressure checks should take place.

If hypertension exists, it is essential to take the prescribed medications and make recommended lifestyle modifications. Lifestyle modifications often are effective in improving blood pressure and sometimes make it possible for people with mild to moderate hypertension to reduce or stop taking antihypertensive medications; this should be done only under a physician's supervision. Suddenly stopping some blood pressure medications can result in serious health problems including "rebound" hypertension in which the blood pressure suddenly shoots dangerously high.

Hyperlipidemia, Atherosclerosis, and Coronary Artery Disease (CAD)

Hyperlipidemia (elevated levels of blood CHO-LESTEROL or TRIGLYCERIDES) affects an estimated 45 percent of African Americans, who tend to have hyperlipidemia at younger ages. Scientists believe the reason is a combination of lifestyle factors, primarily diet and EXERCISE. However, recent research suggests there is a possible genetic component in the function of the body's smallest blood vessels. Hyperlipidemia leads to atherosclerosis, in which excess lipids become deposited along the inner walls of the arteries and narrow the passage through which blood flows. Coronary artery disease exists when atherosclerosis affects the arteries that supply the heart muscle. Restricted blood flow through the coronary arteries causes ANGINA and is a significant risk for heart attack. Blockage of one or more coronary arteries interrupts the flow of blood to the heart, thereby causing heart attack. Coronary artery disease is the primary cause of heart attack.

Lifestyle modifications, including low-fat diet, smoking cessation, and regular EXERCISE, along with medical interventions such as lipid-lowering medications, can improve hyperlipidemia. Over time, these approaches can also improve atherosclerosis. Often surgical intervention such as ANGIOPLASTY or CORONARY ARTERY BYPASS GRAFT (CABG) is necessary to treat coronary artery disease, with lifestyle modifications helpful in preventing its return.

Diabetes

Twice as many African Americans as other ethnicities except Hispanics have type 2 diabetes, although many are undiagnosed. Elevated or significant fluctuations in blood sugar levels cause damage to the sensitive cells of the smallest blood vessels, arterioles and capillaries. This contributes to a cascade of health problems including impaired peripheral circulation (particularly to the feet and hands) and damage to the heart itself. Cardiovascular disease is the leading complication of diabetes; most prevalent are hypertension, atherosclerosis, and coronary artery disease (CAD). Diabetes is the leading cause of kidney disease and kidney failure among African Americans, with the number one cause being hypertension. Appropriate medical intervention and lifestyle modifications are essential to control diabetes.

Heart Attack and Stroke

African Americans between the ages of 35 and 54 are four times more likely than white Americans to have a stroke, and three times more likely between the ages of 55 and 64. At any age, African Americans are twice as likely as people of other ethnicities to die from stroke. This increased risk is due to multiple factors, key among them being the higher rate of hypertension (especially untreated hypertension) and atherosclerosis among African Americans. Cigarette smoking, obesity, and sickle-cell ANEMIA are additional contributing factors. The increased risk for hypertension and coronary artery disease correspondingly increase the risk for heart attack and stroke among African Americans.

Obesity

In 2001 the Centers for Disease Control and the National Institutes of Health released reports identifying that two-thirds of African Americans were overweight. These findings were so alarming that then-Surgeon General Dr. David Satcher issued a public call to action encouraging all Americans to lose weight to improve health and reduce the risk of serious diseases such as heart disease, diabetes, and cancer.

Weight loss alone improves cardiovascular health exponentially; that is, even a loss as small as 10 to 20 pounds can lower systolic blood pressure by 10mm Hg or more and measurably improve the heart's pumping efficiency. Many people are able to reduce or eliminate the need for medications to treat hypertension (high blood pressure) through modest weight loss. Weight loss also improves chronic health conditions such as heart failure, reduces blood lipid levels, and lowers the risk for heart attack and stroke.

Prevention Strategies

Education and lifestyle modification are the key approaches to preventing heart disease regardless of ethnicity. Despite widespread public education efforts by health agencies, many people remain unaware of the general risk factors for heart disease as well as their specific risk factors based on lifestyle and family history. Early detection and treatment of heart problems offer the most effective approach to maintaining optimal heart health. Specific heart disease education and prevention efforts targeting African Americans include:

- Community-based screening programs to encourage regular monitoring of blood pressure, blood sugar (to check for diabetes), and blood cholesterol levels.

- Public appearances by celebrities to promote awareness, screening, and treatment. These efforts often represent a collaboration among public and private interests, such as the "State of the Heart" hypertension awareness program that teams the Congressional Black Caucus, pharmaceutical company AstraZeneca, and celebrities such as Football Hall of Famer Deacon Jones.

- Education efforts through the public schools to encourage young people to develop healthy eating and exercise habits.

- Federal and state efforts to improve access to health-care services.

- Formation in 2001 of the NIH Center for Minority Health and Disparities to focus federal research and educational efforts on heart disease prevention and treatment (among other health concerns) among minority populations.

Lifestyle modification remains the single most effective strategy for preventing heart disease. This includes eating a nutritious, low-fat diet; obtaining regular physical exercise; and not smoking. As well, lifestyle modifications are effective in reducing the severity of heart disease that already exists. Early recognition of warning signs for stroke and heart attack, coupled with prompt treatment, vastly improve survival and recovery following stroke or heart attack.

See also LIFESTYLE AND HEART HEALTH; WOMEN AND HEART DISEASE.

aging, cardiovascular changes as result of The cardiovascular system, like all body systems, undergoes changes with aging that affect its ability to function. Scientists do not fully understand what activates the physiological changes that take place as the body ages. These changes occur at the cell level and begin to affect various body systems at different ages. The cardiovascular system reaches its peak functional effectiveness during the second decade of life, at which period the heart muscle and the arteries in a healthy adult are at prime strength and responsiveness, and tissues throughout the body use oxygen with the greatest efficiency. Barring the presence of cardiovascular disease, cardiovascular function diminishes at about 9 percent each decade to age 60; after age 60, cardiovascular function declines by about 2 percent a year.

Age is the single most significant risk factor for cardiovascular disease of any kind. The risk for cardiovascular disease correspondingly increases with each decade of life after age 30. After age 80 or 85, cardiovascular function is diminished enough in otherwise healthy adults, simply as a dimension of aging, that it constitutes a state of cardiovascular disease, typically in the forms of ATHEROSCLEROSIS, ARTERIOSCLEROSIS, CORONARY ARTERY DISEASE (CAD), PERIPHERAL VASCULAR DISEASE (PVD), and HEART FAILURE.

Changes to the Heart

In a person between the ages of 20 and 29 who has a healthy FITNESS LEVEL, the heart is able to reach maximum pumping rate and force in about four minutes and sustain that level of function for 10 to 14 minutes. With increasing age the heart pumps less blood, less forcefully. Both the time it takes to reach the maximum pumping rate and the length of time a person is capable of sustaining this level of function decline steadily over the next decades. By age 80 it takes a healthy person twice as long to reach maximum heart rate, or about eight minutes, which the person can then sustain for half as long, about five minutes. This cycle is called CARDIAC CAPACITY and is a key measure of cardiovascular health.

The heart muscle of a healthy younger person is lean. Its fibers contract in precise coordination, and electrical conductivity is consistent. As a person ages, fatty tissue begins to infiltrate the heart muscle. Muscle fibers also shorten and stiffen, becoming less flexible and less capable of rapid expansion and contraction. These changes reflect other changes that are taking place at the cell level. In combination, they decrease the heart's CONTRACTILITY and conductivity. This causes diminished cardiac capacity.

The heart has considerable ability to meet the body's essential needs even when cardiovascular disease or damage from MYOCARDIAL INFARCTION (HEART ATTACK) compromises its function. Even at 20 percent cardiac capacity, the heart can sustain moderate physical exertion such as climbing three flights of stairs. Regular physical activity, such as walking for 30 minutes three or four times a week, helps to maintain maximum function even in a damaged heart.

Changes to the Blood Vessels

The blood vessels throughout the body, including the CORONARY ARTERIES that supply the heart with blood, undergo changes similar to those that take place in the heart with aging. As a result, arteries become thicker, stiffer, and less flexible—a condition called arteriosclerosis. This increases the resistance for blood flowing through them, to which the heart responds by intensifying its contractions. As well, fatty deposits begin to accumulate along the inside walls of the arteries, which narrows the opening through which blood can pass—a condition called atherosclerosis. Either change alone can cause HYPERTENSION (high BLOOD PRESSURE); when they exist in combination, at least mild hypertension is almost certain.

Changes in the Body's Ability to Use Oxygen

Changes in cell functions throughout the body alter the efficiency with which cells are able to use oxygen, their primary fuel source. The less efficiently cells use oxygen, the more of it they need. This places an increased burden on the heart, which must increase the amount of work it does to meet this need. The most significant effect of this appears during moderate to strenuous exercise, during which the muscles of movement might be unable to obtain enough oxygen.

Menopause

Before menopause, women are significantly less likely than men to develop cardiovascular disease or to have heart attacks or strokes. Scientists believe this is related to ESTROGEN, which appears to have a protective effect on the cardiovascular system. After menopause, however, a woman's risk for heart disease quickly escalates. In the first five years following menopause, a woman is at greater risk for suffering heart attack as well as from dying of heart attack. This risk subsequently levels off to match that of a man's for the same age.

For decades, doctors prescribed HORMONE REPLACEMENT THERAPY (HRT) for postmenopausal women because it was believed that elevating a woman's estrogen level would help to lower her risk for heart disease. Research findings released in 2002 demonstrated that this was not the case. Postmenopausal estrogen replacement has no measurable protective effect on the cardiovascular system, and it is linked with increased risk for other health problems such as breast cancer. Nutritious eating habits and regular physical activity are particularly important health maintenance measures for postmenopausal women, for cardiovascular health as well as to help maintain bone density and strength and prevent osteoporosis.

The Effects of Lifestyle

Lifestyle factors have a significant affect on cardiovascular health, disease, and the aging process. The body of a person who smokes and drinks alcohol to excess ages more rapidly—that is, experiences a more rapid deterioration of functional capability—than does the body of a person who eats a low-fat, nutritionally balanced diet and exercises four times a week. Cigarette smoking does considerable damage to cells within the cardiovascular system, compounding and accelerating changes already taking place due to aging, as well as in the lungs and throughout the body. Excessive alcohol consumption functions as a toxin for many organs including the heart and can result in CARDIOMYOPATHY. Eating habits that supply the body with the nutrients it needs for healthy function and getting regular physical activity are the two most important lifestyle factors that contribute to sustained cardiac health.

Aging and Cardiovascular Disease

The risk for cardiovascular disease increases with age, most significantly after age 65. This is largely due to the changes that take place in the body with aging. Body systems simply lose effectiveness with age, which sets the stage for various health problems to develop. Doctors are beginning to better understand the sequence of events that take place in the body with aging, and to implement therapeutic approaches to minimize risk and damage related to cardiovascular disease. As recently as the 1980s, doctors considered a gradual increase in blood pressure to be a normal part of the aging process that did not warrant medical treatment. They now know that elevated blood pressure threatens the body's health at any age and should be treated. This single intervention is credited with improving the quality of life and extending life for countless people.

See also AEROBIC CAPACITY; EARLY MENOPAUSE AND HEART DISEASE; LIFESTYLE AND HEART HEALTH; MEDICATION MANAGEMENT; MEDICATIONS TO TREAT HEART DISEASE; NUTRITION AND DIET; ORNISH PROGRAM; WOMEN AND HEART DISEASE.

AIDS and heart disease Some of the drugs commonly taken to slow the development and progression of human immune virus (HIV) and acquired immune deficiency disorder (AIDS) also alter the body's lipid mechanisms, contributing to high blood CHOLESTEROL levels. This significantly raises the risk of HEART DISEASE, particularly ANGINA and CORONARY ARTERY DISEASE (CAD), and HEART ATTACK. The HIV/AIDS treatment regimen known as highly active antiretroviral tri-therapy (HAART), which became the standard for early therapeutic intervention in 1996, is linked to elevated low-density lipoprotein (LDL) cholesterol and TRIGLYCERIDES. It is not clear whether HAART establishes these elevations or hastens their progression when they already are present as underlying risk factors. Studies are underway to further evaluate the correlations between HAART and heart disease.

Low-fat diet, regular EXERCISE, stopping smoking, and LIPID-LOWERING MEDICATIONS appear to have the same beneficial effect in people taking HAART as for anyone with heart disease risk factors related to elevated lipid levels. It is sometimes also necessary to adjust the HAART regimen to eliminate or minimize the protease inhibitors more

likely to cause lipid elevations. Ritonavir is more often linked with elevated triglycerides levels, while nelfinavir appears the least likely to affect blood lipid levels. However, it is the therapeutic effect that these drugs have in keeping HIV/AIDS in check that should determine their selection. Anyone on HAART therapy for HIV/AIDS should have regular and frequent blood tests to monitor cholesterol and triglycerides levels.

People who have AIDS are also more vulnerable to other kinds of heart disease as well. These include ARRHYTHMIAS (irregularities in the pattern of the HEARTBEAT); CARDIOMYOPATHY (particularly dilated cardiomyopathy); inflammation affecting the heart muscle (MYOCARDITIS), the lining of the heart (ENDOCARDITIS), or the membrane surrounding the heart (PERICARDITIS); PERICARDIAL EFFUSION (accumulation of fluid around the heart); and PULMONARY HYPERTENSION (elevated pressure within the pulmonary artery and arteries of the lungs). These conditions appear to develop as a consequence of the disease process of AIDS in combination with the side effects of medications used to treat AIDS.

See also NUTRITION AND DIET; SMOKING AND HEART DISEASE.

alcohol consumption and heart disease For several decades, research studies have suggested that moderate alcohol consumption had a protective effect on the HEART and CARDIOVASCULAR SYSTEM. Most of these studies examined the lifestyles and habits of people with good heart health and compared them with those of people with heart disease. In such comparisons, people who consume moderate amounts of alcohol on a regular basis—two or three drinks in a week, with a drink being defined as one 4-ounce glass of wine, 12-ounce glass of beer, or one shot of distilled spirits (hard liquor)—consistently have less heart disease than people who do not drink alcohol at all or who drink alcohol beyond the defined level of moderation. The rate of heart disease was lowest in people who drank red wine, leading to recommendations that people moderately consume red wine in particular among the kinds of alcoholic beverages.

None of these studies provided conclusive explanation for the differences in heart disease rates, however. Some scientists believe that alcohol's anticoagulant effect helps to keep the blood's platelets from sticking together, reducing the risk of blood clots that could lead to stroke or heart attack. Other theories focus on the ANTIOXIDANTS found in alcoholic beverages, particularly the FLAVONOIDS in red wine, that are known to help prevent the natural by-products of metabolism from causing cell and tissue damage. Continuing research has raised doubts as to whether the alcohol or other factors, particularly lifestyle factors such as diet and exercise, might instead be responsible.

Regardless of the benefits of drinking alcohol in moderation, the effects of excessive alcohol consumption on health and on the heart are clear, numerous, and serious. Alcohol is a known factor in liver disease such as cirrhosis, brain disorders, birth defects related to fetal alcohol syndrome, and certain cancers such as liver cancer, colon cancer, and breast cancer. Drunk driving is a leading cause of injuries and deaths in automobile accidents. Excessive alcohol consumption also appears to be a factor in certain heart problems, including hypertension, heart attack, CARDIOMYOPATHY (enlargement of the heart), elevated blood lipid levels (particularly triglycerides), and stroke. Even in moderate amounts, alcohol can have a triggering or exacerbating effect on ARRHYTHMIAS, in particular ATRIAL FIBRILLATION. As well, alcohol is a toxin that destroys cells and tissues within the body, including those of arteries and the heart muscle.

Currently debate continues as to whether moderate drinking offers enough cardiovascular benefit to be a health recommendation. Some health-care professionals believe that moderation is the key, and that an occasional alcoholic drink is not harmful to people otherwise in good health. Others point out that other factors—such as low-fat diet, regular exercise, and not smoking—are demonstrated to provide protective benefits for the heart without adverse consequences or other health risks associated with alcohol consumption. On its Web site (www.americanheart.org), the American Heart Association (AHA) offers this recommendation regarding alcohol consumption and heart health:

> If you drink alcohol, do so in moderation. This means an average of one to two drinks per day for men and one drink per day for women. (A drink is one 12 oz. beer, 4 oz. of wine, 1.5 oz. of 80-proof spirits, or 1 oz. of 100-proof spirits.) Moderate drinkers have lower heart disease risk than nondrinkers. However, drinking more alcohol increases such public health dangers as alcoholism, high blood pressure, obesity, stroke, breast cancer, suicide, and accidents. Given these and other risks, the American Heart Association cautions people NOT to start drinking . . . if they do not already drink alcohol. Consult your doctor on the benefits and risks of consuming alcohol in moderation.

The AHA bases its position and comments on research findings issued in these reports:

- AHA Scientific Statement: "AHA Dietary Guidelines: Revision 2000," #71-0193 *Circulation.* 2000; 102: 2,284–2,299; *Stroke.* 2000; 31: 2,751–2,766.
- AHA Science Advisory: "Alcohol and Heart Disease," #71-0097 *Circulation.* 1996; 94: 3,023–3,025.
- AHA Science Advisory: "Wine and Your Heart," #71-0199 *Circulation.* 2001; 103: 472–475.

See also DIABETES AND HEART DISEASE; LIFESTYLE AND HEART HEALTH; NUTRITION AND DIET.

Aldomet See METHYLDOPA.

allograft Transplanted tissues or organs that come from a donor other than the recipient. HEART valves (aortic and pulmonary) and the heart itself are the primary allografts used to treat HEART DISEASE. They are removed, or harvested, from organ donors using sterile, surgical technique. A DONOR HEART must be transplanted within hours. Donor heart valves can be prepared and stored frozen for several months. The demand for donor hearts takes precedence over the need for donor valves; if an intact heart is appropriate for transplant, the heart will be harvested for that purpose. If not, then the valves are available for harvest.

Allografts are harvested, handled, and distributed according to strict federal regulations under the oversight of the Food and Drug Administration (FDA). Tissues such as heart valves are processed and available through tissue banks located throughout the United States. Because heart valves are more abundant and are treated during their preparation following harvesting to prevent an immune response in the recipient, there is no need to match tissue type and usually no difficulty obtaining them when needed. The surgeon simply places an order and the tissue bank delivers the valve to the hospital.

Donor hearts are extremely limited, and strict criteria govern their availability and allocation through the UNITED NETWORK FOR ORGAN SHARING (UNOS) system. As the heart must be transplanted as living tissue, it cannot be treated to prevent rejection. Hearts for transplant must be closely matched for tissue type between donor and recipient and are at risk for allograft failure.

Even though an allograft is matched as closely as possible to the recipient's tissue type, the recipient's body will view the transplanted tissue as foreign and produce antibodies in an attempt to destroy it. An allograft recipient takes IMMUNOSUPPRESSIVE MEDICATIONS to prevent this from happening. Failure of a heart valve allograft is uncommon, although it might happen as a result of infection or other problems related to the surgery.

See also HEART TRANSPLANT; VALVE REPAIR AND REPLACEMENT; XENOGRAFT.

alpha agonist medications Drugs that bind with, or activate, certain ADRENERGIC RECEPTORS in the HEART, BLOOD vessels, and other smooth muscle tissue throughout the body to simulate the action of EPINEPHRINE. There are two types of adrenergic receptors, alpha and beta, and several subtypes within each. Some drugs that have alpha agonist actions also nonspecifically bind with all adrenergic receptors. Other alpha agonists target alpha-1 or alpha-2 receptors. Because adrenergic receptors often counteract each other, some drugs that have alpha-1 agonist action at the same time have alpha-2 antagonist, or blocking, action.

- Nonspecific adrenergic agonists such as epinephrine (adrenaline), DOPAMINE, and DOBUTAMINE bind with all types and subtypes of adrenergic receptors. These drugs are given during CARDIAC ARREST or, far more commonly, CARDIOGENIC

SHOCK to increase the responsiveness of heart muscle fibers to electrical stimulation. Combined with other measures, this helps to restore the heart's function.

- Medications taken to treat HYPOTENSION (low BLOOD PRESSURE) or orthostatic hypotension (sudden drop in blood pressure with a change in position) typically target alpha-1 receptors. This causes the arterioles (the smallest arteries) to constrict, keeping more blood in the primary arteries. Commonly prescribed alpha-1 agonists include midodrine (ProAmatine).

- Alpha agonist medications taken to treat HYPERTENSION (high blood pressure) typically dilate peripheral arterioles (alpha-1 agonist action) and relax primary arteries (alpha-2 antagonist action). This simultaneously centralizes a higher volume of blood and lowers the resistance blood encounters as it is pumped through the body, reducing blood pressure. Commonly prescribed drugs in this class include CLONIDINE (Catapres), guanabenz (Wytensin), and METHYLDOPA (Aldomet).

Alpha agonist medications also act on the smooth muscle tissues of the genitourinary system and are taken to treat ERECTILE DYSFUNCTION and ejaculation disorders in men and urinary stress incontinence in women. It is important to take any blood pressure medication as prescribed, and to stop taking it only at a physician's direction. Most blood pressure medications should be tapered over at least two weeks; suddenly stopping such a medication can have serious consequences such as rapid or extreme fluctuations in blood pressure.

See also ALPHA ANTAGONIST MEDICATIONS; ANTIHYPERTENSIVE MEDICATIONS; BETA ANTAGONIST MEDICATIONS; MEDICATIONS TO TREAT HEART DISEASE.

alpha antagonist medications Drugs that block the action of certain ADRENERGIC RECEPTORS in the HEART, blood vessels, and other parts of the body to decrease the action of epinephrine. Alpha antagonists are taken primarily to lower BLOOD PRESSURE as treatment for HYPERTENSION, and they work by causing the arteries to relax. This reduces the resistance for BLOOD as it is pumped through the body, lowering blood pressure. These medications are also called alpha antagonists, alpha-adrenergic blockers, or alpha-adrenergic antagonists, and they are classified according to which subtype of alpha receptor they affect. Some alpha blockers also have alpha agonist actions, and others also have beta-blocker actions.

- Commonly prescribed alpha-1 antagonist medications include PRAZOSIN (Minipres), TERAZOSIN (Hytrin), and DOXAZOSIN (Cardura).
- Commonly prescribed alpha-2 antagonist medications include CLONIDINE (Catapres), guanabenz (Wytensin), GUANFACINE (Tenex), and METHYL-DOPA (Aldomet). These drugs also have alpha agonist actions.
- Commonly prescribed alpha-2 antagonist medications that also have beta-blocker actions include LABETALOL (Normodyne) and CARVEDILOL (Coreg).

Alpha antagonist medications affect other smooth muscle tissues in the body as well, most notably those of the genitourinary system. This can result in undesired side effects such as erectile dysfunction in men and urinary stress incontinence in women. It is important to take any blood pressure medication as prescribed, and to stop taking it only at a physician's direction. Most blood pressure medications should be tapered over at least two weeks; suddenly stopping them can have serious consequences such as rapid or extreme fluctuations in blood pressure.

See also ALPHA AGONIST MEDICATIONS; ANTIHYPERTENSIVE MEDICATIONS; BETA ANTAGONIST MEDICATIONS; MEDICATION MANAGEMENT.

alternans See T-WAVE ALTERNANS.

alveolus (alveoli) See PULMONARY SYSTEM.

ambulatory ECG See ELECTROCARDIOGRAM (ECG).

American Heart Association diet (AHA diet) See NUTRITION AND DIET.

Americans with Disabilities Act (ADA) Federal legislation passed in the United States in 1990 and ameneded in 2009 to give persons with disabilities equitable access to employment, housing, transportation, and other opportunities. In brief, the Americans with Disabilities Act (ADA) requires businesses to make reasonable accommodations for qualified individuals with disabilities. There are many interpretations of this, with just as many variations in implementation. In general, the ADA has the broadest implications in the workplace and prohibits employers from firing individuals solely on the basis of disability.

Not surprisingly, HEART DISEASE is an example of a qualifying disability cited in the language of the ADA. Heart disease, including HYPERTENSION (high BLOOD PRESSURE) and STROKE, accounts for disability in 8 million Americans. Many continue to work with varying degrees of limitation. The extent to which the ADA requires an employer to accommodate a person's disability due to heart disease depends on the nature and extent of the disability. Employers may require a person requesting workplace accommodation under the ADA to provide documentation from a physician that a disability exists.

Generally, a disability is a health situation that will not improve. This creates a considerable gray area in terms of interpreting whether the ADA applies to a person with heart disease. Forms of heart disease that are correctable with appropriate treatment and medication generally do not fall under the scope of the ADA. For example, coronary heart disease (blockage of the arteries that supply blood to the heart), repaired through CORONARY ARTERY BYPASS GRAFT (CABG) or ANGIO-PLASTY, and hypertension that is under control with ANTIHYPERTENSIVE MEDICATIONS are conditions generally considered temporary. Employment laws and workplace policies that regulate sick leave determine the employer's legal responsibilities.

Other forms of heart disease such as HEART FAILURE or damage following HEART ATTACK (myocardial infarction) can result in permanent disability, even with appropriate treatment. For example, stroke disables nearly 1 million Americans every year, many of whom lose vital abilities such as speech and mobility. Such conditions generally do fall within the scope of the ADA. A key factor in determining what accommodations the law requires the employer to make is the person's ability to perform the essential functions of the job. There are circumstances under which the employer may offer the person a different job in lieu of making accommodations in the current job. As well, certain classifications of jobs and kinds of employers are exempt from the ADA.

The U.S. Department of Justice oversees enforcement of the ADA and can provide additional information about this legislation and its compliance requirements. For further information contact:

U.S. Department of Justice
950 Pennsylvania Avenue, NW
Civil Rights Division, Disability Rights
   Section—NYA
Washington, D.C. 20530
(800) 514-0301 (voice), or (800) 514-0383 (TTY)
http://www.ada.gov

See also ACTIVITIES OF DAILY LIVING (ADLs); DISABILITY; LIFESTYLE AND HEART HEALTH; STROKE.

amiloride   A POTASSIUM-sparing diuretic taken to treat mild to moderate HYPERTENSION (high BLOOD PRESSURE) and congestive HEART FAILURE. It generally is taken in combination with other DIURETIC MEDICATIONS (water pills) to provide an added diuretic effect as well as to offset the potassium loss that occurs with other kinds of diuretics. Like all diuretics, amiloride causes the kidneys to extract more fluid from the blood that it filters, passing it from the body as urine. This helps to reduce blood volume, which lowers blood pressure, and EDEMA (swelling from fluid retention), which improves congestive heart failure. This also removes SODIUM and potassium from the body. Generally the sodium loss does not create any health concerns because the body maintains a higher store of SODIUM than other salts and because the typical American diet contains more than adequate (and usually excessive) amounts of sodium. The typical diet often does not replace lost potassium, however, and potassium depletion such as occurs with many diuretics can cause heart ARRHYTHMIAS (irregular

heartbeat) and other health problems. A potassium-sparing diuretic such as amiloride helps the kidneys to retain potassium.

Because of amiloride's potassium-sparing effect, people taking amiloride should not use salt substitute products as these typically contain high amounts of potassium. Amiloride causes stomach irritation in some people, which taking it with food or milk generally relieves. Undesired side effects that can occur include DIZZINESS, nausea, loss of appetite, dry mouth, and excessive hair growth. People who are taking ANGIOTENSIN-CONVERTING ENZYME (ACE) INHIBITOR MEDICATIONS, such as CAPTOPRIL (Capoten) and ENALAPRIL (Vasotec), to treat hypertension should take amiloride only with careful monitoring by a physician. Amiloride is sold under the brand name Midamor in the United States.

See also ADJUNCT THERAPY; ANTIHYPERTENSIVE MEDICATIONS; MEDICATIONS TO TREAT HEART DISEASE.

amino acids   Chemical substances that are the basic structures of proteins. Proteins are key to numerous functions that take place within cells, including the synthesis (manufacture) of many substances essential for life. Although there are only about 20 amino acids, they can form into nearly countless structures through the ways in which they align and configure themselves. The body can manufacture 12 amino acids from compounds that exist within it. These are called the nonessential amino acids. The body must acquire the remaining eight amino acids through the diet. Dietary proteins from animal sources, such as meats and dairy products, supply all eight of these amino acids. Dietary proteins from nonanimal sources—vegetables, fruits, grains, nuts, legumes, and beans—supply some of them. Combining different plant-based foods can provide the full range of essential amino acids. Nearly all body processes require amino acids, so it is important to meet the body's dietary needs for them.

An amino acid called HOMOCYSTEINE first gained the attention of researchers in the FRAMINGHAM HEART STUDY, one of the largest and most comprehensive assessments of cardiac health and disease in the United States, who noticed that people who have HEART DISEASE tend to have elevated levels of homocysteine in their blood, while people without heart disease have normal levels. The reason for this is not clear, although at present, researchers believe homocysteine has a role in allowing fatty acids such as cholesterol in the blood to accumulate along the walls of the arteries, and also in causing PLATELETS (blood cells responsible for clotting) to clot.

Amino acids also form numerous proteins that are linked to heart disease, including LIPOPROTEINS (cholesterols) and apolipoprotein B, which form arterial PLAQUE; FIBRINOGEN, which is essential for clotting; and C-REACTIVE PROTEIN, a substance released during inflammatory responses throughout the body. A combination of genetic and environmental factors influences the extent to which these proteins present risks for cardiovascular health.

See also ANGIOGENESIS; ARTERIOSCLEROSIS; ATHEROSCLEROSIS; CHOLESTEROL, BLOOD; EXERCISE; HYPERLIPIDEMIA; INFLAMMATION AND HEART DISEASE; LIFESTYLE AND HEART HEALTH; NUTRITION AND DIET.

amiodarone   See ANTIARRHYTHMIA MEDICATIONS.

amlodipine   A CALCIUM CHANNEL ANTAGONIST MEDICATION taken to treat ANGINA (HEART pain) and HYPERTENSION (high BLOOD PRESSURE). It causes the arteries to dilate (widen), reducing the resistance BLOOD encounters flowing through them. This lowers blood pressure and decreases the heart's workload. Doctors may gradually increase the amlodipine dose or prescribe amlodipine in combination with other MEDICATIONS TO TREAT HEART DISEASE, including additional medications for angina. The goal of amlodipine is to lower the frequency of angina attacks and to make possible a more active lifestyle. Amlodipine is not effective for treating angina attacks when they occur.

Undesired side effects include peripheral edema, constipation, fatigue, sleep disturbances (including vivid dreams), headache, difficulty urinating, and rarely psychosis. Amlodipine is available in the United States under the brand name Norvasc.

See also ALPHA ANTAGONIST MEDICATIONS; ANTIHYPERTENSIVE MEDICATIONS; BETA ANTAGONIST MEDICATIONS; MEDICATION MANAGEMENT; MEDICATION SIDE EFFECTS; MEDICATIONS TO TREAT HEART DISEASE.

amphetamines   See DRUG ABUSE AND HEART DISEASE.

anaerobic exercise   See EXERCISE.

anemia   A condition in which there are not enough red BLOOD cells to meet the body's need for oxygen. Red blood cells contain HEMOGLOBIN, a protein that transports oxygen from the lungs to all of the body's cells and tissues. Anemia develops when the body does not make enough red blood cells or loses too many red blood cells, or there are abnormalities in the red blood cells or in the forms of hemoglobin that they contain.

Studies conducted in the late 1990s and early 2000s confirmed that people who have mild to moderate anemia are less likely to survive a HEART ATTACK. Because OXYGENATION is already compromised with anemia, a serious challenge such as heart attack can push the body beyond its limits in terms of adjusting and compensating. Adequate oxygenation becomes crucial following heart attack as the body struggles to overcome the assault. Giving transfusions to people who are anemic immediately following heart attack boosts the red blood cell count and improves the blood's ability to transport much-needed oxygen.

Symptoms and Diagnostic Path
Anemia can cause symptoms such as tiredness, FATIGUE (especially on exertion), and weakness, or it may cause no symptoms at all and is discovered through routine blood tests done for other purposes. Although anemia is not itself a CARDIOVASCULAR DISEASE, it affects the function of the CARDIOVASCULAR SYSTEM, particularly the heart. When body tissues are not receiving enough oxygen, the heart pumps harder and faster to move higher volumes of blood through the body. When cardiovascular disease such as atherosclerosis impairs blood CIRCULATION, anemia further complicates the situation by further reducing the amount of oxygen body tissues receive.

Various diagnostic tests help to determine what kind of anemia is present. Which tests are ordered depends on what symptoms, if any, are present. Some tests, such as hemoglobin and hematocrit, are part of the general blood-screening test called a complete blood count (CBC). Other tests are ordered to clarify general findings or to further differentiate the type of anemia. Common diagnostic tests for anemia include:

- **Hemoglobin.** A blood test that measures the amount of the protein hemoglobin present in the blood. Hemoglobin binds with, or carries, oxygen in the blood.
- **Hematocrit.** This is the basic blood test to diagnose anemia; it measures the percentage of red blood cells in the blood. The blood of a healthy adult contains about 40 percent red blood cells; 39 percent or lower is considered anemic. Any percentage below that is considered anemia.
- **Serum iron.** A blood test that measures the amount of iron present in the blood. Low levels suggest iron-deficiency anemia; high levels suggest other blood disorders such as HEMOCHROMATOSIS (too much iron).

  ERYTHROPOIETIN **(EPO).** The kidneys are very sensitive to the blood's oxygen levels. When these levels drop, the kidneys release EPO, a hormone that stimulates the marrow to manufacture more red blood cells.
- **Serum ferritin.** Blood components contain this protein, which binds with and stores iron in the body. Measuring the ferritin level helps to determine whether anemia is due to iron deficiency; a low level indicates low iron. An elevated level might suggest hemolytic anemia (anemia caused by the over-destruction of red blood cells). Any inflammation in the body affects the ferritin level, so this test result is not by itself conclusive.
- **Total iron-binding capacity (TIBC).** A protein called transferrin binds with iron to transport it in the blood. This blood test (also called transferrin saturation) measures the percentage of transferrin that is bound to iron. When iron deficiency anemia is present, the TIBC is high and the serum iron level is low. When iron levels are too high, such as in hemochromatosis, the TIBC is normal or even low and the serum iron level is high.
- **Bone marrow biopsy.** In this test, the doctor uses a needle to remove a small amount of marrow, which makes red blood cells, from within the center of a bone such as the hip crest or the sternum (chest bone). The lab then analyzes the types of blood cells and their states of development, which helps to diagnose certain kinds of anemia such as aplastic and pernicious.

Treatment Options and Outlook

Treatment depends on the reason or cause of the anemia. Iron-deficient anemia, the most common type of anemia among adults, generally improves with iron supplementation. When anemia results from underlying health conditions, treatment targets those conditions. Severe anemia (hematocrit below 30 percent) requires blood transfusions. Blood transfusion is sometimes warranted for moderate anemia when other heart disease is present, to improve oxygenation as much as possible.

Risk Factors and Preventive Measures

There are numerous possible causes for anemia. Anemia can result from iron deficiency, which limits the body's ability to manufacture hemoglobin, or as a deficiency of vitamin B12 or folate (folic acid), which limits the body's ability to produce new red blood cells. Treatments for other health conditions, including medications, may deplete the body's supply of red blood cells, as can chronic health conditions such as autoimmune disorders. Ulcerative colitis and bleeding stomach ulcers, which may have no symptoms other than anemia, also deplete red blood cells. Menstruating women whose periods are heavy are often anemic because their bodies do not have time to fully replenish red blood cells lost in one menstrual cycle before the next menstrual bleeding begins. Longstanding, untreated HYPERTENSION also can cause anemia. Preventive treatment with iron supplementation and appropriate treatment for any underlying health condition are the most effective preventive measures. Some less common forms of anemia, such as aplastic anemia and sickle-cell anemia, have genetic components and are not preventable.

See also AFRICAN AMERICANS AND HEART DISEASE; ANTIHYPERTENSIVE MEDICATIONS; NUTRITION AND DIET; THROMBOCYTHEMIA.

anesthesia   See SURGERY TO TREAT CARDIOVASCULAR DISEASE.

aneurysm   A weak place in the wall of an ARTERY that bulges or tears. An aneurysm can occur in any artery and can present a significant risk if it leaks or ruptures. Aneurysms in large arteries or in vital organs such as the brain can be fatal if untreated. Treatment is surgery to strengthen and repair the weakness in the arterial wall.

Symptoms and Diagnostic Path

An aneurysm often has no symptoms; a doctor discovers the aneurysm during a routine physical examination or incidental to another health concern. When symptoms are present, they vary depending on the aneurysm's location. Aneurysms in the brain might cause headache, blurred vision, or other symptoms that are similar to those of STROKE. Aneurysms in other locations might cause pain; abdominal aortic aneurysms sometimes cause bulging in the belly around the umbilicus (belly button).

The most common form of aneurysm is a dissecting aneurysm, in which a small tear in the innermost layer of the artery allows BLOOD to begin seeping between the tissue layers of the artery's wall. This causes the other layers to separate and split, and blood may leak from the artery. Although this process may take months or years to unfold, the threat of a sudden rupture along the weakened area is high. The bigger the dissection becomes, the faster it grows. An untreated small aneurysm can become life-threatening without showing any symptoms. Occasionally the rupture is sudden and severe, and immediate surgery is necessary to stop blood loss and repair the artery. About half of such ruptures are fatal.

Diagnostic tests include ANGIOGRAPHY (dye injected into the arteries and viewed via specialized X-ray), MAGNETIC RESONANCE IMAGING (MRI), and COMPUTED TOMOGRAPHY (CT) SCAN. Echocardiogram can help diagnose aneurysms in the chest area and near the heart.

Treatment Options and Outlook

Repair of an aneurysm is major surgery, generally requiring several days to a week in the hospital. For a large aneurysm, the surgeon must make an incision large enough to provide access to the damaged artery, clamp the artery to prevent blood from flowing through it (sometimes making it necessary to reroute the body's blood supply through a bypass machine), and cut out the damaged section and replace it with a synthetic patch or sleeve called a graft.

A procedure called MINIMALLY INVASIVE CARDIAC SURGERY allows repair of certain aneurysms by inserting a device called a STENT into the aneurysm area. The surgeon makes a small incision to expose an artery in the groin, and then threads the stent through the artery to the location of the aneurysm. Special endoscopic tools allow the surgeon to anchor the stent in place, creating the repair from the inside of the artery rather than removing the damaged portion of the arterial wall. Some aneurysms simply might be removed, depending on their size and location. Most people recover from aneurysm repair surgery and return to full, normal lives.

Sometimes doctors will choose "watchful waiting" with small aneurysms, particularly in elderly people or when surgery is a significant risk because of other health problems. This typically involves regular diagnostic tests such as angiography or MRI to monitor the aneurysm's progression. The greatest risk of untreated aneurysm is rupture, which can cause STROKE, HEART ATTACK, or death.

Risk Factors and Preventive Measures

Most aneurysms are idiopathic; that is, there is no clear reason they develop. Some aneurysms arise as a result of congenital defects in the structure of the affected artery. Family history of aneurysm suggests genetic factors. Cigarette smoking is a significant risk factor for aneurysm because of NICOTINE's action on the arteries. Other risks include ARTERIOSCLEROSIS (accumulation of PLAQUE within the walls of the arteries) and untreated or uncontrolled HYPERTENSION (high BLOOD PRESSURE). Early detection and treatment of aneurysm afford the most positive outcome. Not smoking, lifestyle practices to reduce overall risk for CVD, and appropriate diagnosis and treatment for cardiovascular conditions that do develop are the most effective measures to prevent aneurysm.

See also ABDOMINAL AORTIC ANEURYSM; ANGIOPLASTY; BRAIN ANEURYSM; FAMILY HEALTH HISTORY.

anger and heart health   Some researchers theorize that people who become angry quickly and often are more likely to have early CARDIOVASCULAR DISEASE (CVD), especially HYPERTENSION and CORONARY ARTERY DISEASE (CAD), than are people who are able to manage their EMOTIONS. They are also more likely to experience cardiovascular crises such as HEART ATTACK and STROKE and less likely to recover. The reasons for this remain unclear even after decades of research, although scientists believe there is a correlation to the body's stress hormones and stress response.

Anger and fear are closely related responses that activate the body's "FIGHT-OR-FLIGHT" mechanism, which sets in motion a cascade of events that cause the BLOOD PRESSURE to rise, heart rate to increase, breathing rate to increase, and muscles to become stimulated. The stress response puts increased levels of EPINEPHRINE, NOREPINEPHRINE, and DOPAMINE into the bloodstream. These chemicals are neurotransmitters that intensify nerve signals from the brain to the cardiovascular system. One theory about anger's relationship to heart disease is that continually elevated levels of these hormones eventually damages sensitive control mechanisms in the body, such as that which regulates blood pressure, and perhaps cells in the heart and arteries as well.

Learning to eliminate or diminish the anger response, which includes expressed as well as suppressed anger, through anger management and STRESS REDUCTION TECHNIQUES can mitigate the effect of anger on the cardiovascular system. Anger management focuses on helping a person identify the reasons for his or her anger reactions and learning different methods for addressing these underlying issues. Much anger results from feelings of frustration and lack of control, so anger management methods often target ways to improve a person's sense of control. Psychotherapy is often helpful. Stress management techniques such as meditation and yoga can help a person maintain emotional equilibrium.

Anger is a common reaction to a serious health crisis such as heart attack or stroke, or to a serious chronic health problem such as heart failure that interferes with or limits lifestyle. The same anger management methods and stress reduction techniques can help in these circumstances as well, particularly approaches that restore independence and control.

See also ANXIETY; DENIAL; DEPRESSION; PERSONALITY TYPES.

angina   A sensation of squeezing pressure or pain in the chest. The word means "to choke," which is a good description of this kind of discomfort. It is most commonly a symptom of CORONARY ARTERY DISEASE (CAD) in which arterial PLAQUE deposits block the arteries that supply the HEART muscle (myocardium) with blood. The chest discomfort warns that the myocardium is not receiving enough oxygen and this is the body's signal to decrease the demand on the heart, slowing it down so the oxygen it does receive is adequate. In response to pain, most people stop what they are doing; this typically relieves an angina attack because the heart slows down.

There are varying degrees as well as different types of angina. Most angina comes on or becomes more severe with physical exertion. It can be mild and barely noticeable or severe and completely debilitating. Angina that is present at rest or that fails to improve with medication indicates severe CAD that requires immediate medical attention. Treatments for angina include medications such as NITROGLYCERIN and BETA ANTAGONIST MEDICATIONS or surgery such as ANGIOPLASTY or CORONARY ARTERY BYPASS GRAFT (CABG) to clear the coronary artery occlusions that are the underlying cause of the angina. Severe angina can be a symptom of HEART ATTACK (myocardial infarction), which requires emergency medical treatment.

Angina Pectoris

Angina pectoris ("choking pain of the chest") is the clinical term for common angina that is cardiac in origin. When most people use the term *angina*, they are referring to angina pectoris, although there are other, noncardiac types of angina. Angina, as it is a symptom of underlying cardiovascular disease, becomes more common with increasing age. Many people live with mild to moderate angina as a chronic health condition, controlling its symptoms with medication.

- **Stable angina** is angina that occurs under predictable circumstances, such as physical exertion or emotional stress, and goes away when the person rests or takes nitroglycerin. A person can live with mild to moderate stable angina as a chronic condition for many years. Most people with stable angina can go about their everyday regular activities without restriction or limitation except during an angina attack, when they must rest until the pain subsides. Pain that worsens, either in intensity or in the length of time it is present, requires prompt medical evaluation. Someone who is accustomed to intermittent chest pain might not recognize pain that is actually a sign of a heart attack.
- **Unstable angina** occurs without warning or provocation and is often severe enough to be immediately debilitating. Unstable angina is a medical emergency that requires prompt evaluation for heart attack.

Although doctors treat angina to relieve symptoms or to prevent progression to a heart attack, angina is a symptom of CAD. Treatment must also consider the underlying causes of the pain and attempt to correct those. In addition to being a primary symptom of CAD, angina can indicate other heart problems such as VALVE DISEASE or dysfunction, ISCHEMIC HEART DISEASE (a consequence of CAD), or arrhythmias.

Variant (Prinzmetal) Angina

Arterial spasms cause variant, or Prinzmetal, angina. For reasons doctors do not fully understand, this form of angina generally occurs when the person is sleeping. Because it occurs at rest, it is considered a variation of unstable angina. Because it is predictable in its pattern of occurrence, however, attacks are not necessarily medical emergencies, although

they do signal significant coronary artery occlusion, usually in more than one artery and often in more than one location within each affected artery. For most people with variant angina, coronary artery bypass graft (CABG) is the only treatment that will correct the underlying cause of the pain when that cause is CAD. However, NITRATE MEDICATIONS and calcium channel antagonist medications can relieve the spasm, which often is superimposed on partially included arteries. Angioplasty often is not an option because of the extensiveness of the CAD, though angioplasty with STENT may be the treatment of choice for an isolated STENOSIS (narrowing). It is possible for variant angina to cause spasms in arteries that are not occluded, although this is not very common. When this is the case, treatment targets relaxing the arteries, typically with nitrates and calcium channel blockers.

"Silent" Angina

Some people with moderate to significant coronary artery disease do not feel pain from the lack of oxygen to the heart, even though the CAD seriously compromises the blood supply to the heart. The heart's electrical activity, as measured by electrocardiogram (ECG), shows the same pattern of electrical disturbance as occurs during an angina attack, but the person does not feel these disturbances as pain. Doctors call this "silent" angina because the heart still sends out the message although the brain does not interpret it as pain. A person with angina might feel some shortness of breath with physical exertion, if the coronary blockage is substantial, but often feels nothing at all. Scientists do not know why this disruption in communication takes place, but it can have deadly consequences when heart attack occurs without warning.

When present as pain, angina provides clear warning that the heart is having trouble working properly. When there is no pain, the first sign that there is trouble may be heart attack. Often in someone with silent angina, ECG can detect abnormalities in the heart's function that are the result of CAD and oxygen deprivation if the ECG is performed during an angina attack. Further tests such as echocardiogram and angiography confirm the extent of the blockage, or occlusion, and doctors can recommend appropriate treatment.

Noncardiac Angina

Some chest pain that is called angina has nothing to do with the heart. These kinds of angina might suggest pleurisy (inflammation of the lining of the lungs) and problems involving the lungs; non-heart-related pain, such as that caused by gastric ulcer, gallbladder disease, and liver disease; and exudate angina or angina trachealis, the clinical term for an upper respiratory infection known commonly as croup. Treating the pain associated with these conditions involves identifying and resolving their underlying causes.

Symptoms and Diagnostic Path

The symptoms of angina vary with the type of angina, although commonly include chest pain, chest tightness, and shortness of breath. Finding the cause of angina often requires a combination of tests and procedures. The most simple and least invasive are electrocardiogram (ECG), EXERCISE STRESS TEST (ECG done during closely supervised exercise), and ECHOCARDIOGRAM (ultrasound of the heart). Additional tests might include angiogram (cardiac catheterization), which involves injecting a dye into the arteries and then taking a series of X-rays, or specialized nuclear medicine studies such as thallium uptake. Careful assessment of the person's symptoms—when pain occurs, how long it lasts, what helps it to go away—is also essential in determining the cause of angina.

Treatment Options and Outlook

Medications can keep mild to moderate angina under control in many people and might be the only alternative for people who have complicating circumstances that make other treatments such as surgery too risky. Nitroglycerin is the oldest and most common medication taken to treat angina. It helps to reduce the heart's need for oxygen. It can be used regularly to prevent or reduce the frequency of angina attacks or be taken sublingually (tablets that dissolve when placed under the tongue) during an angina attack. Nitroglycerin comes in several forms, including long-acting or timed-release formulas, skin patches (transdermal), and ointment applied to and absorbed through the skin.

Beta antagonist medications such as METOPROLOL and ATENOLOL often relieve angina by blocking the effects of adrenaline on the heart, slowing the heart's contractions. This means the heart uses and requires less oxygen, which relieves the strain that is causing the angina. Some people cannot take these drugs because of their side effects or because they have other forms of heart disease in which beta-blockers are not appropriate. Calcium channel antagonist medications such as NIFEDIPINE and DILTIAZEM, taken to lower blood pressure, also can relieve angina by reducing the amount of work the heart does. It is not clear whether calcium channel blockers are effective for angina when hypertension is *not* present, and there is controversy about taking these drugs when blood pressure is normal.

Doctors might prescribe these medications in varying combinations to try to treat angina without surgery. People who do not get relief from medications generally require surgery to clear the blocked coronary arteries and restore blood flow to the heart, either angioplasty or coronary artery bypass graft (CABG).

Angina is a message from the heart that it is not receiving enough oxygen. This means the heart is under stress and significantly increases the likelihood of heart attack. When medication controls angina, it is possible to live with it as a chronic condition for a considerable time, even years. When medication cannot control angina, other interventions are necessary to avert inevitable cardiac crisis. Surgery to correct underlying problems, such as restoring blood flow through occluded coronary arteries or repairing or replacing damaged heart valves, can permanently end angina. Most people who undergo such treatments fully recover to enjoy life free from the pain of angina. Everyone with angina should also make appropriate lifestyle changes—eat nutritiously, exercise regularly, and stop smoking.

Risk Factors and Preventive Measures

Cardiovascular disease, in particular CAD, is the key cause of most forms of angina; angina is as much a symptom of underlying heart disease as it is a medical condition itself. Preventive measures to reduce the risk for CAD also reduce the risk for angina. Key among these measures are daily physical EXERCISE, nutritious eating habits, maintaining healthy weight, and controlling blood cholesterol and triglycerides levels.

See also LIFESTYLE AND HEART HEALTH; MEDICATION MANAGEMENT; MEDICATIONS TO TREAT HEART DISEASE; QUALITY OF LIFE.

angiogenesis   The growth of new BLOOD vessels. In cancer, angiogenesis is undesirable because it supports tumor growth and is the target of some forms of treatment. In HEART DISEASES however, angiogenesis offers hope that the HEART muscle can generate new networks of blood vessels as nonsurgical treatment for ISCHEMIC HEART DISEASE (impaired blood flow to the myocardium, or heart muscle) and repair itself after tissue damage resulting from MYOCARDIAL INFARCTION (HEART ATTACK).

Researchers are investigating treatments that use AMINO ACID–based substances called angiogenic factors to stimulate new growth of blood vessels. Scientists discovered the natural occurrence of angiogenic factors in the 1990s and continue to explore therapeutic applications of them. At present, induced therapeutic angiogenesis remains investigational. The two angiogenic factors showing the most promise for treating heart disease are fibrinoblast growth factor (FGH) and vascular endothelial growth factor A (VEGF-A). These factors target cells in the blood vessels, encouraging their reproduction and resulting in new growth of this specific tissue type.

Key challenges of therapeutic angiogenesis include administering the factors and controlling their effects after administration. Because angiogenic factors are amino acid based, the body quickly metabolizes them. In phase I clinical studies, the most consistent results occur when researchers inject the factor directly into the blood vessels where angiogenesis is desired. This requires invasive techniques such as CARDIAC CATHETERIZA-TION; some small studies have tested this approach during ANGIOPLASTY or CORONARY ARTERY BYPASS GRAFT (CABG) surgery. Other methods involve GENE THERAPY, which also is investigational at present, and injectable protein solutions in which the angiogenic growth factor is suspended. These are less precise methods, making it more difficult to regulate the action of the factors. Uncontrolled angiogenesis can cause overgrowth of blood vessels, resulting in various problems that interfere with rather than support proper heart function.

angiography   A diagnostic procedure in which dye is injected into an ARTERY to make it visible by X-ray. Angiography is used to diagnose CORONARY ARTERY DISEASE (CAD; blockage of the arteries supplying the HEART), PERIPHERAL ARTERY DISEASE (PAD; blockages in the arteries supplying other parts of the body such as the arms and legs), ANEURYSM, carotid artery occlusion, ISCHEMIC HEART DISEASE, ischemic STROKE, and other problems involving the CIRCULATION of BLOOD. The procedure is painless, although some people experience mild discomfort when the dye is first injected.

Angiography in which the dye is injected directly into the coronary arteries is part of a cardiac catheterization. In this procedure, the cardiologist inserts a catheter through an artery in the groin or arm and threads it through to the coronary arteries. Once the catheter is in place, the cardiologist injects the dye and uses FLUOROSCOPY to observe the pattern of its flow through the coronary arteries. This highlights any blockages or abnormalities in the coronary arteries.

Angiography may also be computer-assisted, and it is then called digital cardiac angiography (DCA) or digital substraction angiography (DSA). In these imaging procedures, an X-ray machine takes a series of pictures to follow the flow of the injected dye as it travels to the brain or the heart. A computer then compiles the pictures of blood flow. Cardiologists use DCA and DSA to identify stenosis, accumulations of arterial plaque, and other impediments to the flow of blood through the arteries.

Angiography can be performed in the cardiac catheterization facility at a hospital or in a free-standing cardiac catheterization facility. It is important for the facility to have the capacity to respond to a life-threatening emergency should one occur. Occasionally angiography can cause a piece of arterial PLAQUE to break free or for a clot to form and enter the bloodstream, which can result in heart attack or stroke. Because angiography requires puncturing the skin and inserting an object into the body (the catheter), there is a slight risk of bleeding or infection. Angiography generally takes about an hour to conduct, during which time the person is lightly sedated. A local anesthetic numbs the area where the catheter is inserted for coronary angiography.

See also ANGIOPLASTY; CAROTID BRUIT; COMPUTED TOMOGRAPHY (CT) SCAN; POSITRON EMISSION TOMOGRAPHY (PET); SINGLE PHOTON EMISSION COMPUTED TOMOGRAPHY (SPECT) SCAN.

angioplasty A procedure for clearing blockages of the CORONARY ARTERIES to restore the flow of BLOOD to the HEART muscle (myocardium). The correct clinical term for this procedure is percutaneous transluminal coronary angioplasty, or PCTA. People commonly refer to PCTA as balloon angioplasty. This treatment for CORONARY ARTERY DISEASE (CAD) does not require surgery to open the chest and expose the heart, as does CORONARY ARTERY BYPASS GRAFT (CABG), but instead uses an incision into an artery near the skin's surface ("percutaneous") to insert and guide a small, hollow, flexible tube called a catheter ("transluminal," which means through the center of) into the coronary artery.

Angioplasty is an appropriate treatment option for people who have a single occlusion in one or more coronary arteries. Angioplasty typically is *not* an appropriate treatment option for people whose coronary arteries have multiple occlusions, occlusions in locations that are difficult to visualize using FLUOROSCOPY or to place the balloon, have previously had more than two angioplasty procedures in the same location, or who have other heart disease. People who have more extensive coronary artery disease generally need CABG.

Procedure

Angioplasty is performed with local anesthetic to numb the area in the groin where the catheter is inserted and with mild sedation for relaxation, and is done in a hospital that has a CARDIAC CATHETERIZATION facility as well as full surgical facilities for OPEN-HEART SURGERY should it be necessary. The procedure takes about an hour, followed by several hours of close monitoring. Most people stay in the hospital overnight.

During angioplasty, the cardiologist inserts a catheter into the femoral artery in the groin, and then threads the catheter through the femoral artery into the abdominal aorta, into the heart, and into the coronary artery to the location of the blockage, called an occlusion. A kind of X-ray called fluoroscopy allows the cardiologist to visualize the arteries and see the progression of the catheter into the coronary artery. Sometimes the cardiologist instead uses an artery in the arm to thread the catheter into the heart; this determination depends on various factors including the location of the occlusion.

Once the catheter is in place, the cardiologist inserts through it a second catheter that has a tiny, deflated balloon at its tip. When the balloon catheter is at the site of the occlusion, the cardiologist then injects a solution that inflates the balloon, compressing the arterial PLAQUE against the arterial wall to widen the passageway for blood. After ANGIOGRAPHY confirms that the artery is dilated, the cardiologist withdraws the fluid to deflate the balloon, and removes the balloon catheter. The cardiologist chooses whether to leave the guide catheter in place for several hours, until the cardiologist determines that the angioplasty is going to hold and the person is stable, or to remove it immediately following the procedure. The advantage of removing the catheter and suturing the entry incision is that the person then can sit up and even walk within a few hours. There are several kinds of angioplasty.

- **Dilatative or simple angioplasty** is the basic procedure in which the inflated balloon compresses the occlusion to reopen the artery. Simple angioplasty generally treats moderate occlusions (75 to 85 percent) in which there is no increased risk for the occlusion to recur.

- **Ablative angioplasty** involves first removing the occlusion, called ATHERECTOMY. In this procedure, the catheter is threaded into the blocked coronary artery as for simple PCTA. Before inflating the balloon, the cardiologist inserts tiny instruments or a specialized laser through the catheter to ablate, or destroy, the collection of plaque.

- **Stent angioplasty** involves placing a tiny "tunnel" inside the artery at the location of the occlusion. The cardiologist can place the stent after compressing the plaque against the artery's wall, or insert the stent as a "sleeve" over the balloon and place it at the same time the balloon is inflated. When the balloon is deflated to remove it, the stent stays in place. Made of a specialized stainless steel mesh, the stent helps to hold the artery open and prevent plaque from recollecting in the same location. The meshlike structure of the stent encourages the tissues of the arterial wall to attach, helping to hold the stent in place. Stent angioplasty can, and often does, follow ablative angioplasty.

Risks and Complications

Most complications resulting from angioplasty occur fairly immediately. The most serious is the sudden closure of the artery at the site of the occlusion, which occasionally occurs as somewhat of a spasm response in the artery. The cardiologist can usually correct this by reinserting the balloon catheter and deploying a stent, although sometimes CABG is necessary to replace the damaged portion of coronary artery. Other complications include bleeding at the entry site and infection, typical risks of any surgical procedure.

Angioplasty sometimes fails to prevent recurrent narrowing in the coronary artery. This is called restenosis. When this happens, as it does for about one in four people who undergo the procedure, the cardiologist might consider a repeat angioplasty depending on what was done the first time and the suspected reasons for the restenosis. More often, the cardiologist recommends CABG, which is more extensive surgery and recovery but has a higher rate of long-term success.

Outlook and Lifestyle Modifications

Most people (95 percent) fully recover from the angioplasty procedure and are back to normal activities within a few days to a week or two. There might be soreness at the incision site, where the catheter was inserted into the artery, for several days. ANGINA, shortness of breath, and other symptoms of coronary artery disease typically go away immediately following the angioplasty. Factors that can complicate recovery from angioplasty include uncontrolled HYPERTENSION, DIABETES, cigarette smoking, and OBESITY. Depending on the kind of angioplasty, a person might take an ANTICOAGULANT MEDICATION for a short time (six to eight weeks) or other medications. It is important to appropriately treat any other kinds of cardiovascular disease that are also present, such as hypertension.

The best success with angioplasty occurs when the person also makes lifestyle changes to support heart health following the procedure. These include stopping smoking, eating a low-fat, nutritious diet, and getting regular EXERCISE. Most cardiologists recommend a structured CARDIAC REHABILITATION program following angioplasty, which provides a supervised and individualized nutrition and exercise plan.

See also LIFESTYLE AND HEART HEALTH; MEDICATIONS TO TREAT HEART DISEASE; NUTRITION AND DIET; QUALITY OF LIFE; SURGERY TO TREAT, CARDIOVASCULAR DISEASE.

angiotensin-converting enzyme (ACE) inhibitor medications   Drugs taken to lower BLOOD PRESSURE by preventing the action of ANGIOTENSIN-CONVERTING ENZYME (ACE). ACE is a substance the body produces that metabolizes angiotensinogen (angiotensin I), which is inactive in this form, into angiotensin II, which is a powerful VASOCONSTRICTOR. This action is part of the RENIN-ANGIOTENSIN-ALDOSTERONE (RAA) HORMONAL SYSTEM, the body's primary mechanism for regulating blood pressure. Angiotensin II is a potent vasoconstrictor that acts on the smallest of peripheral arteries, the arterioles, causing them to become narrow and more rigid. This increases BLOOD pressure.

ACE inhibitors interfere with the action of ACE to prevent this sequence of events from completion, which keeps blood pressure from rising. ACE inhibitors are sometimes taken for congestive HEART FAILURE and to delay or prevent further kidney damage in diabetes. These drugs also have an effect on the myocardium (HEART muscle) that helps to restore function following HEART ATTACK.

There are numerous ACE inhibitors available in the United States. They include BENAZEPRIL

(Lotensin), CAPTOPRIL (Capoten), ENALAPRIL (Vasotec), FOSINOPRIL (Monopril), LISINOPRIL (Prinivil), MOEXIPRIL (Univasc), RAMIPRIL (Altace), and TRANDOLAPRIL (Mavik). The effects these drugs have on blood pressure are comparable, although individuals might experience better benefit or fewer side effects with one drug over another.

ACE inhibitors have numerous undesired side effects, among them a troubling and persistent cough that often continues even after the person stops taking the ACE inhibitor. People who have problems with cough as a side effect often can switch to another classification of ANTIHYPERTENSIVE MEDICATIONS, ANGIOTENSIN II RECEPTOR ANTAGONIST MEDICATIONS, for a similar effect on blood pressure without this side effect. Other common side effects include headache, DIZZINESS, weakness, and rash. Like many other antihypertensive medications, ACE inhibitors can cause the body to retain POTASSIUM so people taking them should not use salt substitutes that contain potassium. Very rare but very serious side effects are kidney failure, allergic reaction, depleted white blood cells, and EDEMA (fluid retention that results in tissue swelling).

People with mild to moderate hypertension often can control their blood pressure with an ACE inhibitor as monotherapy (the only drug used). Moderate to severe hypertension often requires a combination of medications for control. DIURETIC MEDICATIONS are commonly incorporated as ADJUNCT THERAPY.

See also DIABETES AND HEART DISEASE; HYPERTENSION; MEDICATIONS TO TREAT HEART DISEASE.

angiotensin II receptor A molecular structure on a cell that can receive, or bind with, the molecular structure of an enzyme called angiotensin II. These cells are located primarily in the arterioles, the body's smallest arteries. Angiotensin II is a strong VASOCONSTRICTOR; when it binds with its receptors, it causes the arterioles to contract. This narrows and stiffens these tiny arteries, requiring increased pressure to push blood through them. This in turn raises BLOOD PRESSURE.

The body produces angiotensin II as part of the RENIN-ANGIOTENSIN-ALDOSTERONE (RAA) HOR-

MONAL SYSTEM, which is one of the body's primary mechanisms for regulating blood pressure. Drugs called ANGIOTENSIN II RECEPTOR ANTAGONIST MEDICATIONS can prevent angiotensin II from binding with its receptors, preventing the arterioles from contracting. This keeps the arterioles open, reducing the resistance blood encounters when flowing through them and keeping blood pressure from going up.

See also ANGIOTENSIN-CONVERTING ENZYME; ANGIOTENSIN-CONVERTING ENZYME INHIBITOR MEDICATIONS; ANTIHYPERTENSIVE MEDICATIONS; HYPERTENSION; MEDICATIONS TO TREAT HEART DISEASE.

angiotensin II receptor antagonist medications
ANTIHYPERTENSIVE MEDICATIONS that work by preventing the enzyme angiotensin II from binding with its receptors in the walls of the body's tiniest arteries, the arterioles. Angiotensin II receptor antagonists available in the United States include CANDESARTAN (Atacand), IRBESARTAN (Avapro), LOSARTAN (Cozaar), VALSARTAN (Diovan), TELMISARTAN (Micardis), and EPROSARTAN (Teveten). Losartan also is available in combination with a diuretic, HYDROCHLOROTHIAZIDE, in a product called Hyzaar. The first of these medications, losartan, came into use in the mid-1990s. These medications are sometimes called AIIAs or ARBs.

There do not appear to be significant differences among the different drugs in this classification in terms of their effectiveness in lowering blood pressure, although the body metabolizes them differently. A person might have better benefit from some than from others as a matter of individual response. Adding a diuretic such as hydrochlorothiazide as an ADJUNCT THERAPY to a treatment regimen that includes an angiotensin II receptor antagonist significantly enhances the effect of the latter drug in many people.

Undesired side effects are uncommon, but when they do occur might include stomach upset, diarrhea, DIZZINESS, and headache. Angiotensin II receptor antagonists can cause a buildup of POTASSIUM in the BLOOD, so people taking these drugs should not use salt substitutes that contain potassium. These drugs also are prescribed to help prevent the progression of kidney disease in people with hypertension or DIABETES. Angiotensin II receptor antagonist drugs are known to cause birth defects; women who are pregnant should not take them.

See also ANGIOTENSIN-CONVERTING ENZYME (ACE) INHIBITOR MEDICATIONS; DIURETIC MEDICATIONS; MEDICATIONS TO TREAT HEART DISEASE.

anorexia nervosa See EATING DISORDERS AND HEART DISEASE.

antianxiety medications Drugs that help a person to feel calm and relaxed and that relieve the symptoms of anxiety. Many people feel mild to moderate anxiety following a cardiac crisis such as HEART ATTACK or with conditions such as ANGINA. This can intensify fear and worry, adding emotional stress and interfering with healing, recovery, and return to full activities. For anxiety that persists, antianxiety medications (also called tranquilizers) can provide temporary relief.

There are many antianxiety medications. The most commonly prescribed family of antianxiety medications is the benzodiazepines, whose best-known members include diazepam (Valium) and alprazolam (Xanax). Benzodiazepines act on receptors in the brain to slow nerve signals from the central nervous system (CNS). They typically cause drowsiness, particularly during the first two to six weeks of taking them, and can be addictive when taken inappropriately (in higher-than-prescribed doses or for an extended time). Some ANTIDEPRESSANT MEDICATIONS also have antianxiety effects. These include selective serotonin reuptake inhibitors (SSRIs), such as paroxetine (Paxil) and fluoxetine (Prozac), and tricyclic antidepressants, such as amitriptyline and imipramine. A drug that is in a class of its own as an antianxiety medication is buspirone (Buspar), which acts on serotonin and dopamine receptors in the brain but does not cause sedation or other CNS symptoms. It can cause PALPITATIONS and CHEST PAIN, however.

In most situations, antianxiety medications should be taken for short-term relief. STRESS REDUCTION TECHNIQUES such as MEDITATION and visualization often are helpful in relieving anxiety for the longer term. Antianxiety medications can interact with a broad variety of other medications, so it is important for the prescribing physician to know all of the other medications, including any herbal products, that the person is also taking.

See also DEPRESSION; LIFESTYLE AND HEART HEALTH; MEDICATION MANAGEMENT.

antiarrhythmia medications Drugs that help to restore the normal electrical patterns of the heartbeat. An ARRHYTHMIA is an irregular heartbeat; the kind of irregularity determines the drug that is appropriate to restore the heartbeat to a normal rhythm. Heart rhythm disorders are common, and most of them respond to treatment with medication. However, this does not minimize the significance of arrhythmias. These heart conditions cause many of the deaths that result from sudden cardiac arrest.

Type of Anti-arrhythmic	Taken to Treat	Common Drugs
adenosine	paroxysmal supra-ventricular tachycardia	adenosine (Adenocard)
sodium channel blocking medications (class I)	severe ventricular fibrillation	quinidine (Cardioquin, Quinidex), procainamide (Pronestyl), mexiletine (Mexitil), propafenone (Rythmol)
beta antagonist medications (class II)	atrial fibrillation, ventricular tachycardia	acebutolol (Sectral), atenolol (Tenormin), labetolol (Normodyne), metoprolol (Lopressor), propranolol (Inderal)
potassium channel blocking medications (class III)	atrial tachycardia, atrial fibrillation	amiodarone (Cordarone), ibutilide (Corvert), dofetilide (Tikosyn)
calcium channel blocking medications (class IV)	sinus tachycardia, other sinus arrhythmias	verapamil (Isoptin), diltiazem (Cardizem)

There are several families of drugs within the classification of antiarrhythmia medications. As it is possible for more than one arrhythmia to be present, medication therapy might include two or more antiarrhythmia medications or antiarrhythmics in combination with other heart medications. Some drugs treat arrhythmias as well as other cardiovascular symptoms.

Antiarrhythmia medications do not work consistently among people who have the same diagnosis, and finding the "right" one can be a challenging trial-and-error experience. These drugs also can *cause* arrhythmias. The margin of safety, or therapeutic index, for antiarrhythmia medications is very narrow. Blood tests can monitor the levels of these drugs in the body so the prescribing physician can make necessary adjustments to maintain an appropriate therapeutic level with minimal side effects. Doctors are looking increasingly toward other approaches to managing arrhythmias, including implanted devices and catheter OBLATION.

See also ATRIAL FIBRILLATION; LIVING WITH HEART DISEASE; SUDDEN CARDIAC ARREST.

antibiotic prophylaxis   Antibiotics taken before certain dental, surgical, and medical procedures to prevent infection. People with certain kinds of heart disease are at increased risk for infection involving the HEART, particularly the HEART VALVES and the heart itself (ENDOCARDITIS). Anyone who has heart disease should tell this to each health-care provider (such as doctors, dentists, oral surgeons) who provides health-care services so the provider can determine whether antibiotic prophylaxis is appropriate. It is also critical to identify any antibiotic allergies to each provider each time antibiotics are discussed, just to make sure this vital information does not get overlooked.

People who are at high risk should always have antibiotic prophylaxis for procedures that could introduce bacteria into the body; people at moderate risk should discuss the procedure and its specific risks for their conditions with the provider to determine whether prophylactic antibiotics are necessary. Antibiotics typically are taken by mouth or given by injection shortly before the procedure takes place. The antibiotic used depends on the heart condition, the potential infection risk, and any antibiotic allergies the person might have.

People who have had RHEUMATIC HEART DISEASE, Kawasaki disease, previous heart surgery such as CORONARY ARTERY BYPASS GRAFT (CABG) or SEPTAL DEFECT repair, or PACEMAKER placement and have no residual effects from these procedures typically do not need antibiotic prophylaxis.

See also SURGERY TO TREAT CARDIOVASCULAR DISEASE.

WHO NEEDS ANTIBIOTIC PROPHYLAXIS		
People with These Heart Conditions Have High Risk	**People with These Heart Conditions Have Moderate Risk**	**Should Take Prophylactic Antibiotics for These Procedures**
Artificial heart valves	Other congenital heart conditions	Dental extractions and surgeries including periodontal (gum) and endodontic (root canal) and dental prophylaxis (cleaning) when there is a possibility of bleeding gums
Congenital cyanotic heart disease	Valve disease or dysfunction	
Ever had bacterial infections affecting the heart such as endocarditis	Hypertrophic cardiomyopathy (HCM)	
Surgical pulmonary shunts	Mitral valve prolapse with regurgitation	Any surgery
		Bronchoscopy (rigid scope)
		Genitourinary tract procedures such as cystoscopy and urethral dilation
		Endoscopy and endoscopic procedures including transesophageal echocardiogram
		Uterine D & C
		Placement/removal of contraceptive intra-uterine device

antibiotics and statin medications   There is some concern among health experts that statin medications taken to lower BLOOD cholesterol and TRIGLYC-ERIDES levels can interact with certain antibiotics to cause a very rare but potentially fatal complication called RHABDOMYOLYSIS. Research continues to explore this apparent interaction to determine whether it involves entire classifications of drugs or specific drugs taken in combination. As well, some antibiotics cause higher than normal blood levels of statin medications when taken in combination, such as the antibiotic erythromycin and the statin drug ATORVASTATIN (Lipitor). Erythromycin and the antibiotic clarithromycin are also linked to myositis (inflammation of the muscles). Common statin medications include atorvastatin, SIMVAS-TATIN (Zocor), and PRAVASTATIN (Pravachol). People who take statin medications should tell this to any doctor who prescribes an antibiotic.

See also LIPID-LOWERING MEDICATIONS; MEDICA-TION MANAGEMENT; MEDICATION SIDE EFFECTS; MEDI-CATIONS TO TREAT HEART DISEASE.

anticoagulant medications   Drugs taken to help prevent BLOOD clots from forming. These medications are prescribed for various cardiovascular diseases, including DEEP VEIN THROMBOSIS (DVT), MITRAL VALVE PROLAPSE, ischemic STROKE prophylaxis, ISCHEMIC HEART DISEASE (IHD), and following cardiovascular procedures such as CARDIAC CATHETERIZATION or ANGIOPLASTY with STENT. One of the most common anticoagulants is ASPIRIN. Other anticoagulant medications are HEPARIN, WARFARIN (Coumadin), DIPYRIDAMOLE (Persantine), CLOPI-DOGREL (Plavix), TICLOPIDINE (Ticlid), CILOSTAZOL (Pletal), prasugrel (Effient), and PENTOXIFYLLINE (Trental).

Dietary factors can influence the effectiveness of anticoagulant medications, particularly coumadin. Green vegetables are high in vitamin K, a natural coagulant (substance that encourages blood to clot). Numerous medications interfere with the actions of anticoagulants and can either intensify or minimize their effectiveness. Anticoagulants have similar effects on other drugs. It is important for the prescribing physician and the dispensing pharmacist to know all of the medica-tions a person is taking. Regular blood tests are necessary to monitor the effectiveness of antico-agulant medications.

antidepressant medications   Drugs that elevate mood and relieve DEPRESSION. Antidepressant medications act on neuroreceptors in the brain, altering the balance of NEUROTRANSMITTERS (specialized chemicals involved in carrying signals from nerve cells) in the brain. There are three major classifications or types of prescription antidepressants: monoamine oxidase inhibitors (MAOIs), tricyclics, and selective serotonin reuptake inhibitors (SSRIs). There are also a number of herbal products, sold as dietary supplements in the United States, that many people take for their antidepressant qualities. Each type of antidepressant affects the brain in a different way. Antidepressants can interact with numerous other medications including MEDI-CATIONS TO TREAT HEART DISEASE. As well, medications to treat heart disease can affect the actions of antidepressants.

Although it is normal and common for people to feel a wide range of emotions when diagnosed with a cardiovascular disease or following HEART ATTACK or STROKE, feelings of sadness and futility that continue for more than a few weeks can signal clinical depression, a potentially serious medical condition for which professional assistance is appropriate. Depression is common in people who have had a cardiac event or cardiac crisis, or who have chronic cardiovascular conditions that limit or change their lifestyles such as HEART FAILURE or ISCHEMIC HEART DISEASE (IHD).

Most people should take antidepressants only for a limited time, typically no longer than six months. Many people benefit from psychotherapy to help them understand the reasons for their depression. It is especially important for people with HEART DISEASE who have symptoms of depression to receive prompt medical attention, as depression can affect cardiovascular functions such as BLOOD PRESSURE and HEART RATE and can activate the body's "FIGHT-OR-FLIGHT" stress response mechanism. Antidepressant medications restore the proper balance of chemicals in the brain, helping to suppress the stress response as well as reestablish emotional equilibrium. Undesired side effects from antidepressant medications differ among medications.

Monoamine Oxidase Inhibitors (MAOIs)

Although MAOIs were the first antidepressants available, they are usually the last choice for treating depression today because of their many and sometimes serious side effects, particularly for people with heart disease. Monoamine oxidase is an enzyme that occurs naturally in the body. Its role is to metabolize neurotransmitters in the brain that affect mood such as NOREPINEPHRINE, serotonin, and DOPAMINE. Inhibiting, or blocking, this action elevates the amounts of these neurotransmitters that are present. MAOIs generally are *not* a good choice for people with cardiovascular disease, especially those taking medications for their heart conditions.

MAOIs interfere with numerous medications and should not be taken at the same time, including other antidepressants and many medications taken to treat heart disease including:

- ANTIHYPERTENSIVE MEDICATIONS such as GUANADREL (Hylorel), GUANETHIDINE (Ismelin), HYDRALAZINE, (Apresoline), METHYLDOPA (Aldomet), and RESERPINE (Serpasil)
- Adrenergic agonist medications such as dopamine (Intropin), EPINEPHRINE (adrenaline), isoproterenol (Isuprel), and metaraminol (Aramine)
- Some BETA ANTAGONIST MEDICATIONS and DIURETICS taken to treat hypertension or HEART FAILURE

Other drugs with which MAOIs interfere include medications to treat Parkinson's disease, over-the-counter cough and cold preparations and decongestants, SSRIs, tricyclic antidepressants, antiseizure medications, antianxiety medications, appetite suppression medications, demerol, many anesthetics, and sleeping aids. MAOIs also interact with foods containing the enzyme tyramine. The list of these foods is extensive but generally includes foods that are fermented, such as cheeses and wines; smoked, pickled, or processed meats; and foods that contain the preservative monosodium glutamate (MSG).

Tricyclic Antidepressants

The first tricyclic antidepressants became available in the 1950s. They are called tricyclic because the body metabolizes them in three distinct stages. These drugs affect how neurons in the brain reabsorb the components of key neurotransmitters involved with nerve signals related to mood such as acetylcholine, norepinephrine, serotonin, and dopamine. Tricyclic antidepressants are nonselective in this, which means that they affect this reabsorption, or reuptake. They have numerous potential and common side effects including weakness, fatigue, dry mouth, increased heart rate, and arrhythmias.

People with heart disease, including hypertension, generally should *not* take tricyclic antidepressants. Because tricyclic antidepressants can cause ARRHYTHMIAS, in particular people with heart rhythm disorders such as ATRIAL FIBRILLATION and A-V node disturbances should not take them. These medications interfere with numerous medications taken to treat cardiovascular disease including most antihypertensives and antiarrhythmia medications. Tricyclic antidepressants in combination with quinidine for arrhythmia can cause heart failure.

Selective Serotonin Reuptake Inhibitors (SSRIs)

The SSRIs are the safest type of antidepressant medication for people being treated for heart disease who also need an antidepressant medication, although like all drugs, they are not without risk of potentially serious side effects. SSRIs interact with some other medications, including other antidepressants, oral medications to treat diabetes, and benzodiazepine drugs taken to treat anxiety, such as alprazolam (Xanax) and diazepam (Valium). SSRIs also interfere with the action of certain medications taken to treat cardiovascular disease, in particular:

- DIGOXIN taken to treat arrhythmias or heart failure
- ANTIARRHYTHMIA MEDICATIONS such as MEXILETINE (Mexitil) and PROPAFENONE (Rythmol)
- beta antagonist medications taken to treat hypertension or ANGINA such as metoprolol (Lopressor) and propanolol (Inderal)

• calcium channel blockers including nifedipine (Procardia) and verapamil (Calan)

Unlike other antidepressants, SSRIs can be taken with cardiovascular drugs as long as the blood levels of the cardiovascular drugs are carefully monitored. SSRIs tend to increase the action of these medications, which can intensify their effects. This is potentially dangerous with digoxin in particular, as digoxin has a narrow therapeutic range and can quickly reach toxic levels in the body.

Herbal Antidepressants

In recent years, herbal antidepressants available without a prescription have become popular in the United States. Marketed as dietary supplements, they are widely available. Many people who take them do not think of them as drugs, although in fact they are because they alter the body's chemistry. Because medications taken to treat cardiovascular disease are so potent and can interact with numerous other drugs, it is essential for people taking herbal products to tell their physicians and pharmacists. People who are taking medications for heart conditions should not start taking any herbal product or other over-the-counter medication without first consulting a doctor or pharmacist about possible interactions.

Because herbal products are classified as dietary supplements, they are excluded from the regulations and standards that apply to other drugs. Manufacturing procedures can be inconsistent, so different brands can deliver varying amounts of active ingredients even though the label strengths are the same. As well, manufacturers sometimes blend ingredients to create unique products. It is important to read labels carefully. Do not take herbal antidepressants with prescription antidepressants.

The three most commonly used herbal antidepressant products are Saint-John's-wort (hypericum), borage, and kava kava. A number of clinical studies show that Saint-John's-wort is as effective as SSRIs or tricyclic antidepressants for mild depression with fewer side effects. However, it does interfere with the actions of some cardiovascular drugs including digoxin (taken to treat arrhythmias or heart failure) and the anticoagulant warfarin (Coumadin). It also interacts with CYCLOSPORINE, a drug commonly taken after HEART TRANSPLANT to

---

ANTIDEPRESSANTS AND MEDICATIONS TO TREAT HEART DISEASE

Type of Antidepressant	Common Drugs	Cardiovascular Cautions
Monoamine oxidase inhibitors (MAOIs)	phenelzine (Nardil), seligiline (Eldepryl), tranylcypromine (Parnate)	Can cause tachycardia (rapid heartbeat), rapid elevation of blood pressure, and stroke or heart attack in interaction with tyramine, an enzyme in certain foods
		Interact with many antihypertensive medications, adrenergic agonist medications, beta antagonist medications, and diuretics
Tricyclics	amitriptyline (Elavil), desipramine (Norpramin), imipramine (Tofranil), nortriptyline (Pamelor), trimipramine (Surmontil)	Interfere with nearly all types of anti-hypertensive and anti-arrhythmia medications; can cause arrhythmias; can cause increased heart rate; with quinidine, can cause heart failure
Selective serotonin reuptake inhibitors (SSRIs)	citalopram (Celexa), fluoxetine (Prozac), fluvoxamine (Luvox), paroxetine (Paxil), sertraline (Zoloft)	Interact with digoxin; interact with some anti-arrhythmia medications; interact with beta-blockers and calcium channel blockers (anti-hypertensives)
Herbal products	Saint-John's-wort (hypericum), kava kava	Saint-John's-wort interferes with the action of cyclosporine (taken following organ transplant to prevent rejection, digoxin (taken for arrhythmias and heart failure), and warfarin (taken to prevent blood clots)

prevent rejection of the donor heart. Borage contains high amounts of POTASSIUM, which can cause problems for people who are taking potassium-sparing diuretics to treat hypertension or heart failure. Kava kava can cause serious liver damage or liver failure; the National Institutes of Health (NIH) has issued a warning advising against taking products containing kava kava for any reason.

See also ANTIANXIETY MEDICATIONS; ANXIETY; COLD/FLU MEDICATIONS AND HYPERTENSION; HERBAL REMEDIES; MEDITATION; QUALITY OF LIFE; STRESS REDUCTION TECHNIQUES; YOGA.

antihypertensive medications Drugs taken to lower BLOOD PRESSURE as treatment for HYPERTENSION (high blood pressure). There are numerous classifications, or types, of these medications, each of which acts by different mechanisms to lower blood pressure. Because hypertension is a complex condition, it is common for people to take two or more medications of different types and actions to bring and keep blood pressure under control. Each type of antihypertensive medication has unique benefits and potential side effects. Some of these drugs are taken to treat cardiovascular conditions other than, or in addition to, hypertension. The most effective therapeutic approach for most people combines antihypertensive medications with LIFESTYLE modifications such as increased physical activity and EXERCISE, WEIGHT MANAGEMENT, and nutritious eating habits (lowering the amounts of fat and salt in the diet).

Drugs That Reduce Fluid Volume: Diuretics

People often refer to DIURETIC MEDICATIONS as "water pills" because they act to increase the amount of fluid the kidneys extract from the BLOOD. This reduces the volume of blood flow, lowering the amount of pressure required to circulate the blood supply through the body. There are several types of diuretics; the choice depends on numerous factors including other cardiovascular disease, other medications, and potential side effects. Diuretics are often the first line of medication therapy for mild to moderate hypertension and are taken in combination with other kinds of antihypertensive medications for serious hypertension. The types of diuretics have different

characteristics and actions in the body, and doctors sometimes prescribe more than one type of diuretic to get maximum benefit.

Drugs That Block Adrenergic Activity: Alpha and Beta Antagonists

The cells of the myocardium (heart muscle) and the muscle fibers in the walls of the arteries contain ADRENERGIC RECEPTORS. Epinephrine binds with these receptors to set in motion a sequence of events that constricts (narrows and stiffens) the walls of the arteries and intensifies the pumping action of the heart. The result is an increase in blood pressure. Drugs that interfere with adrenergic binding cause the arteries to relax, reducing resistance for blood flowing through the arteries and lowering blood pressure. There are two main types of adrenergic receptors in the heart and blood vessels, denoted as alpha and beta. Each type has multiple subtypes. Antihypertensives target one or more of these types or subtypes, and are classified accordingly.

- ALPHA ANTAGONIST MEDICATIONS block alpha-1, alpha-2, or alpha-1 and alpha-2 receptors. Doctors generally reserve alpha blockers for hypertension that does not respond to other treatment efforts. Alpha blockers affect other smooth muscle tissues in the body that have alpha-adrenergic receptors including the genitourinary system. Undesired side effects such as erectile dysfunction in men and urinary stress incontinence in women are unfortunately common with these drugs.

- BETA ANTAGONIST MEDICATIONS block beta-1, beta-2, or beta-1 and beta-2 receptors. They also relieve mild anxiety. Response to these medications is highly individual and it can take some time to identify the appropriate dose. Tiredness upon exertion is a sign that the dose is too high. Among the most common side effects of beta-blockers are fatigue and reduced libido (sex drive) in men and women.

- Alpha+beta antagonist medications block both alpha and beta receptors. These drugs lower blood pressure by simultaneously relaxing the arteries and slowing the heart rate.

Drugs that block adrenergic activity also are taken to treat ARRHYTHMIAS and migraine headaches.

Drugs That Inhibit the Renin-Angiotensin-Aldosterone (RAA) Hormone System

The RENIN-ANGIOTENSIN-ALDOSTERONE (RAA) HORMONE SYSTEM is the body mechanism primarily responsible for regulating blood pressure. Specialized cells in the kidneys are highly sensitive to minute changes in blood pressure. When blood pressure drops, these cells respond by releasing an enzyme called renin. Once in circulation in the bloodstream, renin acts to metabolize the protein angiotensinogen (to angiotensin I), which the liver produces and is converted into angiotensin II by ACE.

Angiotensinogen is inert; that is, it has no activity in the body. However, its end product angiotensin II is a powerful vasoconstrictor. Angiotensin II binds with receptors that line the body's tiny arteries, the arterioles, and causes them to constrict. It also signals the adrenal glands to release the hormone aldosterone. Aldosterone causes the kidneys to release less sodium, which draws fluid into the blood and increases blood volume, causing blood pressure to rise. Interfering with this cycle blocks blood pressure from rising. In the 1990s two new types of drugs came on the market that do just that using different approaches.

- ANGIOTENSIN II RECEPTOR ANTAGONIST MEDICATIONS, the first antihypertensive drugs to target the RAA hormone system, work by preventing angiotensin II from binding with its receptors. This keeps the arterioles open and relaxed.

- ANGIOTENSIN-CONVERTING ENZYME (ACE) INHIBITOR MEDICATIONS work by preventing ACE from converting or metabolizing angiotensin I into angiotensin II. Without this chemical messenger to signal the adrenal glands, aldosterone levels remain unchanged.

These two classifications of drugs are similarly effective in lowering blood pressure. A key difference is in their potential side effects. ACE inhibitors have a tendency to cause a dry, persistent cough that can continue for four to six weeks after stopping the drug. Switching to an angiotensin II receptor inhibitor typically provides the same level of blood pressure control without the cough. Very rare but very serious side effects with ACE inhibitors are kidney failure, a lowered WHITE BLOOD CELL count, and angioedema (fluid retention that results in tissue swelling), an allergic reaction.

Calcium Channel Blocking Medications

CALCIUM CHANNEL ANTAGONIST MEDICATIONS work by slowing muscle contractions. This relaxes the arteries and the heart, providing an open passage for blood and some slow the heart rate. The combined effect causes lower blood pressure as the heart does not have to work as hard to circulate blood through the body. These drugs also are taken to treat arrhythmias.

Drugs That Open the Arteries: Vasodilators

VASODILATOR MEDICATIONS are drugs that act on the muscles of the walls of the arteries to cause them to relax. This opens the arteries and allows an increased volume of blood to flow through with less pressure. The end result is that overall blood pressure drops. Many medications taken to treat hypertension that act on smooth muscle in some way have vasodilator effects.

Calcium channel antagonist medications, alpha antagonist medications, angiotensin receptor antagonist medications, angiotensin-converting enzyme (ACE) inhibitor medications, and NITRATE MEDICATIONS all have vasodilating properties.

Other Antihypertensive Medications

Some medications taken to treat hypertension do not fit into specific categories or classifications. Among them are:

- RAUWOLFIA alkaloid (Reserpine, Serpasil) is a peripheral adrenergic antagonist that blocks the action of NOREPINEPHRINE, serotonin, and DOPAMINE in tissues throughout the body including the brain. This causes general relaxation as well as relaxation of the arteries. Because rauwolfia also affects brain activity, it often causes drowsiness. It has many side effects, some of which are serious.

See also ACUPUNCTURE; MEDICATIONS TO TREAT HEART DISEASE; NUTRITION AND DIET.

Type or Classification	Common Drugs
Alpha antagonists (blockers)	prazosin (Minipres), terazosin (Hytrin), doxazosin (Cardura), clonidine (Catapres), guanabenz (Wytensin), guanfacine (Tenex), methyldopa (Aldomet)
Alpha+beta antago- nists (blockers) Angiotensin-converting enzyme (ACE) inhibitors	labetalol (Normodyne), carvedilol (Coreg) benazepril (Lotensin), captopril (Capoten), enalapril (Vasotec), fosinopril (Monopril), lisinopril (Prinivil), moexipril (Univasc), ramipril (Altace), trandolapril (Mavik)
Angiotensin II receptor antagonists (blockers)	candesartan (Atacand), eprosartan (Teveten), irbesartan (Avapro), losartan (Cozaar), valsartan (Diovan), telmisar- tan (Micardis), olmesartan (Benicar)
Beta antagonists (blockers)	atenolol (Tenormin), propranolol (Inderal), nadolol (Corgard), metopro- lol (Lopressor), timolol (Blocadren), pindolol (Visken), sotalol (Betapace), bisoprolo (Zebeta), esmolol (Brevibloc)
Calcium channel blockers	nifedipine (Procardia), verapamil (Calan), diltiazem (Cardizem), felodipine (Plendil), amlodipine (Norvasc)
Diuretics	chlorothiazide (Diuril), chlorthalidone (Hygroton), methyclothiazide (Aquatensen, Enduron), metolazone (Zaroxolyn), polythiazide (Renese), quinethazone (Hydromox), furosemide (Lasix), bumetanide (Bumex), hydrochlorothiazide (HydroDIURIL)
Other antihypertensives	rauwolfia (Reserpine, Serpasil)
Vasodilators	hydralazine (Apresoline), minoxidil (Loniten), diazoxide (Proglycem)

antioxidant A substance that counters oxidation. Oxidation is a by-product of metabolism that many health experts believe causes damage to cells and tissues. Scientists have demonstrated that oxidation damages the genetic structure, or DNA, of cells, and that this is how many disease processes such as heart disease and cancer begin. Although the concept of using antioxidants to prevent oxidation damage and the disease process that occurs as a result is intriguing, so far studies have failed to demonstrate that this is effective.

Studies of the antioxidants vitamin C, vitamin E, and BETA CAROTENE, which many people take to help prevent heart disease, have provided contradictory findings. Observational studies in which researchers gather information about lifestyle habits including nutrition typically find lower rates of heart disease in people who eat high amounts of fruits and vegetables, which are naturally high in antioxidants. Many health-conscious people also take vitamin supplements that increase their antioxidant intakes. Controlled clinical studies, by contrast, so far have shown no direct correlation between antioxidants and heart disease. These results lead many health experts to conclude that overall lifestyle is a more significant factor, includ-ing nutritional diet and regular exercise. Researchers continue to study the role that antioxidants might play in preventing cardiovascular disease.

See also COENZYME Q-10; FOLIC ACID; LIFESTYLE AND HEART HEALTH; NUTRITION AND DIET.

antiphospholipid syndrome (APLS) A rare AUTO-IMMUNE DISORDER in which the body forms antibodies that attack metabolized fatty acids called phospholipids. This causes the phospholipids to clump together, forming clots in the blood. Primary antiphospholipid syndrome (APLS) can be familial (hereditary) or idiopathic (reason unknown). Other autoimmune conditions such as lupus erythematosus can cause secondary APLS. About a third of the people who have primary APLS also have growths on their HEART VALVES that cause the valves to become thick-ened and deformed, ultimately requiring surgery to replace them with mechanical valves.

Treatment for APLS consists of prophylactic ANTICOAGULANT MEDICATIONS to minimize clot for-mation, and intensive anticoagulant therapy to dissolve clots that do form. Sometimes corticoste-roids are necessary to suppress the body's immune response, helping to limit the antibody response.

Eating a low-fat, nutritious diet and getting regular EXERCISE help keep BLOOD lipid levels low, which lessens the antibody response. Researchers do not yet know what causes APLS, which usually affects people under age 45, to develop. In women, recurrent loss of pregnancy is one of the early symptoms. People with APLS have a high risk of DEEP VEIN THROMBOSIS (DVT), STROKE, and HEART ATTACK.

See also CHOLESTEROL, BLOOD; HYPERLIPIDEMIA; LIPIDS; TRIGLYCERIDES.

aorta See HEART.

aortic aneurysm See ABDOMINAL AORTIC ANEURYSM.

aortic regurgitation Improper closure of the aortic valve that allows BLOOD to leak back into the left ventricle after being pumped into the aorta. In about two-thirds of the people who have aortic regurgitation, the valve damage follows RHEUMATIC FEVER (bacterial infection followed by an autoimmune reaction that affects the joints and the HEART valves). Aortic regurgitation also can develop when there is a defect in the aortic valve's structure such as a congenital malformation in which the valve is bicuspid (has two flaps) instead of the normal tricuspid (three flaps), or as a consequence of conditions such as AORTIC STENOSIS and MARFAN SYNDROME that affect the base of the aorta where it enters the heart. Aortic regurgitation also may result when a deformed aortic valve becomes infected.

Mild aortic regurgitation often shows no symptoms and requires no medical care beyond regular monitoring. More extensive aortic regurgitation puts extra stress on the heart, which often causes changes that cause the valve dysfunction to worsen over time. The blood that flows back into the ventricle adds to the volume of blood that is entering the ventricle to be pumped out. The ventricle gradually enlarges to accommodate the extra volume, which further distorts the valve.

Symptoms of moderate aortic regurgitation include rapid tiring with exertion, EDEMA (swelling) especially at the ankles, shortness of breath, and chest pain (ANGINA). Some people also have ARRHYTHMIAS (irregular HEARTBEAT), and nearly always the doctor can hear a HEART MURMUR (a characteristic sound that the blood makes when it flows back into the ventricle) with a STETHOSCOPE. At this stage the doctor might prescribe DIURETIC MEDICATIONS to remove excess fluid and medications to strengthen the heartbeat.

As aortic regurgitation worsens, it begins to behave like HEART FAILURE. The heart's pumping efficiency significantly diminishes, and the left ventricle continues to enlarge as it struggles to pump hard enough to send blood out into the body as well as contain the increasing volume of blood leaking back through the aortic valve. At this stage, the optimal treatment for most people is replacing the damaged valve, usually with a prosthetic (artificial) valve. For most people, this is a permanent solution for the aortic regurgitation. However, having a prosthetic valve means taking anticoagulant medications to help keep clots from forming in the valve mechanisms.

People who have aortic regurgitation or who have had valve replacement surgery to treat aortic regurgitation have an increased risk for infection involving the valves, and they should receive prophylactic antibiotics before dental and surgical procedures. Prompt treatment of strep throat in children and young adults with appropriate antibiotics also is essential, as untreated strep infection is associated with rheumatic fever, which can eventually result in aortic regurgitation. Tests that help diagnose aortic regurgitation include ECHOCARDIOGRAM; DOPPLER ULTRASOUND, and CARDIAC CATHETERIZATION.

See also ANTIBIOTIC PROPHYLAXIS; AUSCULTATION; CARDIOVASCULAR SYSTEM; CONGENITAL HEART DISEASE; LIVING WITH HEART DISEASE; SURGERY TO TREAT CARDIOVASCULAR DISEASE; VALVE REPAIR AND REPLACEMENT.

aortic stenosis Narrowing of the aorta (the body's largest artery) near where it joins the HEART or of the aortic valve, restricting the flow of oxygenated BLOOD from the heart into the body. Aortic stenosis can be congenital (present from birth), which accounts for most aortic stenosis, or acquired (developed as a result of disease or infection). In either circumstance, most people do not experience symptoms until middle age, by which time the strain of the extra work the heart has been doing to pump blood out of the left ventricle begins to wear on other structures of the heart. Over time, the left ventricle enlarges and thickens to compensate for the extra effort it takes to pump blood through the constricted area.

Symptoms and Diagnostic Path

When symptoms of aortic stenosis do develop, they are similar to those of ISCHEMIC HEART DISEASE, HEART FAILURE, AORTIC REGURGITATION, and CORONARY ARTERY DISEASE (CAD) and include CHEST PAIN (ANGINA), shortness of breath, dizziness, and fainting (SYNCOPE) with physical activity. The doctor hears a murmur or might hear clicks and other sounds of valve dysfunction through the stethoscope, with or without other symptoms. Diagnostic procedures such as ELECTROCARDIOGRAM (ECG), ECHOCARDIOGRAM, DOPPLER ULTRASOUND, and CARDIAC CATHETERIZATION help make the appropriate diagnosis. Treatment with medications used for heart failure can relieve symptoms of moderate aortic stenosis, holding the disease in check for years in many people. However, the stenosis and the secondary damage that it causes tend to worsen with increasing age, leading to surgery to repair or replace the defective valve or portion of the aorta that is the site of the stenosis.

Treatment Options and Outlook

When congenital aortic stenosis causes symptoms in infancy or childhood, the constriction or deformity generally is severe and requires surgical correction, usually by ANGIOPLASTY or valvuloplasty. Both are open-heart surgeries that require exposing the heart. A less invasive procedure that can correct some kinds of congenital aortic stenosis in infants is balloon valvuloplasty, in which the cardiologist threads a specialized catheter to the heart through an incision into a peripheral artery in the groin and inflates a tiny balloon inside the valve to gently stretch it. This generally provides temporary relief, however, with additional treatment becoming necessary in adulthood.

Risk Factors and Preventive Measures

The major risk associated with undetected aortic stenosis is SUDDEN CARDIAC ARREST (SCA) in young athletes. Although sudden cardiac arrest is very rare in young people, aortic stenosis is its most common cause. Children who have asymptomatic aortic stenosis should receive regular cardiac checkups to monitor the condition's status.

See also BICUSPID AORTIC VALVE; COARCTATION OF THE AORTA; MITRAL VALVE PROLAPSE; VENTRICULAR SEPTAL DEFECT.

aphasia Damage to the brain's speech center as a consequence of STROKE or other brain injury. Aphasia can also occur following HEART ATTACK if lack of oxygen to the brain causes damage in the area of the speech center. The degree of aphasia and correspondingly the likelihood for recovery depend on the extent of damage. With aggressive speech therapy, many people with aphasia can recover adequate and sometimes full speech function. Early intervention is critical to preserve as much function as possible; speech therapy with a speech/language pathologist (health-care professional with specialized training) should begin as soon as the person's physical condition permits. The speech/language pathologist conducts a comprehensive examination to evaluate the extent of damage and assess the strengths of remaining language skills. Exercises then focus on reinforcing and adapting strengths to accommodate for lost or weakened skills.

A person with aphasia might be unable to speak, unable to write, unable to understand what they hear or read, or have a combination of these problems. Aphasia is very frustrating for people because they know what they want to say or write but cannot get it out. Although aphasia primarily affects the brain functions related to speech, often there is other damage from the brain injury (whether stroke or another trauma) that affects the muscles of the throat and face. This can result in swallowing difficulties as well as physical limitations in forming words and breath control to move air through the vocal cords.

See also ACTIVITIES OF DAILY LIVING (ADLs); AMERICANS WITH DISABILITIES ACT (ADA); BREATHING EXERCISES; TAI CHI; YOGA.

apple body shape See BODY SHAPE AND HEART DISEASE.

Apresoline   See HYDRALAZINE.

arrhythmia   Any abnormality in the electrical coordination of the HEART's contractions. Heart rhythm abnormalities are generally categorized by their effect on the HEART RATE. Symptoms from arrhythmias span a very wide range. Some arrhythmias can be totally asymptomatic, and others can be quickly fatal.

Broad classes of arrhythmias (also called dysrhythmias) include:

- slowing of the heart rate (bradycardia)
- rapid heart rate (TACHYCARDIA)
- any condition in which the contractions of cardiac chambers are out of synch with each other or are irregular, which may or may not affect the overall heart rate

Cardiologists further categorize bradycardias by identity of the anatomic location of the problem, which generally involves either the sinus node (where the normal HEARTBEAT initiates), the atrioventricular (AV) node (which connects the atria to the ventricles), or the His-Purkinje system, which normally delivers coordinated electrical signals to the ventricles.

Further categorization of tachydysrhythmias identifies the anatomic location, which is either supraventricular (atrial or AV nodal) or ventricular, and the mechanism of the tachycardia (either ectopic/automatic, reentrant, or fibrillatory). The main causes of supraventricular tachycardia include focal ectopic atrial tachycardia, junctional ectopic tachycardia, atrioventricular nodal reentrant tachycardia, atrioventricular reentrant tachycardia, atrial flutter, and atrial fibrillation. The main causes of ventricular arrhythmias include ventricular tachycardia and ventricular FIBRILLATION.

There are several methods for evaluating and diagnosing cardiac arrhythmias:

- Electrocardiogram (ECG), which produces a "snapshot" recording of the heart's electrical activity, is the first step but may not show any disturbances if the arrhythmia is not happening at the time of the ECG. An ECG is done in the doctor's office and takes just a few minutes.
- A HOLTER MONITOR provides ECG recording over a 24-hour period. This involves wearing electrodes and a recording device (the Holter monitor) while going about the regular activities of living.
- Event monitoring can capture arrhythmias that occur without regular patterns. The person wears a device that resembles a watch or a pager and can dial a telephone number to send a signal of an event. The device also has a short-term memory function so the person can record the event and then send the recording via telephone.
- Electrophysiological studies use cardiac catheterization to send patterned electrical impulses to the heart. This allows the cardiologist to construct a map to indicate where and how the signals affect the heart.

Bradycardia

Bradycardia, or slow heart rate, affects the entire heart and occurs mostly in older people. It generally is a condition of the heart's conduction system, in which the heart's electrical impulses are slowed. The most common treatment is an implanted PACEMAKER that augments the heart's natural pacing with supplemental electrical impulses when the heart rate falls below a certain point. Athletes in top condition might have resting heart rates that would be considered bradycardia in people without such extraordinary aerobic fitness. They do not require treatment unless the bradycardia causes symptoms such as LIGHT-HEADEDNESS or fainting, indicating that the body is not receiving adequate OXYGENATION.

Atrial (Supraventricular) Arrhythmias

Atrial arrhythmias (fibrillation, multifocal ectopic beats, flutter) affect the heart's upper chambers, and occur when the muscle fibers contract independently of one another. This establishes a chaotic, discordant discharge of activity that reduces the atrium's effectiveness in pumping BLOOD to the ventricle. The most significant risk is that this can allow blood to pool in the atrium, making it possible for clots to form. When these clots finally make it through the ventricle, they can lodge in the lung (pulmonary embolus), the brain (STROKE), or the coronary arteries (HEART ATTACK). People with atrial arrhythmias often take anticoagulant medications to help keep clots from forming. Atrial arrhythmias almost always are disturbances of the heart's conduction system and usually respond to treatment with ANTIARRHYTHMIA MEDICATIONS.

Ventricular Arrhythmias

Ventricular arrhythmias affect the heart's lower chambers and are generally more serious than atrial arrhythmias because they affect the flow of blood from the heart to the lungs and to the body. They can be electrical or mechanical in origin and often accompany cardiac crisis such as heart attack or severe ANGINA. Treatment targets the underlying condition as well as the arrhythmia and usually includes medications to stabilize heart rate.

Common causes of ventricular tachycardia include hypertrophic cardiomyopathy (HCM), MYOCARDITIS (inflammation of the heart muscle), CORONARY ARTERY DISEASE (CAD), ISCHEMIC HEART DISEASE, and myocardial infarction (HEART ATTACK). Ventricular tachycardia that persists can become ventricular fibrillation, which is life-threatening. While in ventricular tachycardia the heartbeat is rapid, it is still putting blood into circulation. In ventricular fibrillation the ventricle's contractions are uncoordinated and ineffective. DEFIBRILLATION (electrical shock) and emergency cardiac medications are necessary to restore normal rhythm.

Extra Beats

Nearly everyone experiences occasional extra or ectopic beats. When they are infrequent, these "cardiac hiccups" are harmless and meaningless. When they are persistent, however, they can signal problems with the heart's conductive system. One of the most common arrhythmias caused by extra beats is premature ventricular contraction (PVC). In this arrhythmia, the ventricle experiences an extra contraction slightly ahead of its regular contraction. Occasional PVCs are common and can be brought on by stimulants such as caffeine. Persistent PVCs signal a more serious problem with the heart's conduction system and warrant further investigation. Antiarrhythmia medications usually control PVCs.

Arrhythmias of Cocaine Use

Many substances, among them alcohol, legal medications, and illicit drugs, can affect the heart's function. COCAINE is particularly dangerous because it can cause sudden and fatal interruptions of the heart's electrical impulses, even at first use of the drug, causing sudden cardiac arrest. It causes ventricular tachycardia that quickly progresses to ventricular fibrillation, which the heart can sustain for only a few minutes before going into complete cardiac arrest. Even if the person receives immediate emergency medical attention, the likelihood of survival is slim because the drugs doctors typically administer to restore the heart's rhythm do not work.

See also CARDIOMYOPATHY; HEART BLOCK; MEDICATIONS TO TREAT HEART DISEASE; SICK SINUS SYNDROME; RADIOFREQUENCY ABLATION; STOKES-ADAMS DISEASE; SUDDEN CARDIAC ARREST; SURGERY TO TREAT CARDIOVASCULAR DISEASE.

arrhythmic right ventricular cardiomyopathy (ARVC)   See CARDIOMYOPATHY.

arterial plaque   See PLAQUE, ARTERIAL.

arterial switch procedure   Major reconstructive surgery of the HEART and its arteries to correct TRANSPOSITION OF THE GREAT ARTERIES (TGA), a form of CYANOTIC CONGENITAL HEART DISEASE in which the aorta and the pulmonary artery are reversed. This means the heart fails to pump BLOOD through the lungs before pumping it out into the body, so the blood does not carry oxygen. TGA is a life-threatening heart defect that generally becomes apparent within hours of birth. The arterial switch procedure usually must be done immediately.

In a normal heart, the pulmonary artery comes out of the right ventricle and carries blood to the lungs to become oxygenated. The oxygenated blood returns to the heart via the left atrium, which pumps it to the left ventricle. The aorta comes out of the left ventricle and carries the oxygenated blood out into the body. This forms a single loop of blood circulation that exchanges the oxygen-depleted blood that comes back from the body for oxygen-rich blood that comes from the lungs.

When these arteries are reversed as in TGA, they form two closed loops of CIRCULATION. Oxygen-rich blood circulates only through the lungs and the right side of the heart, while oxygen-depleted blood circulates only through the body and the left side of the heart. The pulmonary artery comes from the left ventricle and continuously circulates blood through the lungs. The aorta comes from the right ventricle and pumps unoxygenated blood through the body. The infant's skin quickly takes on the dusky, bluish hue characteristic of CYANOSIS.

Most TGA is diagnosed within minutes to hours of birth. The examining neonatologist (physician specializing in the care of newborns) or pediatrician usually can detect unusual heart sounds upon AUSCULTATION. An ELECTROCARDIOGRAM (ECG), which records the heart's electrical activity, and an ECHOCARDIOGRAM, which uses ultrasound to create images of the structures of the heart, often can conclusively diagnose TGA. If there is any question, the pediatric cardiologist does a cardiac catheterization, which uses dye to make the structures of the heart visible with X-ray, to examine in detail the heart's structure and the flow of blood through the heart.

Procedure

The arterial switch procedure is OPEN-HEART SURGERY. The surgeon places the infant on a HEART-LUNG BYPASS MACHINE that takes over the heart's functions during surgery, pumping blood through the lungs and through the body so the surgeon can stop the heart to perform the necessary repairs. The surgeon then cuts the aorta and the pulmonary artery where each attaches to the heart, reconnects them to the proper ventricles, and properly connects the coronary arteries to the aorta. Because the coronary arteries branch off the aorta, which is displaced in TGA, they also often have deformities that the surgeon corrects during the arterial switch procedure. If there are other heart defects such as septal defect or patent ductus arteriosus present, which is common, the surgeon repairs these, too.

Risks and Complications

The arterial switch procedure is a complex operation. Among its risks are those associated with any surgery, such as excessive blood loss, reaction to anesthesia, and postoperative infection. Because each infant's heart anomalies are unique, the skill and experience of the surgical team are crucial to the operation's success. Other complications may include difficulty coming off cardiopulmonary bypass or restarting the heart. After surgery, the infant requires highly specialized care in the intensive care unit (ICU) and may remain on mechanical ventilation (breathing machine) for several days. The total length of hospital stay varies depending on the severity of the deformities and the complexity of the repairs. After recovery from the operation, complications that may develop include ARRHYTHMIAS (irregularities in the HEARTBEAT), heart valve problems, and narrowing of the arteries at the surgical sites.

Outlook and Lifestyle Modifications

Although the surgery is extensive and complex, it restores the heart's structure and function to normal. After recovering from the surgery, most infants grow and develop normally and have no greater than normal risk for heart disease as adults.

See also HEART DISEASE IN CHILDREN; OXYGENATION; PULMONARY STENOSIS; SURGERY TO TREAT CARDIOVASCULAR DISEASE.

arteriogram See ANGIOGRAPHY.

arterioplasty See ANGIOPLASTY.

arteriosclerosis CARDIOVASCULAR DISEASE in which the walls of the arteries thicken and become less resilient. This increases the resistance BLOOD encounters when flowing through them, causing BLOOD PRESSURE to rise. People sometimes call arteriosclerosis "hardening of the arteries." There are various forms of arteriosclerosis; it is common to have more than one of them as they are inter-related. Treatment depends on a number of variables including the types of arteriosclerosis and other health conditions including cardiovascular diseases such as HYPERTENSION (high blood pressure) and HEART FAILURE.

Age-Related Arteriosclerosis

Much arteriosclerosis develops as a consequence of the changes that take place with aging and affects the inner layer of the arterial wall. Lifestyle factors, most notably cigarette smoking, influence the rate at which arteriosclerosis develops as well as its severity. Age-related arteriosclerosis tends to affect the arteries throughout the body rather than an isolated artery. It is a leading cause of age-related dementia (impaired memory and cognitive functions). The most effective treatment is prevention, through lifestyle habits such as nutritious diet and regular EXERCISE that help to maintain overall cardiovascular health and to keep blood pressure within normal ranges. Arteriosclerosis often causes hypertension, as the narrowed and rigid arteries increase the resistance blood encounters in flowing through them.

Mönckeberg's Arteriosclerosis (Medial Calcific Arteriosclerosis)

This form of arteriosclerosis is the least common. It affects the middle layer of the arterial wall, with damage to the muscle and connective tissues that give the artery its flexibility. Calcium deposits accumulate in the damaged areas, increasing the stiffness of the artery. This type of arteriosclerosis can increase the risk for STROKE when it affects the carotid or other arteries that supply blood to the brain. Depending on the location and severity, ANGIOPLASTY is sometimes a treatment option.

Atherosclerosis

ATHEROSCLEROSIS is the most common form of arteriosclerosis among Americans. Because of this, many people use the terms *arteriosclerosis* and *atherosclerosis* interchangeably. In atherosclerosis, it is an accumulation of fatty deposits along the inside walls of the arteries that causes the arteries to thicken and stiffen.

Lifestyle is a major factor in the development of atherosclerosis. Health experts estimate that lifestyle modification could eliminate 80 percent or more of heart disease resulting from atherosclerosis. Eating a nutritious, low-fat diet and exercising regularly to maintain a healthy weight helps to reduce overall blood lipid levels and prevent atherosclerosis.

Lifestyle modification (low-fat diet, regular exercise, and SMOKING CESSATION) and LIPID-LOW-ERING MEDICATIONS can help to control the spread of atherosclerosis. Once atherosclerosis develops, however, generally surgical intervention such as angioplasty or CORONARY ARTERY BYPASS GRAFT (CABG) is the preferred treatment.

Arteriolosclerosis (Arteriolar Sclerosis)

This form of arteriosclerosis is a consequence of untreated or uncontrolled hypertension (high blood pressure) and affects the smallest arteries in the body, the arterioles. The repeated battering that these fragile blood vessels take from high blood pressure causes the structure of their walls to deteriorate. Microscopic calcium deposits collect in the damaged areas, causing the walls to become stiff and rigid. These changes in the walls of the arteries further increase resistance, signaling the body to raise the blood pressure even more. Bringing blood pressure under control with medications is the first priority in treatment.

See also ANTIHYPERTENSIVE MEDICATIONS; CAROTID ENDARTERECTOMY; LIFESTYLE AND HEART HEALTH; MEDICATIONS TO TREAT HEART DISEASE.

artery   See CARDIOVASCULAR SYSTEM.

artificial heart   See HEART, ARTIFICIAL.

aspirin   A common over-the-counter pain reliever that has mild anticoagulant (anticlotting) effects, which research demonstrates can prevent HEART ATTACK and STROKE by keeping platelets (blood cells responsible for forming clots) from clumping together. Aspirin suppresses the body's production of PROSTAGLANDINS; hormones that play key roles in numerous functions including pain perception and blood clotting. Heart experts recommend that men over age 40 and women past menopause take the equivalent of one-half regular strength aspirin daily (162mg).

People who are taking prescription ANTICOAGU-LANT MEDICATIONS such as WARFARIN (Coumadin), DIPYRIDAMOLE (Persantine), or CLOPIDOGREL (Plavix) should check with their doctors before taking aspirin. Recent studies suggest that taking NONSTEROIDAL ANTI-INFLAMMATORY DRUGS (NSAIDs) significantly reduces and might even negate the anticoagulant effects of aspirin, even when several hours separate doses of each. Aspirin can cause gastrointestinal upset, including irritation of the stomach lining that is serious enough to result in bleeding or ulcers. Enteric-coated aspirin dissolves in the intestine rather than the stomach, helping to prevent this side effect.

There also is evidence that taking one regular-strength aspirin when there are symptoms of heart attack such as chest pain or shortness of breath can reduce the amount of damage if indeed a heart attack or stroke is taking place.

See also MEDICATIONS TO TREAT HEART DISEASE; THROMBOSIS; THROMBOLYSIS; TISSUE PLASMINOGEN ACTIVATOR.

Atacand See CANDESARTAN.

atenolol A BETA ANTAGONIST MEDICATION taken to treat HYPERTENSION (high BLOOD PRESSURE). Doctors also sometimes prescribe atenolol to treat ANGINA, mild ANXIETY that is causing PALPITATIONS, migraine headaches, and following HEART ATTACK (MYOCARDIAL INFARCTION) to help strengthen and stabilize HEART functions. The common brand-name product available in the United States is Tenormin. Doctors often prescribe atenolol and other ANTIHYPERTENSIVE MEDICATIONS in combination.

Atenolol's most common undesired side effects are tiredness, weakness, and loss of libido (interest in sex). Switching to a different beta-blocker can sometimes alleviate these effects, although some people find it necessary to change to a different type of antihypertensive altogether. As with all beta-blockers, one should not stop taking atenolol abruptly. This can cause a HYPERTENSIVE CRISIS in which the blood pressure shoots up. Most people should gradually taper the dose over two weeks, according to physician or pharmacist instruction.

See also ANGIOTENSIN-CONVERTING ENZYME (ACE) INHIBITOR MEDICATIONS; ALPHA ANTAGONIST MEDICATIONS; ANGIOTENSIN II RECEPTOR ANTAGONIST MEDICATIONS; MEDICATIONS TO TREAT HEART DISEASE.

atherectomy A procedure to remove collections of accumulated PLAQUE, called ATHEROMAS, from the insides of arteries. Most atherectomies clear the coronary arteries, although cardiologists can use the procedure to clear plaque accumulations in other arteries. With coronary atherectomy done to treat CORONARY ARTERY DISEASE (CAD), sometimes the cardiologist also performs as balloon ANGIOPLASTY and might place a STENT to help the artery remain open and help prevent the reaccumulation of plaque.

Procedure

Atherectomy takes one to two hours, during which the person is awake but sedated. The cardiologist uses a local anesthetic to numb the area in the groin or arm where the catheters will be inserted. During CARDIAC CATHETERIZATION, the cardiologist inserts either a specialized laser or a tiny rotary scalpel through the catheter to the point of the accumulation. The laser vaporizes the accumulation; the rotary scalpel shaves it away. This reopens the artery for unobstructed BLOOD flow. The catheter collects any plaque fragments, which are then removed when the cardiologist pulls the catheter from the artery at the end of the procedure.

Following atherectomy, most people stay in the hospital for one or two nights, depending on the extensiveness of the plaque removal, concerns for RESTENOSIS (reclosure of the artery), and the length of time the cardiologist wants to leave the catheters in place (in case additional treatment becomes necessary).

Risks and Complications

Risks of atherectomy include postoperative bleeding at the locations of catheter insertion, soreness at the insertion site that may persist for several days, and the formation of blood clots within the arteries at the sites where the atheromas were removed. Clots that break away and enter the blood circulation can cause STROKE or HEART ATTACK. There is also the possibility that the atheroma may recur (restenosis) or that new atheromas may develop when significant ARTERIOSCLEROSIS exists.

Outlook and Lifestyle Modifications

Most people return to full and normal activities within a week of the procedure. Many people experience relief from ANGINA, intermittent CLAUDICA-

TION, or other symptoms of arterial blockage, and may be able to stop taking medications to treat these symptoms. Lifestyle modifications for heart health, such as nutritious eating and daily physical exercise, may slow the progression of underlying arteriosclerosis and CAD. The cardiologist may also prescribe lipid-lowering medications to aid this effort.

While the catheters are in place, the person must lie flat in bed without bending the groin where the catheter enters the artery.

See also ANTICOAGULANT MEDICATIONS; CAROTID ENDARTERECTOMY; CORONARY ARTERY BYPASS GRAFT (CABG); SURGERY TO TREAT CARDIOVASCULAR DISEASE.

atheroma   An accumulation of fatty acids and other substances that forms along the inner wall of an ARTERY, causing a narrowing of the passageway for BLOOD. The term comes from the Greek words for "porridge" and "tumor," which is an apt description of this accumulation that has the consistency of cream cheese. The condition of having atheromas is called atherosclerosis. Atheromas can develop in any artery but are most common at the junctions where arteries branch off in different directions. They begin when excess lipids in the bloodstream, particularly CHOLESTEROL, stick to white blood cells that have attached to the arterial wall. Once an atheroma begins, it attracts further materials, such as blood cells and calcium from the bloodstream, that attach to it, increasing its size.

Atheromas present two primary risks, OCCLUSION and THROMBOSIS. An atheroma that occludes, or blocks, the artery reduces or even cuts off blood flow through the artery. This can cause HEART ATTACK when the occlusion is in the coronary arteries or stroke when it is in the carotid arteries. Atheromas also can rupture or break apart, sending fragments of debris through the arteries, causing heart attack or stroke.

A diagnostic procedure called superfast CT scan can detect and measure the amounts of calcium that are present in the walls of the arteries, providing a fairly accurate method of assessing the extent to which atheromas have developed. ANGIOGRAPHY, in which doctors inject dye into the arteries and then watch the dye's movement through the blood vessels using specialized X-rays, shows precisely where atheromas are located and how much they occlude the arteries.

See also CAROTID ENDARTERECTOMY; CORONARY ARTERY DISEASE (CAD); FLUOROSCOPY.

atherosclerosis   See ARTERIOSCLEROSIS.

atorvastatin   A LIPID-LOWERING MEDICATION that helps to lower BLOOD cholesterol and blood TRIGLYCERIDE levels. The common brand name in the United States for this drug is Lipitor. Like other statin medications, atorvastatin is an HMG CoA REDUCTASE INHIBITOR that works by inhibiting, or slowing, the action of HMG CoA reductase (3-hydroxy-3-methylglutaryl coenzyme A), the enzyme necessary for the body to manufacture cholesterol and other lipoproteins such as apo-B. Statin medications such as atorvastatin also appear to provide significant protection following HEART ATTACK (myocardial infarction), helping the heart to restore its functions.

Common side effects are minor, such as headache and flatulence (gas). Less common but more serious is interference with liver function, which can result in liver damage. People taking atorvastatin or other HMG CoA reductase inhibitors should have regular blood tests (annual unless there are elevations) to monitor liver enzyme levels. Atorvastatin can increase the action of digoxin, so people taking both drugs should have regular blood tests to monitor DIGOXIN levels as well. A very rare but potentially fatal side effect is RHABDOMYOLYSIS, in which muscle tissue breaks down. The excessive amounts of protein that subsequently flood the bloodstream are very damaging to the kidneys and can quickly cause kidney failure. Early symptoms of rhabdomyolysis are muscle pain and weakness.

See also FLUVASTATIN; LOVASTATIN; MEDICATIONS TO TREAT HEART DISEASE; PRAVASTATIN; SIMVASTATIN.

atrial fibrillation   An ARRHYTHMIA involving the atria (the heart's upper chambers), in which atrial contractions are rapid and uncoordinated. This results in incomplete atrial emptying, which allows BLOOD to pool. Consequently, the ventricles pump less blood and the HEART works harder to meet the body's needs. The pooling of blood that occurs also presents a great risk for clots to form and break free to enter the bloodstream, correspondingly causing a heightened risk for STROKE. Atrial fibrillation tends to more often involve the right atrium, though it may involve both atria, and is the most common arrhythmia.

Electrical dysfunctions in the heart's conduction pathway are responsible for atrial fibrillation. Researchers believe many of these dysfunctions develop as a consequence of age-related degenerative changes in the heart. Other forms of HEART DISEASE can also cause atrial fibrillation. Among them are HYPERTENSION (high BLOOD PRESSURE), heart VALVE DISEASE, HEART FAILURE, TACHYCARDIA-BRADYCARDIA SYNDROME, heart surgery, infections, and sleep apnea. Paroxysmal atrial fibrillation (PAT) occurs intermittently; chronic atrial fibrillation is continually present. A milder form of this arrhythmia is atrial flutter, in which the atrial contractions are not as rapid and chaotic as in atrial fibrillation; atrial flutter often progresses to atrial fibrillation.

Symptoms and Diagnostic Path

Some people have no symptoms of atrial fibrillation. Other people feel the sensation of skipped heartbeats, may experience FATIGUE, and may have PALPITATIONS. LIGHT-HEADEDNESS, DIZZINESS, mental confusion, difficulty breathing (DYSPNEA), and CHEST PAIN (ANGINA) may also occur. Atrial fibrillation often is apparent when taking the pulse, which is irregular. Electrocardiogram (ECG) or HOLTER MONITOR can document the errant electrical activity to confirm the diagnosis. When there is question of underlying heart disease, the doctor may also perform blood tests, echocardiogram, chest X-ray, or other diagnostic procedures depending on symptoms and health history.

Treatment Options and Outlook

When an underlying heart condition is causing the atrial fibrillation, treating the condition usually eliminates the atrial fibrillation. When atrial fibrillation is not caused by another heart condition, the first objective of treatment is to restore the heart's natural rhythm. This is called CARDIOVERSION and can be done either with ANTIARRHYTHMIA MEDICA-

TIONS, given in a hospital with ECG monitoring of heart activity, or through the administration of an electrical shock, done under anesthesia. Some people require ongoing treatment with antiarrhythmia or other medications such as DIGOXIN to regulate the heart rate. Increasingly, ABLATION is the treatment of choice to permanently destroy the areas of cells responsible for errant electrical activity. Most people with atrial fibrillation also take an ANTICOAGULATION MEDICATION, such as WARFARIN, to lower the risk for blood clots. Although all of these treatment options can be highly effective, atrial fibrillation requires ongoing monitoring and evaluation.

Risk Factors and Preventive Measures

Atrial fibrillation becomes increasingly common with advancing age; some experts believe as many as 5 percent of Americans over age 65 and 10 percent over age 80 have atrial fibrillation. Men are somewhat more likely to develop atrial fibrillation. Treating other forms of heart disease helps to lower the risk for atrial fibrillation that might be associated with them.

See also ACCESSORY PATHWAY; AGING, CARDIOVASCULAR CHANGES THAT OCCUR WITH; COAGULATION; LIVING WITH HEART DISEASE; MEDICATIONS TO TREAT HEART DISEASE; SLEEP DISTURBANCES; SURGERY TO TREAT CARDIOVASCULAR DISEASE.

atrial tachycardia See ARRHYTHMIA.

atrioventricular (AV) canal defect A congenital HEART defect (present at birth) in which there is an opening in the septum, or wall, of the heart separating the atrium from the ventricle. This condition is also called atrioventricular (AV) septal defect or endocardial cushion defect (because the defect occurs when embryonic structures called the endocardial cushions fail to properly develop). The defect may be complete, partial, or transitional. It is one of the most common forms of congenital HEART DISEASE.

Often there are structural valve defects as well, involving the mitral valve between the left atrium and ventricle, the triscuspid valve between the right atrium and ventricle, or both valves if the

AV canal defect is complete (occurs at the base of the atria and the ventricles, affecting all four heart chambers).

Symptoms and Diagnostic Path

With an AV canal defect, the heart cannot properly pump blood to the lungs or to the body. This deprives the body of oxygen, causing breathing that is faster and harder than normal. The heart also cannot regulate its pumping force and sends BLOOD to the lungs with the same high pressure used to send blood to the body. The overworked and underefficient heart soon moves into congestive failure. The doctor can sometimes detect AV canal defect shortly following birth. Typically, however, further symptoms develop over the first several months of life and include:

- unusual tiredness
- below average growth
- sweating, especially while breast-feeding
- HEART MURMUR
- difficulty breathing or shortness of breath (DYSPNEA)
- CYANOSIS (bluish tint to the lips, nail beds, and sometimes skin)

The primary diagnostic tool for AV canal defect is ECHOCARDIOGRAM, which is noninvasive and shows both the physical structure and the function of the heart. Other diagnostic procedures might include ELECTROCARDIOGRAM (ECG) and chest X-RAY.

Treatment Options and Outlook

AV canal defect requires surgical repair of the heart, via OPEN-HEART SURGERY, to patch the septal opening and repair or reconstruct any damaged valves. This surgery is typically done between ages three and 18 months. The pediatric cardiologist may prescribe medications, such as diuretics and ANGIOTENSIN-CONVERTING ENZYME (ACE) INHIBITOR MEDICATIONS, to relieve symptoms and improve congestive HEART FAILURE until surgery is feasible. Following surgical repair of the heart, many children with AV canal defect are able to enjoy normal, active lives without restriction. When the repairs are complicated, the cardiologist may recommend limitations for physi-cal activities. If the septal defect (opening) is close to the atrioventricular (AV) node that is the heart's natural pacemaker, it might be necessary to implant a PACEMAKER. Some children may require long-term medications. Long-term complications may include rhythm disturbances of the heart (ARRHYTHMIAS) and incomplete mitral valve function that requires subsequent surgical repair.

Risk Factors and Preventive Measures

AV canal defect accounts for about 5 percent of congenital heart defects and is closely associated with Down syndrome (trisomy 21). About 20 percent of infants with Down syndrome also have AV canal defect. For this reason, the current standard of care for infants who have Down syndrome is to perform an echocardiogram shortly after birth. As well, a woman who herself had AV canal defect is significantly more likely to have a child who has AV canal defect. There are no known measures to prevent AV canal defect.

See also SURGERY TO TREAT CARDIOVASCULAR DISEASE; VALVE REPAIR AND REPLACEMENT.

atrioventricular (AV) node See HEART.

atrium See HEART.

atropine A drug that acts on the parasympathetic nervous system to speed up the HEART RATE as a treatment for bradycardia, an ARRHYTHMIA in which the heart rate drops below 60 beats per minute and may become symptomatic when the heart rate goes below 50 beats per minute. Atropine works by blocking the actions of acetylcholine, a NEUROTRANSMITTER that affects the function of smooth muscle such as that found in the myocardium (HEART muscle), at the synapses of neurons in the VAGUS NERVE. The vagus nerve carries nerve impulses from the brain that instruct the heart to beat slower; interrupting these signals allows the heart to maintain a faster rate.

Atropine typically is given by intravenous injection during a cardiac crisis. It also can be injected directly into the heart (intracardiac) during CARDIAC

ARREST to help restart the heart. Some oral medications taken to treat gastrointestinal conditions such as diarrhea and irritable bowel syndrome, Parkinson's disease, urinary incontinence, motion sickness, pancreatitis, and urinary frequency also contain atropine. Because atropine taken for any reason will have an effect on the heart, people taking any medication for cardiovascular disease should not take medications that have atropine in them. Atropine also interacts with many drugs used to treat heart problems including DIGOXIN and ANTIARRHYTHMIA MEDICATIONS.

See also HEART ATTACK; MEDICATIONS TO TREAT HEART DISEASE.

auscultation   Listening to the sounds of the HEART and lungs with a STETHOSCOPE. Heart sounds provide many clues about heart function, heart health, and HEART DISEASE. Auscultation is an essential and basic component of any physical examination and is a primary means of screening for heart problems as well as detecting the progression of certain kinds of heart disease. Sound patterns characterize specific heart problems. There are four basic kinds of heart sounds.

First and Second Heart Sounds

The first and second heart sounds are the familiar "lubb-dubb" of the heartbeat and are the basic heart sounds present in heart health as well as heart disease. They are the sounds of the valves closing as the heart pumps BLOOD from the atria (upper heart chambers) to the ventricles (lower heart chambers) and from the ventricles into the pulmonary artery and the aorta.

- The first sound, the "lubb," happens when blood enters the ventricles from the atria. It represents the closing of the mitral (left side) and triscuspid (right side) valves.
- The second sound, the "dubb," happens when the ventricles pump blood into the pulmonary (right ventricle) artery and the aorta (left ventricle).

In a healthy heart, the right and left sides of the heart function simultaneously. The mitral and tri-cuspid valves open and close at precisely the same time, so the physician hears them as a single sound. The aortic and pulmonary valves open and close at slightly different times, resulting in a double sound. Damage to the valves generally does not alter the first and second sounds but instead generates other sounds that are abnormal.

Third Heart Sound

The third heart sound is a low-pitched vibration that originates in the muscle fibers as the ventricles fill with blood. Although often a third heart sound is normal in children and young adults, in adults over age 40 a third heart sound may indicate heart failure.

Fourth Heart Sound

A fourth heart sound is always abnormal, and indicates abnormal myocardium (heart muscle). Although it is called the fourth sound, the physician actually hears it as a low-pitched vibration that occurs before the first sound. It reflects a "dead" area in the tonal vibration pattern of the muscle fibers, much like a wet patch on a taut string affects the string's vibrational qualities. A fourth heart sound is prominent following HEART ATTACK (MYOCARDIAL INFARCTION) and also occurs in CARDIOMYOPATHY, HYPERTENSION, and ISCHEMIC HEART DISEASE (IHD).

Clicks, Snaps, and Murmurs

Clicks, snaps, and murmurs are all abnormal sounds, although they do not necessarily signal serious problems.

- Clicks are high-pitched sounds that occur when a valve suddenly stops in the process of closing or opening. Clicks suggest the presence of valve closing problems such as MITRAL VALVE PROLAPSE or tricuspid valve prolapse, and valve opening problems with hypertension, AORTIC STENOSIS, or PULMONARY STENOSIS.
- Snaps are sharp, high-pitched sounds that occur immediately following the second heart sound. They primarily characterize MITRAL STENOSIS.
- Murmurs are common. They are "whooshing" sounds that reflect the turbulence of blood flow-

ing back into the ventricle because of improper valve closure such as in aortic or pulmonary regurgitation; the presence of CONGENITAL HEART DISEASE such as ATRIOVENTRICULAR CANAL DEFECT; or blood flowing back into the atria with mitral or tricuspid valve regurgitation or during the ejection of blood from the ventricles with aortic or pulmonary valve stenosis.

Whether abnormal heart sounds are cause for further investigation and possible treatment depends on their consistency and what other symptoms the person has.

See also AGING, CARDIOVASCULAR CHANGES AS A RESULT OF.

autoimmune heart disease HEART DISEASE that occurs when the body produces antibodies that affect cardiac functions. Evidence began to emerge in the late 1990s connecting certain kinds of heart disease with autoimmune response, particularly congestive HEART FAILURE related to CARDIOMYOPATHY (enlarged HEART). Researchers discovered that people with this form of heart disease produce antibodies that overly excite beta receptors in the heart, causing the HEART RATE to remain at a higher than normal pace. People with heart failure due to ISCHEMIC HEART DISEASE (IHD) or CORONARY ARTERY DISEASE (CAD) do not produce these antibodies. Currently treatment for heart failure includes BETA ANTAGONIST MEDICATIONS to interrupt the activation of beta-blockers and help slow the heart.

See also MEDICATIONS TO TREAT HEART DISEASE.

automated external defibrillator (AED) A device that delivers an electrical shock to stop ventricular fibrillation so that a normal HEART rhythm can restart following HEART ATTACK (myocardial infarction). Automated external defibrillators (AEDs) are small and portable. They have clear and simple instructions printed on them so virtually anyone can use an AED to save a life, although health experts emphasize programs to provide widespread training in AED use. Most courses in CPR (cardiopulmonary resuscitation) also include instruction for using AEDs.

Many businesses and locations where there is broad public access have AED programs, called public access to defibrillation (PAD) programs in place, with staff specially trained in using the devices. The U.S. Health and Human Services (HHS) Department has established guidelines for public use of AEDs, which were designed with collaboration from the American Heart Association and the American Red Cross. Federal law protects those who use AEDs from liability through the Cardiac Arrest Survival Act of 2000.

For more information see these Web sites:

- American Heart Association, http://www.americanheart.org
- American Red Cross, http://www.redcross.org
- HHS, http://www.hhs.gov
- Public Access Defibrillation League (PADL), http://www.padl.org

See also BRUGADA SYNDROME; CHAIN OF SURVIVAL; COMMOTIO CARDIS.

autonomic nervous system The structures and functions of the nervous system that regulate automatic body activities such as breathing, BLOOD PRESSURE, and HEART RATE. The primary physical structures of the autonomic nervous system are the medulla oblongata portion of the brain stem and the spinal nerves. There are two functional components of the autonomic nervous system—the sympathetic nervous system, which conveys signals that stimulate the CARDIOVASCULAR SYSTEM and relax other autonomic functions such as digestion, and the parasympathetic nervous system, which conveys signals that relax the cardiovascular system and stimulate other autonomic functions. These two components work to counterbalance each other according to the body's needs.

Sympathetic Nervous System

The sympathetic nervous system conveys nerve signals, via the neurotransmitters EPINEPHRINE and NOREPINEPHRINE, from the medulla oblongata along a paired pathway of nerve structures that branch from the top of the spinal cord and parallel the spinal cord, called the ganglia chains. These signals cause biochemical and physical actions that intensify the HEARTBEAT (increase its strength and pace), raise blood pressure (by initiating hormonal action through the RENIN-ANGIOTENSIN-ALDOSTE-RONE [RAA] HORMONAL SYSTEM), dilate (open) airways in the lungs, and dilate arteries that supply the muscles. At the same time these signals cause the BLOOD vessels in other parts of the body such as the digestive system to constrict, pushing blood into the body's central arteries. Under normal circumstances, the sympathetic nervous system is dominant during waking hours to accommodate the body's higher level of physical activity.

Parasympathetic Nervous System

The parasympathetic nervous system conveys nerve signals via the neurotransmitter acetylcholine, from the medulla oblongata in a single pathway along the spinal nerves. These signals cause biochemical and physical actions that dilate arteries supplying the digestive system and peripheral structures (such as the skin). At the same time these signals slow the heart rate, lower blood pressure, constrict the airways, and constrict the arteries supplying the muscles to provide an adequate blood supply for body functions such as digestion. Under normal circumstances the parasympathetic nervous system is dominant during sleeping hours, when the body's physical activity is minimal.

Stress Response

One of the key functions of the autonomic nervous system is to direct the body's stress response—the "FIGHT-OR-FLIGHT" response. When physical or emotional stress activates this response, the sympathetic nervous system sends a jolt of nerve signals to the body that cause a "jump" in cardiovascular functions. The rush of epinephrine this releases causes feelings of jitteriness or queasiness,

the heart races, and the breathing quickens. It is the body's biological preparation for survival in the face of crisis. When the perceived crisis passes, the parasympathetic nervous system engages to bring the body's systems back to normal.

The parasympathetic response is not nearly as rapid as the sympathetic response. When stress is persistent or frequent, the body remains in a state of heightened function for prolonged periods of time as it does not have time to return to a state of balance before being jolted into stress response again. Over time, this wears on the body and it begins to adapt by keeping the blood pressure and heart rate elevated as its new "norm." This can result in HYPERTENSION, ARRHYTHMIAS, and other cardiovascular problems.

Role in Cardiovascular Disease

Many MEDICATIONS TO TREAT HEART DISEASE target the functions of the autonomic nervous system by interfering in some way with adrenergic response (release and action of epinephrine and norepinephrine). Among them are ANTIHYPERTEN-SIVE MEDICATIONS such as ALPHA ANTAGONIST MEDI-CATIONS and BETA ANTAGONIST MEDICATIONS, many ANTIARRHYTHMIA MEDICATIONS, and VASODILATOR MEDICATIONS such as HYDRALAZINE (Apresoline) and MINOXIDIL (Loniten).

See also STRESS AND HEART DISEASE; STRESS REDUC-TION TECHNIQUES.

AV block   See HEART BLOCK.

AV canal defect   See ATRIOVENTRICULAR CANAL DEFECT.

AV node   See HEART.

bacterial endocarditis　See ENDOCARDITIS.

bad cholesterol　See CHOLESTEROL, BLOOD.

balloon angioplasty　See ANGIOPLASTY.

Barnard, Christiaan (1922–2001)　The South African surgeon who performed the first human HEART TRANSPLANT on December 3, 1967. Born and raised in South Africa, Barnard studied medicine at the University of Cape Town in South Africa and in 1958 came to the United States for further studies in surgery at the University of Minnesota. The world's first kidney transplant four years earlier had roused much excitement in the medical research community, and Barnard became enthralled with research on early models of the HEART-LUNG BYPASS MACHINE at the University of Minnesota. When he returned to South Africa to establish a private HEART surgery practice, he continued his research with the heart-lung bypass machine and heart transplantations on dogs.

In early December 1967 one family's tragedy became a pioneering triumph in heart surgery. Twenty-five-year-old DENISE DARVALL suffered extensive brain injuries in an automobile accident. Her family donated her organs, and on December 3 Barnard assembled a surgical team of 30 specialists to transplant Darvall's heart into LOUIS WASHKANSKY. Washkansky, a 53-year-old dentist with severe HEART FAILURE as a consequence of diabetes, survived just 18 days with his new heart before succumbing to pneumonia. Barnard continued his work as a heart transplant surgeon until his retirement in 1983, pioneering surgical techniques for attaching a donor heart without removing the original heart and experimenting with XENOGRAFTS using hearts from dogs and pigs.

Barnard's work established the foundation of heart surgery as we know it today. With improvements in IMMUNOSUPPRESSIVE MEDICATIONS, heart transplantation has become a viable treatment option that extends life by years and decades for thousands of people. Heart surgeons in the United States now perform about 2,300 heart transplants a year, a rate that has been fairly constant since 1992.

See also ALLOGRAFT; CARDIOMYOPATHY; CARDIOPULMONARY BYPASS; CLARK, BARNEY; COOLEY, DENTON; DEVRIES, WILLIAM C.; DONOR HEART; HEART, ARTIFICIAL; HEART-LUNG TRANSPLANT; JARVIK, ROBERT; LEFT VENTRICULAR ASSIST DEVICE; SURGERY, CARDIOVASCULAR.

Batista heart failure procedure　An experimental operation to improve HEART function in severe HEART FAILURE. In heart failure, the left ventricle, the heart's primary pumping chamber, enlarges in an effort to compensate for its diminishing effectiveness. As heart failure progresses, however, the increasing enlargement weakens the left ventricle until it can no longer pump enough BLOOD out of the heart to meet the body's oxygen needs. The Brazilian heart surgeon Randas Jose Vilela Batista developed the procedure in 1994 as an alternative for HEART TRANSPLANT in people for whom that procedure had become the final treatment option. Batista's procedure involves removing a wedge of heart muscle from the enlarged ventricle, which requires less sophisticated facilities and surgical expertise than heart transplantation and also relieves reliance on donor organs.

Procedure

The Batista heart failure procedure involves OPEN-HEART SURGERY with general anesthesia and CARDIOPULMONARY BYPASS. The cardiovascular surgeon slices out a wedge of the heart muscle, then pulls together and sutures the edges of the incision. This reduces the size of the ventricle. A more complex modification of the Batista procedure that evolved from 2002 to 2006 as an attempt to improve results, called ventricular remodeling, involves surgical sculpturing of the ventricle to reconfigure it into a more natural shape and size. Either procedure is sometimes done in combination with CORONARY ARTERY BYPASS GRAFT (CABG) to improve blood flow to the heart.

Risks and Complications

The Batista heart failure procedure has many risks and potential complications, due in part to the severity of the underlying heart disease and the person's overall weakened state of health and in part to the invasiveness and extensiveness of the surgery. The numerous risks associated with cardiopulmonary bypass and open-heart surgery include excessive bleeding during and after the operation, the formation of clots in the blood vessels (leading to risk of STROKE and MYOCARDIAL INFARCTION), difficulty weaning from bypass, inability to restart the heart, and death. Risks specific to the Batista procedure include ventricular rupture and fatal ARRHYTHMIAS. As well, there are the risks associated with general anesthesia. Postoperative complications may include BLOOD PRESSURE and HEART RATE irregularities, pneumonia, and infection. The Batista heart failure procedure remains an investigational treatment performed at few cardiac centers.

Outlook and Lifestyle Modifications

Although the Batista heart failure procedure generated much excitement among cardiovascular surgeons in the mid-1990s, it has not produced the decrease in cardiac hospitalizations or deaths that they had hoped to see. Recent studies suggest there is the same or greater benefit from CABG with lower risk. Although the Batista procedure improves heart function as assessed by EJECTION FRACTION and other measures, people who undergo the operation have significant heart disease and require ongoing cardiac care after the surgery. They must continue to take, or need additional, MEDICATIONS TO TREAT HEART DISEASE, and may need other treatments as their heart failure progresses.

See also CARDIOMYOPATHY; HEART, ARTIFICIAL; INVESTIGATIONAL TREATMENTS; LEFT VENTRICULAR ASSIST DEVICE (LVAD); SURGERY TO TREAT CARDIOVASCULAR DISEASE.

benazepril An ANGIOTENSIN-CONVERTING ENZYME (ACE) INHIBITOR MEDICATION taken to treat HYPERTENSION (high BLOOD PRESSURE). Common brand names include Lotensin. Doctors typically prescribe benazepril to treat moderate hypertension and may prescribe it as monotherapy (taken by itself) or in combination with other ANTIHYPERTENSIVE MEDICATIONS such as DIURETIC MEDICATIONS. Some people experience headache, DIZZINESS, nausea, and LIGHTHEADEDNESS when they first begin taking benzepril; these side effects usually go away within six to eight weeks.

As with other ACEs, peripheral EDEMA (swelling of the hands, feet, and lips and mouth) is a rare but potentially serious adverse reaction, particularly when it involves the face, when taking benazepril. Women who are pregnant or breast-feeding should not take benazepril; like other ACEs, it can harm or cause the death of the unborn baby. A woman who is taking benazepril and becomes pregnant should notify her doctor immediately to switch to a different antihypertensive medication.

See also ALPHA ANTAGONIST MEDICATIONS; ANGIOTENSIN II RECEPTOR ANTAGONIST MEDICATIONS; BETA ANTAGONIST MEDICATIONS; CALCIUM CHANNEL ANTAGONIST MEDICATIONS; COLD/FLU MEDICATION AND HYPERTENSION; MEDICATIONS TO TREAT HEART DISEASE; SODIUM CHANNEL BLOCKING MEDICATIONS; VASOCONSTRICTOR MEDICATIONS.

bepridil A CALCIUM CHANNEL ANTAGONIST MEDICATION taken to relieve the symptoms of ANGINA. Common brand names include Vasocor. Doctors sometimes prescribe bepridil in combination with BETA ANTAGONIST MEDICATIONS and/or NITRATE MEDICATIONS. Like other calcium channel blockers, bepridil works by interfering with the contraction of smooth muscle cells, causing artery walls to relax. This allows more BLOOD to flow through the coronary arteries that supply the heart, improving its supply of oxygen and relieving the pain of angina.

Bepridil also slows nerve activity in the muscle cells of the heart, which affects the heart's rhythm. This can improve certain ARRHYTHMIAS (irregular heartbeats), but it also can worsen other kinds of arrhythmias and cause new arrhythmias, particularly following a HEART ATTACK (myocardial infarction). A rare but serious side effect is agranulocytosis, a condition in which the white blood cell count drops rapidly and precipitously. Because of these potentially serious adverse reactions doctors typically prescribe bepridil only after other medications have failed to control angina symptoms; doctors in the U.S. rarely prescribe bepridil. Common side effects include nausea and gastrointestinal disturbances. Bepridil can interact with various other medications including tricyclic antidepressants, certain diuretics, QUINIDINE, and PROCAINAMIDE.

See also ANTIDEPRESSANT MEDICATIONS; BETA ANTAGONIST MEDICATIONS; MEDICATIONS TO TREAT HEART DISEASE; HEART BLOCK; HYPERTENSION; SICK SINUS SYNDROME.

beta antagonist medications A classification of medications prescribed to treat HYPERTENSION (high BLOOD PRESSURE), ANGINA, ARRHYTHMIAS such as LONG DT SYNDROME (LQTS), HEART FAILURE, and after a HEART ATTACK to prevent additional heart attacks. Commonly prescribed medications include PROPANOLOL (Inderal), NADOLOL (Corgard), bisoprolol (Zebeta), ATENOLOL (Tenormin), and METOPROLOL (Lopressor).

These medications, often called beta-blockers, work by keeping EPINEPHRINE from binding with receptors in cardiac and smooth muscle cells such as in the HEART and the ARTERIES. Epinephrine stimulates the contraction of these cells. Inhibiting epinephrine's ability to bind, or chemically connect, with adrenergic receptors in the cells slows the contractions of these cells and relaxes the muscle structures they comprise. Arteries dilate, allowing higher volumes of blood to flow through them

with less pressure, lowering blood pressure. When its contractions are slowed, the heart requires less oxygen and can pump more efficiently, which relieves the pressure and pain of angina.

There are three general categories of beta antagonist medications:

- **Beta-1 blockers.** Beta-1 receptors are present in cardiac muscle and nerve cells that regulate the strength and rate of the heartbeat. Medications that selectively block beta-1 receptors help to slow and stabilize the heart's rhythm, reducing the amount of work the heart must do to pump blood through the body.

- **Beta-2 blockers.** Beta-2 receptors are present in the cells of smooth muscle such as the walls of arteries and bronchi (airway passages in the lungs). Medications that block beta-2 receptors constrict smooth muscle tissue. This narrows the arteries and relieves migraine headache symptoms in some people. Doctors do not know the precise mechanisms by which beta-blocking medications decrease blood pressure; proposed mechanisms include a central nervous system effect, inhibition of RENIN, and a reduction in CARDIAC OUTPUT. Beta-2 blockers also inhibit some bodily responses related to anxiety, such as sweating, and are sometimes prescribed to treat mild ANXIETY and panic attack.

- **Nonselective beta-blockers.** Nonselective beta-blockers were the first of the beta-blocking medications to come onto the market. They block both beta-1 and beta-2 receptors. They have the combined effects of slowing the heart rate and regulating the heart's rhythm. They also reduce blood pressure by various mechanisms.

Common side effects with beta-blockers include tiredness, weakness, occasional orthostatic HYPOTENSION (a sudden drop in blood pressure when changing position from lying down or sitting to standing), sleep disturbances (including vivid dreams), and SEXUAL DYSFUNCTION (diminished libido, ERECTILE DYSFUNCTION). Sometimes changing to a different beta-blocker medication reduces or eliminates most side effects. Beta-blockers also can interfere with various other medications and mask

COMMONLY PRESCRIBED BETA ANTAGONIST MEDICATIONS

Medication	Common Brands	Beta-1	Beta-2	Nonselective
acebutolol	Sectral	X		
atenolol	Tenormin	X		
betaxolol	Kerlone	X		
bisoprolol	Zebeta	X		
carteolol	Cartrol	X	X	
carvidolol	Coreg	X	X	
labetalol	Normodyne, Trandate	X	X	
metoprolol	Lopressor, Toprol-XL	X		
nadolol	Corgard	X	X	
penbutolol	Levatol	X	X	
pindolol	Visken	X	X	
propanolol	Inderal, Inderal-LA			X
sotalol	Betapace			X
timolol	Blocadren	X	X	

early signs of low blood sugar in people who take medications to treat diabetes (oral or insulin).

Some beta-blocker medications are primarily beta-1 blockers but will block beta-2 receptors as well at higher doses, such as acebuterol and betaxolol. A few beta-blocker medications also block alpha adrenergic receptors (alpha-blocking activity), such as CARVEDILOL and LABETALOL. Doctors might prescribe a combination of medications, such as a beta antagonist with a diuretic ("water pill"), to control severe hypertension or hypertension that does not respond to a single medication. People who take medications to treat asthma should not take beta-blockers that have beta-2 actions as these drugs constrict (tighten) the airways, which can trigger asthma attacks or counteract the effects of beta-agonist medications (drugs that activate adrenergic receptors) taken to prevent asthma attacks.

See also ALPHA ANTAGONIST MEDICATIONS; CALCIUM CHANNEL ANTAGONIST MEDICATIONS; LIFESTYLE AND HEART HEALTH; MEDICATIONS TO TREAT HEART DISEASE; SODIUM.

beta carotene A natural biochemical found in foods such as carrots and sweet potatoes that the body converts to vitamin A. Beta carotene is an ANTIOXIDANT, a chemical substance that combats the potentially damaging effects of the oxidation that is a natural by-product of METABOLISM in the body. For many years, observational studies showed that people who ate diets high in fruits and vegetables also had an increased intake of antioxidants and seemed to have a lower risk for health problems such as HEART DISEASE and cancer. It became a prevailing perspective that antioxidants, particularly beta carotene and tocopherol (the active chemical family in vitamin E), helped protect against these health problems. Extensive research studies, some conducted over 10 to 12 years, failed to substantiate this premise, however. Although health experts believe a diet high in fruits, vegetables, and whole grains supports overall good health, there remains no conclusive evidence that increased beta carotene intake has any effect on reducing the risk of heart disease.

See also COENZYME Q-10; EXERCISE; FOLIC ACID; LIFESTYLE AND HEART HEALTH; NUTRITION AND DIET.

Betapace See SOTALOL.

betaxolol A BETA ANTAGONIST MEDICATION taken to treat HYPERTENSION (high BLOOD PRESSURE) and ANGINA. Common brand names include Kerlone. Doctors may prescribe betaxolol in combination with other ANTIHYPERTENSIVE MEDICATIONS, such as DIURETIC MEDICATIONS, to more effectively control high blood pressure. Over-the-counter or prescription NSAIDs, such as ibuprofen can lessen betaxolol's effectiveness. Mild side effects might include headache, nausea, dizziness, orthostatic HYPOTENSION (sudden drop in blood pressure when standing from a lying or sitting position), and SEXUAL DYSFUNCTION. Women who are pregnant or who become pregnant while taking betaxolol should not take this medication, as it has not been proven safe for the unborn child. When stopping this medication, it is important to taper the dose down over two weeks; stopping suddenly can cause unexpected and potentially dangerous spikes in blood pressure.

See also ALPHA ANTAGONIST MEDICATIONS; ANGIO-
TENSIN-CONVERTING ENZYME (ACE) INHIBITOR MEDI-
CATIONS; ANGIOTENSIN II RECEPTOR ANTAGONIST
MEDICATIONS; CALCIUM CHANNEL ANTAGONIST MEDI-
CATIONS; CORONARY ARTERY DISEASE (CAD); MEDICA-
TIONS TO TREAT HEART DISEASE.

bicuspid aortic valve   A congenital abnormality
of the valve between the aorta and the heart's left
ventricle in which the valve has two cusps or flaps
rather than the normal three (tricuspid). The aortic
valve opens to allow BLOOD to leave the left ventricle for circulation through the body, and closes
behind each ventricular contraction to keep the
blood from flowing back into the ventricle. The
pressure on the valve is considerable, and the normal tricuspid structure of the aortic valve is stronger than a bicuspid structure, which eventually
weakens and can stiffen or fail to close properly.
Bicuspid aortic valve affects as many as 2 percent of
people, making it one of the most common HEART
abnormalities. Doctors might suspect a bicuspid
valve if they can hear a MURMUR when listening to
the heart with a STETHOSCOPE; this is the sound of
blood flowing out of the heart during ejection (SYS-
TOLE) or back into the left ventricle, during filling
(DIASTOLE). Imaging procedures such as ECHOCAR-
DIOGRAM and cardiac catheterization can confirm
the diagnosis and show the extent to which the
abnormal valve affects heart function.

Sometimes the bicuspid aortic valve structure
functions improperly from birth and doctors diagnose the deformity in infancy or early childhood.
Often, people who have bicuspid aortic valve do
not know it until later in life when the deformed
valve begins to fail. Treatment in either circumstance is surgery to replace the valve. Symptoms of
aortic valve failure might include dizziness or light-
headedness and ANGINA (CHEST PAIN), although it
is common to have no symptoms. An untreated
bicuspid aortic valve that malfunctions allows
blood to return to the heart, which causes the heart
to work harder to pump an adequate supply of
oxygenated blood out to the body. It can result in
HEART FAILURE and CARDIOMEGALY (enlarged heart).
Bicuspid aortic valves may calcify and result in
aortic stenosis (narrowing of the orifice), increas-

ing the heart's workload per beat which can lead
to major complications. The abnormal (bicuspid)
anatomy of the valve may increase the risk for bacterial ENDOCARDITIS (infection of the heart). People
diagnosed with bicuspid aortic valve should check
with their doctors about prophylactic antibiotics
before dental procedures, certain gynecological
procedures, and other surgical procedures that
could introduce bacteria into the body. The doctor
will determine whether the person's circumstances
meet the criteria for antibiotic prophylaxis. People
who have bicuspid aortic valves have a greater
incidence of vascular disease, in particular complications of HYPERTENSION, and should receive aggressive preventive medical care.

See also ANTICOAGULANT MEDICATIONS; AOR-
TIC REGURGITATION; AORTIC STENOSIS; CARDIOPUL-
MONARY BYPASS; CARDIOVASCULAR SYSTEM; HEART
DISEASE; HEART DISEASE IN CHILDREN; SURGERY TO
TREAT CARDIOVASCULAR DISEASE; VALVE REPAIR AND
REPLACEMENT.

bidirectional Glenn procedure   An OPEN-HEART
SURGERY to repair serious congenital HEART malformations such as TRICUSPID ATRESIA, PULMONARY
ATRESIA, HYPOPLASTIC LEFT HEART SYNDROME (HLHS),
and SINGLE VENTRICLE, in which the heart does
not properly pump BLOOD through the lungs and
into the body. It often follows a BLALOCK-TAUSSIG
PROCEDURE (surgery to correct blood vessel malformations so blood goes to and from the lungs and
heart) and is typically one of several surgeries performed as a series within the first three years of life.
It is sometimes called a partial FONTAN PROCEDURE
or a bidirectional cavopulmonary anastamosis.

In a healthy, correctly formed heart two large
veins, the superior (upper) vena cava and inferior
(lower) vena cava, receive blood from the body
before it enters into the heart. This deoxygenated
blood flows into the right atrium and then into the
right ventricle, which pumps it through the pulmonary artery to the lungs. Oxygenated blood returns
to the heart through the pulmonary veins to the
left atrium and into the left ventricle, which pumps
it into the body through the aorta. In the serious
heart malformations that require the bidirectional
Glenn procedure, the heart's structure is deformed

and typically there is just one functioning ventricle. Little blood goes to and from the lungs, so the blood the heart pumps into the body does not carry enough oxygen to meet the body's needs.

Procedure

The bidirectional Glenn procedure reconfigures the heart's structure so that the heart's single functioning ventricle pumps blood only to the body, not to the lungs and then to the body. The surgeon joins the pulmonary artery and the superior vena cava to each other, which allows deoxygenated blood returning to the heart to flow instead directly into the lungs. The blood that then enters the heart is partially oxygenated, which the heart then pumps out to the body. Although oxygenation still is less than normal, it is adequate to meet the body's basic needs for the short term. Additional surgery within the child's first three years of life must either reconstruct or transplant the heart, depending on the nature and complexity of the heart's malformations.

Risks and Complications

The risks and complications of the bidirectional Glenn procedure include those of open-heart surgery, anesthesia, and cardiopulmonary bypass as well as those related to the procedure. The most significant procedural risks are excessive bleeding, failure of the anastamosis (joining of the blood vessels), and continued inadequate oxygenation (HYPOXIA) after the operation. Postoperative infection, blood clots, and pneumonia are also concerns. Because the underlying heart defects are so severe and the child's health is poor, death is also a significant risk. About a third of children develop COLLATERAL CIRCULATION, that in some cases becomes capable of bypassing the anastamosis, by the time of their next operations. Additional complications may develop due to the underlying heart defects and the continued abnormal function of the heart. These complications include PULMONARY HYPERTENSION, ARRHYTHMIAS, and congestive HEART FAILURE.

Outlook and Lifestyle Modifications

Because the bidirectional Glenn procedure immediately improves the heart's ability to circulate oxygenated blood, there is usually immediate and pronounced improvement in the child's condition.

Most children stay one to three days in the intensive care unit and up to a week in the hospital when postoperative recovery is without complications. The bidirectional Glenn procedure is palliative rather than corrective, intended to provide temporary relief until the child is able to undergo the extensive operations required to reconstruct the defective heart. So although the child's condition improves, the heart's function remains limited and abnormal. Medications are necessary to help strengthen the heart's contractions (commonly DIGOXIN), control BLOOD PRESSURE (typically ANGIOTENSIN-CONVERTING [ACE] INHIBITOR MEDICATIONS), and prevent clotting (ANTICOAGULANT MEDICATIONS such as Coumadin [warfarin]). Further operations, and possibly heart transplant, are necessary to achieve more normal cardiac function. Until the sequence of operations is complete, the child is likely to have slow growth, limited physical strength and energy, and restrictions on activity.

See also CARDIO-PULMONARY BYPASS; HEART DISEASE IN CHILDREN; HEART TRANSPLANT; NORWOOD PROCEDURE; PALLIATION, STAGED.

bile acid sequestrants See LIPID-LOWERING MEDICATIONS.

biofeedback A mind-body therapy that can help to reduce STRESS, lower BLOOD PRESSURE, and slow HEART RATE. Biofeedback uses monitoring equipment to help identify physiological responses such as body temperature, heart rate, breathing rate, and electrical activity in muscle groups. The person learns techniques to affect body responses under the guidance of a therapist trained to use and teach biofeedback. Eventually the person can do the techniques without the monitoring equipment. Biofeedback is sometimes called psychophysiological interaction or neurobiofeedback. Most people can learn biofeedback techniques for relaxation and stress reduction, which causes blood pressure and heart rate to drop. Many people can also learn to specifically influence blood pressure and heart rate. Competitive athletes sometimes use biofeedback to help achieve ideal heart rates for maximum physical performance during strenuous activity.

See also COMPLEMENTARY THERAPIES; MEDITATION; MINDFULNESS; ORNISH PROGRAM; YOGA.

birth control pills   See ORAL CONTRACEPTIVES.

biventricular assist device (BVAD)   See MECHANICAL CIRCULATORY SUPPORT.

biventricular pacing   See CARDIAC RESYNCHRONIZATION THERAPY (CRT).

black cohosh   A herb women sometimes take to relieve hot flashes and other discomforts of menopause. Black cohosh is also called bugbane, bugwort, and black snakeroot. It is available without a prescription in various forms including tea, powder, and capsules. Because black cohosh is classified and sold as a food product, it is not subject to U.S. Food and Drug Administration (FDA) requirements and inspections. It is also included as an ingredient in numerous combination products marketed to relieve menopause discomforts.

Most health experts agree, and some studies support the claim, that when used as directed on the package label black cohosh can be effective in relieving menopausal discomforts. However, some research suggests that taking higher than recommended doses of black cohosh can slow the HEART RATE. Women who have diagnosed HEART conditions or who take any medications for heart conditions, particularly ARRHYTHMIAS (irregular heartbeat), should check with their doctors before taking black cohosh. Because the risk for HEART DISEASE increases with age and, for women, after menopause, it is prudent for a woman to discuss taking black cohosh with her doctor. A general cardiac examination can determine whether there are existing heart problems that could be a problem when taking black cohosh.

See also HORMONE REPLACEMENT THERAPY (HRT); WOMEN AND HEART DISEASE.

Blalock, Alfred (1899–1964)   The cardiac surgeon who, in collaboration with pediatric cardiologist HELEN TAUSSIG, developed the Blalock-Taussig procedure to restore BLOOD flow between the lungs and the HEART. Blalock performed the first such surgery in 1944; the surgery has since become a standard treatment for "blue baby" heart defects, such as TETRALOGY OF FALLOT. Blalock started his career as a researcher at Vanderbilt University. There his work proved that the blood loss during surgery caused shock. The discovery prompted the use of BLOOD TRANSFUSIONS as routine treatment for surgical shock. In 1941 Blalock went to Johns Hopkins University, from which he had received his medical degree, to continue his surgical research. With the advent of antibiotics, effective anesthesia, and the HEART-LUNG BYPASS MACHINE, the time was ripe for rapid advances. History credits Blalock with developing numerous surgical procedures to correct heart malformations.

See also BIDIRECTIONAL GLENN PROCEDURE; BLALOCK-TAUSSIG PROCEDURE; HEART DISEASE IN CHILDREN; SURGERY TO TREAT CARDIOVASCULAR DISEASE; HYPOPLASTIC LEFT HEART SYNDROME (HLHS); NORWOOD PROCEDURE; THOMAS, VIVIEN.

Blalock-Taussig procedure   A surgery to correct congenital malformations of the heart's great vessels or the heart's ventricles, such as TETRALOGY OF FALLOT, that prevent oxygenated BLOOD from moving from the lungs to the HEART or from the heart to circulation through the body. Developed by cardiac surgeon ALFRED BLALOCK and pediatric cardiologist HELEN TAUSSIG in 1944, the surgery uses the superior vena cava to create an anastamosis (joining) of the aorta and the pulmonary artery. This procedure routes oxygenated blood from the lungs to the heart so the heart can pump it out to the body. It usually is done shortly following birth.

Procedure

The Blalock-Taussig procedure was one of the first heart operations to improve cardiac health and life expectancy for children with congenitally malformed hearts, and today often is the first of multiple surgeries for infants born with serious heart malformations. The operation is done while the heart is beating; it does not require CARDIOPULMONARY BYPASS. The surgeon makes an incision through the rib cage under the left arm to gain access to the heart and its major vessels. The surgeon then connects the appropriate blood vessels either directly or with a synthetic shunt and closes the incision.

Risks and Complications

Although the Blalock-Taussig procedure restores the flow of oxygenated blood, it does not correct underlying malformations or deformities. The risks and complications of the Blalock-Taussig procedure include those of surgery and anesthesia in general as well as those related to the procedure. Key among these are excessive bleeding, failure of the shunt that requires reoperation, ARRHYTHMIAS, blood clots, infection, and pneumonia. Because the underlying heart defects are so severe, death is also a risk. Additional complications may develop due to the underlying heart defects and the continued abnormal function of the heart. Additional operations are necessary to correct the malformations and establish more normal heart function.

Outlook and Lifestyle Modifications

Because the Blalock-Taussig procedure immediately improves the heart's ability to circulate oxygenated blood, there is usually immediate and pronounced improvement in the child's condition. Most noticeable is the disappearance of CYANOSIS as adequate oxygen reaches the tissues. Most children stay one to three days in the intensive care unit and up to a week in the hospital when postoperative recovery is without complications. Medications are often necessary to help strengthen the heart's contractions, control BLOOD PRESSURE, and prevent clotting. Until the sequence of staged operations to reconstruct the heart is complete, the child has slow growth, limited physical energy and strength, and restrictions on activities.

See also BIDIRECTIONAL GLENN PROCEDURE; CARDIOPULMONARY BYPASS; FONTAN PROCEDURE; HEART DISEASE IN CHILDREN; HYPOPLASTIC LEFT HEART SYNDROME; NORWOOD PROCEDURE; PULMONARY ATRESIA; SURGERY TO TREAT CARDIOVASCULAR DISEASE; THOMAS, VIVIEN; TRICUSPID ATRESIA.

Blocadren   See TIMOLOL.

blood   The viscous fluid that transports oxygen and nutrients throughout the body via the CARDIOVASCULAR SYSTEM. Blood contains four basic components:

- plasma, the straw-colored liquid that is about 90 percent water, which transports blood cells and other substances and comprises about 55 percent of blood volume
- platelets, which facilitate clotting; they comprise about 1 percent of blood volume
- red blood cells, which ferry oxygen and other nutrients to body cells and carbon dioxide and other waste from body cells; they comprise about 40 percent of blood volume
- white blood cells, which maintain the body's immune system and fight infection; they comprise about 4 percent of blood volume

Blood also carries various and numerous dissolved or suspended substances such as sugars, salts (ELECTROLYTES), LIPIDS (fatty acids), proteins and enzymes, HORMONES, and other chemicals. The typical adult human body contains 10 pints of blood which, when the body is at rest, the heart pumps through its network of blood vessels once each minute. During EXERCISE or strenuous physical activity, the HEART can pump 20 times that volume each minute to carry vital nutrients to tissues and remove wastes from them. Blood travels through a structure of arteries, veins, and capillaries that, if stretched out, would cover nearly 100,000 miles.

Blood Composition

Red blood cells, or erythrocytes, are the most abundant cells in the blood. Their role is to transport oxygen and nutrients to cells throughout the body and return waste products for excretion through the kidneys and the lungs. Red blood cells are rich in a protein called hemoglobin, which contains iron to bind with oxygen molecules. Red blood cells are somewhat doughnut-shaped, with a thick wall-like rim and a flat, thin center. This structure makes the cells flexible enough to pass through the arterioles, the body's microscopically small arteries where the oxygen/carbon dioxide exchange between body cells and red blood cells takes place.

It takes about five days for the bone marrow to manufacture a red blood cell; the marrow produces millions of them each day. A red blood cell newly released from the marrow into the bloodstream, called a reticulocyte, is not yet mature enough to participate in oxygen/carbon dioxide transport. It takes about 48 to 72 hours for it to come of age. Red blood cells typically live for about 120 days (four months), at the end of which their structure begins to deteriorate and they become less flexible. The spleen contains a network of small blood vessels that trap aged red blood cells, holding them for white blood cells called macrophages to destroy.

White blood cells are the largest cells in the blood and are responsible for preventing and fighting infection. In general white blood cells are known as leukocytes; there are also specific types and subtypes of white cells that have specialized functions. Granulocytes and monocytes attack and consume bacteria and other invading organisms; the bone marrow produces them and they have a lifespan of just a few days. The lymphatic system, a component of the immune system, produces lymphocytes, which circulate in the blood and in the lymph.

Platelets, also called thrombocytes, are the smallest cells in the blood. The bone marrow produces them, and they circulate through the bloodstream for about 10 days. Their only function is to cause blood to clot; they remain inert unless activated by chemical messengers released when there is bleeding. When activated they become sticky and change shape; they clump together with each other and with other cells in the blood to form clots.

The fatty acid deposits that accumulate along the insides of arterial walls when blood lipid levels are elevated cause microscopic damage to the artery, releasing tiny amounts of the chemicals that activate platelets. Although not enough to initiate a full-blown clotting process in most circumstances, it is enough to snag a few passing platelets that adhere to the artery wall along with the fatty deposits. Over time, this debris pile builds up and can block the artery or break away. Either scenario can result in STROKE or HEART ATTACK, depending on what artery is involved.

Blood Types

Red blood cells contain proteins that mark them as "native" to protect them from attack by white blood cells. There are two general types of these markers, also called antigens, that can exist in one of four presentations—A, B, AB (both A and B), and O (neither A nor B). These antigens represent the basic four blood types and are not compatible with each other; when they come in contact with each other (as might occur during transfusions), antibodies in the native blood will attack the "invading" red blood cells.

A second aspect of blood type is the Rhesus factor, which is either positive (the antigen, called factor D, is present) or negative (the antigen is not present). Positive and negative Rhesus factors are also incompatible. About 85 percent of people are Rhesus positive. A person's blood type can be A positive or A negative, B positive or B negative, AB positive or AB negative, or O positive or O negative. Type and cross-match for transfusion must consider both antigen factors.

Blood Circulation Through the Body

New cells join the blood and old cells leave the closed network of the circulation on a regular basis. Through the kidneys the body extracts water to increase blood volume or excretes water to decrease blood volume on an ever-shifting basis according to its needs for maintaining BLOOD PRESSURE but keeping a fairly constant level of about 10 pints. Blood transports everything that body tissues need to function.

Blood Manufacture and Maintenance

The bone marrow—a spongy tissue in the inner core of the body's long bones, hip bones, and sternum—manufactures all blood cells except lymphocytes from foundation cells called stem cells. The spleen's primary function is to destroy worn-out red blood cells, returning their chemical components to the body for use in making new red blood cells. It also contains lymph tissue that manufactures some white blood cells, mostly lymphocytes, that help fight infections as well as participate in destroying aged red blood cells.

Blood Disorders

Numerous disorders affect the manufacture and function of blood cells. One of the most common is iron-deficient ANEMIA, which limits the capacity of the hemoglobin in red blood cells to carry oxygen. Chronic anemia causes the heart to work harder in an effort to increase the oxygen supply that reaches body tissues, increasing the force and rate of contractions to move blood more quickly through the body. Other blood disorders, such as THROMBOCYTOPENIA and THROMBOCYTHEMIA affect the blood's ability to clot.

See also ANTICOAGULANT; COLLATERAL CIRCULATION; DEEP VEIN THROMBOSIS (DVT); EMBOLISM; HEMOCHROMATOSIS; POLYCYTHEMIA; THROMBOLYTIC MEDICATIONS.

blood clot　See EMBOLISM.

blood gases　Measurements of the oxygen, carbon dioxide, and acidity (pH) levels in BLOOD samples drawn from an artery near the surface of the body, such as the femoral (in the groin) or radial (in the wrist). Blood gases help to determine whether enough oxygen is getting into the blood and if the oxygenated blood is circulating through the body. This laboratory test also detects whether oxygen levels are too high, as might occur with oxygen therapy or when a person is on MECHANICAL VENTILATION (breathing machine). Because arteries are deeper than veins and their structure contains more layers and nerves, the needle puncture into the artery can cause a quick, sharp pain. The person doing the draw may use a local anesthetic to numb the skin and surface tissue to minimize discomfort. Normal values vary depending on the person's age and other factors. Other blood values are also important. Although blood gases are usually drawn when HEART ATTACK is suspected, blood gases cannot tell a doctor whether a heart attack or other cardiac crisis has occurred. However, they do provide useful information about the effectiveness of the heart and lungs in various clinical conditions.

See also BLOOD TESTS TO DETECT HEART ATTACK; CHRONIC OBSTRUCTIVE PULMONARY DISEASE (COPD); PULMONARY SYSTEM; PULSE OXIMETRY.

bloodless surgery　Surgery performed without administering BLOOD TRANSFUSIONS or other BLOOD products. Some people refuse blood transfusions

and BLOOD products because of their religious beliefs, and others because they fear infection or other health risks associated with receiving living cells from donors. Bloodless surgery techniques emphasize minimal blood loss and sometimes require innovative methods, particularly for operations on structures of the CARDIOVASCULAR SYSTEM that transport blood. The many and subtle variations in anatomy among individuals makes it challenging for surgeons to avoid every circumstance in which they might encounter unexpected bleeding. Advances in imaging technology such as MAGNETIC RESONANCE IMAGING (MRI) and ANGIOGRAPHY help surgeons to discover any anatomical anomalies before surgery, so they are better prepared to manage them. Other technologies such as laser scalpels and argon beam coagulators seal bleeding tissues instantly, and cell collectors allow surgeons to salvage any blood that is lost and administer it back to the person.

See also CARDIOPULMONARY BYPASS; SURGERY TO TREAT CARDIOVASCULAR DISEASE.

blood pressure　The amount of pressure the flow of BLOOD exerts on the walls of the arteries as it travels through them, usually expressed in millimeters of mercury (mm/Hg) as a ratio between systolic and diastolic pressures. Systolic pressure, the top or first number in a blood pressure reading, measures the peak of the heart's ventricular contraction that sends blood into the aorta for circulation through the body. It also reflects the pressure of the aorta's recoil response as blood surges into this largest of arteries in the body, which is the greatest pressure against a blood vessel that the contracting heart exerts. Diastolic pressure, the bottom or second number in a blood pressure reading, measures the pressure in the peripheral arteries when the ventricles are relaxed between contractions. Many variables influence blood pressure, from physical exertion to emotional tension such as fear or anxiety.

The Body's Blood Pressure Regulatory Mechanisms
Several mechanisms in the body share regulatory control of blood pressure. Structures within the BRAIN STEM signal the HEART to increase or decrease

the force and frequency of its contractions, which correspondingly raises or lowers blood pressure. Fluid and electrolyte levels in the blood as the blood passes through the kidneys influence the RENIN-ANGIOTENSIN-ALDOSTERONE (RAA) HORMONAL SYSTEM, through which the kidneys produce chemicals that initiate a sequence of events to constrict the body's tiniest arteries, the arterioles, and correspondingly raise blood pressure. Nerve clusters in the major arteries, primarily the aorta and the carotid arteries going to the head, sense the pressure of blood as it flows past them and send signals to the brain when the pressure is too high, which causes the brain (primarily the brain stem) to direct the heart to beat more slowly and with less force to lower blood pressure. These mechanisms work both in concert with one another and independently of each other, the body's redundancy to make sure there is always some means of regulating the vital actions of blood pressure. These systems respond to continual minute changes as well as significant physiological events such as SHOCK (such as from extensive blood loss), HEART ATTACK, and STROKE.

Measuring Blood Pressure

The device used to measure blood pressure is called a SPHYGMOMANOMETER, which is sometimes a dial gauge though more often an electronic device with a digital readout. A cuff wrapped around the arm is inflated to a pressure that constricts the arteries and stops blood flow, and then is released while the health-care provider listens to a pulse point in the artery using a STETHOSCOPE. The first detectable beat is the systolic pressure; the last detectable beat is the diastolic pressure. Automated machines also can provide blood pressure readings, such as in the operating suite or in the cardiac care unit when it is important to regularly monitor blood pressure.

Although there is a general perception that a blood pressure reading of 120/70 mm Hg is "normal," healthy, or optimal, blood pressure spans a range of readings and relates to some extent to other factors of health such as physical fitness. A person who is very athletic and has a high level of physical fitness might have a blood pressure and corresponding pulse rate that is lower than what doctors typically consider healthy, yet for this person such readings are within the healthy range. Generally the range of acceptable or normal blood pressure is a systolic pressure of 120 to 130 mm Hg and a diastolic pressure of less than 80 to 89 mm Hg. Pressures that are consistently over these levels—systolic, diastolic, or both—are considered hypertensive. For decades doctors primarily paid attention to the diastolic (bottom) figure in determining whether HYPERTENSION (high blood pressure) was present; research in recent years demonstrates that an elevated systolic pressure carries the greatest risk to health.

Blood Pressure and Cardiovascular Health

Consistently elevated blood pressure—hypertension—is itself a cardiovascular health condition as well as a risk factor for multiple forms of CARDIOVASCULAR DISEASE. Untreated hypertension is the leading cause of STROKE, a key factor in HEART ATTACK, and a contributing factor in HEART FAILURE and kidney failure. Disease conditions affecting the arteries and their ability to contract and dilate, such as ATHEROSCLEROSIS and ARTERIOSCLEROSIS, increase the resistance blood encounters in flowing through them, which causes blood pressure to increase. Obesity also increases arterial resistance, with the same result. Consistently low blood pressure—HYPOTENSION—can result in inadequate oxygenation of vital body tissues such as the brain and liver.

Lifestyle factors are key to maintaining blood pressure within healthy limits. Multiple studies show that even mild exercise done regularly, such as walking for 15 minutes every day, can reduce systolic blood pressure by 10 mm/Hg; moderate exercise done regularly, such as walking for 30 to 60 minutes a day at a brisk pace, can lower blood pressure even further.

See also AFRICAN AMERICANS AND CARDIOVASCULAR DISEASE; ANTIHYPERTENSIVE MEDICATIONS; DIABETES AND HEART DISEASE; DIASTOLIC DYSFUNCTION; HEART ATTACK; LIFESTYLE AND HEART HEALTH; PULSE; STROKE; SYSTOLIC DYSFUNCTION.

blood tests to detect heart attack   Several BLOOD tests can help determine whether a person is having or has had a HEART ATTACK by detecting changes in certain enzymes and proteins that signal damage to the MYOCARDIUM (HEART muscle). Because early treatment establishes the best likelihood of recovery, blood tests should be performed as soon as possible whenever there is a possibility of heart attack, even if symptoms are inconclusive. These tests include:

- cTnT (cardiac troponin T) and cTnI (cardiac troponin I)—These proteins regulate the balance of two enzymes, actin and myosin, that cause myocardial muscle fibers to contract. Elevated levels of cTnT and cTnI in the blood signal increased contraction activity, a sign of damage to the myocardium. Elevation begins within two to three hours of the heart attack, with levels peaking at about 14 hours. The levels of cTnT and cTnI remain elevated for up to seven days.

- creatine kinase (CK)—The myocardium releases increased amounts of this enzyme beginning about six hours after the heart attack. The CK level peaks 18 to 20 hours after the heart attack and generally returns to normal 36 hours after the heart attack. The more significant the damage the higher the CK level, and the longer it takes for the CK level to peak and then return to normal.

- creatine kinase mb (CK-MB)—CK-MB is a component of CK. Elevated levels of both CK and CK-MB strongly suggest heart attack. Like CK, CK-MB returns to normal about 36 hours following the heart attack.

- MYOGLOBIN—This oxygen-transport protein is present in all striated muscle fibers (skeletal muscles and cardiac muscle). Injury to muscle tissue, including heart attack, releases additional myoglobin into the bloodstream within minutes of the injury. Although myoglobin levels are not specific to heart damage, continuing elevation is a solid early indicator that a heart attack is under way or has occurred. Other lab tests are necessary to corroborate this indication. When a heart attack is taking place, myoglobin levels generally double every hour or two; when the injury is to other muscle tissue, the levels generally return to normal in three or four hours.

Other changes in blood chemistry often occur following heart attack but are not conclusive for diagnosis. Doctors typically do other diagnostic tests as well, including ELECTROCARDIOGRAM (ECG) and sometimes ECHOCARDIOGRAM or ANGIOGRAPHY, to determine whether a heart attack has occurred. See also CARDIAC ENZYMES.

blood thinner   See ANTICOAGULANT MEDICATIONS.

blood transfusion   The replacement of large amounts of BLOOD from serious bleeding such as might occur as a result of traumatic injury, due to a ruptured ANEURYSM, or during surgery, with donor blood or blood products. Transfusions also are sometimes necessary to treat severe ANEMIA. Transfused blood products are given by intravenous flow into a vein, usually in the arm. For all blood products except plasma and white cells, the donor blood must match the blood type and Rh factor of the recipient. A laboratory test called a type and cross match confirms this.

Whole Blood Transfusion

Whole blood contains all the components of blood and comes from donors. After donation, whole blood can be refrigerated for up to four weeks. Doctors administer whole blood transfusions when there is significant blood loss and the need to replace blood cells as well as fluid volume. The body must have an appropriate volume of fluid in circulation to maintain blood pressure and to circulate oxygen and vital nutrients to body tissues. The blood type and Rh factor of the whole blood being administered must match the recipient's.

Red Cell Transfusion

Red blood cell transfusions contain either packed cells with most of the plasma removed or washed red cells, a blood product that has the white blood cells and plasma proteins removed. A red cell transfusion delivers the hemoglobin capacity of red blood cells (the ability to transport oxygen) without adding very much fluid volume. This is particularly important for people who have both chronic anemia and heart failure; the additional fluid volume of whole blood worsens heart failure. Packed or washed red blood cells, like whole blood, can be refrigerated and stored for up to four weeks. Red blood cells are also called erythrocytes. A donor can give blood about every six to eight weeks under normal circumstances, although people with rare blood types often donate more frequently.

Platelet Transfusion

Platelets, also called thrombocytes, are cells in the blood that are necessary for clotting. Doctors might administer platelet transfusions during surgery in which there has been significant bleeding, and to treat blood disorders in which there is a shortage of platelets such as THROMBOCYTOPENIA. Platelets can be extracted from whole blood or obtained from donors through a process called apheresis, in which the platelets are removed immediately and the rest of the blood is returned to the donor. This allows platelet donors to donate as often as twice a week if needed.

White Cell Transfusion

Some health conditions cause depletion of white blood cells, which fight infection. This might happen following chemotherapy (treatment for cancer) or a serious infection. A transfusion of white blood cells (primarily granulocytes) can boost the recipient's immune system enough to allow antibiotics to work more effectively. White blood cells live just 24 hours, however, so multiple white cell transfusions might be necessary. White blood cells are extracted from whole blood donations.

Plasma and Plasma Product Transfusion

Plasma separated from whole blood can be frozen for extended periods of time. It can be thawed, warmed, and administered to treat a variety of bleeding and clotting disorders. The primary protein of plasma, albumin, also can be separated into a concentrated solution that can be stored in ready-to-use form. Doctors use albumin transfusions to treat shock and substantial blood loss when the correct type of whole blood is unavailable or the person's blood has not yet been typed. Albumin transfusions are also given for certain kinds of kidney disorders.

Clotting Factor Transfusion

Whole blood contains numerous proteins that initiate or otherwise participate in clotting. These pro-

teins, called clotting factors, are missing in bleeding disorders such as hemophilia. The amount of clotting factors in a single unit of blood is small; to get enough to transfuse, it is necessary to combine clotting factors from multiple donors. Clotting factor products generally are autoclaved or otherwise treated to prevent them from transmitting viruses and other infectious agents.

Side Effects and Complications

Serious adverse effects, including shock and kidney failure, can result when there is a mismatch of blood types in blood products containing cells, as antibodies on the surface of the cells initiate an immune response that attacks the "invading" blood cells in the recipient's body. Less serious side effects such as fever, chills, and rash can occur even when blood types match, as the person receiving the blood can react to numerous proteins and antigens in the donor blood. Other risks associated with blood transfusion, although minimal because of extensive testing and screening procedures, include infection from viruses such as hepatitis and HIV/AIDS. It also is possible for a person to have an allergic reaction to allergens in a blood transfusion.

See also ANEMIA; BLOODLESS SURGERY.

blood type   See BLOOD.

body image   The perception a person has about the appearance of his or her body. Some people who have OPEN-HEART SURGERY, in which the surgeon makes an incision that runs the length of the sternum (breastbone), feel the extensive chest scar that results is unattractive. They might be uncomfortable wearing clothing that exposes it, or in situations where the scar is visible, such as swimming or undressing in front of a spouse or partner. It helps when others can reassure the person that the scar is instead a reason for joy and celebration of health restored. Many people find that their scars fade over time as healing becomes complete, reducing their awareness of the scar's presence. Other factors that can affect body image include OBESITY, particularly if this is a contributing factor to the person's HEART DISEASE.

Engaging in lifestyle activities that further promote health, such as good nutrition and regular exercise, often results in positive changes like weight loss and improved physical fitness. When such changes occur the person generally feels better physically and emotionally, which helps to improve body image and self-esteem. MEDITATION, YOGA, and other practices that encourage inward focus and relaxation are also helpful.

See also DEPRESSION; LIFESTYLE AND HEART HEALTH; NUTRITION AND DIET; PHYSICAL FITNESS.

body mass index (BMI) A mathematic calculation that provides a measure for assessing the health risks associated with body weight. Numerous research studies confirm that body size below and particularly above a defined range increases the risk for health problems such as HEART DISEASE, as well as DIABETES and cancer. The body mass index (BMI) provides a representation of body fat; the greater amount of body fat a person has, the higher the health risks. Health experts consider excess body weight from body fat the leading modifiable risk factor for heart disease.

This table gives whole value BMI figures by height and weight. Find height in inches in the left column, move across the row to closest weight, and read the BMI across the top row. For example, a person who is five-feet nine-inches tall is 69 inches. At a weight of 155 the BMI is 23. A person who is the same 69 inches tall but weighs 215 pounds has a BMI of about 32. Men and women of the same height and weight have the same BMI.

A healthy BMI is 18.5 to 24.9. This reflects a ratio between weight and height that presents no

BODY MASS INDEX (BMI)																	
BMI	**19**	**20**	**21**	**22**	**23**	**24**	**25**	**26**	**27**	**28**	**29**	**30**	**31**	**32**	**33**	**34**	**35**
Height (inches)						**Body Weight (pounds)**											
58	91	96	100	105	110	115	119	124	129	134	138	143	148	153	158	162	167
59	94	99	104	109	114	119	124	128	133	138	143	148	153	158	163	168	173
60	97	102	107	112	118	123	128	133	138	143	148	153	158	163	168	174	179
61	100	106	111	116	122	127	132	137	143	148	153	158	164	169	174	180	185
62	104	109	115	120	126	131	136	142	147	153	158	164	169	175	180	186	191
63	107	113	118	124	130	135	141	146	152	158	163	169	175	180	186	191	197
64	110	116	122	128	134	140	145	151	157	163	169	174	180	186	192	197	204
65	114	120	126	132	138	144	150	156	162	168	174	180	186	192	198	204	210
66	118	124	130	136	142	148	155	161	167	173	179	186	192	198	204	210	216
67	121	127	134	140	146	153	159	166	172	178	185	191	198	204	211	217	223
68	125	131	138	144	151	158	164	171	177	184	190	197	203	210	216	223	230
69	128	135	142	149	155	162	169	176	182	189	196	203	209	216	222	230	236
70	132	139	146	153	160	167	174	181	188	195	202	209	216	222	229	236	243
71	136	143	150	157	165	172	179	186	193	200	208	215	222	229	236	243	250
72	140	147	154	162	169	177	184	191	199	206	213	221	228	235	242	250	258
73	144	151	159	166	174	182	189	197	204	212	219	227	235	242	250	257	265
74	148	155	163	171	179	186	194	202	210	218	225	233	241	249	256	264	272
75	152	160	168	176	184	192	200	208	216	224	232	240	248	256	264	272	279
76	156	164	172	180	189	197	205	213	221	230	238	246	254	263	271	279	287

Source: Chart derived from the U.S. National Institute of Health's National Heart, Lung, and Blood Institute (NHLBI)

BMI	Reflects	Effect on Cardiovascular Health Risks
less than 18.5	underweight	increased
18.5 to 24.9	healthy weight	none
25 to 29.9	overweight	moderately increased
30 to 34.9	obese	significantly increased
35 and greater	severely obese	severely increased with health problems related to body fat likely present

greater than the typical risks of health problems. A BMI below 18.5 reflects an increased risk of health problems associated with being underweight. A BMI from 25 to 29.9 reflects body weight that is 10 percent to 15 percent above what is healthy and double the risk for HYPERTENSION. A BMI over 30 reflects body weight that is 20 percent or more above healthy weight and two to six times the risk for cardiovascular disease of any kind. A BMI over 35 reflects nearly certain health problems related to obesity, most of which are cardiovascular such as hypertension, HYPERCHOLESTEROLEMIA or HYPER-LIPIDEMIA, CORONARY ARTERY DISEASE (CAD) and HEART FAILURE.

Some people are in between the whole number BMI figures, are at the border between health risk classifications, or are not on the chart. In such situations, it is more effective to calculate the precise BMI by following these steps:

- Determine body weight in pounds (without clothing)
- Measure height in inches
- Multiply height in inches by itself (gives height in inches^2)
- Divide body weight in pounds by height in inches^2
- Multiply the answer by 703
- Result is BMI

BMI is one of numerous health indicators. People with BMIs in the "healthy weight" range can still have hypertension, coronary artery disease, and other cardiovascular conditions. Con-versely, people with BMIs in ranges associated with increased risk for heart disease can have healthy cardiovascular systems. BMI is not accurate for certain people—athletes with high muscle mass, pregnant women, people under age 18, and the very elderly. However, the correlation between BMI and cardiac health is strong. Body weight, or more appropriately body fat, is a modifiable risk factor. To the extent possible, it is desirable for cardiovascular health (and health overall) to manage weight through nutrition, diet, and physical activity to maintain a BMI in the "healthy weight" range.

See also BODY SHAPE AND HEART DISEASE; EXER-CISE; LIFESTYLE AND HEART HEALTH; NUTRITION AND DIET; WAIST CIRCUMFERENCE; WAIST-TO-HIP RATIO; WEIGHT MANAGEMENT.

body shape and heart disease Research over recent decades has established a correlation between body shape, as it represents distribution of body fat, and HEART DISEASE. There are two general body shapes, commonly referred to as "apple" and "pear." People with apple-shaped bodies, in which body fat accumulates in the torso, have a significantly higher risk for developing heart disease than people with pear-shaped bodies, in which body fat collects in the hips and thighs. Excess body fat is the primary concern; a WAIST CIRCUMFERENCE greater than 35 inches for women and 40 inches for men is a strong indicator of increased risk of heart disease. However, the WAIST-TO-HIP RATIO (greater than 0.80 for women and 1.0 for men) may reflect as substantial an increased risk for heart disease even when body weight is within healthy parameters.

The apple body shape features what doctors call abdominal adiposity. Although the outward appearance of a "beer belly" or "spare tire" is what most people notice, the real danger comes from the body fat that collects internally around the organs in the abdomen and chest. In this body fat distribution pattern, these fatty deposits put pressure on the HEART, lungs, liver, spleen, and other organs. This increases the resistance that BLOOD encounters in flowing through the arteries to these organs and also increases the workload of the heart as it encounters both this pressure on itself and the need to use greater force to pump blood through the arteries to the organs. As well, fat cells infiltrate the MYOCARDIUM (heart muscle), weakening its pumping strength and capacity. The combined effect, when it persists over time, can produce HYPERTENSION (high BLOOD PRESSURE), ARRHYTHMIAS (irregular heartbeats), HEART FAILURE, and CARDIO-MYOPATHY (enlarged heart). Although medications can relieve many of the symptoms of these problems, restoring cardiac health requires weight loss to reduce the amount of fatty tissue.

The pear body shape represents a more benign pattern of fat accumulation but still bears increased risk for heart disease when there is excess body fat. Any excess body fat, no matter its distribution pattern, increases the risk for numerous health conditions including DIABETES (a leading cause of heart disease), CORONARY ARTERY DISEASE (CAD), HYPERTENSION (high blood pressure), heart failure, and HEART ATTACK or STROKE. A method of calculation called BODY MASS INDEX (BMI) stratifies the increased risk levels and provides a consistent means of evaluating health risk related to body size.

See also EXERCISE; LIFESTYLE AND HEART HEALTH; NUTRITION AND DIET; OBESITY; WEIGHT MANAGEMENT.

bradycardia See ARRHYTHMIA.

brain aneurysm A weakening, bulge, or rupture in the wall of an artery within the brain, also called an intracranial aneurysm. If BLOOD leaks from the aneurysm into the surrounding brain tissue, it often results in a hemorrhagic, or bleeding, STROKE. The extent of damage this causes depends on the amount of bleeding, its location, and the pressure it creates. The increased pressure from the extra fluid within the skull can cause brain cells to die as well.

Symptoms and Diagnostic Path

A bulging aneurysm that has not ruptured can put pressure on structures of the brain, causing problems such as visual disturbances, seizures, or severe headaches. Often, however, there are no symptoms until a brain aneurysm bleeds or ruptures, at which

time the situation becomes a surgical emergency. Doctors diagnose brain aneurysms using imaging procedures such as COMPUTED TOMOGRAPHY (CT) SCAN, MAGNETIC RESONANCE IMAGING (MRI), and ANGIOGRAPHY. Once the aneurysm is confirmed and its location pinpointed, doctors decide the best course of treatment.

Treatment Options and Outlook

Occasionally, as when the aneurysm is very small or in a location where other structures will keep it from rupturing, treatment might consist of watchful waiting. More often, brain aneurysm requires some form of surgical intervention. Which surgical procedure is appropriate depends on many factors, including the person's age, the location and extent of the aneurysm, the suspected cause of the aneurysm, and any symptoms the person might be experiencing.

- **Microclipping.** The neurosurgeon drills a small hole through the skull and uses an operating microscope to place a tiny clip at the edge of the aneurysm to seal it off at the point where it arises from the artery. This collapses the aneurysm and allows blood to continue flowing through the artery.

- **Embolization.** The neurosurgeon inserts a catheter into the femoral artery through a small incision in the groin and threads the catheter through the body's arteries until it reaches the point of the aneurysm in the brain. The neurosurgeon then releases tiny steel coils or a tiny balloon into the aneurysm, which "plugs" it off from the artery. This has the same effect as microclipping but is done without entering the skull.

- **Arterial occlusion and bypass.** This major neurosurgery involves opening the skull, removing the damaged segment of arterial wall, and crafting a bypass, using either existing blood vessels or an arterial graft.

Risk Factors and Preventive Measures

Brain aneurysms, like aneurysms in any other part of the body, often develop for no known reason. Doctors believe they form at congenital weaknesses in the walls of arteries and develop as a result of the repeated, long-term stress of blood coursing through the artery. Brain aneurysms are most likely to make their presence known in people who are in their 40s and 50s. A specific congenital deformity called arteriovenous malformation, in which there is a twisted tangle of blood vessels instead of the normal structures of arteries and veins, accounts for about one in 10 brain aneurysms. There are no known measures to prevent brain aneurysm.

See also ABDOMINAL AORTIC ANEURYSM; CARDIO-VASCULAR SYSTEM, HEART.

brain attack See STROKE.

brain stem The most primitive portion, structurally and functionally, of the brain. The brain stem is beneath the brain and above the spinal cord, connecting the two. About three inches long, the brain stem regulates the basic functions of life, including breathing, HEART RATE, and BLOOD PRESSURE. The centers that control these vital activities are located in the medulla, the lowest part of the brain stem that connects with the spinal cord, and in the reticular formation, a network of nerves that forms the core of the brain stem. The 10th cranial nerve pair, the vagus nerves, convey nerve signals between the medulla and key CARDIOPULMONARY organs—the HEART and lungs.

The brain stem functions without conscious direction or awareness. Damage to the brain stem can cause impaired cardiopulmonary function and death. STROKE is a common cause of such damage; other causes include oxygen deprivation (such as from HEART ATTACK that causes the heart to stop beating and BLOOD CIRCULATION to cease), trauma (injury), and tumors. Irreversible loss of brain-stem function is a key criterion for establishing "brain death," which becomes significant for donating organs such as the heart and lungs that must be harvested immediately to remain viable.

See also HEART TRANSPLANT.

bran See NUTRITION AND DIET.

breathing exercises Intentional breathing patterns that help to increase LUNG CAPACITY and airflow, to reduce STRESS and encourage relaxation, and to maintain adequate oxygenation and open airways following surgery. Breathing exercises can be done anywhere, at any time, and as often as desired.

Breathing Exercises for Stress Reduction and Relaxation

Focused, controlled breathing is one of the most effective methods for reducing stress and allowing the body and mind to relax. There are many techniques for this, from BIOFEEDBACK to YOGA. Many MEDITATION methods also incorporate breath control.

- **Deep, slow breathing.** For this technique, sit or stand so the lungs and chest can fully expand. Breathe in slowly and steadily over a count of 10, letting the lungs fill completely. Hold the breath for a count of five, and then let it out slowly and steadily over a count of 10. Repeat in sets of six as often as desired.
- **Full body breathing.** For this technique, sit upright or lie down in a prone position. With eyes closed, begin to take a breath in. Envision the breath entering the body through the toes and traveling up the legs and torso into the lungs, and then continuing on through the neck and out the top of the head. Envision that as the breath passes through the body, it picks up and carries with it a piece of tension or stress. Exhale slowly, releasing the tension with the breath. Repeat in sets of six as often as desired.
- **Belly breathing.** For this technique, sit upright or lie down in a prone position. With eyes closed, place one hand on the belly. Begin to take a breath in. Feel the air filling the abdominal cavity from the belly up. Feel the belly extend as it fills with air, and then let the air move upward to fill the lungs from the bottom up. Keep the shoulders level. When the lungs are filled, slowly let the breath out. Feel it move down through the lungs and into the belly, and feel the belly flatten as the air leaves the abdomen. Repeat in sets of six as often as desired.

Breathing exercises are effective for relieving stress when it occurs as well as for helping to prevent the accumulation of stress. They also can be integrated into meditation exercises for more focused stress management.

Breathing Exercises for Lung Capacity and Airflow

The lungs love a good workout. Allowing them to stretch toward their capacity by filling them with air increases the surface area for gas exchange and more rapidly and effectively gets oxygen into and CARBON DIOXIDE out of the bloodstream. This expansion also helps to clear the lungs of microscopic debris that enter with each breath, such as dust particles, and to maintain the pressure that allows efficient return of oxygenated blood to the heart. The deep breathing exercises that help to reduce stress also increase lung capacity and airflow. Various YOGA breathing exercises do so as well.

Regular physical activity improves AEROBIC CAPACITY—the maximum amount of oxygen the body can consume during EXERCISE—by increasing the rate and depth of breathing. The higher the body's aerobic capacity, the better its cardiovascular fitness. It also improves aerobic fitness—the efficiency with which the body uses oxygen as fuel—for improved cardiac and pulmonary health and better health overall. Patterned breathing improves physical performance during exercise, at any level of physical fitness. Breathing exercises teach pacing and control, so putting an increased demand on the lungs can occur without discomfort or breathlessness.

Nearly everyone, even people who have significant heart disease, can engage in deep breathing and physical activities that expand lung capacity. People with known cardiovascular conditions (including high blood cholesterol levels), who have a family history of heart disease, who smoke, or who have not had a complete physical examination within two years should consult their physicians before entering into any program of physical activity or exercise, whether structured or self-designed.

Breathing Exercises Following Surgery

Deep breathing following a surgical procedure, especially if the surgery required general anesthe-

sia, is an important aspect of recovery. It helps to expand the small airways in the lungs to keep fluid from accumulating. Deep breathing infuses the blood with oxygen, a vital fuel for cells, which the body needs for effective healing. INCENTIVE SPIROMETRY is one form of deep breathing into a handheld device, with the goal of moving a small floating ball from one tube to another. This expands the forcefulness of both inhalation (taking air into the lungs) and exhalation (releasing air from the lungs), moving larger volumes of air and improving oxygenation. Deep breathing following surgical procedures can also incorporate conventional deep breathing techniques such as slowly taking in a breath until it feels like it fills the lungs, holding it for a count of five, and slowly letting the breath out until it feels like the lungs are completely empty. It is important to sit as upright as possible to allow the lungs to fully expand.

Incentive spirometry and deep breathing can be uncomfortable in the first hours and days following surgery, particularly open-heart surgery because the extensive incision through the sternum causes soreness. The lungs obtain the resistance air movement requires by pushing against the structures of the rib cage, and the healing sternum is sensitive to this pressure. Holding a pillow firmly against the incision area when taking deep breaths provides additional support. The sensitivity rapidly diminishes as healing progresses and breathing can return to normal without discomfort, usually within four or five days.

See also PULMONARY SYSTEM; STRESS AND HEART DISEASE; STRESS REDUCTION TECHNIQUES.

Brugada syndrome A condition in which defects in the sodium ion channels in the HEART allow erratic electrical activity, increasing the risk of SUDDEN CARDIAC ARREST (SCA) These defects result from mutations in the genes that encode (direct) their functions and are usually inherited.

Symptoms and Diagnostic Path

Most people have no symptoms until they experience cardiac arrest. The condition may be first detected incidentally on an ELECTROCARDIOGRAM (ECG) done for other reasons. When symptoms are present, they include palpitations and SYNCOPE (fainting). Diagnosis is by ECG, which reveals the specific pattern of irregularity in the heart's electrical cycle called the Brugada sign.

Treatment Options and Outlook

Treatment for people who survive an SCA event or who have syncope and ECG evidence of Brugada sign is an IMPLANTABLE CARDIOVERTER-DEFIBRILLATOR (ICD), which automatically shocks the heart when the ventricles go into fibrillation. Some cardiologists think people who are diagnosed by ECG but have no symptoms should also receive ICD, while others think it is appropriate to carefully monitor such people without further treatment until they experience symptoms. Because the first symptom could be sudden cardiac arrest, this approach is controversial. However, ICD is not without risk itself. The person in this situation should consider a consultation with a cardiologist specializing in clinical cardiac electrophysiology.

Risk Factors and Preventive Measures

The most significant risk factor for Brugada syndrome is family history. Genetic testing can identify those who carry the gene mutations. Other risk factors include being male and being Asian. Electrolyte imbalance and certain prescription medications (notably sodium channel blocking medications, tricyclic antidepressant medications, and lithium) can also cause Brugada syndrome. Because Brugada syndrome is primarily genetic, there are no preventive measures.

See also ANTIARRHYTHMIA MEDICATIONS; MEDICATION SIDE EFFECTS; LONG QT SYNDROME; SURGERY TO TREAT CARDIOVASCULAR DISEASE.

bumetanide A DIURETIC MEDICATION taken to relieve or prevent EDEMA (fluid accumulation) in HEART FAILURE. Common brand names include Bumex. Bumetanide is a loop diuretic, which means it acts on a structure in the kidney called the loop of Henle. This structure functions to extract water from the blood that passes through the kidney; bumetanide works by preventing the loop of Henle from reabsorbing SODIUM and POTASSIUM, which in turn restricts the kidney's ability to pull

water back into the bloodstream. This sodium- and potassium-depleting action can cause the body's levels of these ELECTROLYTES to drop precipitously, affecting the heart's rhythm. Doctors sometimes prescribe sodium and/or potassium supplements for people taking bumetanide long-term, or recommend dietary sources such as bananas. Occasionally doctors prescribe bumetanide to treat HYPERTENSION (high BLOOD PRESSURE), especially in people who have kidney disease. Sodium, and especially potassium, depletion can have potentially serious consequences, particularly if ARRHYTHMIAS already exist.

The most noticeable effect of bumetanide and other diuretics is increased urination. Common side effects include DIZZINESS, LIGHT-HEADEDNESS, orthostatic HYPOTENSION (sudden drop in blood pressure upon rising), and headache. Often these side effects diminish or disappear over time. Bumetanide interacts with various other medications including some ANTIHYPERTENSIVES (medications to treat high blood pressure) and lithium (taken to treat bipolar disorder).

See also EXERCISE; FUROSEMIDE; LIFESTYLE AND HEART HEALTH; MEDICATIONS TO TREAT HEART DISEASE; NUTRITION AND DIET.

Bumex See BUMETANIDE.

bundle branch See HEART.

bundle branch block An interruption of the His-Purkinje system, or "wiring" of the HEART. This system is responsible for delivering electrical impulses to the heart muscle to initiate a HEARTBEAT and to help synchronize the contraction of the ventricles. Beginning at the atrioventricular (AV) node, this system starts as a single bundle of cells before splitting into the left and right branches, which usually conduct electrical impulses at roughly the same speed. A block in one of these bundles (when the electrical impulse fails to fully conduct) disrupts the heart's timing and may cause the affected ventricle to beat out of synchrony with the unaffected ventricle.

Symptoms and Diagnostic Path

Most people who have bundle branch block do not have any symptoms; doctors detect the bundle branch block during an ELECTROCARDIOGRAM (ECG). If both bundles become blocked at the same time the person might experience sensations of feeling faint or actually fainting (syncope), especially upon exertion when the heart's rhythm cannot support the demand for increased CARDIAC OUTPUT. When both bundle branches are blocked (complete heart block), total heart block results and can cause the heart to stop beating.

Treatment Options and Outlook

Often, no treatment is necessary for right or left bundle branch block that causes no symptoms and when no other heart disease exists. Medications sometimes help to restore appropriate cardiac rhythm when ARRHYTHMIAS develop. For bundle branch block that causes symptoms, when other heart disease is present, or when bundle branch block develops following a heart attack (alternating right and left bundle branch block, transient right and left bundle branch block, or complete heart block), doctors implant a PACEMAKER to deliver electrical impulses past the point of the block and directly to the affected ventricle. This restores a normal heart rate and pumping action.

Risk Factors and Preventive Measures

There is some correlation between left bundle branch block and an increased likelihood of developing other HEART DISEASE. Right bundle branch block is more likely to exist without symptoms and independent of other heart problems.

See also ATRIOVENTRICULAR (A-V) CANAL DEFECT; ATRIOVENTRICULAR (A-V) NODE; CARDIOVASCULAR SYSTEM; HEART BLOCK; SINOATRIAL (SA) NODE.

bundle of His   See HEART.

caffeine A chemical stimulant that occurs naturally in numerous foods and drinks, including coffee, tea, colas, many energy drinks, and chocolate. Caffeine acts on the brain and central nervous system, increasing alertness and focus. Hundreds of medications contain caffeine, which has the effect of potentiating, or enhancing, the effect of pain relief medications. Caffeine also acts as a mild diuretic, increasing the amount of fluid the kidneys withdraw from the BLOOD and pass as urine.

There is much debate over the effects of caffeine on general health and on cardiac health in particular. Most health experts agree that mild to moderate caffeine consumption, up to 250 mg a day (the equivalent of three 8-ounce cups of coffee), likely is benign. Too much caffeine—which is largely a subjective measure—causes feelings of jitteriness and edginess and is suspected of causing irregularities in heart rhythm called PREMATURE VENTRICULAR CONTRACTIONS (PVCs). These are extra beats that make the HEART feel as though it is "jumping." Although PVCs are generally harmless, they cause considerable anxiety. Caffeine also stimulates the adrenal glands to produce EPINEPHRINE and NOREPINEPHRINE, HORMONES that increase muscle contractions, including the HEART RATE and blood vessel tone. This can cause BLOOD PRESSURE to rise. And there is some evidence that caffeine allows the body to more rapidly metabolize fatty acids from stored body fat.

Many cardiologists recommend that people with diagnosed HEART conditions restrict or eliminate their caffeine intake because of caffeine's stimulant effects. Heavy coffee, tea, or cola drinkers need to taper down their consumption rather than just stopping; suddenly withdrawing caffeine can result in headache and other discomforts.

See also NUTRITION AND DIET; PALPITATIONS; PULSE; SLEEP DISTURBANCES.

Calan See VERAPAMIL.

calcium and arterial plaque Recent research studies suggest that there is a strong correlation between the amount of calcium contained in the deposits that collect along the inside walls of the arteries and the risk for HEART ATTACK. Arterial plaque contains varying substances, typically including fatty acids (LIPIDS), BLOOD cells, platelets, proteins, and minerals such as calcium. Over time, the calcium accumulation causes the arterial plaque to become thick and stiff. The rate of calcification varies among individuals; researchers do not fully understand what factors contribute to this. They do know, however, that people who have mild CORONARY ARTERY DISEASE (CAD; accumulated arterial deposits in the arteries that supply the heart with blood) with high calcification are significantly more likely to have heart attacks than people who have moderate to even serious coronary artery disease with low calcification. A noninvasive radiology procedure called ELECTRON BEAM COMPUTED TOMOGRAPHY (EBCT) SCAN can detect arterial plaque calcification, allowing doctors to determine whether it poses a significant risk for heart attack and to plan appropriate therapeutic intervention such as ANGIOPLASTY or CORONARY ARTERY BYPASS GRAFT (CABG) surgery.

See also ARTERIOSCLEROSIS; ATHERECTOMY; ATHEROSCLEROSIS; INFLAMMATION AND HEART DISEASE; PLAQUE, ARTERIAL.

calcium channel antagonist medications A classification of medications to treat HYPERTENSION, ANGINA, and certain ARRHYTHMIAS. They work by blockading the ion channels that carry calcium. Calcium is necessary for muscle contraction; this blockade of the calcium ion channels helps blood vessels to relax. Two calcium channel antagonists, DILTIAZEM and VERAPAMIL, affect the heart muscle directly. These two drugs slow the force and rate of the HEART's contractions, lowering the pressure under which blood from the heart enters the aorta for circulation through the body. Calcium channel blockers became available in the mid-1980s for use when other medications for hypertension, such as DIURETIC MEDICATIONS and BETA ANTAGONIST MEDICATIONS, could not adequately lower blood pressure.

Common side effects that often improve over time or with a change to a different calcium channel blocker include nausea, headache, CONSTIPATION, peripheral EDEMA, DIZZINESS, SLEEP DISTURBANCES, and anxiety. Serious but rare side effects include arrhythmias, HEART FAILURE, and HEART ATTACK (myocardial infarction). GRAPEFRUIT AND GRAPEFRUIT JUICE interfere with some calcium channel blockers. Each medication in this classification has unique side effects and precautions. For some of the calcium channel blockers, use depends on the medication's form—regular release or long-acting. Calcium channel blockers are not usually the first medications of choice for hypertension or angina, but rather become options when other medications do not control symptoms or have unacceptable side effects. Doctors often prescribe calcium channel blockers in combination with other MEDICATIONS TO TREAT HEART DISEASE, such as beta antagonist medications and diuretics.

In the mid-1990s, about a decade after calcium channel blockers had been in use, concerns arose that some medications in this classification increased the risk of heart attack (myocardial infarction) and unexpected arrhythmias resulting in CARDIAC ARREST and SUDDEN CARDIAC ARREST. Though several large clinical trials have not confirmed these concerns, several calcium channel blocker medications were removed from the American market as a result, and restrictions or recommendations to limit prescribing were issued about others. In general people with heart failure or moderate to advanced HEART BLOCK should not take calcium channel blockers, although certain of these medications are currently in CLINICAL RESEARCH STUDIES to evaluate their effectiveness in heart failure.

See also ANGIOTENSIN-CONVERTING ENZYME (ACE) INHIBITOR MEDICATIONS; ANGIOTENSIN II RECEPTOR ANTAGONIST MEDICATIONS; ANTIHYPERTENSIVE MEDICATIONS; CALCIUM CYCLE; MEDICATION MANAGEMENT; MEDICATIONS TO TREAT HEART DISEASE; SODIUM CHANNEL BLOCKING MEDICATIONS.

CALCIUM CHANNEL ANTAGONIST MEDICATIONS

Medication	Common Brand Names	Prescribed to Treat
amlodipine	Norvasc	chronic stable angina, Prinzmetal's (variant) angina, hypertension
bepridil	Vascor	chronic stable angina
diltiazem	Cardizem, Cardizem CD, Cardizem CR, Cartia XT, Dilacor XR	chronic stable angina, Prinzmetal's (variant) angina, hypertension
felodipine	Plendil	hypertension
isradipine	DynaCirc, DynaCirc, CR	hypertension
nicardipine	Cardene, Cardene SR	chronic stable angina, hypertension
nifedipine	Procardia, Procardia XL, Adalat, Adalat CC, Adalat PA	chronic stable angina, Prinzmetal's (variant) angina, hypertension
nislodipine	Sular	hypertension
verapamil	Calan, Calan SR, Isoptin, Isoptin SR, Covera HS, Verelan, Verelan PM	chronic stable angina, Prinzmetal's (variant) angina, hypertension, supraventricular tachycardia, atrial fibrillation, atrial flutter

calcium cycle The process of calcium retention and release that regulates the contractions of the HEART. Calcium is the most abundant mineral in the human body, with 99 percent of it located in the bones and teeth. The remaining 1 percent is in nerve cells, where it facilitates the transmission of nerve signals, and in the muscle cells, where it facilitates contraction and relaxation of the muscle fibers. Calcium is an electrolyte, or ion—a chemical capable of carrying an electrical charge.

Each myocardial cell in the heart contains a stored supply of calcium. When the heart's electrical system discharges an electrical impulse, it activates the release of calcium into electrochemical pathways called ion channels. This sets in motion the release of proteins and other chemicals that cause myocardial cells to contract, initiating a CARDIAC CYCLE. A protein released at the end of this chain is phospholamban (PLN), which causes the calcium to return to its microscopic storage reservoir within the cell, and the contraction ends. From the initial release of calcium to its return is the calcium cycle.

The calcium cycle is susceptible to malfunctions at numerous points, most of which allow the level of calcium within the heart cell to remain high. This keeps the cell in a state of contraction. When this affects a measurable segment of heart fibers, it diminishes the ability of the heart's chambers to fill completely before the state of contraction forces blood out of the heart. The heart begins to pump harder and faster in response to signals of inadequate oxygenation from body tissues, attempting to compensate. The consequences can include HYPERTENSION (high BLOOD PRESSURE) and HEART FAILURE.

See also ANTIHYPERTENSIVE MEDICATIONS; CALCIUM CHANNEL ANTAGONIST MEDICATIONS; MEDICATIONS TO TREAT HEART DISEASE; POTASSIUM; SODIUM; SINO-ATRIAL (S-A) NODE.

cancer of the heart Malignancies in the HEART are rare and almost always arise as metastases from cancers that originate in other parts of the body such as the lung or the liver. This is because cancer develops when cells reproduce, and the cells of the heart do not reproduce except to replace damaged cells. The heart's location within the protective confines of the rib cage minimizes external trauma to the heart; internal trauma occurs primarily as a result of HEART ATTACK or myocardial infarction (death of myocardial cells) from CORONARY ARTERY DISEASE (CAD). The few cancers that arise as primary malignancies of the heart are usually rhabdomyosarcomas (cancers of muscle tissue) or cardiac angiosarcomas (cancers of the BLOOD vessels of the heart). An asbestos-caused cancer, mesothelioma, can form in the pericardium (membrane that surrounds the heart) as a primary site.

Symptoms and Diagnostic Path
Often there are no symptoms of cancer involving the heart until the malignancy and its metastases are quite advanced. When there are symptoms, they might include pain similar to ANGINA, EDEMA (fluid retention) around the heart, and ARRHYTHMIAS. Cancers that infiltrate the MYOCARDIUM or the heart's valves can prevent the heart from properly pumping blood, causing an array of cardiovascular problems to develop.

Diagnostic imaging procedures such as MAGNETIC RESONANCE IMAGING (MRI), COMPUTED TOMOGRAPHY (CT) SCAN, or ECHOCARDIOGRAM often raise the suspicion of malignancy, which is then confirmed through biopsy. Usually a thoracic or cardiac surgeon then performs a thoracotomy to open the chest to expose the tumor and remove it if possible. Pathological analysis of the tumor's cells determines whether the tumor is cancerous.

Treatment Options and Outlook
Treatment for cancers involving the heart might include surgery to remove the tumor, if it is intact and discreet, followed by chemotherapy to kill any remaining cancer cells. Diffuse tumors that have infiltrated the myocardium are difficult to remove surgically without causing significant damage to the heart; chemotherapy is the treatment option for such malignancies. Chemotherapy agents can be infused directly into the pericardium to combat cancer cells directly. Radiation therapy is not usually a treatment option for malignancies of the heart as it is likely to cause irreparable damage to the myocardium. HEART TRANSPLANT is not an option, either, when cancer is present.

Risk Factors and Preventive Measures
Cancer of the heart, either primary or secondary, is extremely rare. Most cancer of the heart is secondary; it metastasizes (spreads) from other locations in the body. Sarcomas (soft tissue cancers) and melanomas (particularly aggressive cancers that often start in the skin) are the kinds of cancers most likely to metastasize to the heart; lymphoma may also sometimes cause cancerous tumors in the heart. Having any of these cancers establishes the risk for metastasis to the heart. Exposure to asbestos is the sole risk factor for mesothelioma.

candesartan An ANGIOTENSIN II RECEPTOR ANTAGONIST MEDICATION taken to treat HYPERTENSION (high BLOOD PRESSURE). Common brand names include Atacand. Candesartan works by blocking the actions of angiotensin II, an enzyme the kidneys produce as part of the RENIN-ANGIOTENSIN-ALDOSTERONE (RAA) HORMONE SYSTEM that regulates blood pressure. Angiotensin II causes arteries to constrict, increasing the resistance encountered by blood flowing through the arteries and causing blood pressure to increase. Blocking its actions prevents arterial constriction, helping to lower blood pressure. Like other ANTIHYPERTENSIVE MEDICATIONS in this classification, candesartan can cause nausea, diarrhea, headache, and DIZZINESS. Angiotensin II blockers can cause serious health problems, including kidney failure and death in an unborn child when taken during pregnancy, so women who are pregnant should not take them.

See also ANGIOTENSIN-CONVERTING ENZYME (ACE); INHIBITOR MEDICATIONS; MEDICATIONS TO TREAT HEART DISEASE.

capillary See CARDIOVASCULAR SYSTEM.

Capoten See CAPTOPRIL.

captopril An ANGIOTENSIN-CONVERTING ENZYME (ACE) INHIBITOR MEDICATION taken to treat HYPERTENSION (high BLOOD PRESSURE) or HEART FAILURE, and to stabilize the HEART following HEART ATTACK (myocardial infarction). Common brand names include Capoten. Captopril, like other ACE inhibitors, prevents angiotensin-converting enzyme from converting angiotensin I, which is inert, into angiotensin II. Angiotensin II constricts the arterioles (the body's tiniest arteries) to raise blood pressure. Doctors often prescribe captopril in combination with diuretics to maintain stable control of blood pressure. Captopril can cause nausea, diarrhea, headache, and DIZZINESS. It also is known to cause serious health problems in an unborn child when taken during pregnancy. Women who are pregnant should not take captopril or other ACE inhibitors.

See also ANGIOTENSIN II RECEPTOR ANTAGONIST MEDICATIONS; MEDICATIONS TO TREAT HEART DISEASE.

carbohydrate See NUTRITION AND DIET.

carbon dioxide A gas that is a natural waste by-product of METABOLISM in the body. One role of the CARDIOVASCULAR SYSTEM is to retrieve carbon dioxide when it delivers oxygen, the body's key fuel for energy production, to cells and return it to the lungs for release from the body. Metabolic functions that generate energy produce the highest levels of carbon dioxide. Carbon dioxide levels in the bloodstream help to determine the rate of respiration (breathing). During strenuous exercise the body's energy production activities are high, which generates high amounts of carbon dioxide—breathing becomes rapid and deep to increase the exchange of oxygen and carbon dioxide in the lungs. At rest, the body's energy production is low and so, correspondingly, are carbon dioxide levels—breathing slows.

Elevated BLOOD carbon dioxide levels, as measured by arterial BLOOD GASES, suggest the HEART is not pumping effectively enough to maintain adequate circulation and cardiovascular function. There are numerous causes for this, from congenital heart malformations to various forms of heart disease. Generally there are other symptoms of this inadequacy as well that help to focus diagnostic efforts and treatment approaches. Chronic pulmonary diseases such as CHRONIC OBSTRUCTIVE PULMONARY DISEASE (COPD) and emphysema also result in elevated blood carbon dioxide levels, as damage to the lungs prevents adequate oxygen/carbon dioxide exchange. Carbon dioxide levels can drop too low in the bloodstream, as well, which has the effect of slowing respiration. Low carbon dioxide levels might occur during oxygen therapy or when a person is on mechanical ventilation, such as following a major HEART ATTACK or OPEN-HEART SURGERY. Mechanical ventilators have sensors that measure the carbon dioxide with exhalation to monitor this.

See also CARBON MONOXIDE; MECHANICAL VENTILATION; OXYGENATION; PULSE OXIMETRY.

carbon monoxide A poisonous gas that binds more easily than oxygen with HEMOGLOBIN in the BLOOD, preventing oxygenation. Carbon monoxide is a waste by-product of numerous energy-producing processes that use fossil fuels such as coal, natural gas or propane, and oil. This includes industrial processes as well as home appliances such as furnaces. Combustion engine exhaust—cars, trucks, buses, airplanes—is a leading source of carbon monoxide. Carbon monoxide is a significant environmental pollutant in heavily populated areas. Small amounts of carbon monoxide are always in the air; carbon monoxide becomes a problem only when it accumulates to such levels that it begins to replace oxygen in the body. Cigarette smoke also contains high amounts of carbon monoxide. For about 20 minutes after smoking a cigarette, the body experiences a drop in oxygen levels.

Carbon monoxide poisoning most commonly occurs through exposure to faulty or improperly vented furnaces or other appliances, and from using propane stoves or charcoal grills indoors. It is especially dangerous because of its insidious progression. Most people do not know they are being exposed to toxic levels of carbon monoxide; the gas has no odor. As the binding process is cumulative, symptoms come on gradually and are indistinct. The brain, with its high need for oxygen, is the first organ to experience the effect. Nausea, DIZZINESS, headache, and confusion are common early symptoms. As more of the brain becomes affected, so do the functions of consciousness. Carbon monoxide poisoning can cause permanent damage to the brain and other organs, and death. The first course of action for suspected carbon monoxide poisoning is to get the person into fresh air. Artificial respiration is necessary if the person has stopped breathing and full CPR if there also is no pulse, followed by emergency medical treatment.

See also CARBON DIOXIDE; CPR.

Cardene See NICARDIPINE.

cardiac ablation See ABLATION.

cardiac arrest A suddenly occurring, life-threatening situation in which the HEART stops beating. Cardiac arrest results from a dangerous ARRHYTHMIA in the ventricle of the heart, either ventricular FIBRILLATION or ventricular TACHYCARDIA. HEART ATTACK (MYOCARDIAL INFARCTION) and preexisting HEART FAILURE are the most common provocations of such arrhythmias, although they can occur without apparent cause. Other causes of cardiac arrest include severe BLOOD loss, electrical shock that disrupts the heart's electrical system, severe hypothermia (body temperature below 90°F), certain drugs, and respiratory failure such as from drowning or suffocation.

When cardiac arrest occurs, all cardiovascular function ceases. Body tissues can continue to function for as long as their oxygen supplies last. Damage to vital and sensitive organs such as the brain and kidneys begins almost immediately; they have almost no oxygen stores. Other organs may have five to seven minutes. Damage becomes irreversible and widespread at about six minutes after the heart stops. Blood that stops moving through the blood vessels begins to clot. At 10 minutes, survival is highly unlikely (except in situations of hypothermia, which slows metabolism and reduces oxygen needs).

Symptoms and Diagnostic Path

Some people may feel a rapid HEARTBEAT or DIZZINESS, though often there are no symptoms before cardiac arrest occurs. The primary indication of cardiac arrest is a very rapid, erratic, or nonexistent pulse. The person is usually unconscious and not breathing. An automated external defibrillator (AED), if available, can confirm the arrhythmia and also initiate treatment.

Treatment Options and Outlook

Cardiac arrest requires immediate intervention and rapid emergency medical attention. It is essential to begin cardiopulmonary resuscitation (CPR) and call 911, and when an AED is available, to initiate DEFIBRILLATION. Time is crucial; according to the American Heart Association (AHA), every minute without resuscitative efforts reduces the likelihood of survival by 7 to 10 percent. Unfortunately, only about 5 percent of people who go into cardiac arrest receive immediate intervention; about a third of them ultimately survive. Recovery to the previous quality of life depends on the extent of damage to the heart, brain, kidneys, and other organs and systems of the body and might require considerable rehabilitation. Residual health problems are common.

The AHA estimates that at least 250,000 Americans die from cardiac arrest each year. One reason this number is so high is that the "typical" cardiac arrest victim is not who people expect: More than half of cardiac arrests occur in people who are in their late 50s to early 60s and have no history of heart disease. Young people are also at risk for cardiac arrest.

Risk Factors and Preventive Measures

Key risk factors for cardiac arrest include CORONARY ARTERY DISEASE (CAD), heart failure, CARDIOMYOPATHY, and arrhythmia disorders. People who survive cardiac arrest are at significantly increased risk for another; it is important to identify the cause of the cardiac arrest and take appropriate treatment measures. An IMPLANTABLE CARDIOVERTER-DEFIBRILLATOR (ICD) can prevent cardiac arrest in people with certain cardiac conditions. Lifestyle measures to reduce overall risk for cardiovascular disease (CVD) and prompt diagnosis and treatment for CVD that does develop can significantly reduce the likelihood of cardiac arrest, although cannot prevent it. Increasing the number of teens and adults who are trained in CPR and the availability of AEDs in locations where people gather are measures that could improve the chance for survival when cardiac arrest does occur.

See also BRUGADA SYNDROME; CARDIAC INTENSIVE CARE UNIT; CARDIAC REHABILITATION; SUDDEN CARDIAC ARREST.

cardiac capacity   The ability of the CARDIOVASCULAR SYSTEM to meet demands for increased CARDIAC OUTPUT, such as with EXERCISE. It reflects the HEART's ability to rapidly increase the volume of BLOOD it pumps relative to the rate at which it pumps. Cardiac capacity is closely related to aerobic fitness (the efficiency with which the body uses oxygen to generate energy). Cardiac capacity improves with regular EXERCISE, even if the exercise is modest. Younger people generally have a higher cardiac capacity than older people, although an individual's level of physical activity can compensate for natural decreases that occur with aging. CARDIOVASCULAR DISEASE (CVD) also affects cardiac capacity.

Doctors use exercise stress testing (or pharmaceutical stress testing when a person is unable or unwilling to do an EXERCISE STRESS TEST) to evaluate cardiac capacity. Studies reported in 2002 and 2003 that cardiac capacity is a significant independent factor for predicting the likelihood of death from CVD among people who have no symptoms of CVD. These studies further suggest that the heart's ability to accommodate moderate to intense exercise is especially important for cardiovascular health in women.

See also AEROBIC CAPACITY; FITNESS LEVEL; HEART RATE; LIFESTYLE AND HEART HEALTH; NUTRITION AND DIET, WOMEN AND HEART DISEASE.

cardiac catheterization   A procedure in which a CARDIOLOGIST inserts a catheter (a long, very thin, and flexible tube) into an artery near the skin's surface (usually in the groin or the arm) and threads it through the artery into the HEART. X-rays help the cardiologist to guide the catheter. Cardiac catheterization is the base procedure for diagnostic studies such as ANGIOGRAPHY as well as for therapeutic applications such as ANGIOPLASTY. Cardiac catheterization is done under sterile conditions in a hospital or cardiac catheterization facility where emergency resuscitative equipment and staff, including surgery facilities, are available. Any time there is an invasive procedure involving the heart, there is a risk of unanticipated complications. The procedure can take up to several hours, depending on what is being done. Because cardiac catheterization is an invasive procedure that involves entering the body through an incision, it is considered a surgical procedure. It requires INFORMED CONSENT and often insurance preauthorization.

Procedure

Cardiac catheterization is done with the person sedated but awake, with a local anesthetic to numb the area on the skin where the cardiologist will make a small incision and insert the catheter. The person feels pressure at the insertion site but cannot feel the catheter being moved through the BLOOD vessels and into the heart. Once the catheter is in place, the cardiologist can inject contrast material (dye) into the coronary arteries and visualize its movement through them with X-rays to determine the extent to which they are occluded; this is called an angiogram and it is done to evaluate CORONARY ARTERY DISEASE (CAD).

The cardiologist also might perform angioplasty (removing an occlusion) or place a STENT (a spring-like device to hold the walls of the artery apart). Other procedures using cardiac catheterization can let the cardiologist examine the actions of the heart valves and the flow of BLOOD through the chambers of the heart. Cardiac catheterization presents a means for the cardiologist to see many of the inner workings of the heart without an operation. When the procedure is finished, the cardiologist withdraws the catheter and places a pressure dressing over the insertion site to make sure there is no bleeding.

Risks and Complications

Typically following a cardiac catheterization the person must lie flat in bed for six to eight hours so an adequate clot can form at the insertion site. It is not unusual for the cardiologist to want the person to stay overnight in the hospital, particularly if the catheterization is done later in the day, so the person can gradually return to regular activities under supervision. Discomfort generally is mild and mostly involves pain at the insertion site; pain medications can relieve this. Some people feel light-headed or nauseated as a result of the dyes and sedatives; this goes away within a few hours. Most people also feel chilled after the catheterization; this is a normal response and the recovery staff will offer heated blankets to help maintain warmth. This also goes away within a few hours. It generally takes a week or two for the insertion site to heal completely; during the healing process there can be considerable bruising and some swelling. Any fresh bleeding or increase in swelling after the first 24 hours requires immediate medical attention. Most people return to their regular activities within several days.

Outlook and Lifestyle Modifications

Because cardiac catheterization is a diagnostic procedure, lifestyle changes and outlook depend on the underlying condition and any resulting treatments. Most people fully recover from the catheterization without any residual effects.

See also ATHEROSCLEROSIS; COMPUTED TOMOGRAPHY (CT) SCAN; ECHOCARDIOGRAM; ELECTRON BEAM COMPUTED TOMOGRAPHY (EBCT) SCAN; LIGHT-HEADEDNESS; PLAQUE, ARTERIAL.

cardiac cycle The sequence of events that generates a HEARTBEAT. A cardiac cycle begins when the heart's upper chambers, the right atrium and the left atrium, receive BLOOD and ends when the heart's left ventricle sends oxygenated blood out through the aorta for circulation through the body. The right atrium receives deoxygenated blood from the superior vena cava (blood returning from the upper body) and the inferior vena cava (blood returning from the lower body). Simultaneously, the left atrium receives oxygenated blood from the lungs via the pulmonary vein. The atria contract in unison: the right atrium sends its volume of blood through the tricuspid valve into the right ventricle and the left atrium sends its volume of blood through the mitral valve into the left ventricle. The ventricles then contract in unison. The right ventricle sends its blood through the pulmonary valve into the pulmonary artery, which carries it to the lungs for oxygenation. The left ventricle sends its blood through the aortic valve into the aorta under tremendous pressure; the aorta carries the blood into systemic (body) circulation. The cardiac cycle repeats about 70 times a minute in the typical adult at rest, which is detected as the heartbeat or the PULSE rate.

See also BLOOD PRESSURE; CARDIOVASCULAR SYSTEM CONDUCTION SYSTEM; HEART; HEART RATE.

cardiac enzymes   Protein-based substances (sometimes referred to as cardiac proteins) released by the myocardium (HEART muscle) during the normal CARDIAC CYCLE. When there is damage to the heart, as in HEART ATTACK, cardiac enzyme levels in the BLOOD rise. Measuring these enzymes is one means of determining whether a heart attack is taking, or has taken, place. Some enzymes rise within hours and fall back to normal again within hours to days, while others take days to rise and can remain elevated for a week or longer. The rate of rise and the level help to provide a "ballpark" assessment of the seriousness of the damage, although further diagnostic tests are required.

The cardiologist evaluates cardiac enzymes measured in a sample of blood drawn from a vein. Among the enzymes this evaluation might include are:

• Cardiac troponin, which is a protein complex that facilitates contraction of myocardial cells in the cardiac cycle. Cardiac troponin has three component proteins: cardiac troponin C (cTnC), cardiac troponin I (cTnI), and cardiac troponin T (cTnT). Within two to three hours of damage to the heart, such as myocardial infarction, there is a significant release of cTnI and cTnT, which act on the enzymes that initiate myocardial cell contraction and relaxation respectively, into the bloodstream. The presence of cTnI and cTnT, which normally are present in the blood at almost immeasurable levels, is one of the earliest indicators to confirm damage to the heart. Their levels peak at 12 to 14 hours and remain elevated for seven to 10 days.

• Creatine kinase (CK), also called phosphocreatine kinase (PCK), is an enzyme that muscle cells, including those of the heart, release into the bloodstream when they experience damage. In the circumstance of the heart, this occurs with the death of myocardial cells due to myocardial infarction. CK levels begin to rise within six hours of the onset of damage and remain elevated for about 36 hours. CK levels also rise with RHABDOMYOLYSIS, a very rare but potentially fatal complication of certain LIPID-LOWERING MEDICATIONS (HMG CoA REDUCTASE INHIBITOR MEDICATIONS) in which skeletal muscle deteriorates. The CK level is sometimes called total CK or total PCK.

• Creatine kinase MK (CK-MK), also called phosphocreatine kinase MK (PCK-MK), is a component of CK that is especially abundant in the heart muscle. Like cardiac troponin, CK-MK is normally almost undetectable in the blood. Its blood level rises in two to six hours following damage to the heart and peaks at 12 to 24 hours. CK-MK usually returns to normal within three days; its failure to do so signals that there is continuing damage to the heart.

• Myoglobin is a protein in the muscles throughout the body, including the heart, that is closely related to hemoglobin. It stores and releases oxygen in muscle cells to meet their increased energy demands during activity and EXERCISE when muscle contractions intensify. Damaged muscle cells, including myocardial cells, release myoglobin into the bloodstream. Myoglobin is also excreted in the urine, turning the urine brownish in color. Like CK, elevated myoglobin levels occur in rhabdomyolysis.

Measurement of cTnI, cTnT, and CK-MK are specific for damage to the heart muscle, though their levels must be considered in the context of the overall presentation of symptoms to determine the kind of damage. While the most common circumstance is myocardial infarction, damage to the heart muscle also may occur with MYOCARDITIS, CARDIOMYOPATHY, severe CORONARY ARTERY DISEASE (CAD), and following heart procedures including surgery.

See also BLOOD TESTS TO DETECT HEART ATTACK; CARDIAC CATHETERIZATION; ECHOCARDIOGRAM; ELECTROCARDIOGRAM.

cardiac intensive care unit (CICU)   An inpatient unit within a hospital that provides care for people who have had HEART ATTACKS or are recovering from cardiovascular surgery. CICUs are segregated from the rest of the hospital, with regulated visiting procedures and hours to give the recovering person enough rest. CICU staff have advanced training in cardiovascular disease treatments, and resuscitation methods. Patients in the CICU are closely monitored both through personal observation by staff and various items of equipment that measure and record body functions such as HEART RATE, BLOOD PRESSURE, respiratory rate, BLOOD GASES, pressures within the HEART, and other clinically significant functions. Some CICUs care for both medical (heart attack) and surgical (post-operative) patients, and others care for one or the other.

Hospitalization in a CICU can be a frightening experience for patients and loved ones. There are numerous monitors and items of equipment, and the people who are hospitalized in the CICU are critically ill. The atmosphere is one of no-nonsense attentiveness to medical needs, which are extensive for many CICU patients, and family members can find this intimidating. Staff might request that families designate a single representative to receive updates on the person's condition and status. It is important for loved ones to respect CICU visiting procedures, as these are structured to allow staff to provide necessary care and for the recovering person to get adequate rest. A person is admitted to a CICU only when his or her medical needs are more extensive than a regular hospital unit's staff can manage; although many people in the CICU recover from their cardiac crises, they are very sick at the time they are in the CICU. Many hospitals also have cardiac step-down units, which provide care that is not quite as extensive as the CICU but more complex than a regular hospital unit can handle.

See also CARDIAC REHABILITATION; STROKE; SURGERY TO TREAT CARDIOVASCULAR DISEASE.

cardiac output The volume of BLOOD the HEART's left ventricle pumps in a minute, measured as mathematical calculation that multiplies HEART RATE (the number of beats) by STROKE VOLUME (the volume of blood each beat, or contraction, moves). For the average adult, a resting cardiac output roughly equals the volume of blood in the body—about five liters (10 pints)—with the body's

blood supply circulating from the heart through the body and back to the heart once a minute. During activity cardiac output can increase significantly, depending on fitness level. The higher the fitness level, the greater the cardiac output. An athlete in peak condition, such as a bicyclist or swimmer, can generate a cardiac output that is six times greater than resting cardiac output. Aerobic exercise conditions the heart and improves cardiac output. Cardiac output is one measure of the heart's pumping efficiency.

See also EXERCISE; LEFT VENTRICULAR EJECTION FRACTION.

cardiac rehabilitation A multifaceted, structured, medically supervised approach to facilitate recovery from a HEART ATTACK, heart operation, or other cardiac event. Many hospitals that provide cardiovascular care also offer outpatient cardiac rehabilitation programs, often through on-site cardiac rehabilitation centers that have the appropriate facilities, equipment, and specialty staff under the direction of a cardiologist. Most medical insurance pays for at least a portion of such a program with a doctor's prescription, although there might be preauthorization requirements.

Cardiac rehabilitation typically integrates a progressive physical activity and EXERCISE component, NUTRITION AND DIET counseling, STRESS REDUCTION TECHNIQUES, education about cardiovascular health and disease, lifestyle and behavior modification, and smoking cessation. Components are adapted to the person's individual health situation and needs and generally change as the person's cardiovascular status improves. A cardiac rehabilitation program might include registered nurses (RNs), exercise physiologists, occupational therapists, dietitians, and psychologists on its staff. Many programs also have support groups so people with heart conditions can talk with each other about their experiences.

The goal of cardiac rehabilitation is to provide instruction and understanding about lifestyle factors affecting cardiovascular health, including adaptations for any limitations resulting from CARDIOVASCULAR DISEASE (CVD) as well as changes to reduce the risk for future cardiovascular conditions. This includes a comprehensive assessment of the person's medical and family histories, including the presence of other medical conditions such as diabetes, hypertension (high blood pressure), or elevated blood lipids (HYPERCHOLESTEROLEMIA or HYPERLIPIDEMIA). The intent is for the person to leave the cardiac rehabilitation program capable of integrating its measures into his or her normal lifestyle and daily activities for improved quality of life, and to continue the core components of the program as part of everyday living. Some cardiac rehabilitation programs offer follow-up services for people to stay in contact with the structure of the program. A number of community organizations such as the YMCA offer ongoing exercise and fitness programs specifically geared toward maintaining cardiac health. The cardiologist should approve such a program for a person's specific individual needs. The program also should be customized for the person's needs and have staff on-site at all times who are trained in cardiopulmonary resuscitation (CPR) to respond to any cardiac crisis.

See also LIFESTYLE AND HEART HEALTH; MEDICATION MANAGEMENT; WEIGHT MANAGEMENT.

cardiac resynchronization therapy (CRT) The use of implanted pacing wires to deliver coordinated electrical stimulation to both the left and right ventricles, a technique also called biventricular pacing. CRT is used to treat HEART FAILURE when the electrical signals of the HEART become poorly coordinated due to damage to the heart muscle and the CONDUCTION PATHWAY. CRT may also incorporate automatic DEFIBRILLATION, in which case it is called CRTD (cardiac resynchronization therapy with defibrillation).

Implanting the CRT is a surgical procedure, done with IV sedation and local anesthetic, in which the cardiologist punctures a large vein such as the subclavian vein under the clavicle (collarbone) and threads the leads through the vein into the heart, watching their progress via FLUOROSCOPY and also with ELECTROCARDIOGRAM (ECG) monitoring. The cardiologist also makes a small pocket under the skin, usually on the chest, which will hold the CRT device. When the leads are in place, the cardiologist connects them to the device and sets the appropriate pacing. Often the person stays overnight in the hospital after the implantation to make sure the device is working properly.

The surgical incision sites heal in about four weeks, during which it is usually okay to return to most regular activities. It is best to delay return to activities that stress the upper chest—such as heavy lifting, swimming, golfing, tennis, rowing, and bowling—for about six weeks. After healing is complete, the CRT device imparts no restrictions on activity. A CRT device uses batteries that last six to eight years; batteries in a CRT device last about half that. Most cardiologists want to check the CRT every three to six months.

See also IMPLANTABLE CARDIOVERTER DEFIBRILLATOR (ICD); LIVING WITH HEART DISEASE.

cardiac revascularization See CARDIAC CATHETERIZATION.

cardiogenic shock An inability of the HEART to pump enough BLOOD to sustain the body's needs, resulting in cardiovascular collapse and life-threatening medical crisis. Cardiogenic shock most often occurs following MYOCARDIAL INFARCTION (HEART ATTACK) that severely damages the heart's ventricles, particularly the left ventricle. With appropriate treatment, about half of people who experience cardiogenic shock survive. Without immediate medical treatment, cardiogenic shock is fatal.

Symptoms and Diagnostic Path

The person in cardiogenic shock is often unconscious. The HEARTBEAT may be rapid and irregular, the pulse weak, the breathing shallow and fast, and the person's skin clammy and pale. BLOOD PRESSURE is usually very low, and the ELECTROCARDIOGRAM (ECG) shows abnormal heart activity. With heart attack, CARDIAC ENZYMES, BLOOD GASES, and ELECTROLYTES are also abnormal. ECHOCARDIOGRAM or ANGIOGRAPHY is typically done to more precisely assess the heart's damage. Diagnostic angiography offers the advantage of also performing immediate ANGIOPLASTY to open occluded CORONARY ARTERIES or to place an intra-aortic balloon pump (IABP) to assist the heart and relieve some of its workload.

Treatment Options and Outlook

Prompt EMERGENCY CARDIOVASCULAR CARE (ECC) response and appropriate medical treatment offer the best chance for survival. Time is critical. Treatment may include CPR (CARDIOPULMONARY RESUSCITATION), administration of IV fluids, and medications to help stabilize and strengthen the heart so it can more effectively pump blood to the lungs and the body. Emergency surgery to clear or bypass blocked CORONARY ARTERIES, such as ANGIO-PLASTY or CORONARY ARTERY BYPASS GRAFT (CBAG), or VALVE REPAIR AND REPLACEMENT SURGERY when the underlying cardiovascular condition is valvular, is often necessary. Those who survive may face a long road of recovery and require ongoing treatment for heart disease, although they may eventually be able to return to normal activities. The risk for another heart attack is high; preventive measures to reduce this risk often include medications as well as lifestyle modifications. Depending on the extent of damage to the heart, further surgery including implantation of a left VENTRICULAR ASSIST DEVICE (LVAD) or HEART TRANSPLANT might become necessary.

Risk Factors and Preventive Measures

Heart attack is the most common cause of cardiogenic shock, typically resulting from CORONARY ARTERY DISEASE (CAD), and is the most significant risk factor. Although rapid medical response to heart attack affords the best possible prognosis, such response alone is not enough to prevent cardiogenic shock when the heart suffers significant damage. The most important preventive measures are those that reduce the risk for heart disease in general, to decrease the risk for heart attack. Other causes include serious ARRHYTHMIAS, cardiac TAMPONADE, MYOCARDITIS, ENDOCARDITIS, serious VALVE DISEASE, and pulmonary embolism (blood clot in the lungs that prevents oxygenation of the blood). Measures to prevent further subsequent heart attacks and heart disease are important after cardiogenic shock has occurred.

See also BLOOD TESTS TO DETECT HEART ATTACK; LIFESTYLE AND HEART HEALTH; INTRA-AORTIC BALLOON PUMP (IABP) COUNTERPULSATION; LIVING WITH HEART DISEASE; MEDICATIONS TO TREAT HEART DISEASE; SURGERY TO TREAT CARDIOVASCULAR DISEASE.

cardiologist   A physician with extensive specialized training in treating CARDIOVASCULAR DISEASE. A cardiologist completes an additional five to seven years of training following medical school. Cardiologists must pass the written and oral examinations to become board-certified in INTERNAL MEDICINE as well as CARDIOLOGY. This training is required for any doctor to be designated as a cardiologist. Those who choose to belong to the American College of Cardiology (ACC) and meet this professional organization's educational and experience requirements can earn the designation of "Fellow," entitling them to place the initials F.A.C.C. after their names. This means they have achieved the highest level of professional expertise in cardiology. About half of the cardiologists who practice in the United States are ACC Fellows. Cardiologists typically see only patients who are referred to them by other physicians and who need specialized care for their heart conditions.

cardiomyopathy   A diminishment of the heart's ability and capacity to pump BLOOD, often accompanied by enlargement of the HEART. Most forms of cardiomyopathy strike people who are middle-aged or older, although some forms can affect people of all ages. A primary consequence of cardiomyopathy is HEART FAILURE. People with cardiomyopathy generally take medications to help manage the condition; in some situations, HEART TRANSPLANT is the only treatment alternative. With proper medical and lifestyle management cardiomyopathy can remain stable for many years; although it may improve it usually does not become "cured." Cardiomyopathy does not usually show any symptoms until it is quite advanced, which is one of the major challenges in treating it. For many people who have cardiomyopathy, detection comes too late to prevent serious loss of CARDIAC CAPACITY and cardiovascular function. Cardiomyopathy is a key cause of SUDDEN CARDIAC ARREST, particularly in younger people.

Arrhythmogenic Right Ventricular Cardiomyopathy (ARVC)

Also called arrhythmogenic right ventricular dysplasia (ARVD), this form of cardiomyopathy affects primarily people under the age of 40. Fibrous tissue and fat replace the right ventricle's muscle tissue, interfering with the ventricle's ability to conduct the electrical impulses necessary for synchronized contractions. The loss of muscle tissue reduces the ventricle's strength. As a result, the ventricle experiences ARRHYTHMIAS that the person might feel as PALPITATIONS and might cause episodes of (LIGHT-HEADEDNESS or syncope fainting) because the ventricle cannot adequately pump blood to the lungs for oxygenation so blood that circulates out of the heart and into the body does not contain enough oxygen to meet the body's needs. Episodes can be brief and unnoticed or can correspond with strenuous physical activity. Rarely, ARVC can cause sudden cardiac arrest.

Because ARVC's symptoms are transient—they come and go without apparent correlation to activity or circumstance—the condition can be difficult to diagnose. A chest X-ray can show whether the heart is enlarged, a common symptom of cardiomyopathy in general. Imaging procedures such as ECHO-CARDIOGRAM, MAGNETIC RESONANCE IMAGING (MRI), and MULTI-UNIT GATED ACQUISITION (MUGA) SCAN can sometimes detect the changes in the structure of the ventricle's wall. In other situations, definitive diagnosis requires more invasive procedures such as cardiac catheterization to visualize the ventricle or endomyocardial biopsy (removing a small piece of ventricular tissue for pathological evaluation) to examine the tissue structure for abnormal fat and fibrous tissues. ELECTROCARDIOGRAM (ECG) and use of a HOLTER MONITOR can help to detect the premature ventricular contractions (PVCs) or ventricular tachycardia that are key indicators of ARVC.

Doctors are unsure what causes ARVC, although there appears to be a genetic link. Recent research has identified several genetic abnormalities in those who have ARVC. There is no cure for ARVC, which can be progressive and involve the left ventricle as well as the right (and occasionally the atria, particularly if untreated). Some people respond to treatment with ANTIARRHYTHMIA MEDICATIONS, although many who have ARVC require an implantable pacing defibrillator that can regulate the ventricle's electrical impulses and automatically deliver a shock to restore normal rhythm when necessary. Cardiologists generally recommend that people with ARVC avoid strenuous exercise, such as athletic competition.

Dilated Cardiomyopathy

Dilated cardiomyopathy is the most common form of cardiomyopathy, in which the walls of the heart become thinned and stretch, or dilate, when the heart contracts. Dilated cardiomyopathy can affect the right atrium and ventricle (upper and lower pumping chambers) of the heart, the left atrium and ventricle, or the entire heart. The condition develops over time, typically producing symptoms in middle age. Untreated dilated cardiomyopathy often leads to heart failure (and is the most common cause of heart failure among Americans). The inability of the heart to pump blood efficiently allows fluid to build up in the lungs, establishing congestion. Dilated cardiomyopathy that has progressed to this level of severity is often called congestive cardiomyopathy. With early diagnosis and appropriate treatment, it is possible to stop the progression of, and sometimes even reverse, dilated cardiomyopathy.

Most people with dilated cardiomyopathy have no symptoms until the condition is fairly advanced, at which time they have symptoms of heart failure such as being short of breath and arrhythmias (commonly atrial fibrillation). Diagnosis uses electrocardiogram (ECG), echocardiogram, chest X-ray, imaging procedures such as magnetic resonance imaging (MRI), and sometimes cardiac catheterization. Most often there is no identifiable cause for dilated cardiomyopathy, in which case the diagnosis is idiopathic dilated cardiomyopathy. Among the known causes of dilated cardiomyopathy are:

- **Infection and inflammation (myocarditis).** Viruses and bacteria can cause infections of the heart tissue. More often than not this myocarditis causes no symptoms but can nonetheless wreak serious damage on the heart that continues even after the myocarditis goes away. The symptoms of dilated cardiomyopathy may not show up until years or even decades later. By then the damage to the heart is often extensive, having progressed to heart failure.

- **Pregnancy.** Rarely, a woman's heart becomes inflamed late in pregnancy. The reasons for this generally are unknown; some researchers believe it is a combination of factors that become potentiated by the stress pregnancy places on the woman's body and cardiovascular functions. Most of the time dilated cardiomyopathy that is pregnancy-related goes away within a few months following the baby's birth. There might be residual enlargement, but the condition usually does not progress.

- **Chronic, long-term substance abuse.** Alcohol has a highly toxic effect on the cells of the heart. Over time, heavy alcohol consumption causes myocardial cells to become dysfunctional or to die off. This weakens the heart, allowing the walls of its chambers to become thin. Abuse of other substances such as cocaine also causes dilated cardiomyopathy, among a plethora of cardiovascular problems.

- **Vitamin B₁ deficiency.** Sometimes this is a component of dilated cardiomyopathy that results from alcoholism, as heavy alcohol consumption interferes with the body's absorption of the B vitamins. Poor nutrition in general is also a factor in long-term chronic alcoholism.

- **Chronic, severe obesity.** Severe OBESITY (BMI over 40, or 50 percent or greater above healthy weight) places an extraordinary burden on the heart in several ways. One is that there is more body mass that requires blood, increasing the amount of work the heart must do. Another is that excess body fat wraps around and exerts pressure on internal structures and the blood vessels that supply them, increasing the amount of force the heart must use to pump blood through the body. The person who is severely obese generally has poor AEROBIC CAPACITY AND CARDIAC CAPACITY as a result of physical inactivity, making the heart's pumping actions significantly less efficient.

Treatment focuses on lightening the heart's workload. This might include lifestyle changes such as weight loss or stopping alcohol consumption if that is a factor. Most people with moderate dilated cardiomyopathy need medications to improve the heart's pumping efficiency and to treat related symptoms such as arrhythmias. Those commonly prescribed include ANGIOTENSIN-CONVERTING ENZYME (ACE) INHIBITOR MEDICATIONS, BETA ANTAGONIST MEDICATIONS, antiarrhythmia medications such as AMIODARONE and DIGOXIN, and DIURETIC MEDICATIONS to prevent EDEMA (fluid accumulation). For most people with dilated cardiomyopathy, medical treatment combined with lifestyle modifications such as weight loss restore a quality of life the same as or better than before diagnosis. For the small percentage of people for whom medical treatment fails to control the condition and it progresses, heart transplant becomes an option for those who meet the criteria.

Hypertrophic Cardiomyopathy

Hypertrophic means "overgrown." In hypertrophic cardiomyopathy the walls of the heart become so thick that they intrude into the ventricular chambers, reducing the volume of blood they can hold. This thickness also stiffens the heart's walls, making them less efficient at contracting and relaxing during the cardiac cycle. In some people the wall separating the ventricles, called the septum, also thickens and distorts into one of the ventricles, usually the left. This combination of stiff, thick walls and a displaced septum can cause the valves between the atrium and the ventricle to operate improperly, further impeding the flow of blood. Hypertrophic cardiomyopathy appears to be primarily an inherited genetic defect. Because of this, it can show up at any age. There are at least six known mutations found in people with hypertrophic cardiomyopathy that affect the way the heart muscle responds to CARDIAC ENZYMES such as myosin and cardiac tropotin T (CTNT) that are essential to the cardiac cycle. Hypertrophic cardiomyopathy is sometimes called idiopathic hypertrophic subaortic stemosis (IHSS).

As with other cardiomyopathies, there are usually no symptoms of hypertrophic cardiomyopathy until it becomes advanced. Sometimes the condition is diagnosed incidentally, getting detected on a chest X-ray or during physical examination. ECG and echocardiogram generally are sufficient to make the diagnosis once the condition is suspected. Endomyocardial biopsy provides a conclusive diagnosis, as the normal alignment of the myocardial cells is distorted in hypertrophic cardiomyopathy into random arrangements in a pattern called myocardial disarray.

Treatment focuses on relieving symptoms and maintaining normal electrical activity and contractions in the heart. Medications are able to accomplish this for many people with hypertrophic cardiomyopathy, particularly in the early stages of the condition. Those commonly prescribed include CALCIUM CHANNEL ANTAGONIST MEDICATIONS to make the walls of the heart more flexible, beta-blockers to slow the rate and force of the heartbeat, and antiarrhythmia medications. Persistent arrhythmias might require a PACEMAKER or IMPLANTABLE CARDIOVERTER DEFIBRILLATOR (ICD). In some cases where the septum becomes so thickened that it prevents proper valve operation, a cardiovascular surgeon might reshape it to remove the protruding tissue. This is called myectomy. Cardiologists also can reduce the septal thickness by catheterizing the artery that supplies blood to it, then injecting alcohol to necrotize (kill) some of the extra muscle. A person with severe, advanced hypertrophic cardiomyopathy might be a candidate for HEART TRANSPLANT.

Ischemic Cardiomyopathy

Ischemic cardiomyopathy develops when coronary artery disease reduces the flow of blood to a portion of the heart muscle and generally affects people in middle age and older. This causes the myocardial cells in the area to become weakened, dysfunctional, or die. The heart muscle in the area then becomes weakened and is unable to contract with the force necessary to move blood appropriately. Symptoms, when they occur, might include ANGINA. Treatment requires addressing the coronary artery disease, usually through angioplasty or coronary artery bypass graft (CABG), followed with medications to moderate and maintain the pumping force and strength of the heart. Damage from the ischemia is usually permanent. If the heart cannot compensate, heart transplant becomes a treatment option.

Restrictive Cardiomyopathy

Restrictive cardiomyopathy is relatively uncommon, and is most often a consequence of other medical conditions such as HEMOCHROMATOSIS (hereditary disorder in which iron accumulates in the blood and becomes deposited in organs such as the heart) and amyloidosis (deposits of protein that infiltrate myocardial tissues). The walls of the heart stiffen (without thickening), which limits blood volume in the atria and the ventricles. Symptoms include weakness, shortness of breath, edema, arrhythmias, and HEART BLOCK (a disruption of the heart's electrical system). As with other cardiomyopathies, diagnosis involves ECG, echocardiogram, and other diagnostic procedures as necessary. Treatment targets management of symptoms through medications and lifestyle changes (reduced strenuous physical activity). When medical approaches fail, heart transplant becomes an option for those who meet the criteria.

Living with Cardiomyopathy

Untreated cardiomyopathy progressively worsens until it results in life-threatening arrhythmias, heart failure, and other complications. With early diagnosis and appropriate treatment, cardiomyopathy might have little effect on the quality of life beyond limiting strenuous or competitive activities. Everyone with cardiomyopathy benefits from lifestyle changes that include nutritious eating and regular (even if moderate) physical activity to improve cardiac fitness. Weight management also is important.

See also ALCOHOL CONSUMPTION AND HEART DISEASE; BATISTA HEART FAILURE PROCEDURE; CARDIAC RESYNCHRONIZATION THERAPY; CARDIOMYOPLASTY; INFLAMMATION AND HEART DISEASE; MEDICATIONS TO TREAT HEART DISEASE.

cardiomyoplasty An operative procedure to improve the heart's efficiency in people who have severe HEART FAILURE that has not responded to other treatments.

Procedure

The cardiovascular surgeon creates a pedicle graft using a long skeletal muscle from the person's back, usually the latissimus dorsi, and bands it around the myocardium, or HEART muscle. This procedure leaves the latissimus dorsi muscle connected at its base, which maintains its blood supply. The surgeon then attaches wires from an implanted PACEMAKER to the graft. The pacemaker sends mild electrical signals to the muscle, causing it to contract in synchronization with the contractions of the heart's ventricles. The effect is that of a dynamic "girdle," adding strength and support to the heart's pumping action. The repeated stimulation from the pacemaker gradually alters the skeletal muscle's contraction pattern to accommodate perpetual contractions without becoming fatigued.

Risks and Complications

The key risks and complications of cardiomyoplasty are those common to surgery and anesthesia and include excessive bleeding and postoperative infection. As well, there is the possibility that the graft could fail, causing the procedure to be ineffective, or the procedure might simply not work or provide the desired relief.

Outlook and Lifestyle Modifications

Surgeons first performed cardiomyoplasty in 1985 as an alternative for people with end-stage heart failure who were not candidates for HEART TRANSPLANT. The most successful outcomes at present are among people who have dilated CARDIOMYOPATHY, in which the walls of the heart muscle have become so weakened that they balloon out with each ventricular contraction. Many variables affect outcome. In some people, even though heart function improves, their quality of life changes very little. Other people are able to return to everyday activities they have been unable to enjoy for years. Currently cardiomyoplasty remains experimental.

See also BATISTA HEART FAILURE PROCEDURE.

cardiopulmonary bypass Mechanical replacement for the body's cardiopulmonary functions during OPEN-HEART SURGERY. This is done so the cardiovascular surgeon can stop the HEART for surgery. Cardiopulmonary bypass makes possible most of the sophisticated heart operations performed today, from CORONARY ARTERY BYPASS GRAFT (CABG), the most commonly done heart operation, to the repair and reconstruction of congenital malformations and HEART TRANSPLANT. Cardiopulmonary bypass is also called extracorporeal ("out of the body") perfusion. The American Heart Association reports that more than 500,000 Americans undergo cardiovascular surgeries requiring cardiopulmonary bypass each year.

The first HEART-LUNG BYPASS MACHINES that made cardiopulmonary bypass possible were developed in the 1950s and were so large that they required priming with 10 pints of BLOOD, the same amount of blood circulating in the adult human body, and occupied a full room adjacent to the operating suite where the surgery was taking place. Through the decades since, computer technology has made it possible to construct smaller, more efficient units that require minimal priming with blood. Sophisticated electronics continually monitor the blood's oxygen and CARBON DIOXIDE levels, blood chemistries, and temperature. A filter screens out air bubbles before the blood returns to the body.

Procedure

Although it seems a simple premise to redirect blood to an external source for oxygenation and then to return it to the body, the process is very precise. Large tubes called cannulas collect the blood that normally flows into the right atrium from the superior vena cava and the inferior vena cava, the two large veins that bring deoxygenated blood back to the heart for circulation to the lungs. Other cannulas collect the oxygenated blood that returns from the heart and pass it, under pressure, back into the aorta for circulation into the body. Typically the body is cooled to slow its metabolic functions, reducing its need for oxygen during the procedure. Any blood lost during the operation is collected and returned to the bypass machine.

Risk and Complications

The risk of complications rises with the length of time cardiopulmonary bypass is in use and can include disturbances of the blood's normal clotting mechanisms, oxygen transfer in the peripheral arterioles, damage to red blood cells, and reduced hemoglobin capacity. As the body's metabolism is slowed, other body processes that otherwise would affect the blood, such as glucose conversion, become altered. Cells throughout the body receive adequate but not optimal oxygen and nutrients.

Outlook and Lifestyle Modifications

There is some concern among cardiologists and cardiovascular surgeons that the brain's sensitivity to even minuscule changes in blood composition may result in cognitive problems such as memory loss and confusion following surgery; studies are under way to assess the nature of these observances. Because many people who undergo open-heart surgery with cardiopulmonary bypass have already had a cardiovascular crisis that could have deprived the brain of oxygen, it is difficult to assess the source of any cognitive problems following surgery. Most people who recover completely from their operations also recover from any adverse effects of cardiopulmonary bypass.

See also BARNARD, CHRISTIAAN; CARDIAC REHABILITATION; HEART-LUNG TRANSPLANT; STROKE.

cardiorenal syndrome A correlation between HEART FAILURE and renal (kidney) failure in which having one increases the likelihood of having the other. The kidneys play an essential role in the regulation of BLOOD PRESSURE through the control of BLOOD fluid volume, filtration of ELECTROLYTES, and the actions of the RENIN-ANGIOTENSIN-ALDO-STERONE (RAA) HORMONE SYSTEM. Damage to the kidneys, notably in late-stage diabetes though also in other forms of kidney disease, disturbs these regulatory mechanisms in ways that adversely affect cardiovascular function. Conversely, late-stage heart failure and the medications to treat it put an extraordinary strain on these mechanisms.

In either scenario, the resulting symptoms become intertwined and require a coordinated and aggressive approach to treatment. About 25 percent of people with either heart failure or renal failure develop cardiorenal syndrome. Treatment approaches include medications to draw excessive fluid from the body (DIURETIC MEDICATIONS), strengthen and support the pumping efficiency of the HEART, and restore proper electrolyte balance. Renal (kidney) dialysis is also necessary to treat kidney failure. Because both conditions—heart failure and kidney failure—have reached end-stage disease when cardiorenal syndrome develops, cardiorenal syndrome is quite difficult to successfully treat, other body systems become impaired, and the outlook is poor.

See also DIABETES AND HEART DISEASE; MEDICATIONS TO TREAT HEART DISEASE.

cardiovascular disease (CVD) A collective term for a wide range of health problems related to dysfunctions and medical conditions involving the HEART and BLOOD vessels. It incorporates conditions such as HYPERTENSION, CORONARY ARTERY DISEASE (CAD), ARRHYTHMIAS, congenital heart malformations, ATHEROSCLEROSIS, ARTERIOSCLEROSIS, CARDIOMYOPATHY, HEART BLOCK, HYPOTENSION, BUNDLE BRANCH BLOCK, STROKE, TRANSIENT ISCHEMIC ATTACK (TIA), HYPERCHOLESTEROLEMIA, HYPERLIPIDEMIA, structural malformations and damage to the heart and blood vessels, ANEURYSM, PERIPHERAL VASCULAR DISEASE (PVD), valve disorders and damage, ion channelopathies, ISCHEMIC HEART DISEASE (IHD), and RHEUMATIC HEART DISEASE.

Cardiovascular disease is the leading cause of death in the United States, accounting for nearly 700,000 deaths each year. Health experts believe that 90 percent or more of these deaths—and the heart disease that causes them—could be prevented through lifestyle modifications that include nutritious eating habits, regular physical EXERCISE, WEIGHT MANAGEMENT, and smoking cessation. According to the Centers for Disease Control (CDC), nearly 6 million cardiovascular operations are performed in the United States each year, making them the most common kind of surgery (excluding obstetric procedures). The costs to treat cardiovascular disease extend into the billions just for medical care; the costs of lost productivity and other factors are almost impossible to estimate. It is the goal of numerous health organizations and initiatives, including Healthy People 2010, the CDC, the National Institutes of Health (NIH), and the American Heart Association, among others, to significantly reduce the numbers of deaths related to heart disease through education and awareness of prevention and early warning signs.

See also HEART DISEASE; LIFESTYLE AND HEART HEALTH; NUTRITION AND DIET.

cardiovascular event A catchall term denoting a circumstance of unusual or other than normal activity involving the heart or blood vessels. A cardiovascular event can range in severity from mild episodes of ANGINA or ARRHYTHMIA to

TRANSIENT ISCHEMIC ATTACK (TIA), HEART ATTACK, CARDIAC ARREST, or STROKE. It might be as nondescript as chest pain or LIGHT-HEADEDNESS if heart function or CARDIOVASCULAR DISEASE is suspected as a cause. Suspected or known cardiovascular events should be evaluated by a doctor. A person experiencing any warning signs of heart attack or stroke should seek emergency medical treatment without delay.

See also CORONARY ARTERY DISEASE (CAD); HYPERTENSION.

cardiovascular system The network of organs, structures, and functions responsible for circulating BLOOD throughout the body. "Cardio" means HEART and "vascular" means vessel; the main features of the cardiovascular system are the heart and a complex network of about 100,000 miles-worth of blood vessels—arteries, veins, and capillaries. The cardiovascular system intimately integrates with the lungs and the PULMONARY SYSTEM for the exchange of oxygen (the body's primary source of cellular energy) and CARBON DIOXIDE (the body's primary cellular waste by-product). The cardiovascular system is a closed, pressurized system; the blood that it recirculates contains components all of which are manufactured within the body (by contrast, the pulmonary system functions as a constant exchange of substances that come from outside the body).

HEART VALVES

Valve	Location	Function
tricuspid valve	between right atrium and right ventricle	prevents blood from backflowing into right atrium
mitral valve	between left atrium and left ventricle	prevents blood from backflowing into left atrium
pulmonary valve	between right ventricle and pulmonary artery	prevents blood from backflowing into right ventricle
aortic valve	between left ventricle and aorta	prevents blood from backflowing into left ventricle

Heart

The heart is the core of the cardiovascular system. It collects and pumps blood, completing more than 100,000 CARDIAC CYCLES and circulating about 3,000 gallons of blood every 24 hours. The heart has four chambers—two atria and two ventricles. The atria (right atrium and left atrium) are the upper chambers; they collect blood that comes into the heart.

Arteries

Arteries carry oxygenated blood from the heart to other parts of the body. The exception is the pulmonary artery, which is the body's only artery that carries deoxygenated blood; it transports deoxygenated blood from the heart to the lungs. The body's largest artery is the aorta, which can be an inch or more across at its widest point near its juncture with the left ventricle. Blood moves through the arteries under pressure, so the arteries can rapidly deliver the oxygen the blood carries to the cells throughout the body that need it. Arteries are muscular and flexible, and pulsate in waves that are synchronized with the heart's contractions. The arteries generally follow the body's bones, which help to protect them from injury and damage. The body's tiniest arteries are called arterioles; they merge into the capillary beds. The arterioles also play a role in lowering, maintaining, and raising blood pressure.

Veins

Veins carry deoxygenated blood from the body back to the heart. The pulmonary vein is the only vein in the body that carries oxygenated blood; it brings blood to the heart from the lungs. Veins are less muscular and more flexible than arteries and generally have thinner walls. They also have valves in them, to keep blood flowing in just one direction. The force of blood going through the arteries maintains enough pressure within the veins to assist blood flow to the heart. The tiniest veins are called venules; they arise from the capillary beds. The veins generally parallel the arteries.

Capillary Beds

In many respects, capillaries are where the action takes place. These microscopic blood vessels, often

THE BODY'S MAIN ARTERIES

Artery	Location	Function
aorta	arises from the heart's left ventricle	primary conduit carrying blood from the heart; the body's other major arteries branch from it
aortic arch	first few inches of aorta as it leaves heart	carries blood to upper part of the body; gives rise to the brachi- ocephalic, left common carotid, and left subclavian arteries
descending aorta	aorta as it drops over the back of the heart	carries blood to lower part of the body
thoracic aorta	aorta as it passes through the chest	gives rise to arteries that supply the lungs
abdominal aorta	aorta as it passes through the central abdomen	gives rise to the celiac, renal, mesenteric, and iliac arteries
brachiocephalic	arises from the aortic arch	carries blood to the right side of the upper body; gives rise to the right carotid and right brachial arteries
brachial, right and left	upper arm along the humerus bone	carries blood to arms and hands; branches into the radial and ulnar arteries
carotid, right and left	neck	carries blood to the head, brain, and face
celiac	upper abdomen	carries blood to the stomach, duodenum, liver, spleen, pancreas
femoral, right and left	thigh along the femur bone	carries blood to the thighs and legs
iliac, right and left	branches from abdominal aorta in lower abdomen	carries blood to organs of lower abdomen; gives rise to femoral artery
mesenteric, superior and inferior	intestines	carries blood to the large and small intestines
popliteal, right and left	behind the knee	carries blood to the legs; branches into tibials
pulmonary, central, right, and left	leads from heart's right ventricle to the lungs	carries blood from the heart to the lungs for oxygenation; central branches into right and left shortly after leaving the heart
radial, right and left	thumb-side of forearm, along the radius bone	carries blood to forearm, hand, thumb, and forefinger
renal, right and left	kidney	carries blood into and to supply the kidneys
subclavian, right and left	beneath the collarbone (clavicle)	carries blood to the arm
tibial, anterior right and left, posterior right and left	leg, along front and back of the tibia bone	carries blood to the legs and feet
ulnar, right and left	little finger side of arm, alongthe ulna bone	carries blood to the arm, hand, and middle, ring, and little fingers

only the width of a cell, are the end of the line for arterial transport and the start of the return trip to the heart. They represent a merging of arterioles and venules in meshlike configurations throughout the body. The walls of the capillaries are very thin and porous. As red blood cells file through the capillaries, they exchange the oxygen they are carrying for carbon dioxide and other waste by-products of metabolism that other cells in the body generate. The deoxygenated red blood cells

THE BODY'S MAIN VEINS

Vein	Location	Function
brachial, right and left	arm	carries blood from the arm to the subclavian vein
femoral, right and left	thigh along the femur bone	carries blood from the thigh to the iliac vein
iliac, right and left	lower abdomen	carries blood from the lower abdomen to the inferior vena cava
jugular, right and left	neck	carries blood from the head, face, and brain to the subclavian vein
portal	liver	carries blood from the liver to the inferior vena cava
pulmonary, right, left, and central	right and left lung, merging into central pulmonary vein which enters the heart's left atrium	carries blood from the lungs
renal vein, right and left	kidneyjcarries blood from the kidney to the inferior vena cava	
sapphenous, right and left	leg	carries blood from the foot and leg to the femoral vein
subclavian, right and left	beneath the collarbone (clavicle)	carries blood from the arm to the superior vena cava
vena cava, inferior	enters heart's right atrium from the bottom	carries blood from the lower body to the heart
vena cava, superior	enters heart's right atrium from the top	carries blood from the upper body to the heart

then enter the venules, which transport them to the veins.

Blood Pressure and Heart Rate

The cardiovascular system is a closed network and relies on pressure to function against the force of gravity. HEART RATE is the number of times each minute that the heart contracts, or completes a cardiac cycle. A healthy adult heart at rest has a heart rate of 60 to 80 beats per minute; during intense exercise heart rate can double or triple. The PULSE rate is the measure of the heart rate. Numerous factors influence heart rate; the BRAIN STEM assimilates them and sends the signals that then regulate heart rate. Several interdependent mechanisms cooperate to regulate BLOOD PRESSURE, which is an interplay between the heart's rate and strength of contractions. In a healthy heart, there is close coordination between heart rate and contraction force that collaborates to regulate the volume of blood each contraction generates. Various disease conditions, such as HYPERTENSION (high blood pressure) and ARRHYTHMIAS (irregular heartbeat), alter this balance.

See also ACCESSORY PATHWAY; CARDIOVASCULAR DISEASE; CIRCULATION; CONDUCTION SYSTEM; OXYGENATION; VAGUS NERVE; VALVE DISEASE; VASOVAGAL SYNCOPE; VITAL SIGNS.

cardioversion Therapeutic delivery of an electrical shock to the HEART to correct an ARRHYTHMIA and restore a normal SINUS RHYTHM (pattern of electrical discharge within the heart). A CARDIOLOGIST performs cardioversion in a hospital setting with full resuscitative facilities and equipment at the ready. After the person receives a sedative or a general anesthetic, the cardiologist positions defibrillator paddles on the person's chest and delivers a controlled electrical impulse, timed with the heart's natural rhythm, that momentarily disrupts the heart's electrical activity. The interruption is brief, and when the heart recovers it restores itself to normal electrical signals. It sometimes takes more than one shock to accomplish sustainable normal rhythm. After the procedure the person remains under supervision until the sedative or anesthesia wears off and it is clear that the heart is maintaining its normal rhythm. For the majority of people who are undergoing scheduled cardioversion, the procedure is done on an outpatient basis and they go home the same day.

Cardiologists use cardioversion primarily for ATRIAL FIBRILLATION, episodes of rapid and uncontrolled beating of the atria (heart's upper chambers). Atrial fibrillation is fairly common and typically responds to treatment with ANTIARRHYTHMIA MEDICATIONS following cardioversion. Atrial fibrillation carries a risk for blood clots to develop in the blood that pool in the atrium because the atrium is not effective in pumping it out. Clots can dislodge, enter the bloodstream, and get carried along until they reach a point where they are too big for the blood vessel and they create a blockage. This can cause HEART ATTACK or STROKE. The cardiologist might prescribe anticoagulant medications for the person to take for a defined period of time before and after the cardioversion.

See also CONDUCTION PATHWAY; CPR; DEFIBRILLATION; EMBOLISM; IMPLANTABLE CARDIOVERTER DEFIBRILLATOR; THROMBOSIS.

Cardizem   See DILTIAZEM.

carotid artery   See CARDIOVASCULAR SYSTEM.

carotid bruit   An abnormal sound the doctor can hear through a STETHOSCOPE placed over the carotid artery in the neck. The word *bruit* means "noise." What the doctor hears is the sound of BLOOD rushing past a buildup of arterial plaque that creates a narrowing of the artery's interior passage. A carotid bruit is an indication of ATHEROSCLEROSIS (fatty deposits along the inside walls of the arteries) and CAROTID STENOSIS (narrowing of the carotid artery's interior passage). Atherosclerosis in the carotid arteries, which carry blood to the head and brain, presents a significant risk for STROKE and TRANSIENT ISCHEMIC ATTACK (TIA).

There is one carotid artery on each side of the neck; either or both can have bruits and corresponding atherosclerosis. There is no treatment for carotid bruit, as it is a sign rather than a disease. Treatment targets the underlying atherosclerosis. Further diagnostic tests are necessary to determine the extent of risk of the OCCLUSION versus the risk of procedures to remove it, as those risks also include stroke and TIA. Decisions about testing and treatment should take into consideration other factors in addition to the potential severity of the atherosclerosis, including the age of the person and any other cardiovascular disease or health problems that exist.

See also CAROTID ENDARTERECTOMY; CAROTID PHONOANGIOGRAPHY; LIPID-LOWERING MEDICATIONS; PLAQUE, ARTERIAL.

carotid endarterectomy   A procedure to remove an arterial OCCLUSION from the carotid artery to relieve CAROTID STENOSIS and improve BLOOD flow to the brain.

When arterial PLAQUE constricts 75 percent or greater of the artery's channel, the risk for spontaneous STROKE skyrockets. Blood moves through the carotid arteries at substantial velocity, pumped against gravity to make it to the brain. This force continuously batters the occlusion, with the risk that fragments of it will break away to become lodged in the small arteries of the brain. The interrupted blood flow that results—a stroke—can have serious consequences depending on what part of the brain it affects. The decision to undergo carotid endarterectomy first should consider all other possible alternatives as well as weigh the potential risks against the potential benefits.

Procedure

Carotid endarterectomy involves making an incision in the carotid artery where the occlusion is located and using rotoblade devices to whittle the arterial plaque from the arterial wall. It is done under general anesthetic, with the person completely asleep, in a hospital operating room, and takes up to several hours. The person generally stays several nights in the hospital following the surgery, often the first night in a surgical intensive care unit (SICU) under continual medical observation to make sure there is no bleeding from the incision site and there are no adverse effects.

Risks and Complications

Carotid endarterectomy is a fairly high-risk surgery in that it can cause the very problems it is intended to prevent, stroke and TRANSIENT ISCHEMIC ATTACK (TIA). Carotid artery occlusions often are brittle and break away when disturbed by surgical intervention; the only direction they can travel is toward the brain. Studies suggest that the risk of the procedure outweighs the benefits unless the artery is 50 percent or more occluded (blocked). Because of the high risk that carotid endarterectomy can cause stroke, the American Heart Association recommends this operative procedure as an option when the carotid artery is more than 60 percent occluded. Many cardiovascular surgeons prefer to delay the operation until the occlusion exceeds 75 percent or is causing significant symptoms.

In addition to the risks of stroke or TIA during surgery, other problems that can arise during carotid endarterectomy include HEART ATTACK (myocardial infarction) if fragments of the arterial plaque break away and lodge in the coronary arteries and cardiovascular problems from uncontrolled HYPERTENSION (high BLOOD PRESSURE). One of the most serious surgical risks of carotid endarterectomy is a reaction called postendarterectomy hyperperfusion syndrome. Carotid stenosis develops over time, usually decades. This allows the vascular structures of the brain to adapt to the gradual restriction of blood flow through various mechanisms to help maintain adequate blood flow to brain tissues. One such adaptation is that the arterioles eventually become and remain fully dilated. This is called impaired hemodynamics; these tiny vital arteries no longer contract and dilate to regulate the volume of blood that flows through them. When the surgeon removes the carotid occlusion and restores free blood flow through the carotid artery to the brain, these arterioles do not "remember" how to respond to the suddenly increased blood flow and they cannot respond to limit it. The arteriole network floods with blood, which causes intracerebral hemorrhage—a stroke. The damage can be extensive enough to cause death. There is no way for surgeons to predict whether this will happen or to intervene once it begins.

Outlook and Lifestyle Modifications

Although surgery can remove the atherosclerotic deposits creating the carotid occlusion, lifestyle changes following recovery from the surgery are important to maintain optimal cardiovascular health following the operation. Key among these changes are a low-fat diet and daily physical EXERCISE, along with close monitoring of blood lipid levels (blood CHOLESTEROL and TRIGLYCERIDES) with appropriate LIPID-LOWERING MEDICATIONS when lifestyle alone is not enough to maintain the desired levels. Even after surgery, the risk for stroke remains higher than for people without carotid occlusions.

See also ATHERECTOMY; CAROTID STENT; SURGERY TO TREAT CARDIOVASCULAR DISEASE.

carotid hypersensitivity syndrome An overreaction of the body's baroreceptor response that results in a brief, temporary cessation of electrical activity in the HEART (called a cardioinhibition response) causing a sudden, rapid drop in HEART RATE (bradycardia). Less commonly the result is a sudden, rapid drop in BLOOD PRESSURE (HYPOTENSION), called a vasodepressor response. Baroceptors are specialized cells, called carotid sinus receptors, located in the walls of the interior carotid arteries near the base of the neck, that monitor the movement of the walls of these arteries. Constriction, or tightening, of the arterial wall tells the baroreceptors that blood pressure is dropping; dilation, or expanding, of the arterial wall indicates rising blood pressure. The baroreceptors constantly send signals to the BRAIN STEM to minutely adjust the many physiologic interactions responsible for keeping blood pressure at the appropriate level.

For reasons doctors do not understand, these baroreceptors become overly sensitive in some people such that touching the neck or twisting the neck, or even normal fluctuations in cardiac contraction strength, causes the baroreceptors to falsely perceive the artery wall is expanding. This can trigger an overreaction by the brain stem to drop the blood pressure via the vagus nerve and other nervous system mechanisms, potentially resulting in SYNCOPE (fainting) due to inadequate blood supply to the brain.

Symptoms and Diagnostic Path

Most people come to the doctor because they have experienced syncope, sometimes causing a fall or a traffic accident (if the person was driving at the time), or episodes of DIZZINESS. The diagnostic path includes ELECTROCARDIOGRAM (ECG) and often HOLTER MONITOR, as well as AUSCULTATION of the carotid arteries (listening to the arteries through a STETHOSCOPE). When the doctor suspects carotid hypersensitivity, he or she may also conduct a TILT TABLE TEST and carotid massage. Typically the carotid massage will evoke cardioinhibition, and sometimes a syncopal episode, which helps to confirm the diagnosis. Sometimes further diagnostic procedures, such as EXERCISE STRESS test or pharmacologic stress test (ADENOSINE, DIPYRIDAMOLE, or DOBUTAMINE), are necessary when the person may have other CARDIO-VASCULAR DISEASE (CVD) as well.

Treatment Options and Outlook

Treatment focuses first on avoiding movements and activities that produce symptoms. If this is not successful or the episodes of syncope have caused falls or other problems, the doctor may recommend a PACEMAKER to prevent the bradycardia. However, pacing does not affect carotid hypersensitivity that is vasodepressive. Although some medications have been tried, they do not produce consistent or reliable results. Treatment with a pacemaker dramatically decreases the likelihood for subsequent syncopal episodes, though does not entirely prevent them.

Risk Factors and Preventive Measures

Underlying HEART DISEASE, especially HYPERTEN-SION (high blood pressure) and CORONARY ARTERY DISEASE (CAD), is the most significant risk factor for carotid hypersensitivity. Some MEDICATIONS TO TREAT HEART DISEASE, such as DIGITALIS, also can cause carotid hypersensitivity. Preventive measures to lower the overall risk for heart disease are also effective for lowering the risk for carotid hypersensitivity syndrome.

See also CAROTID STENOSIS; LIVING WITH HEART DISEASE.

carotid phonoangiography   A noninvasive means of assessing the degree of carotid ATHEROSCLEROSIS (a buildup of arterial plaque in one or both of the carotid arteries in the neck). A highly sensitive microphone placed over the carotid artery amplifies and records any CAROTID BRUIT, helping to identify whether atherosclerosis is present and to what degree. Carotid phonoangiography is one of several diagnostic procedures that help to measure a person's risk for stroke. It is a painless procedure that takes less than 30 minutes to perform and is done on an outpatient, scheduled basis.

See also DIGITAL SUBTRACTION ANGIOGRAPHY (DSA); DOPPLER ULTRASOUND; PLAQUE, ARTERIAL.

carotid stenosis   Narrowing of the interior passage of the carotid artery in the neck as a consequence of accumulated arterial plaque (ATHEROSCLEROSIS). Doctors can detect carotid stenosis by listening with a STETHOSCOPE to the carotid artery in the neck. Carotid stenosis produces a characteristic abnormal sound called a CAROTID BRUIT. Carotid stenosis becomes more common with advancing age. The narrowing carotid stenosis in the artery's interior passage reduces the flow of BLOOD to the brain, raising the risk for STROKE and TRANSIENT ISCHEMIC ATTACK (TIA) as well as for impaired cognitive function and other lapses in conscious function. When carotid stenosis creates an occlusion greater than 75 percent of the artery's interior passage, the risk for STROKE jumps significantly. Once such an occlusion develops, the most effective correction is CAROTID ENDARTERECTOMY. Although this procedure can remove the occlusion, it has significant risks. Another surgical option being investigated is a CAROTID STENT, a tiny springlike device inserted into the artery at the location of the occlusion to compress the arterial plaque and widen the artery's interior passage.

See also INFLAMMATION AND HEART DISEASE; PLAQUE, ARTERIAL.

carvedilol   A medication taken to treat HYPERTEN-SION (high BLOOD PRESSURE) and in combination with other medications to treat mild to moderate HEART FAILURE. Common brand names include Coreg. Carvedilol has both alpha adrenergic antagonist and beta adrenergic antagonist functions—it acts as an alpha and beta-blocker to inhibit the heart's response to EPINEPHRINE. This slows the heart rate and the force of the heart's contractions. Carvedilol also acts on the RENIN-ANGIOTENSIN-ALDOSTERONE (RAA) HORMONAL SYSTEM, the body's primary mechanism for regulating blood pressure.

Like other medications with beta-blocking actions, carvedilol can interfere with the actions of insulin and oral medications taken to treat diabetes. Women who are pregnant or nursing should not take carvedilol. Common side effects that often go away after taking carvedilol over time include dizziness, orthostatic HYPOTENSION (sudden drop in blood pressure upon standing), headache, and nausea. More serious side effects include arrhythmias; people with SICK SINUS SYNDROME or HEART BLOCK generally should not take carvedilol.

See also ALPHA ANTAGONIST MEDICATIONS; ANTIHYPERTENSIVE MEDICATIONS; BETA ANTAGONIST MEDICATIONS; MEDICATIONS TO TREAT HEART DISEASE.

Catapres   See CLONIDINE.

catecholamines   Biochemicals in the body that are compounds of catechol and amine. The body produces catecholamines from the amino acid tyrosine. The three major catecholamines are DOPAMINE, EPINEPHRINE, and NOREPINEPHRINE. They can bind with receptors in nerve cells, in which case they are called neurotransmitters, or with receptors in cells of other tissues in the body, in which case they are called HORMONES. Dopamine is a norepinephrine precursor, which means the body can convert dopamine into norepinephrine. Similarly, norepinephrine is an epinephrine precursor.

Catecholamines play key roles in regulating HEART RATE, BLOOD PRESSURE, and other cardiovascular functions. They act directly on myocardial cells and on nerve cells in the arteries. Rising catecholamine levels signal the HEART to increase the rate and force of its contractions to boost CARDIAC OUTPUT (the amount of blood pumped into the body during each CARDIAC CYCLE). Many factors can trigger catecholamines, including stress. Catecholamine levels typically are elevated in people with moderate to serious HEART FAILURE and with HYPER-

TENSION (high blood pressure), indicating that the heart is working harder than normal. Medications such as ALPHA ANTAGONIST MEDICATIONS and BETA ANTAGONIST MEDICATIONS that inhibit the actions of epinephrine by binding with adrenergic receptors help to lower catecholamine levels, reducing the heart's workload and improving these conditions.

Catecholamines increase in response to physical exertion, serving to raise blood pressure and heart rate to meet the body's increased needs for oxygen. The higher a person's aerobic fitness level, the less of an increase is necessary. The body's stress reaction also causes the release of catecholamines. Doctors administer dopamine and epinephrine in the form of injectable drugs during cardiac crisis, to stimulate heart action.

See also BRAIN STEM; HEART ATTACK.

cerebrovascular accident (CVA)   See STROKE.

chain of survival   A metaphor to increase public awareness of the need for early recognition and intervention in cardiac crisis. It has four links:

- Early access to care—call 911 or emergency aid
- Early CPR—initiate CARDIOPULMONARY RESUSCITATION to restore the flow of oxygenated BLOOD
- Early DEFIBRILLATION—use AUTOMATED EXTERNAL DEFIBRILLATOR (AED) to restore normal heart rhythm
- Early advanced cardiovascular care—transport to a hospital

The emphasis with the chain of survival is to begin intervention as soon as there is suspicion of a cardiac crisis. When intervention starts soon enough, it can interrupt the HEART ATTACK and prevent it from fully unfolding. Current THROMBOLYTIC MEDICATIONS ("clot-busters") can dissolve occlusions in the coronary arteries, restoring the flow of blood to the heart before any permanent damage to the myocardium takes place. The window of time during which this treatment has the highest success rate is within the first hour of the heart attack. However, symptoms during this window of opportunity are often vague and not clearly cardiac in origin. Many people delay seeking treatment, or even telling others that they are not feeling well, until the signs of heart attack are unmistakable. By that time, the process of damage is well under way. Immediate treatment will still mitigate further damage and can help to reverse some of the damage that has already taken place.

The American Heart Association reports that 80 percent of CARDIAC ARRESTS (complete stoppage of the heart) take place at home, and 60 percent in front of witnesses. Yet only 5 percent of those receive early intervention that allows them to survive long enough to reach a hospital. Many people who do initiate early response begin with CPR (cardiopulmonary resuscitation), which has long been the standard, but research over the past decade demonstrates that people who reach a hospital emergency department that can administer advanced cardiac care are far more likely to survive. The American Heart Association and other organizations urge people to first dial 911 (or the local emergency access number) and then begin CPR. The few seconds it takes to place the call get help on the way minutes sooner yet do not make a difference for the effectiveness of CPR.

The chain of survival metaphor also targets hospital emergency departments, encouraging staff to perform preliminary cardiac assessment including BLOOD TESTS TO DETECT HEART ATTACK. Levels of certain CARDIAC ENZYMES, particularly CTnI (cardiac troponin I) and CTnT (cardiac troponin T), begin to rise very early in the process of a heart attack, providing important clues that a cardiac event is under way. Other tests such as ELECTROCARDIO-GRAM (ECG) might show subtle aberrations that, taken into consideration with blood test findings, corroborate the suspicion of heart attack and indicate appropriate clinical intervention.

See also CARDIOVASCULAR EVENT; CHEST PAIN.

chelation therapy Intravenous injection of a chemical substance that binds with metals and minerals in the body and draws them into the bloodstream, after which the kidney filters the bound compounds and sends them for excretion in the urine. Chelation therapy is a legitimate therapeutic treatment for poisoning with metals such as lead and mercury. The chelating agent commonly used for such treatment, ethylenediamine tetraacetic acid (EDTA), also chelates calcium, drawing it from the body as well. This has led to speculation that chelation therapy could draw the calcium from arterial plaque, returning plaque accumulations to fatty deposits that the blood could wash away. This was seen as a potential treatment for ATHEROSCLEROSIS. However, there are no CLINICAL RESEARCH STUDIES that support this hypothesis. The few studies that have been done show no change in the calcium content of arterial plaque following chelation.

Numerous professional and health organizations—among them the U.S. Food and Drug Administration (FDA), the American Medical Association (AMA), the American College of Cardiology (ACC), the American Heart Association (AHA), and the National Heart, Lung, and Blood Institute (NHLBI)—have taken the position that EDTA chelation therapy as a treatment for atherosclerosis, CORONARY ARTERY DISEASE (CAD), and related CARDIOVASCULAR DISEASE (CVD) is inappropriate because it is untested and unproven. The perception that chelation therapy is safe may not be accurate; EDTA is known to cause damage to the kidneys. As well, doctors are concerned that people who undergo chelation therapy might believe that this treatment "cures" their atherosclerosis, generating a false sense of security that keeps them from seeking conventional medical treatments that actually can improve their cardiovascular disease.

In 2003 the NHLBI and the National Center for Complementary and Alternative Medicine (NCCAM) launched a cooperative CLINICAL RESEARCH STUDY to examine chelation therapy's effects on atherosclerosis and related cardiovascular disease. The study, called Trial to Assess Chelation Therapy (TACT), has enrolled 2,300 participants through 100 research sites across the United States. The research team expects to report its findings in 2010.

See also LIFESTYLE AND HEART HEALTH; LIPID-LOWERING MEDICATIONS; PLAQUE, ARTERIAL.

chest pain Discomfort originating from the chest area that can be cardiac or noncardiac in nature.

Noncardiac causes of chest pain can include gastroesophageal reflux disorder (GERD), pancreatitis, stomach ulcers, and injury to the ribs or spleen. Although gallbladder disease more typically produces pain on the right side of the chest, it can refer to (be felt on) the left side. Gallbladder pain also can be intense enough to cause some of the symptoms characteristic of HEART ATTACK, such as diaphoresis (profuse sweating) and pain that radiates through the shoulder and into the neck region. A thoracic aortic aneurysm or an ABDOMINAL AORTIC ANEURYSM (AAA) that is fairly high might cause chest pain, as can a BLOOD clot in the lung (pulmonary embolism) if it results in a pulmonary infarct.

Cardiac causes of chest pain can include ANGINA from CORONARY ARTERY DISEASE (CAD) or ISCHEMIC HEART DISEASE (IHD) and myocardial infarction (heart attack). There is a common perception that heart attack pain is characteristically severe and crushing; although this can be the case, more often than not the pain can range from discomfort resembling indigestion to intermittent sharp stabs. PERICARDITIS, an inflammation or infection of the pericardium (the membranous sac surrounding the heart), and ENDOCARDITIS, an inflammation or infection of the lining and valves of the heart, also can cause chest pain. A doctor should evaluate all chest pain; early intervention is essential when the problem is the heart. Although much chest pain turns out to be noncardiac, often there is no clear way to know whether this is the case based on the chest pain alone.

See also CHAIN OF SURVIVAL.

chest percussion Patterned tapping on the outside of the chest. Chest percussion can be done for diagnostic or therapeutic purposes. During diagnostic chest percussion, the doctor listens to the quality of tones that result from tapping on certain areas of the chest. There are characteristic changes from the normal sounds that indicate particular disease states. The area over the lungs normally produces a resonant sound, for example, when air fills the lungs. When fluid collects in the lungs, as happens with moderate to advanced congestive HEART FAILURE, the percussed tone turns dull and flat above the fluid-filled areas. Percussed

tones also change with HEART enlargement (as in CARDIOMYOPATHY) and structural malformations of the heart that affect the flow and accumulation of blood. This basic diagnostic method can help the doctor decide what further tests and procedures are necessary.

In therapeutic chest percussion, a clinical specialist taps on the chest to loosen secretions within the lungs so the person can bring them up. People with chronic lung conditions such as CHRONIC OBSTRUCTIVE PULMONARY DISEASE (COPD) and emphysema often accumulate large quantities of sputum and mucus within the lower bronchi (breathing tubes). These accumulations often are sticky and hard to dislodge. The person might have limited cough capability, or coughing alone might generate insufficient force. Therapeutic chest percussion, sometimes called clapping, helps to jar the accumulations free so coughing is more effective in bringing them up.

See also AUSCULTATION; CORVISART, JEAN-NICHOLAS.

Cheyne-Stokes respiration An abnormal pattern of breathing in which 20- to 30-second periods of apnea (no breathing) alternate with 20- to 30-second periods of hyperpnea (rapid breathing). It often develops in people who have moderate to severe congestive HEART FAILURE and is sometimes a symptom of brain-stem lesion or other neurological disorders. Cheyne-Stokes respiration occasionally occurs in people who are extremely obese. Researchers believe it results from a delayed response in the respiratory centers of the brain to changes in blood oxygen and blood CARBON DIOXIDE levels. The breathing pattern was originally reported by two physicians in Dublin, Ireland, John Cheyne (1777–1836) and William Stokes (1804–78). There is no treatment for Cheyne-Stokes respiration, which itself is not damaging but signals serious underlying medical problems. BREATHING EXERCISES can help to improve overall pulmonary capacity.

See also BRAIN STEM; MEDICATIONS TO TREAT HEART DISEASE; PULMONARY EDEMA; STOKES-ADAMS DISEASE.

childhood heart disease See HEART DISEASE IN CHILDREN.

chlorothiazide A DIURETIC MEDICATION taken to treat HYPERTENSION (high BLOOD PRESSURE) and EDEMA caused by HEART FAILURE. Common brand names include Diuril and Diurigen. Chlorothiazide belongs to a classification of diuretics called thiazides; these all have similar pharmacological activity. Thiazides work by causing the kidneys to release more fluid to pass from the body as urine, earning these medications the nickname "water pills." This action reduces the volume of BLOOD, lowering the amount of work the HEART must do to circulate it through the body. This in turn lowers blood pressure. Frequent urination is common when someone first starts to take chlorothiazide but usually goes away after a few weeks.

Chlorothiazide can increase the skin's sensitivity to sunlight, making it more susceptible to sunburn. Chlorothiazide interacts with the LIPID-LOWERING MEDICATIONS CHOLESTYRAMINE and COLESTIPOL; people taking both chlorothiazide and either of these medications should separate their doses by at least an hour. Chlorothiazide also causes the kidneys to excrete more POTASSIUM. Doctors generally recommend that people taking chlorothiazide eat foods high in potassium such as bananas and raisins. With higher doses of chlorothiazide, the doctor might also prescribe a potassium supplement.

See also ANTIHYPERTENSIVE MEDICATIONS; MEDICATIONS TO TREAT HEART DISEASE.

cholesterol, bad See CHOLESTEROL, BLOOD.

cholesterol, blood One of several lipids, or fatty acids, the liver manufactures and the body uses to produce HORMONES, make bile, repair cells, and help transport other fats through the bloodstream. The common perception is that cholesterol is "bad" for health; this is not true. Cholesterol is essential for health and for the body to function properly. It becomes a health problem only when there is more of it circulating in the bloodstream than the body can use. Excess cholesterol and other fatty acids end up as accumulations along the interior walls of the arteries, a condition called ATHEROSCLEROSIS. Over time these accumulations become hard and brittle and extend out into the artery enough to

slow or block the flow of blood. Elevated blood cholesterol levels are an indicator of the risk for or presence of CARDIOVASCULAR DISEASE, particularly CORONARY ARTERY DISEASE (CAD).

The liver manufactures the cholesterol in the body. Dietary cholesterol can be a source of the "building block" materials the liver uses for this purpose, but other dietary fats, especially saturated fats, provide most of the source material for cholesterol manufacturing. Blood cholesterol levels can rise to unhealthy levels because as long as the liver has the ingredients to make cholesterol, it keeps doing so. There is no mechanism to tell the liver the body has enough cholesterol. The liver also destroys cholesterol that returns to it, as part of the liver's role in filtering waste substances from the blood. It dismantles cholesterol into particles that it either recycles for use in creating new cholesterol or sends back into the bloodstream for the kidneys to catch and filter out to be excreted in the urine.

As a fatty acid, cholesterol cannot dissolve in the BLOOD. Instead, protein carriers called lipoproteins envelop cholesterol particles. The lipoproteins are suspended in the blood, which carries them to where the body needs them. There are various forms of lipoproteins. Blood tests that measure blood cholesterol levels measure the cholesterol carried by low-density lipoproteins (LDL) and high-density lipoproteins (HDL). Some tests also measure another form of LDL cholesterol, very low-density lipoprotein VLDL. High levels of VLDL are associated with certain patterns of HYPERCHOLESTEROLEMIA and HYPERLIPIDEMIA that tend to be familial in nature.

LDL cholesterol is thick and sticky. It is the primary form of cholesterol in arterial plaque, the fatty deposits that accumulate along the walls of the arteries. It drops easily out of the bloodstream, and it has an affinity for other LDL particles. The higher the LDL blood level, the greater the risk for heart disease. HDL cholesterol is not as thick or sticky as LDL cholesterol, and it stays suspended in the bloodstream long enough for transport back to the liver, where the liver dismantles it. There is some evidence that HDL can attract LDL, carrying it along to the liver as well so the liver can dispose of it, too. The higher the HDL level, the lower the risk

BLOOD CHOLESTEROL LEVELS

CVD Risk	Total Cholesterol	HDL Cholesterol	LDL Cholesterol	Total: HDL Ratio
Desirable	less than 200	45 or higher	less than 100	3 or less
Borderline High Risk	200 to 239	36 to 45	100 to 159	3 to 4
High Risk	240 or higher	35 or lower	160 or higher	greater than 4

for heart disease. Researchers do not know what causes the liver to produce LDL instead of HDL.

Blood tests to measure blood cholesterol levels typically measure total cholesterol, HDL cholesterol, and LDL cholesterol. It is important to know the relationships among the forms of cholesterol to assess how they might affect health. It is possible to have a total cholesterol in the "desirable" range yet have a dangerously high LDL level. Generally, a high LDL cholesterol level accompanies a high total blood cholesterol level. Blood tests generally report total cholesterol, HDL cholesterol, LDL cholesterol, and the ratio between total and HDL.

Doctors recommend lifestyle changes including increased exercise and nutritious eating habits (with 30 percent or fewer calories coming from fat) to improve blood cholesterol readings that fall into the "borderline high risk" category. When blood cholesterol readings are in the "high risk" category, doctors recommend LIPID-LOWERING MEDICATIONS in addition to lifestyle changes. Doctors also often prescribe lipid-lowering medications when the LDL level is in the "high" category or even into the high end of the "moderate" category, regardless of the other levels. LDL seems to be the most significant factor, among the components of blood cholesterol, for heart disease.

High blood cholesterol levels become particularly dangerous when they coexist with HYPERTENSION (high BLOOD PRESSURE). Arterial plaque becomes brittle over time, and under constant battering from the flow of blood, fragments of it easily break away. These fragments can become lodged in the arteries that supply the brain, causing STROKE, or in the heart, causing HEART ATTACK. They also can lodge elsewhere in the body, causing occlusions that block the flow of blood to other organs. Although normal blood cholesterol levels are no guarantee of heart health or that a person will not have a heart attack, blood cholesterol is among the

risk factors for heart disease that can be controlled for most people.

See also CAROTID ENDARTERECTOMY; CHOLESTYRAMINE; COLESTIPOL; CORONARY ARTERY BYPASS GRAFT (CABG); CORONARY RISK PROFILE; EXERCISE; LIFESTYLE AND HEART HEALTH; NUTRITION AND DIET; PLAQUE, ARTERIAL.

cholesterol, dietary See NUTRITION AND DIET.

cholesterol-lowering medications See LIPID-LOWERING MEDICATIONS.

cholestyramine A LIPID-LOWERING MEDICATION taken to reduce the total BLOOD cholesterol level. Common brand names include Questran. Cholestyramine was among the first of the medications to become available for treating HYPERCHOLESTEROLEMIA and is a bile-acid sequestrant (sometimes called a bile-binding resin). It works by binding with bile in the intestinal tract, which prevents the body from digesting fats. This reduces the amount of cholesterol the body absorbs from dietary sources. Cholestyramine lowers total cholesterol and LDL cholesterol; it has no effect on other lipids. It comes in a powder that can be mixed with various liquids and soft foods such as oatmeal and soups.

Cholestyramine can cause numerous gastrointestinal side effects including dyspepsia (heartburn), nausea, abdominal cramping, flatulence (gas), and diarrhea or constipation. Constipation can become severe enough to cause fecal impaction and intestinal obstruction, which is a medical emergency. A doctor should evaluate abdominal pain that persists for longer than 24 hours. Cholestyramine interacts with numerous medications including BETA ANTAGONIST MEDICATIONS taken to treat HYPERTENSION, ANTICOAGULANT MEDICATIONS taken to prevent blood clots, some ANTI-ARRHYTHMIA MEDICATIONS, thiazide and loop DIURETIC MEDICATIONS taken to treat hypertension and HEART FAILURE, some antibiotics taken to treat infections, and thyroid medications.

Cholestyramine can lower total blood cholesterol and LDL appreciably, 15 to 30 percent. Many people cannot tolerate the gastrointestinal side effects, however, particularly older people. Newer lipid-lowering medications have fewer such problems and provide more effective blood lipid level regulation. Occasionally doctors prescribe cholestyramine in combination with statins, another classification of lipid-lowering medication. There is evidence that bile sequestrants can reduce the risk for subsequent heart attack (myocardial infarction) in people who have already had one HEART ATTACK.

See also CHOLESTEROL, BLOOD; CHOLESTEROL, DIETARY; COLESEVELAM; COLESTIPOL; EXERCISE; HYPERLIPIDEMIA; LIFESTYLE AND HEART HEALTH; NUTRITION AND DIET; TRIGLYCERIDES.

chronic obstructive pulmonary disease (COPD)
A progressive condition that destroys lung tissue and reduces the ability of the lungs to oxygenate the BLOOD. The World Health Organization (WHO) reports COPD as the fourth-leading cause of death worldwide; it is the fourth-leading cause of death in the United States as well. The vast majority of COPD results from cigarette smoking. About 16 million Americans have COPD, which can take the form of emphysema (destruction of the alveoli, the tiny air sacs deep in the lungs where oxygen/carbon dioxide exchange takes place), chronic bronchitis (inflammation and irritation of the airways that over time causes the airways to become constricted or to collapse), or a combination of these conditions.

HEART FAILURE, particularly congestive heart failure and right heart failure, commonly accompanies moderate to severe COPD. Typically the right ventricle does not have to pump against much resistance to get BLOOD through the pulmonary artery and into the lungs. When COPD scars the lungs, resistance increases. There is less lung tissue available to participate in the oxygen/CARBON DIOX-IDE exchange, and blood that returns to the heart does not carry as much oxygen as it should. The HEART attempts to compensate by increasing the rate and force of its contractions, trying to move blood through the body faster. Over time, this takes a tremendous toll on the heart, which begins to enlarge to handle the increased workload. This soon becomes counterproductive, and the heart becomes less effective. The result is heart failure. In congestive heart failure, fluid accumulates in the lungs. This further increases the resistance the right ventricle faces in pumping blood to the lungs and in turn increases the degree of right heart failure.

Symptoms and Diagnostic Path
Because COPD develops over time, its early symptoms are subtle. They include a nagging cough and feeling winded or out of breath with moderate exertion such as climbing a flight of stairs or running to catch a bus. As the condition advances to moderate disease, symptoms become more persistent and intrusive. The cough increases in persistence, and there are sudden coughing episodes that often bring up mucus (called COPD exacerbations or flare-ups). Shortness of breath (DYSPNEA) begins to limit physical activity. In advanced COPD, dyspnea is constant, coughing brings up an abundance of mucus, and there is often CYANOSIS (bluish tint to the lips and skin) and peripheral EDEMA (fluid accumulation). When congestive heart failure is present, its symptoms are similar, which compounds their intensity.

The diagnostic path typically begins with AUSCULTATION (listening to the heart and lungs with a STETHOSCOPE), chest X-ray, and general blood tests. The doctor may also request ELECTROCARDIOGRAM (ECG) and ECHOCARDIOGRAM to evaluate heart function. Various tests can assess CARDIAC CAPACITY, to further assess heart involvement, and LUNG CAPACITY to measure lung function. Some procedures and tests that seem unrelated to COPD are nonetheless essential for ruling out potential cardiovascular conditions. As well, COPD often coexists with CARDIOVASCULAR DISEASE (CVD), so it is important to obtain a comprehensive diagnostic picture.

A simple test called spirometry, which measures how much air a person can exhale, provides an accurate assessment of lung function. Spirometry produces two results, FEV1 (forced expiratory volume in one second), which is the volume of air that a person can exhale in one second, and FVC (forced vital capacity), which is the volume of air that a person can exhale after taking a deep breath and pushing air out for as long as possible. FEV1 is the more important measure for COPD and is given as a percentage. Doctors use FEV1, along with symptoms, to stage COPD. Staging determines treatment and prognosis (outlook). FEV1 also helps to assess the effectiveness of treatment approaches as well as the progression of lung damage as the disease advances.

Treatment Options and Outlook

Because there is no cure for COPD, treatment focuses on managing both the progression of the disease and the symptoms. A very important factor is to stop smoking and avoid areas where other people smoke. The two main types of medications to help reduce symptoms are:

- bronchodilators, which relax the airways so more air can enter the lungs. Bronchodilators may be short- or long-acting and come in oral and inhaler forms. They may be anticholinergic medications such as ipratropium and tiotropium, or beta-2 antagonist medications such as albuterol and formoterol. Some products combine these kinds of medications.

- corticosteroids, which reduce inflammation and swelling. These come in oral (prednisone) and inhaled (fluticasone propionate, beclomethasone) forms. Some products combine a corticosteroid and a beta-2 antagonist (fluticasone and salmeterol, better known by its brand name Advair).

When there is cardiovascular involvement (congestive heart failure), DIURETIC MEDICATIONS are often added to help control fluid accumulation in the body (peripheral edema) and in the lungs. As COPD advances and oxygenation decreases, OXYGEN THERAPY can get more oxygen into the lungs with each breath. As damage to the lungs becomes severe, hospitalization for treatment with mechanical ventilation to assist with breathing and improve oxygenation may be necessary.

When COPD and heart failure are both moderate, the conventional treatments for each are

COPD Stage	FEV1	Symptoms	Treatment
Stage 1	80 percent or greater	cough that comes and goes; mucus with coughing; mild shortness of breath with exertion	primarily lifestyle: stop smoking and avoid areas where others smoke; minimize exposure to air pollution; develop healthy eating habits; breathing exercises; daily physical activity to the extent possible medical: may start using an inhaled brochodilator
Stage 2	50 to 79 percent	persistent, frequent cough with occasional episodes of significant coughing (flare-ups); much mucus with coughing; occasional wheezing; shortness of breath with modest activity; mild peripheral edema	inhaled and oral bronchodilator medications; breathing exercises; occasional corticosteroid medications
Stage 3	30 to 49 percent	increasingly persistent cough with much mucus; more frequent and more severe flare- ups; fairly constant wheezing; accumulation of fluid in the lungs; frequent bacterial bronchitis and pneumonia; weight loss	inhaled and oral bronchodilator medications; oral corticosteroid medications; diuretic medications; antibiotic medications when infection is present; oxygen therapy; frequent hospitalizations; possible mechanical ventilation
Stage 4	less than 30 percent	very difficult breathing; intense and potentially life-threatening coughing episodes; very limited physical activity; mental confusion	frequent or lengthy hospitalization; intravenous medications; mechanical ventilation; hospice

typically effective. However, as both conditions progress, the conventional treatments that are appropriate for either condition can cause problems with the other condition. Nonspecific beta antagonist medications commonly prescribed for heart failure, for example, can cause bronchial constriction which worsens the COPD. Effective treatment management requires close coordination between the pulmonologist (lung specialist) and the cardiologist (heart specialist).

The earlier treatment begins, the more effective it is at slowing the progression of the lung damage and heart involvement. Many people are able to enjoy good QUALITY OF LIFE for many years. However, COPD is progressive and eventually treatment is no longer effective at managing symptoms. It is beneficial for the person who has COPD as well as for family members and loved ones for the person to establish ADVANCE DIRECTIVES to specify end-of-life care desires.

Risk Factors and Preventive Measures

Cigarette smoking is the leading cause of COPD. Studies suggest that about half of people who begin smoking in their teens or early 20s have COPD by the time they are in their mid-40s, although they may not have symptoms for another 10 to 20 years. COPD may also develop as a result of chronic exposure to air pollutants such as dust and fumes. And sometimes the cause is unknown.

Not smoking, or smoking cessation for those who do smoke, is a key preventive measure for both COPD and congestive heart failure. It is also important to avoid exposure to pollutants and to wear appropriate protective gear in job situations in which such exposure is unavoidable. Regular physical activity, as can be tolerated, and nutritious eating habits are additional lifestyle measures that can improve symptoms, especially in the earlier stages of disease.

See also CARDIOMYOPATHY; PULMONARY SYSTEM; TOBACCO USE.

chronotropic incompetence A dysfunction of the heart's electrical system in which the HEART loses its ability to increase HEART RATE in response to exertion or EXERCISE. Chronotropic incompe-tence is associated with HEART FAILURE and is a key risk factor for SUDDEN CARDIAC ARREST. It can cause symptoms of fatigue and weakness, and can severely limit physical activity. When it does so, the cardiologist may choose to implant a PACEMAKER to help the heart maintain an appropriate heart rate. The presence of chronotropic incompetence more often is a factor the cardiologist considers in determining the appropriate course of treatment for underlying heart conditions. An EXERCISE STRESS TEST can confirm chronotropic incompetence.

See also LIVING WITH HEART DISEASE.

cigarette smoking See TOBACCO USE.

cilostazol An ANTICOAGULANT MEDICATION taken to treat INTERMITTENT CLAUDICATION, a condition in which painful cramps develop in the lower legs with exertion such as walking. Common brand names include Pletal. Cilostazol works by inhibit-ing platelet aggregation, the first stage in the clot-ting process in which platelets become "sticky" and clump together. This helps BLOOD to flow more smoothly through the arteries in the legs that have become narrowed as a consequence of peripheral vascular disease (PVD), a form of CARDIOVASCULAR DISEASE (CVD) that affects the arteries distant from the heart. ATHEROSCLEROSIS (fatty deposits along the interior walls of the arteries) and ARTERIOSCLE-ROSIS (loss of flexibility of the artery due to changes in the muscle fibers of the arterial wall) are the primary causes of PVD.

GRAPEFRUIT AND GRAPEFRUIT JUICE prevent the liver from producing the enzymes that metabo-lize cilostazol, causing high levels of cilostazol to accumulate in the blood. People taking cilostazol should avoid grapefruit and grapefruit juice (other citrus fruits do not cause this interaction). Cilostazol interacts with some antibiotics and CALCIUM CHAN-NEL ANTAGONIST MEDICATIONS. Common side effects are primarily gastrointestinal and include nausea, flatulence (gas), and diarrhea. Rare but serious side effects include ARRHYTHMIAS and HEART FAILURE or worsening of existing heart failure. People diag-nosed with heart failure should not take cilostazol.

See also PENTOXIFYLLINE.

circulation The path and pattern that BLOOD follows as it flows through the arteries, veins, and capillaries of the body. The circulatory path starts and concludes with the HEART. Oxygenated blood leaves the heart to nourish the tissues of the body and returns to the heart bearing the waste by-products of cellular metabolism. The body's volume of blood, about 10 pints (five liters), makes the full circuit of the body about once every minute.

Although ancient physicians recognized that blood and the heartbeat were essential to life, they lacked understanding of the body's structures and functions. The Greek physician Hippocrates (460–377 B.C.), credited by history as the "father of modern medicine" and an advanced thinker by the standards of his time, was the first to refute the long-standing belief that the heart was the center of thought and reason. However, he held with his colleagues the perception that although the arteries arose from the heart they carried air—wrong on the anatomy front but not altogether incorrect from the point of function, as arterial blood is responsible for oxygenating the body. Veins, medical wisdom of this ancient time held, arose from the liver to carry bile—which was not a digestive liquid but rather one of the humors, or essential elements, vital to life.

It was another 500 years before the Roman physician Galen (A.D. 130–200) connected the functions of the heart, lungs, and blood, although he too perpetuated some of the mistaken notions of his time. Galen put forth the premise that digestion produced bile, which flowed to the liver where it became converted to blood. As blood then moved through the body, Galen believed, it became the "food" that fed its tissues. Galen recognized that blood moved through the heart but perpetuated also the belief that the arteries transported air. Despite its complex and often contradictory presentations of structure and function, Galen's postulations formed the foundation of medical practice and understanding of the cardiovascular system for 14 centuries.

A clear comprehension of the body's circulatory network remained obscure until WILLIAM HARVEY (1578–1657), an English physician, published his landmark manuscript *Exercitatio Anatomica De Motu Cordis et Sanguinis in Animalibus* in 1628 (English translation: *An Anatomical Treatise on the Motion of the Heart and Blood in Animals*). Somewhat heretical in its time, *De Motu Cordis*, as the manuscript is commonly known, redefined understanding of the human body and the direction of medicine. Harvey correctly identified the relationships among heart, lungs, arteries, and veins and suspected, though could not prove in the pre-microscope time in which he lived, the structure and function of capillaries. The most revolutionary of Harvey's postulations was that it was the beating of the heart that sent blood through the arteries and veins of the body.

Harvey's presentation of circulation as a mechanical process became the launching pad for centuries of study and exploration, with advances in technology spurring new discoveries even through modern times. Researchers continue to investigate the functioning of the circulatory network, learning through work with genetics, sophisticated cardiovascular imaging techniques and technologies, and molecular studies.

See also CARDIOVASCULAR SYSTEM.

circulatory system See CARDIOVASCULAR SYSTEM.

Clark, Barney A retired dentist with severe HEART FAILURE who became the world's first total ARTIFICIAL HEART recipient. On December 1, 1982, cardiovascular surgeon WILLIAM DEVRIES and his surgical team at the University of Utah cut away the severely damaged ventricles of Clark's HEART and replaced them with a dual-pump mechanical heart, the Jarvik-7 designed by researcher Robert Jarvik. Although the pumps were small enough to fit into the cavity left by removing the diseased ventricles, they required a large external compressor connected by seven feet of tubing to keep them pumping. The tubes extended out of Clark's chest to the compressor. For the 112 days that Clark lived following the heart implant, those tubes tethered him to a washing-machine sized pumping unit at his bedside.

Numerous complications plagued Clark following the surgery, and he had to have several additional operations to fix problems with the Jarvik-7. Clark had seizures, STROKES, and constant nosebleeds related to the medications he had to take to prevent his blood from clotting. DeVries, Jarvik, and Clark all made history on that December day, as much for the accomplishments of the surgery as for the debate that arose as the world witnessed the restricted quality of life that marked the final weeks of Clark's life. Critics were harsh, and the event marked a turning point in artificial heart research. It became clear to researchers that only a self-contained pumping device was a viable option, and research attention shifted to devising pumps that could assist, rather than replace, a diseased heart. Barney Clark died on March 23, 1983.

See also BARNARD, CHRISTIAAN; COOLEY, DENTON; DEBAKEY, MICHAEL; HEART, ARTIFICIAL; JARVIK, ROBERT; LEFT VENTRICULAR ASSIST DEVICE (LVAD); WASHKANSKY, LOUIS.

claudication A cramping pain in the legs caused by PERIPHERAL VASCULAR DISEASE (PVD), a form of ATHEROSCLEROSIS. Claudication occurs when the arteries in the legs become so narrowed and hardened that they are unable to allow increased BLOOD flow to the muscles in the lower extremities during EXERCISE. Doctors generally view claudication as both a condition in its own right and a symptom of underlying CARDIOVASCULAR DISEASE (CVD). CLAUDICATION comes from the Latin word *claudicare*, which means "to limp."

Symptoms and Diagnostic Path

The primary symptom of claudication is cramping pain in the muscles of the legs or feet, commonly the thigh or calf, that occurs during exercise. It may affect one leg or both legs and ranges from achy tiredness to sharp pain that forces immediate cessation of activity. Although the pain occurs most often with exercise, when the underlying PVD is severe claudication may occur even at rest. Diagnosis includes blood tests to measure blood lipids (CHOLESTEROL and TRIGLYCERIDES), taking the pulses along various points of the legs and feet, and blood pressure readings for the legs. DOPPLER ULTRASOUND and MAGNETIC RESONANCE IMAGING (MRI), or less commonly ANGIOGRAPHY, of the legs can provide detailed information about the volume and rate of blood flow in the legs.

Treatment Options and Outlook

As for other forms of atherosclerosis, treatment for claudication combines lifestyle modifications and medications. Doctors typically recommend aspirin therapy (taking low-dose ASPIRIN daily for the anticoagulant and anti-inflammatory effects), or may prescribe a platelet inhibitor medication such as CLOPIDOGREL (Plaxil), CILOSTAZOL (Pletal), or PENTOXAFYLLINE (Trental) to slow the blood-clotting process. Lifestyle modifications include smoking cessation, low-fat eating habits, and daily physical activity that exercises the legs such as walking, bicycling, and swimming. WEIGHT MANAGEMENT, including weight loss if appropriate, is essential.

Surgery becomes an option when leg arteries are severely occluded or other treatment fails to bring relief. Surgical treatment options include peripheral percutaneous balloon ANGIOPLASTY to compress the occlusion and place a STENT, an arterial bypass graft, and ATHEROTOMY. Though the atherosclerotic damage to the arteries is permanent by the time claudication develops, treatment can significantly reduce symptoms. It is also important to treat the other forms of CVD, such as HYPERTENSION and CORONARY ARTERY DISEASE (CAD), that are likely present.

Risk Factors and Preventive Measures

Cigarette smoking, HYPERLIPIDEMIA, DIABETES, and OBESITY are key risk factors for claudication. Inactivity and family history are also contributing factors. The risk for claudication, as with most forms of heart disease, increases with age. Preventive measures focus on lifestyle factors such as nutritious eating habits, daily exercise, and maintaining a healthy weight.

See also DIABETES AND HEART DISEASE; LIFESTYLE AND HEART HEALTH; MEDICATIONS TO TREAT HEART DISEASE; SURGERY TO TREAT CARDIOVASCULAR DISEASE.

clinical research studies Scientific investigations conducted under strictly controlled conditions to assess the effectiveness of new treatments and drugs. Clinical research studies might involve new drugs (in which case they might be called clinical pharmacology studies or trials), devices such as HEART valves or ventricular assist devices (VADs), treatment approaches, lifestyle interventions, and surgical procedures. In the United States federal regulations establish the legal and ethical guidelines that researchers must follow. Although all clinical research involves some risk, these guidelines attempt to safeguard participant health, safety, and well-being to the extent possible. Anyone who participates in a clinical research study should receive full and comprehensive information about the study's goals, methods, and risks. Federal guidelines require all research participants to sign a statement of INFORMED CONSENT that acknowledges the participant's understanding and acceptance of the study's risks and defines the researcher's responsibilities, including any medical treatment made necessary by study participation.

Clinical research studies can be privately or publicly funded and directed. Dozens of studies are under way at any given time, conducted at or under the auspices of government agencies such as the National Institutes of Health (NIH), university-based research facilities, medical centers and hospitals, and cardiology practice groups throughout the country. The NIH maintains a Web site, www.clinicaltrials.gov, that provides information about the current status of clinical research studies, including recruitment parameters and contact information.

The NIH identifies four primary classifications of clinical research studies:

- **Treatment studies** investigate new treatment options such as medications or medication regimens, devices, and operative procedures for people who already have heart disease.
- **Prevention studies** test methods to prevent people from developing heart disease. These investigations might explore lifestyle factors such as diet and exercise, the preventive effects of drugs such as LIPID-LOWERING MEDICATIONS when taken prophylactically, or the effectiveness of ANTIOXIDANT therapy. Prevention trials typically look at not only the method's effectiveness in reducing the risks of heart disease but also the willingness of participants to comply with the method.

- **Screening studies** attempt to find practical ways to identify the presence of heart disease in its earliest stages, before there are symptoms and while any damage is still reversible. Many experts believe that nearly all heart disease in adults results from lifestyle factors that cause damage to develop over decades and preventing this process through lifestyle changes could nearly eradicate heart disease.
- **QUALITY OF LIFE studies** look at the consequences of treatment on happiness and ability to enjoy pleasurable activities, aside from health status, for people who have chronic heart disease or who have undergone significant intervention such as HEART TRANSPLANT. The saga of BARNEY CLARK, who received the world's first artificial heart in 1982, drew scrutiny to this dimension of medical technology as television brought to the public's view Clark's severely restricted life following his landmark operation.

Most clinical research studies take place over months or years, and complete four progressive phases of investigation. Human volunteers participate in phases 2 and 3; phase 4 is the ongoing collection of data after the method, medication, or device receives approval for use and is no longer considered investigational. Typically, people who enroll in clinical research studies continue to receive all other medical care through their regular doctors. It is important for all doctors to know of a person's participation in a clinical research study, and to consult with researchers before making any changes in the person's medical care (including medications).

See also INVESTIGATIONAL TREATMENTS; FRAMINGHAM HEART STUDY; HELSINKI HEART STUDY; LIFESTYLE AND HEART HEALTH; LYON DIET HEART STUDY; NATIONAL CHOLESTEROL EDUCATION PROGRAM; NURSES' HEALTH STUDY; WOMEN'S HEALTH INITIATIVE.

clonidine A medication taken to treat HYPERTENSION (high BLOOD PRESSURE). Common brand names include Catapres and Duraclon and are available in tablet form or as a transdermal (skin) patch. Some products, such as Combipres, combine clonidine with a thiazide DIURETIC medication. Clonidine slows the HEART RATE and lowers both systolic (during contraction) and diastolic (during relaxation) pressures. Side effects include drowsiness, dry mouth, constipation, headache, and ARRHYTHMIAS. Transdermal patches can cause skin irritation, rash, and other forms of contact dermatitis. Tricyclic ANTIDEPRESSANT MEDICATIONS can reduce clonidine's effectiveness. Some people experience relief from migraine headaches with clonidine.

See also ANTIHYPERTENSION MEDICATIONS; BETA ANTAGONIST MEDICATIONS; CALCIUM CHANNEL ANTAGONIST MEDICATIONS; MEDICATIONS TO TREAT HEART DISEASE.

clopidogrel An ANTICOAGULANT MEDICATION taken to reduce the formation of BLOOD clots (thrombi). Common brand names include Plavix. Clopidogrel works by inhibiting adenosine triphosphate (ATP) binding, a key process in allowing PLATELETS to aggregate (clump together). Preventing this binding inhibits platelet aggregation and reduces the blood's ability to clot (thrombose), lowering the risk of repeat STROKE and HEART ATTACK. Side effects include gastrointestinal distress, dizziness, and skin irritation. Doctors often prescribe clopidogrel in combination with aspirin immediately before and following ANGIOPLASTY to reduce the risk of clot formation; following a stroke; and following a heart attack.

In March 2010 the U.S. Food and Drug Administration (FDA) added a "black box" warning to clopidogrel labeling because recent studies showed that people with reduced functioning of the liver enzyme CYP & C19 cannot fully metabolize clopidogrel. This means that in such people, clopidogrel is less effective. There are tests to determine whether CYP2C19 function is a concern.

See also ASPIRIN; COAGULATION; MEDICATIONS TO TREAT HEART DISEASE; TICLOPIDINE; WARFARIN.

clot See COAGULATION.

clot-busting medications See THROMBOLYTIC MEDICATIONS.

coagulation The formation of BLOOD clots (thrombosis). The coagulation process begins when there is damage to blood vessels. This damage can be microscopic, as in inflammation that irritates the interior walls of the arteries, or apparent, as in a cut or wound, and activates a sequence of events (sometimes referred to as the "coagulation cascade") that culminates with the formation of fibrin. Coagulation is an essential dimension of hemostasis, the body's efforts to maintain the equilibrium of its blood supply by preventing blood loss.

Coagulation begins when damaged blood vessels release the enzyme thromboplastin. When thromboplastin enters the bloodstream it interacts with calcium and the inactive enzyme prothrombin, which are already circulating in the blood. This interaction converts prothrombin to the enzyme thrombin, the presence of which attracts and activates platelets in the bloodstream. The platelets change from a smooth, round shape to jagged, stringy structures that stick to each other. Activated platelets release additional thromboplastin.

Additional chemical changes cause reactions that convert inactive substances into active ones called factors. Each of the 13 identified factors has a specific role in coagulation; the absence or dysfunction of any one or more of them causes bleeding disorders such as hemophilia. These factors, in combination with thrombin, convert the enzyme fibrinogen to fibrin, a sticky, threadlike substance that forms a microscopic mesh. This mesh traps additional platelets as well as other blood cells, which form a clump. As the coagulation cascade continues, other chemical interactions extract the fluid from the clump, causing it to tighten and harden. This becomes the familiar structure of a "clot" (thrombus). As healing takes place, specialized white blood cells dismantle and dissolve the fibrin structure.

Clots form more easily on surfaces that are irregular or rough. Arterial plaque causes the insides of the arterial walls to become rough and irregular and also causes irritation and inflammation that activate the coagulation process. This encourages clots to develop and adhere to the walls of the arteries, where they can restrict or occlude the flow of blood. Such a clot is called a thrombus; its formation is called thrombosis. Because the inflammation along the arterial walls is chronic, clots continue to form. They are susceptible to breaking away and moving to different locations (thromboembolus) as blood surges against them, possibly causing HEART ATTACK or STROKE. Clots also form when blood comes in contact with surfaces such as metals and plastics, the materials of which prosthetic HEART VALVES are made. For this reason, people who have had operations to replace diseased or malformed natural heart valves with prosthetic ones typically take ANTICOAGULANT MEDICATIONS to reduce the risk of clots forming. Some medications, such as oral contraceptives (birth control pills), cause higher amounts of clotting factors in the blood which can increase the blood's tendency to clot.

See also ASPIRIN; CLOPIDOGREL; CORONARY ARTERY DISEASE (CAD); DEEP VEIN THROMBOSIS; EMBOLISM; INFLAMMATION AND HEART DISEASE; THROMBOLYTIC MEDICATIONS; WARFARIN.

coarctation of the aorta A congenital malformation in which the aorta, the artery carrying BLOOD from the HEART to the body, is narrowed and constricted. Most commonly the narrowing occurs in the segment of the aorta at or near the ligamentum arteriosum, the part of the aorta after the left subclavian artery branches off to carry blood to the head and upper extremities. Blood supply to the upper body is normal but to the lower body is restricted.

Symptoms and Diagnostic Path

Generally there are few, if any, symptoms in infancy, unless there are other heart malformations present as well. Doctors usually diagnose coarctation of the aorta in childhood, adolescence, or early adulthood during routine physical examination that detects HYPERTENSION (high BLOOD PRESSURE) in the upper body and normal or low blood pressure in the lower extremities. Diagnostic procedures such as chest X-ray, ANGIOGRAM, ECHOCARDIOGRAM, ELECTROCARDIOGRAM (ECG), DOPPLER ULTRASOUND, and MAGNETIC RESONANCE IMAGING (MRI) can confirm the diagnosis.

Treatment Options and Outlook

Treatment requires intervention, usually an operation to cut out or replace with a graft the narrowed segment of the aorta, or to resect the accessible part of the stenosis and replace it with a patch to widen the coarctated aortic segment to improve the flow of blood to the lower body and restore normal blood pressure. In younger people, balloon dilation is sometimes effective. The longer coarctation of the aorta remains untreated, however, the greater the likelihood that hypertension will persist even after circulation returns to normal. Coarctation of the aorta that continues into later adulthood increases the heart's workload and can result in aortic aneurysm (ballooning of the aorta), STROKE or HEART ATTACK as a consequence of high blood pressure, and HEART FAILURE.

Risk Factors and Preventive Measures

Coarctation of the aorta develops at the location on the aorta where the ductus arteriosus, a blood vessel present before birth, inserts. In the fetus, the ductus arteriosus joins the aorta and the pulmonary artery, establishing a shunt around the nonfunctioning lungs. Shortly after birth, the ductus arteriosus closes off. Some doctors believe that coarctation of the aorta occurs when the ductus arteriosus does not completely contract or has extra tissue that extends into the aorta. There is a high incidence of coarctation of the aorta with the chromosomal disorder Turner's syndrome, in which one of the X chromosomes denoting female sex is significantly damaged or missing. Aside from this, coarctation of the aorta is more common in boys. There are no known preventive measures for coarctation of the aorta.

See also ANGIOPLASTY; HEART DISEASE; HEART DISEASE IN CHILDREN; PATENT DUCTUS ARTERIOSUS; SURGERY TO TREAT CARDIOVASCULAR DISEASE; STENOSIS.

cocaine and heart attack Research links illicit use of the narcotic cocaine with an increased risk of HEART DISEASE and HEART ATTACK, with some studies suggesting that the risk of heart attack within the first hour after using cocaine increases 20-fold or greater. Cocaine activates the body's inflammatory response, which can affect the arteries and accelerate the development of CORONARY ARTERY DISEASE (CAD). It also interferes with the blood's normal clotting mechanisms, increasing the blood's tendency to form clots. Nearly immediately following ingestion, cocaine causes a significant jump in BLOOD PRESSURE and HEART RATE and also increases the pumping force of the heart's ventricles. The risk of heart attack is highest in people who have diagnosed or undetected heart disease such as CAD. The presence of CAD further increases the risk for heart attack and CARDIAC ARREST. The risk for STROKE also increases. Although these risks increase with continued cocaine use, even the first use, regardless of age, can cause a fatal heart attack.

See also DRUG ABUSE AND HEART DISEASE; HYPERTENSION.

coenzyme Q-10   An ANTIOXIDANT that some research studies suggest supports health and inhibits diseases such as HEART DISEASE and cancer that result from chronic, long-term damage to cells and tissues. Coenzyme Q-10 exists naturally in numerous foods, including beef, soybeans, peanuts, salmon, and spinach, and also is available as a nutritional supplement. People with chronic heart conditions such as HEART FAILURE and HYPERTENSION tend to have lower levels of coenzyme Q-10 than people without heart disease. Researchers do not know, however, whether boosting coenzyme Q-10 levels through diet or supplementation can slow, halt, or reverse heart disease. There is some question about whether coenzyme Q-10 interferes with ANTICOAGULANT MEDICATIONS.

See also NUTRITION AND DIET.

coffee consumption   See CAFFEINE.

cognitive function   The intellectual and memory activities of the brain. CARDIOVASCULAR DISEASE that affects the flow of BLOOD to the brain and interferes with the amount of oxygen and other nutrients can alter cognitive function. The blood flow might be intermittent, as can happen with occluded carotid arteries (arterial plaque deposits in the arteries of the neck). ATHEROSCLEROSIS (deposits along the inner walls of the arteries) and HYPERTENSION (high BLOOD PRESSURE) can result in fragments of arterial PLAQUE and blood clots being

dislodged and traveling embolized to the brain, where they can block the small arteries and cause brain cells to die. Depending on the extent of the damage, the noticeable effect might be minimal, such as occasional lapses in memory or thought processes, or significant, such as loss of the ability to read, write, manage mathematical and logical processes, and memory loss that interferes with everyday activities.

Heart Surgery and Cognitive Function

There is some evidence that some people who undergo OPEN-HEART SURGERY and HEART TRANSPLANT experience disturbances of cognitive function, ranging from behavior changes such as emotional volatility to loss of memory and intellectual capacity, following surgery. Most people who notice such disturbances find that cognitive function gradually improves as they recover from the surgery, usually returning to the level it was before surgery. Some people, however, appear to have permanent changes in cognitive function. Researchers are studying this to determine the extent to which extracorporeal perfusion (oxygenating the blood outside the body using a HEART-LUNG BYPASS MACHINE) accounts for these disturbances, as a result of tiny clots in the blood that some researchers believe cause miniscule interruptions to the blood flow to the brain.

Heart Attack and Cognitive Function

A HEART ATTACK may disrupt the heart's ability to pump blood. The length of time this disruption lasts can interrupt blood flow to the brain, damaging delicate brain cells and neurological connections. Unstable emotions, volatile behavior, and disturbed memory and cognition are common following heart attack that results in cardiac arrest (the heart stops beating). Brain cells can survive only three to five minutes without oxygen, and they do not regenerate. For many people, cognitive function gradually returns to what it had been before the heart attack. If the brain goes without blood flow for long enough for substantial damage to occur, cognitive changes and dysfunction can be permanent.

Stroke and Cognitive Function

STROKE is the leading cause of damage to the brain that results in physical and cognitive dysfunction, and hypertension is the leading cause of stroke. Stroke occurs when a blood clot or fragment of arterial plaque lodges in an artery in the brain and blocks the flow of blood, or when there is a hemorrhage, depriving brain tissue of the oxygen and glucose it requires to support its activities. Damage that occurs during such deprivation generally is permanent and irreversible, although supportive therapies such as physical therapy, occupational therapy, and speech pathology can help restore lost functions by teaching other parts of the brain to perform them.

Estrogen and Cognitive Function

Before menopause, women have a significantly lower risk for HEART DISEASE than men of the same age, which appears to be a protective effect of estrogen. After menopause, a woman's risk for heart disease gradually increases to equal that of the risk of a man of the same age. For many years doctors believed that estrogen replacement therapy (ERT) extended estrogen's protection beyond menopause, and that estrogen supplementation helped to minimize the cognitive decline of aging as well. Studies in the 1990s began to cast doubt on this premise, and in 2002 researchers reported clear evidence that not only did postmenopausal estrogen supplementation fail to extend protection against heart disease but also that it raised a woman's risk for breast cancer and uterine cancer. Although there was some evidence that women taking estrogen supplementation after menopause were less likely to develop Alzheimer's disease (a degenerative condition marked by progressive loss of cognitive function), recent studies suggest that estrogen has no protective effect on cognitive function in women after menopause, either. Current medical recommendations no longer support estrogen supplementation—estrogen replacement therapy (ERT) or HORMONE REPLACEMENT THERAPY (HRT)—to maintain cognitive function in women past menopause.

Aging and Cognitive Function

The brain loses a certain level of cognitive function with advanced age. Typically a convergence of circumstances accounts for this. Brain cells become damaged and die over time, as do the arterioles (tiny arteries) that carry oxygen and vital nutrients to brain tissues. Chronic cardiovascular conditions such as atherosclerosis and ARTERIOSCLEROSIS (stiffening and thickening of the arteries) can cause diminished or inconsistent blood flow, further reducing the supply of oxygen to the brain. TRANSIENT ISCHEMIC ATTACKS (TIAs), or "ministrokes," become more common with increasing age. Although TIAs might have few obvious symptoms, their effects are cumulative. Other risks that affect cognitive function increase with advancing age as well, from degenerative neurological conditions such as Alzheimer's disease and Parkinson's disease to cardiovascular conditions such as CAROTID ARTERY STENOSIS and CORONARY ARTERY DISEASE (CAD).

Maintaining Cognitive Function

Most medical experts agree that the most effective way to maintain cognitive function is to stay involved in activities that require logical thinking and memory. Reading, writing (letters and journals), arithmetic, solving crossword puzzles and word games, and even putting together jigsaw puzzles are among the activities that exercise cognitive skills. When stroke, heart attack, and other health problems disrupt cognitive function, prompt and consistent therapy (physical therapy, occupational therapy, and speech pathology as appropriate) helps to train undamaged parts of the brain to take over some of the lost functions.

See also AGING; ANEURYSM; WOMEN'S HEALTH INITIATIVE.

cold/flu medication and hypertension Medications that contain decongestants such as pseudoephedrine act as stimulants that raise BLOOD PRESSURE and HEART RATE and can cause ARRHYTHMIAS (irregular heartbeat). These drugs are chemically similar to EPINEPHRINE (adrenaline), a cardiovascular stimulant, and act in similar ways in the body. For someone who already has HYPERTENSION (high blood pressure), cold and flu medications can cause dangerous elevations in blood pressure. Decongestants, and medication products that contain them, also can reduce the effectiveness of medications taken to treat hypertension. People who have hypertension, even if it is well-controlled with medication, should check with their doctors before taking any over-the-counter products to relieve cold and flu symptoms.

Antihistamines such as diphenhydramine and chlorpheniramine, also common ingredients in medications for cold and flu, do not affect blood pressure and heart rate and generally do not interfere with medications taken to treat hypertension. Although antihistamines do not relieve nasal and sinus congestion common with colds and flu, they can help dry secretions and reduce sneezing and itching. Some cold/flu medications that are decongestant-free carry special labeling identifying them as such. It is still a good idea to check with a doctor or pharmacist before taking these products, particularly for people who are taking antihypertensive medications.

See also MEDICATION SIDE EFFECTS; MEDICATIONS TO TREAT HEART DISEASE.

colesevelam　A LIPID-LOWERING MEDICATION taken to reduce blood CHOLESTEROL levels. Common brand names include WelChol. Colesevelam is a bile acid sequestrant; it works by binding with bile acids the liver manufactures from cholesterol circulating in the bloodstream. This lowers blood cholesterol levels by using up the cholesterol in the blood. Doctors sometimes prescribe colesevelam in combination with statins (a different classification of lipid-lowering medications). Colesevelam comes in tablets that should be taken with plenty of non-caffeinated liquids. Common side effects, which usually diminish or go away after taking the medication for a few weeks, include gastrointestinal upset, constipation, and headache. Colesevelam is most effective for lowering low-density lipoproteins (LDL cholesterol), the "bad" cholesterol, and modestly lowers total blood cholesterol.

See also ATHEROSCLEROSIS; CHOLESTYRAMINE; COLESTIPOL.

Colestid　See COLESTIPOL.

colestipol　A LIPID-LOWERING MEDICATION taken to reduce blood CHOLESTEROL levels. Common brand names include Colestid. Colestipol is a bile acid sequestrant; it binds with bile acids the liver manufactures from cholesterol circulating in the bloodstream. This binding prevents the small intestine from absorbing the bile acids, which in turn stimulates the liver to manufacture more bile acids. This uses increased amounts of cholesterol, lowering blood cholesterol levels. Colestipol comes in packets of granules that can be mixed with water, juice, or soft foods; and in tablets. It is important to drink plenty of non-caffeinated fluids when taking colestipol.

Colestipol can interfere with the absorption of some medications taken to treat HEART DISEASE, especially HYPERTENSION (high BLOOD PRESSURE), including thiazide DIURETICS, FUROSEMIDE (Lasix), and PROPANOLOL (Inderal). It also reduces the absorption of the antibiotic tetracycline, thyroid replacement hormones such as levothyroxine and other thyroid supplements, and fat-soluble vitamins (vitamins A, D, E, and K). Common side effects include digestive discomfort (gas and bloating) and constipation. These generally go away after taking colestipol for several weeks.

See also ATHEROSCLEROSIS; CHOLESTEROL, BLOOD; CHOLESTYRAMINE; COLESEVELAM.

collateral circulation　Small arteries, ordinarily nonfunctional, that open to route BLOOD around a blockage in an artery. Collateral arteries generally are small (arterioles) and appear to exist as normal structures that the body can activate as a reserve network to maintain crucial circulation. Doctors and researchers have observed collateral circulation in many locations in the body, including the HEART, brain, kidneys, and peripheral circulatory system, but it remains something of a mystery. Researchers are not sure what happens to activate collateral circulation, as it does not function in everyone. Many people with long-standing, and usually severe, CORONARY ARTERY DISEASE (CAD) have some degree of collateral circulation, which helps to get blood past blockages in the CORONARY ARTERIES to deliver oxygen to the myocardium (heart muscle). It appears that activation of collateral arteries takes place over time. Some researchers believe that while competent collateral circulation improves blood supply to the myocardium, it also allows

CAD to develop to a more significant degree before causing symptoms, resulting in an increased risk of "silent" heart attack. More research is necessary to determine whether there are ways to stimulate collateral circulation as a means of delaying the need for surgical interventions, and whether doing so provides a therapeutic advantage.

See also ANGIOGENESIS; ANGIOPLASTY; CORONARY ARTERY BYPASS GRAFT (CABG); GENE THERAPY.

commotio cordis   A rare and usually fatal sudden ventricular FIBRILLATION that results from a blunt blow to the chest directly over the HEART. The most common circumstance of commotio cordis is during sports such as baseball, softball, lacrosse, and hockey when a ball or puck hits a player in the chest. Commotio cordis also may occur as a result of a collision between players or between a player and a stationary object. Because commotio cordis is difficult to definitively diagnose, researchers believe it is more common than the number of reported cases suggests. More than half of documented cases are in boys age 14 and under.

Researchers believe commotio cordis results from a "perfect storm" of events in which the blow intersects with the precise moment at which the heart's electrical activity is vulnerable to interruption, although why this vulnerability exists remains unknown. Animal studies suggest this intersection is a 15-millisecond window when the blow strikes over a particular area of the left ventricle during a stage of the heart's electrical cycle called the T-wave upstroke, which is when the ventricles have completed contracting and are repolarizing (recharging). The prevailing belief is that the blow disrupts this process and the ventricles instead are thrown into early depolarization (discharging), establishing electrical chaos that sends the ventricles into immediate fibrillation.

Symptoms and Diagnostic Path

More than half of those who experience commotio cordis collapse and lose consciousness nearly immediately. Others may seem dazed and unsteady or appear fine and suddenly drop. Among those who survive, there are seldom any abnormalities to explain the event. Similarly, among those who do not survive, there is no evidence of what happened within the heart or of CARDIOVASCULAR DISEASE (CVD).

Treatment Options and Outlook

Treatment is immediate CARDIOPULMONARY RESUSCITATION (CPR) and electrical DEFIBRILLATION. Those who survive usually receive defibrillation within three minutes. However, it is uncommon that CPR begins soon enough because there is often a lag between the onset of ventricular fibrillation and the realization that the person is in crisis. Among documented cases of commotio cordis, only 15 percent have survived.

Risk Factors and Preventive Measures

Commotio cordis is a life-threatening crisis in which seconds matter. Because rapid defibrillation appears the key to survival, medical experts strongly urge the presence of AUTOMATED EXTERNAL DEFIBRILLATORS (AEDs) at locations where sporting events take place, no matter the level of event and especially for youth recreational sports. Research has shown that slower, softer objects, such as safety baseballs in youth games, are less likely to cause commotio cordis. Educational efforts to encourage coaches, parents, and spectators to react immediately when a player receives a blow to the chest, rather than waiting to see if the player is all right, could help get emergency aid to those who need it in time to save their lives.

See also CARDIOMYOPATHY; CONDUCTION SYSTEM; ELECTROCARDIOGRAM (ECG); SUDDEN CARDIAC ARREST.

computed tomography (CT) scan   A noninvasive, sophisticated imaging technology that combines X-rays with computers to generate two-dimensional views of internal body structures. During a computed tomography (CT) scan, the person lies on a narrow table that slides into a ring-shaped X-ray machine. An X-ray beam rotates inside the ring, targeting the specified body region. A computer then assembles the resulting "slices" into images that are displayed on the computer screen and can be printed or developed on X-ray film. A conventional CT scan is useful for detecting damage to the myocardium (heart muscle) such as that which might follow a HEART ATTACK resulting from severe CAD. It also shows the major vessels leaving and entering the heart, the lungs, and other soft tissue structures of the chest, and can help to determine whether symptoms such as shortness of breath or pain result from heart disease (CAD or HEART FAILURE), inflammation or infection such as ENDO-CARDITIS or PERICARDITIS, or lung problems. CT scan also helps to diagnose CARDIOMYOPATHY (enlarged heart), valve disease, and congenital malformations of the heart and its blood vessels.

Doctors also use CT scan to identify ANEURYSMS in the central body and in the brain, and to evaluate cardiovascular disease in other parts of the body such as CAROTID STENOSIS (atherosclerosis affecting the carotid arteries in the neck); peripheral vascular disease (PVD; atherosclerosis affecting the arteries in the legs, feet, arms, or hands); the occurrence of transient ISCHEMIC ATTACKS (TIAs) or "ministrokes" affecting the brain; and the extent of damage to the brain following STROKE. CT scan can be done with or without contrast dye injection. Contrast dye enhances cardiovascular structures.

CT scan causes no physical discomfort and takes 30 minutes to an hour, depending on the parts of the body being scanned. Contrast dye injection can cause stinging at the injection site; people who have allergies to seafood or iodine should alert the radiologist as some dye solutions contain iodine. When contrast dye is to be used, the cardiologist generally has the person refrain from drinking or eating for four hours before the scan to reduce the potential for nausea and vomiting. Some people experience anxiety, particularly if they are claustrophobic; the cardiologist can give a mild sedative just before the scan when this is the case.

See also ANGIOGRAPHY; DIPYRIDAMOLE STRESS TEST; DOPPLER ULTRASOUND; ECHOCARDIOGRAM; ELECTRO-CARDIOGRAM; ELECTRON BEAM COMPUTED TOMOGRAPHY (EBCT) SCAN; MAGNETIC RESONANCE IMAGING (MRI); MULTI-UNIT GATED ACQUISITION SCAN; POSITRON EMIS-SION TOMOGRAPHY (PET); SINGLE PHOTON EMISSION COMPUTED TOMOGRAPHY (SPECT) SCAN; ULTRASOUND.

conduction system   The mechanisms by which the HEART generates and manages electrical activity. The conduction system of the normal, healthy heart is a straightforward, orderly, and precise biochemical process. The SINOATRIAL (SA) NODE, a cluster of specialized cells located on the back wall of the right atrium near the entrance of the vena cava (the large vein bringing BLOOD from the body to the heart), initiates an electrical impulse. This impulse, called an action potential, spreads through the myocardial cells of both atria simultaneously, "igniting" them in a wavelike pattern (called excitation) along specialized pathways that results in synchronized contraction of the atria. The ATRIO-VENTRICULAR (AV) NODE, located at the junction of the atria and the ventricles, momentarily halts, gathers, and refocuses the impulses, releasing them as a unified stream that travels along a network of conductive fibers called the HIS-PURKINJE SYSTEM, that run through the interventricular septum (wall of heart muscle that separates the two ventricles). At the apex, or bottom point, of the heart, the eletrical impulse stream splits and travels up the walls of each ventricle in wavelike patterns that cause synchronized contraction of the ventricles. This pattern repeats with each cardiac cycle.

See also ACCESSORY PATHWAY; ARRHYTHMIA.

congenital heart disease   See HEART DISEASE.

congestive heart failure   See HEART FAILURE.

constipation   Difficult bowel movements. Constipation is common and can result from many causes, most often dietary. The most effective remedy for constipation is prevention—eating foods that are high in fiber, drinking plenty of water, and getting regular exercise. Fiber draws fluid into the intestines and adds bulk to the stool. A doctor should evaluate chronic constipation to make sure there are no underlying medical causes.

Constipation is common following surgery, as the drugs administered during surgery slow smooth muscle function, reduce bowel activity, and diminish movements of gastrointestinal fluids. Narcotic pain relievers and reduced physical activity during post-operative recovery can further exacerbate postsurgical constipation. It can take a week or so for bowel function to return to normal after surgery. Doctors often prescribe stool softeners or a mild laxative to help the bowels get back on track. Some medications, such as antidepressants and antihypertensives (medications taken to treat high blood pressure), also can cause constipation. Some fiber products such as psyllium can interfere with the absorption of medications. It is important to talk with a doctor or pharmacist before using such products.

Constipation often causes people to feel that they must strain to have bowel movements. Straining exerts pressure on the cardiovascular system and can cause a variety of problems from varicose veins to potentially dangerous spikes in BLOOD PRESSURE. Straining increases the heart's workload, which can exacerbate ANGINA and other symptoms of HEART FAILURE.

See also ANTIDEPRESSANT MEDICATIONS; ANTIHYPERTENSIVE MEDICATIONS; DIET AND NUTRITION; EXERCISE; VALSALVA MANEUVER.

contractility The extent to which a muscle cell can contract, or shorten. Contractility is an essential aspect of the HEART's ability to pump BLOOD, and represents an intricate integration of chemical and electrical events among heart cells. Decreased contractility reduces the heart's force and efficiency, correspondingly increasing the effort necessary to meet the body's circulatory needs. Decreased contractility is a physiological hallmark of HEART FAILURE and CARDIOMYOPATHY. ECHOCARDIOGRAM, an ultrasound examination of the myocardium (heart muscle), can help to identify decreased contractility. Some medications taken to treat heart failure act to improve myocardial contractility, increasing the efficiency and force of each heartbeat to lessen the heart's overall workload. Some degree of reduction in contractility occurs naturally with aging. Cardiovascular conditions such as CORONARY ARTERY DISEASE (CAD) and (HEART ATTACK) as well as damage to the heart that results from long-term chronic alcohol abuse, also diminish contractility. Aerobic fitness through regular EXERCISE helps to maintain maximum contractility.

See also ALCOHOL CONSUMPTION AND HEART DISEASE; CARDIAC OUTPUT; LEFT VENTRICULAR EJECTION FRACTION (LVEF); STROKE VOLUME.

Cooley, Denton A., M.D. (1920–) A pioneering HEART surgeon who founded the Texas Heart Institute in Houston, Texas. As a young surgery resident, Cooley assisted in the historic first "blue baby" operation performed by pediatric heart surgeon Alfred Blalock, M.D., correcting an infant's congenital heart defects to restore proper circulation and oxygenation. In 1968 Cooley performed the first heart transplant conducted in the United States, and in 1969 he implanted the first artificial heart in a human being. During a career in which Cooley performed or participated in more than 90,000 heart operations, he developed numerous procedures and technologies that helped to set the standards for modern cardiovascular surgery. Cooley's numerous awards include the National Medal of Technology (1998), the National Medal of Freedom (1984), and the international René Leriche Prize (1967).

See also BARNARD, CHRISTIAAN; BLALOCK, ALFRED; DEVRIES, WILLIAM C.; JARVIK, ROBERT; TAUSSIG, HELEN.

Cordarone See AMIODARONE.

Coreg See CARVEDILOL.

coronary arteries The arteries that wrap around the HEART, supplying the myocardium (heart muscle) with BLOOD. The word *coronary* comes from the Latin word that means "to crown" or "encircle." The adult heart has four major coronary arteries that branch into a network of smaller arteries to form a weblike structure around the heart. The right coronary artery and the left coronary artery arise from the aorta (the major artery carrying oxygenated blood from the heart to the body) as it leaves the heart.

• The **right coronary artery** supplies the right side of the heart, which receives blood from the body (right atrium) and pumps it to the lungs for oxygenation (right ventricle). It branches into the **right posterior descending artery,** which carries blood to the back of the heart, and the

acute marginal artery, which supplies blood to the heart's natural pacemaker, the SINOATRIAL (SA) NODE.

- The **left coronary artery,** which supplies the workhorse left side of the heart, is substantially larger than the right coronary artery and branches into two major arteries, the **left anterior descending artery,** which supplies blood to the front portion of the left ventricle, and the **circumflex artery,** which wraps all the way around the heart. These arteries further divide into the **oblique marginal artery** and smaller arteries called **diagonals.**

ATHEROSCLEROSIS (buildup of arterial plaque) can affect any or all of the coronary arteries and usually does involve all of the coronary arteries to some degree. The seriousness of the resulting CORONARY ARTERY DISEASE (CAD) depends on the extent of narrowing (called STENOSIS) or occlusion that exists and what symptoms the person experiences. There is not necessarily a direct correlation between the amount of occlusion and the severity of symptoms, however. The heart's oxygen needs are nearly twice those of other tissues in the body; the heart takes about 70 percent of the oxygen from the blood that circulates through the coronary artery network. Because of this, any interruption of blood flow can cause the death of myocardial cells (MYOCARDIAL INFARCTION) and the disruption of heart function.

See also ANGINA; ANGIOPLASTY; COLLATERAL CIRCULATION; CORONARY ARTERY BYPASS GRAFT (CABG); PLAQUE, ARTERIAL; STENT.

coronary artery bypass graft (CABG) An operation to replace occluded (blocked) arteries that supply BLOOD to the HEART as a treatment for CORONARY ARTERY DISEASE (CAD). CAD is the most common form of heart disease in the United States and the leading cause of heart-related deaths. One of the most commonly performed operations in the United States today, coronary artery bypass graft (CABG) saves thousands of lives each year.

Conventional CABG is an OPEN-HEART SURGERY in which the surgeon stops the heart from pumping, temporarily rerouting the blood through a HEART-LUNG BYPASS MACHINE during the procedure. During a CABG the surgeon constructs replacement arteries, called grafts, that carry blood around the occluded CORONARY ARTERIES to restore the heart's blood supply. The surgeon typically constructs the grafts from artery segments harvested from the person's chest (internal mammary artery) and forearm (radial artery), and a segment from the large sapphenous vein in the thigh. These donor blood vessels are nonessential; the body quickly adapts to use other blood vessels to handle their functions.

CABG is a major invasion of the body. Although it saves thousands of lives each year, the extent of this invasion, coupled with the complexity of the procedure, carries significant risk of complications, including death. Surgeons are exploring minimally invasive procedures and techniques to reduce the risks and provide less traumatic intervention for CAD. At present these procedures, which typically use fiberoptic scopes (flexible, lighted tubes) and instruments the surgeon inserts into the cardiac cavity through small incisions, remain investigational, although they show great promise. As with most cardiovascular disease, prevention remains the optimal treatment. Medical experts believe nearly all ATHEROSCLEROSIS, including coronary artery disease, is preventable through smoking cessation, nutritional diet, regular physical EXERCISE, and WEIGHT MANAGEMENT.

Determining Whether CABG Is the Appropriate Treatment Option

CABG generally is the treatment of choice when there is a minimum 70 percent occlusion of one or more coronary arteries; most people who undergo CABG have 80 percent or greater occlusion in two or more coronary arteries. Diagnostic procedures such as ANGIOGRAM help to determine the extent of occlusion (also called STENOSIS). Other factors that come under consideration include the person's overall health status (including smoking and body weight), the presence of any other significant medical conditions such as CHRONIC OBSTRUCTIVE PULMONARY DISEASE (COPD) OR DIABETES, the existence of other cardiovascular disease such as HYPERTENSION OR HEART FAILURE, and the person's age. The surgeon will assess the potential for the success of other treatment options such as lifestyle modification, LIPID-LOWERING MEDICATIONS, and ANGIOPLASTY with or without STENT. Nonintervention (watchful waiting or doing nothing) always remains the person's choice.

What to Expect

Most people who undergo CABG spend five to seven days in the hospital and six to eight weeks recovering at home. The surgery itself lasts two to six hours, depending on the number of grafts. The person often checks into the hospital the night before surgery to allow for preoperative preparation including ELECTROCARDIOGRAM (ECG), blood tests, any other tests the surgeon requests, and shaving the chest and leg where operation will be done.

After the operation the person spends several hours in the recovery room, then transfers to the coronary intensive care unit (CICU). Most people stay two or three days in the CICU under close observation, then transfer to the regular surgical unit until the surgeon approves discharge to home. Nursing staff will encourage regular and frequent sitting, standing, and walking to help prevent blood clots from forming, clear the lungs of fluid that accumulates from the anesthesia, and get the recovery process under way.

Procedure

After the person receives general anesthesia, one surgeon harvests and prepares the donor blood vessels while another opens the chest to expose and prepare the heart. CABG might be "on-pump," diverting the body's oxygenation and circulatory functions to extracorporeal perfusion via heart-lung machine to stop the heart for the surgeon to operate on it, or "off-pump," in which the heart continues beating during the operation. The surgeon makes this determination based on various clinical factors; the surgical team generally prepares for either option. The surgeons suture (sew) the grafts onto the myocardium (heart muscle), attaching them to the aorta before and after the coronary artery occlusion to create the bypass. The surgeons repeat this procedure for each occluded coronary artery. When the grafts are all in place, the surgeons restore full circulation to the heart and restart its pumping. After observing the heart

in action to make sure there is no bleeding, the surgeons close the chest and the anesthesiologist allows the person to awaken.

Risks and Complications

Death during or immediately following the operation is the most significant complication, and occurs in about three of 100 CABG surgeries (1 to 3 percent mortality rate). Other potential complications include STROKE (from dislodged blood clots or arterial plaque fragments that lodge in arteries in the brain), peripheral thromboembolism (blood clots in the legs, feet, arms, or hands), kidney dysfunction or failure, lung or breathing problems from the anesthesia, and infection. Many people experience some degree of cognitive dysfunction (difficulty with memory and intellectual processes) for a few weeks to a few months after surgery; in some people, this dysfunction becomes permanent. Researchers are not sure why this happens.

Although a CABG may permanently relieve symptoms of CAD, atherosclerosis can develop in the grafts. It also is possible for the grafts to fail (for various reasons) or to release blood clots during the healing process. Surgeons prescribe ANTICOAGULANT MEDICATIONS to help prevent clotting problems. A person who has CABG relatively early in life (before age 60) might require repeat CABG later in life.

Long-Term Prognosis

Recovery at home following CABG is a progressive return to regular activities. Generally the surgeon restricts activities such as lifting and driving for six to eight weeks, to allow the sternum to heal completely. Physical activity such as walking is important. The person usually can return to most normal functions, including sex, when he or she feels capable of them. The surgeon may suggest delaying return to competitive athletics, particularly contact sports, and activities such as diving and bicycling. Most people benefit from a structured CARDIAC REHABILITATION program that provides nutritional guidance, monitored exercise, and emotional support. The surgeon or hospital can recommend reputable programs that operate under physician oversight.

More than 90 percent of people who undergo CABG return to full and productive lives, enjoying favorite activities within three to six months.

Studies show that 80 percent have no CAD symptoms five years following surgery, and 60 percent remain symptom-free 10 years following surgery. Lifestyle modifications—smoking cessation, nutritious diet, regular physical EXERCISE, and stress reduction—help establish and maintain cardiovascular health.

See also ANGIOGENESIS; COGNITIVE FUNCTION; COLLATERAL CIRCULATION; LIFESTYLE AND HEART HEALTH; MINIMALLY INVASIVE SURGERY; TOBACCO USE.

coronary artery disease (CAD)   The most common form of HEART DISEASE, in which the arteries that supply the HEART with BLOOD become occluded (clogged) by atherosclerotic plaque deposits that impede and sometimes cut off the flow of blood. About 13 to 16 million Americans have coronary artery disease (CAD), which is the leading cause of HEART ATTACK, CARDIAC ARREST, and death due to CARDIOVASCULAR DISEASE (CVD) in the United States. Doctors most commonly diagnose CAD in middle age or later, when it begins to cause symptoms such as CHEST PAIN (ANGINA). Women before menopause are less likely to develop CAD than are men of comparable age, although within 10 years following menopause the risk becomes the same for women and men. Many people are unaware they have CAD until they have heart attacks. CAD often coexists with other kinds of heart disease such as HYPERTENSION (high BLOOD PRESSURE).

CAD develops over time, typically decades, as excess lipids in the bloodstream accumulate on the inner walls of the CORONARY ARTERIES and begin to harden into arterial plaque. These deposits irritate the walls of the arteries, which causes inflammation and activates the body's immune response. This process draws blood cells to the area, where they become entrapped in the deposits. Rather than relieving the problem, the body's inflammatory response ends up contributing to it. Many health experts believe that CAD begins as early as childhood or adolescence as a consequence of high-fat diet and sedentary lifestyle. CAD can cause symptoms with blockages of 50 to 60 percent, although many people can remain symptom-free even with occlusions as high as 90 to 95 percent. CAD can be significantly worse in one coronary artery, but typically once it develops CAD affects all of the coronary arteries to some degree.

Factors That Contribute to CAD

Age, family history, and lifestyle are the three significant factors that contribute to CAD. Lifestyle is the most significant modifiable contributing factor for CAD. The key lifestyle elements that influence the development and severity of CAD include:

- TOBACCO USE, particularly cigarette smoking
- Overweight, particularly OBESITY (more than 20 percent above healthy body weight)
- High-fat diet
- Physical inactivity

Additional contributing factors are:

- DIABETES
- hypertension (high blood pressure)

For many people these elements exist in combination, which compounds their effects. There is a growing body of evidence that obesity is at least as significant a contributing factor for CAD as cigarette smoking. A certain degree of CAD appears to develop as a normal consequence of advanced age; the extent to which age is an independent contributor to CAD is difficult to separate from lifestyle elements. Some people are genetically predisposed to elevated blood lipid (CHOLESTEROL and TRIGLYCERIDES) levels, putting them at increased risk for developing CAD, and CAD that is more severe, at earlier ages.

Symptoms and Diagnostic Path

Many people who have CAD have no symptoms until heart attack occurs. When symptoms are present, they may include

- pressure or tightness in the chest
- chest pain (angina pectoris)
- shortness of breath or difficulty breathing

Symptoms may be present only during, or worsen with, exertion. Some people may feel vague discomfort that seems gastrointestinal or that appears after eating a heavy meal (resulting from the diversion of blood to handle digestion).

Diagnosing CAD

Various diagnostic procedures can determine whether, and the extent to which, CAD is present. These include:

- ELECTROCARDIOGRAM (ECG), which records the heart's electrical activity; moderate to severe CAD that disrupts the heart's blood flow can cause ARRHYTHMIAS (irregular HEARTBEATS) and changes in the normal profile of the heart's electrical activity that show up on ECG.

- ECHOCARDIOGRAM, which uses ultrasound (sound waves) to generate an image of the beating heart; this can reveal enlargement and thickening of the left ventricle (which happens when the heart's workload becomes increased for a length of time). Decreased blood flow to the heart muscle may result in irregularities of the walls of the heart, which suggest CAD.

- Imaging scans such as ELECTRON BEAM COMPUTED TOMOGRAPHY (EBCT), which reveals the presence of calcium in the coronary arteries (a key sign of arterial plaque accumulation), and POSITRON EMISSION TOMOGRAPHY (PET), which looks at the biochemical functioning of myocardial cells to assess whether heart function is efficient.

- ANGIOGRAM, in which the cardiologist inserts a catheter into the heart and injects dye into the coronary arteries to illuminate the flow of blood through them; this detects narrowing (stenosis) and blockages that impede blood movement.

Personal health history and general physical examination, including lab tests to measure blood lipid levels, also contribute to the diagnostic process.

Treatment Options and Outlook

Treatment with medications is often appropriate for mild to moderate CAD. More significant CAD (typically when any of the coronary occlusions exceeds 80 percent) requires surgical intervention for the most effective relief of symptoms.

Medical (Noninvasive) Treatments for CAD. The primary symptom of CAD, when symptoms are present, is chest pain or pressure (angina pectoris), which reflects the heart's inability to obtain enough oxygen and typically occurs with physical exertion or emotional stress. Most medical (medication-based) treatment approaches target symptom relief. Medications containing NITROGLYCERIN relieve angina for many people; nitroglycerin is available in numerous formulations. BETA ANTAGONIST MEDICATIONS inhibit epinephrine binding, reducing the heart's response to biochemical signals to increase its rate and output. This relieves angina and also helps to lessen stress on the heart. CALCIUM CHANNEL ANTAGONIST MEDICATIONS decrease the contraction of smooth muscle fibers that comprise arterial walls, helping to relax the arteries and increase the amount of blood that can flow through them. ANTIARRHYTHMIA MEDICATIONS regulate the rate and force of the heartbeat.

LIPID-LOWERING MEDICATIONS target the source of CAD by reducing the amount of fatty acids (CHOLESTEROL and TRIGLYCERIDES) circulating in the bloodstream. Although these medications cannot remove arterial plaque accumulations that already exist, they can help to prevent the accumulations from growing. There is some evidence that nonsurgical approaches to raise high-density lipoprotein ("good" cholesterol) and lower low-density lipoprotein ("bad" cholesterol) do help the body to remove existing arterial plaque; such approaches generally combine lipid-lowering medications with lifestyle modifications.

Surgical (Invasive) Treatments for CAD. Once CAD becomes established, surgical intervention is the only way to address its cause. Angioplasty is the less invasive surgical approach in which the cardiologist manipulates the occlusion through a catheter threaded into the coronary artery from a peripheral artery in the groin or arm. The cardiologist can use specialized rotating blades to "shave" away arterial plaque, or inflate a tiny balloon to press the plaque tightly against the artery's wall so it no longer blocks blood flow. The cardiologist may choose to place a STENT, a small springlike device, at the area of the occlusion to hold it open.

CORONARY ARTERY BYPASS GRAFT (CABG) is the more invasive but also more successful surgical treatment for CAD in terms of long-term results. It involves open chest, OPEN-HEART SURGERY, during which the surgeon stops the heart from beating, to insert grafts or replacement arteries that bypass the heart's occluded arteries. CABG is often the surgical treatment of choice when more than one coronary artery is significantly occluded, or when angioplasty has failed to maintain open coronary arteries.

Risk Factors and Preventive Measures

Lifestyle modifications can reduce the risk for CAD and sometimes can halt and even reverse existing CAD. These modifications include smoking cessation, low-fat diet, regular physical activity, and weight loss if appropriate. Activities that promote stress relief, such as MEDITATION or YOGA, also are valuable. Many health experts believe it is possible to prevent CAD from developing in the first place through the proper lifestyle choices, but these choices often run counter to convention in Western society, making them difficult for people to accept and follow. Even modest changes can have a significant effect. Doctors and other health-care providers encourage people to make whatever changes they can. Most people can reduce dietary fat to 20 percent or less of daily calories and walk for 30 to 60 minutes a day four days a week, minimal changes that demonstrably improve cardiovascular health.

See also CALCIUM AND ARTERIAL PLAQUE; DEATHS FROM HEART DISEASE; LIFESTYLE AND HEART HEALTH; NUTRITION AND DIET; ORNISH PROGRAM; PLAQUE, ARTERIAL; STROKE; SURGERY TO TREAT CARDIOVASCULAR DISEASE.

coronary artery occlusion   See CORONARY ARTERY DISEASE (CAD).

coronary artery spasm   Prolonged contraction of an artery supplying the HEART with BLOOD that results in limiting or interrupting the flow of blood through the artery. Coronary artery spasms can result in pain from myocardial ischemia (inadequate oxygen supply), in which case the condition often is called variant or Prinzmetal's ANGINA, or the ischemia can be "silent" (without noticeable symptoms). Coronary artery spasms can cause ARRHYTHMIAS (irregularities in the HEARTBEAT) and,

if they continue for an extended time, HEART ATTACK (MYOCARDIAL INFARCTION). Coronary artery spasms often affect arteries in which there are significant arterial plaque accumulations. Cigarette smoking and cocaine are known to initiate coronary artery spasms. CALCIUM CHANNEL ANTAGONIST MEDICATIONS and NITROGLYCERIN often are effective in relieving and preventing the spasms and their associated symptoms and signs, although it is important to identify and treat any underlying cardiovascular disease. ANGIOPLASTY or CORONARY ARTERY BYPASS GRAFT (CABG) might be necessary to treat CORONARY ARTERY DISEASE (CAD) if it exists. Coronary artery spasms reflect an increased risk for heart attack and CARDIAC ARREST.

See also CHEST PAIN; COCAINE AND HEART ATTACK; MEDICATIONS TO TREAT HEART DISEASE; PLAQUE, ARTERIAL; TOBACCO USE.

coronary heart attack   See HEART ATTACK.

Coronary Primary Prevention Trial (CPPT)   The first of several significant CLINICAL RESEARCH STUDIES to identify the correlation between blood cholesterol levels and CARDIOVASCULAR DISEASE, it confirmed the therapeutic value of using LIPID-LOWERING MEDICATIONS to reduce blood cholesterol levels. The Coronary Primary Prevention Trial (CPPT) followed 3,800 American men with high blood cholesterol levels at 12 medical centers across the United States for 10 years, from 1973 to 1983. All of the study participants ate what was at the time a low fat, low cholesterol diet. Half of the group took the lipid-lowering medication CHOLESTYRAMINE. At the end of the study period, the group of men taking cholestyramine had significantly lower blood cholesterol levels, particularly low-density lipoprotein (LDL) cholesterol, and less cardiovascular disease (including fewer HEART ATTACKS) than the group of men using diet alone.

See also CHOLESTEROL, BLOOD; CORONARY RISK PROFILE; FRAMINGHAM HEART STUDY; HELSINKI HEART STUDY; LIFESTYLE AND HEART HEALTH; NUTRITION AND DIET; NATIONAL CHOLESTEROL EDUCATION PROGRAM; NURSES' HEALTH STUDY; WOMEN'S HEALTH INITIATIVE (WHI).

coronary risk profile A means of assessing the likelihood of CORONARY ARTERY DISEASE (CAD) and the potential for HEART ATTACK based on known CAD risk factors. Although many factors contribute to CAD and other kinds of CARDIOVASCULAR DISEASE, elevated blood levels of CHOLESTEROL and TRIGLYCERIDES (collectively known as lipids or fatty acids) provide nearly certain evidence that some degree of CAD exists. The purpose of establishing a coronary risk profile is to make this identification as early as possible in the course of disease, while it is possible to change the course of events before there is permanent damage. Elevated blood lipids are among the modifiable risk factors for HEART DISEASE (the other significant modifiable risk factors are physical inactivity and TOBACCO use, primarily cigarette smoking). Interventions typically include lifestyle modifications (low fat diet, increased physical activity, weight loss if appropriate) for mild to moderate risk, adding LIPID-LOWERING MEDICATIONS for moderate to high risk. Numerous studies support the premise that such interventions can substantially improve an individual's coronary risk profile.

See also CHOLESTEROL, BLOOD; FRAMINGHAM HEART STUDY; LIFESTYLE AND HEART HEALTH; NUTRITION AND DIET.

Corvisart, Jean-Nicholas (1755–1821) Physician who pioneered the technique of chest percussion (tapping on the chest and listening to the sounds) as a means of diagnosing HEART and lung conditions. Corvisart was French ruler Napoleon Bonaparte's personal physician and a professor who translated the writings of Austrian physician Leopold Auenbrugg that described the techniques and applications of chest percussion as a diagnostic tool. This generated renewed interest in Auenbrugg's methods and led the French physician René Laënnec in 1816 to develop the STETHOSCOPE to localize and amplify chest sounds. Corvisart's own text book, *Essay on the Diseases and Organic Lesions of the Heart and Large Vessels,* published in 1806, remained instrumental in medical college curricula for many years.

See also AUSCULTATION; HEART DISEASE.

Coumadin See WARFARIN.

Cozaar See LOSARTAN.

CPR A lifesaving method for maintaining BLOOD oxygenation and circulation for a person who has stopped breathing and whose HEART is not beating. When cardiac arrest occurs, survival depends on immediate response. Cell death begins after four to six minutes without oxygen, resulting in tissue and organ damage that can be permanent or cause death. CPR (cardiopulmonary resuscitation) initiated within three to four minutes of the heart's stopping gives the best chance of survival.

Artificial respiration (rescue breathing) was the first element of CPR to come into use, typically applied to drowning victims pulled from the water who clearly had stopped breathing. As advances in technology and medical understanding expanded and new therapies (medical and surgical) made it possible to treat cardiovascular diseases effectively, emergency medical response personnel began adding chest compressions to resuscitative efforts in the 1960s. In 1974 the American Heart Association issued the first formal guidelines for such efforts, outlining the procedures to sustain respirations and circulation during cardiovascular failure. Updated guidelines were issued in 2005 and remain in effect.

Training is required to learn proper CPR techniques and responses may differ for newborns and children. The following overview is provided for informational purposes.

CPR combines external (closed) chest compressions to push blood through the heart and circulatory system and artificial respiration to force air into the lungs. Health experts strongly urge those giving CPR to **first call for medical aid** and then begin CPR; this summons trained medical personnel to the scene with minimal delay. In most parts of the United States this takes only a telephone call to 911; the few seconds diverted to making this call get help on the way minutes sooner yet do not reduce the effectiveness of CPR. Studies show that people who receive advanced cardiovascular support in a hospital emergency department within the first hour following cardiac arrest are far more likely to survive.

CPR is appropriate only for people who are unconscious and unresponsive, are not breathing, and do not have a heartbeat (pulse). First call for medical help, and then:

1. **Determine responsiveness.** Touch or shake the person, and loudly ask the person if he or she is "okay" (nearly everyone, regardless of language spoken, understands the word *okay*).
2. **Determine breathing.** For five to ten seconds watch for the person's chest to rise and fall, however shallowly, and feel for air moving out of the person's nose or mouth. If appropriate, move the person to lie on his or her back with chin thrusting upward, to open the airway.

CPR is best learned through classes that teach proper methods and allow opportunity for supervised practice. It consists of these basic steps:

- Begin CPR with two breaths, watching or feeling for the person's chest to rise to make sure air is getting into the lungs. Pinch the person's nose closed and breathe into the mouth, forming a mouth-to-mouth seal. Give each rescue breath over one second.
- Immediately begin chest compressions. Push forcefully on the breastbone (sternum) the distance of two finger-widths up from the notch where the ribs join the sternum near the belly. Use only the heel of the palm, and keep the pressure centered on the breastbone. Kneel to be directly over the person, and push straight down with elbows locked. The breastbone should move down about two inches with each compression. Give 30 compressions at a rate of 100 per minute.
- After each series of 30 compressions, give two steady, deep breaths.
- Continue CPR until medical help arrives.

Many factors influence CPR's effectiveness, including the reason the person's cardiopulmonary functions have stopped, what damage to the heart and brain might have occurred, and how quickly CPR begins. Only a physician can determine whether it is appropriate to stop CPR.

The American Heart Association continues to establish the standards that health-care organizations and professionals follow for CPR and provides a curriculum for health educators to use when teaching community-based CPR classes. Fire and emergency aid departments, hospitals, community health centers, American Red Cross offices, and other facilities offer CPR classes to the general public at nominal or no charge. People who require certification in CPR should make sure the classes they choose meet the certification requirements.

See also AUTOMATED EXTERNAL DEFIBRILLATOR (AED); CHAIN OF SURVIVAL; HEART ATTACK; HEIMLICH MANEUVER.

C-reactive protein   A chemical substance body tissues release when they are injured, as by trauma or inflammation. The presence of C-reactive protein in the BLOOD signals an inflammatory process somewhere in the body. Recent research studies have linked elevated C-reactive protein levels with HEART ATTACK that results from CORONARY ARTERY DISEASE (CAD). In CAD, arterial plaque accumulates along the inner walls of the arteries that supply the heart. These plaques are irritating to the tissues of the artery wall, initiating a mild inflammatory response. This releases C-reactive protein into the bloodstream. However, the body releases C-reactive protein in response to inflammation that is noncardiovascular, as well, such as the inflammation of rheumatoid arthritis.

Researchers have demonstrated that the correlation between C-reactive protein levels and arterial inflammation is a strong predictor of heart attack resulting from arterial plaque deposits that occlude the arteries. LIPID-LOWERING MEDICATIONS that reduce the fatty acid accumulations that become arterial plaque also cause C-reactive protein levels to drop, suggesting there is interplay between this protein and fatty acids. Among participants in the WOMEN'S HEALTH INITIATIVE, an extensive ongoing research study that is following 27,000 women to assess heart disease risk factors, those who have cardiac events often have elevated C-reactive protein levels as well as elevated low-density lipoprotein (LDL) levels. The latter is a known risk factor for cardiovascular disease, particularly coronary artery disease. Researchers are now exploring whether these two levels in combination might be among the most accurate predictors yet for heart attack. Much research is under way to further evaluate the purpose and clinical usefulness of learning C-reactive protein levels with regard to predicting heart attack.

See also CALCIUM AND ARTERIAL PLAQUE; CHOLESTEROL, BLOOD; ELECTRON BEAM COMPUTED TOMOGRAPHY (EBCT) SCAN; INFLAMMATION AND HEART DISEASE; LIPIDS.

cyanosis A dusky blue color of the skin that signals insufficient oxygen in the BLOOD. It is most pronounced in the lips and the fingernail beds, and with severe HEART DISEASE it can affect the entire body. Cyanosis is a hallmark of "blue baby syndrome"—congenital heart malformations present at birth that prevent proper exchange of oxygen. People in the late stages of HEART FAILURE often have a cyanotic hue, signaling the heart's inability to pump enough blood to meet the body's circulatory needs.

Noncardiovascular causes of cyanosis can include metal toxicity (exposure to lead or silver) and drugs such as the anti-arrhythmia medication AMIODARONE and some antipsychotic medications. Cyanosis also can occur when a person is extremely cold, reflecting the body's response to pull the blood supply to vital organ systems to maintain adequate central oxygenation.

See also BLOOD GASES, ARTERIAL; CYANOTIC CONGENITAL HEART DISEASE; HEART DISEASE IN CHILDREN; PULSE OXIMETRY; RAYNAUD'S SYNDROME.

cyanotic congenital heart disease Collectively, the various HEART malformations that are present at birth. Many manifest as "blue baby syndrome" (denoting the CYANOSIS that marks insufficient oxygenation of the BLOOD) and require immediate to early childhood correction. Others can exist undetected, or without causing obvious symptoms, well into adulthood.

The typical congenital malformation is a SEPTAL DEFECT (opening in the inner heart wall) that allows blood to shunt between the heart's chambers (usually the ventricles), bypassing the lungs. This mixes oxygenated blood with deoxygenated blood, so the blood the heart pumps out to the body delivers at least minimal, and often adequate, oxygen to body tissues. The more substantial the shunt, the less apparent the malformation in infancy, childhood, and even early adulthood. However, PULMONARY HYPERTENSION (increased resistance to blood flow in the lungs that causes elevated pressure in the pulmonary artery) develops early in life as a result and worsens with progressing age. SUDDEN CARDIAC ARREST is a high risk.

Cyanotic congenital heart disease treated by surgery that creates a shunt (as in the BLALOCK-TAUSSIG PROCEDURE) in infancy or childhood can sometimes resurface as a cardiovascular problem later in life, particularly if pulmonary hypertension gained a foothold before surgical corrections could be completed. This is more likely to happen when the congenital malformations are extensive and require multiple operations to repair.

Symptoms and Diagnostic Path

Most forms of cyanotic congenital heart disease not detected in childhood begin to show symptoms by 30 to 40 years of age and may manifest as sudden and severe HEART FAILURE, CARDIOMYOPATHY, cardiomegaly, and ARRHYTHMIAS. Pregnancy, which places a significant strain on the woman's cardiovascular system, often precipitates these manifestations in women. Diminished AEROBIC CAPACITY with physical exertion is a common reason that adults with undiagnosed cyanotic congenital heart disease seek medical evaluation. Procedures such as ELECTROCARDIOGRAM (ECG), ECHOCARDIOGRAM (ultrasound of the heart), and MAGNETIC RESONANCE IMAGING (MRI) can confirm the diagnosis.

Treatment Options and Outlook

When cyanotic congenital heart disease remains untreated into adulthood, there is permanent and usually extensive damage to the blood vessels in the lungs. Because this damage is so extensive, operative repair of the heart malformations usually does not offer improvement. Medications taken to treat heart failure sometimes help relieve symptoms of heart failure such as shortness of breath and ANGINA or CHEST PAIN resulting from inadequate myocardial blood flow. For those with severe cardiopulmonary symptoms, HEART-LUNG TRANSPLANT is sometimes an option.

Risk Factors and Preventive Measures

Researchers do not know what causes the malformations that result in cyanotic congenital heart disease, although exposure to rubella during the first trimester of pregnancy is known to increase the risk for heart defects in the baby. This is one reason public health officials emphasize the importance of immunizations for such diseases; they protect not only the immunized individual but also others who would be exposed to the disease.

See also DOWN SYNDROME, HEART MALFORMATIONS ASSOCIATED WITH; EISENMENGER'S SYNDROME; FONTAN PROCEDURE; HEART DISEASE IN CHILDHOOD; HYPOPLASTIC LEFT HEART SYNDROME (HLHS); NORWOOD PROCEDURE; PALLIATION, STAGED; PULMONARY ATRESIA; SINGLE VENTRICLE; TETRALOGY OF FALLOT; TRICUSPID ATRESIA.

cyclosporine A medication taken to suppress the functions of the immune system to prevent rejection following HEART TRANSPLANT and HEART-LUNG TRANSPLANT. Common brand names include Neoral and Sandimmune. Although both brands contain cyclosporine, these products are not bioequivalent (cannot substitute for one another). A fungus extract, cyclosporine inhibits the functions of T-lymphocytes in the body. The body's immune system views a transplanted organ as a foreign "invader" and sends T-lymphocytes to attack it; cyclosporine prevents this response. A person with a transplanted organ (heart, liver, kidney) must take cyclosporine for the rest of his or her life. Cyclosporine has numerous side effects and interactions with other drugs. Typical antirejection regimens combine cyclosporine with steroid medications. Because cyclosporine suppresses the body's immune response, a person taking this medication is particularly vulnerable to viral and bacterial infections.

See also ALLOGRAFT; BLOOD.

Damus-Kaye-Stansel procedure A surgical procedure to correct TRANSPOSITION OF THE GREAT ARTERIES (TGA), a serious congenital heart malformation in which the aorta and the pulmonary artery are reversed so that the aorta arises from the right ventricle and the pulmonary artery from the left ventricle. This causes the HEART to pump oxygenated BLOOD back to the lungs without sending it through the body, and unoxygenated blood to the body without going through the lungs. As a result, body tissues fail to receive the oxygen they need. Because TGA is such a serious malformation, surgeons typically try to perform the Damus-Kaye-Stansel procedure within the first 30 days to three months of life. Surgeons sometimes perform this operation in conjunction with other reconstructive procedures when the child has multiple heart malformations.

Procedure

The Damus-Kaye-Stansel procedure is an open-heart operation in which the surgeon splits the pulmonary artery into two vessels, routing one to the right ventricle and the other to the ascending aorta. This allows oxygenated blood to mix with unoxygenated blood in the left ventricle so the blood the heart pumps out to the body is partially oxygenated. Surgeons may modify the procedure based on the specific malformations or anomalies that are present.

Risks and Complications

The risks and complications of the Damus-Kaye-Stansel procedure are those of OPEN-HEART SURGERY, anesthesia, and CARDIOPULMONARY BYPASS as well as those related to the procedure. Excessive bleeding, failure of the separated blood vessel to function as desired, and inadequate OXYGENATION (HYPOXIA) that continues even after the procedure are among the key complications. Postoperative infection, blood clots, and pneumonia are also concerns. Because the underlying heart defects are severe and the child is usually very young and weak, death is also a significant risk. Additional complications may develop after surgery due to the underlying heart defects and the continued abnormal function of the heart.

Outlook and Lifestyle Modifications

There is usually immediate and pronounced improvement following surgery because more oxygen gets into the bloodstream and to the organs. Most children stay one to three days in the intensive care unit and up to a week in the hospital, although complications can extend the hospital stay. Medications are often necessary to help strengthen the heart's contractions, regulate BLOOD PRESSURE, and prevent clotting. The long-term success of the Damus-Kaye-Stansel procedure correlates to the complexity of the child's heart malformations. Most children will need additional heart operations, and sometimes HEART TRANSPLANT, later in childhood to establish more normal heart function. Until the sequence of operations is complete, most children are smaller than normal for age, have limited physical strength and energy, and have restrictions on their activities to help preserve the most efficient cardiovascular function possible.

See also ARTERIAL SWITCH PROCEDURE; BIDIRECTIONAL GLENN PROCEDURE; BLALOCK-TAUSSIG PROCEDURE; FONTAN PROCEDURE; NORWOOD PROCEDURE; PALLIATION, STAGED; PULMONARY ARTERY BANDING; SURGERY TO TREAT CARDIOVASCULAR DISEASE.

Darvall, Denise The 25-year-old South African woman who became the donor for the world's first human HEART TRANSPLANT. Darvall and her mother were walking across the street in Cape Town, South Africa, on December 3, 1967, when they were struck by a car. Darvall's mother died instantly, and Darvall suffered severe head injuries. Although doctors placed her on MECHANICAL VENTILATION, Darvall's injuries led to irreversible neurological damage that rapidly led to brain death (cessation of brain activity). Doctors requested permission from her father to take her kidneys for transplant, and because they knew surgeon Dr. CHRISTIAAN BARNARD was searching for a DONOR HEART to perform the first heart transplant also asked to take her heart. Darvall's father agreed, and hours later 55-year-old LOUIS WASHKANSY became the recipient of the first transplanted heart. He survived 18 days, succumbing to pneumonia that developed after drugs given to suppress rejection of the donor heart weakened his immune system.

Although Denise Darvall's place in history is as the first heart donor, the donation of her kidneys also was groundbreaking. In 1967 (and until 1994) apartheid was still in place in South Africa. This practice of racial segregation classified people as white, black, or mixed and established legal restrictions to maintain separation based on race. Darvall was white; the 10-year-old boy who received her kidneys, in an operation also performed by Barnard, was black. The controversy over that operation became further fuel for debate about and aided efforts to end apartheid.

See also CLARK, BARNEY; DONOR HEART; HEART, ARTIFICIAL.

DASH diet   A nutritional plan based on the "Dietary Approaches to Stop Hypertension" clinical study. The plan is broadly high in fruits and vegetables, low in fat, and low in sodium, following these guidelines for daily consumption:

- eight to 10 servings of fruits and vegetables
- one to three servings of low-fat or no-fat dairy products
- seven to eight servings of grain products
- one to two servings of lean meat
- 1,500 mg to 2,400 mg of sodium

- no more than 30 percent fat (of which no more than 10 percent is saturated)

The DASH diet arises from the findings of two studies that the U.S. National Institutes of Health's National Heart, Lung, and Blood Institute (NHLBI) funded: the original DASH study conducted in 1996 and a follow-up study (DASH-Sodium) conducted in 2000. In both studies, participants had Stage 1 or Stage 2 HYPERTENSION (mild to moderate high BLOOD PRESSURE) but were not taking medication. Those who followed nutrition plans that were high in fruits, vegetables, and low-fat dairy products, and low in sodium and fat experienced significant drops in their blood pressures. The DASH-Sodium study expanded on the original DASH study to examine the effects of even lower daily sodium levels. The original DASH study's participants consumed a limit of 3,000 mg of sodium daily; participants in the follow-up DASH-Sodium study consumed a limit of half that amount, 1,500 mg. The drop in blood pressure was even more dramatic in the DASH-Sodium study, matching the level of reduction typical with medications.

Many researchers believe the DASH diet could control blood pressure without medication for many people and prevent as much as 15 percent of hypertension from developing in the first place. Doctors recommend that in particular people with RISK FACTORS FOR HEART DISEASE follow the DASH diet. The parameters of the DASH diet are broad enough to accommodate a wide range of foods and styles and do not inherently exclude any foods. Many processed and convenience foods now are available in low-fat and low-sodium versions.

See also EXERCISE; LIFESTYLE AND HEART HEALTH; NUTRITION AND DIET; WEIGHT MANAGEMENT.

Dean Ornish reversal diet   See ORNISH PROGRAM.

deaths from heart disease   HEART DISEASE—collectively encompassing CARDIOVASCULAR DISEASE (CVD); HYPERTENSION; RHEUMATIC HEART DISEASE; cerebrovascular accident (STROKE); CONGENITAL HEART DISEASE; CORONARY ARTERY DISEASE (CAD); ISCHEMIC HEART DISEASE; and HEART FAILURE—causes more than 16.7 million deaths worldwide each year, according to the World Health Organization (WHO); making it the leading cause of death among developed nations. In the United States heart disease has been the leading cause of death since the 20th century and today accounts for 40 percent of deaths among men and women over age 18 of all races each year, a rate of one death every 37 seconds according to the American Heart Association. In 2005, the most recent year for which mortality statistics were available at the time of this writing, heart disease claimed the lives of 685,000 Americans, accounting for 30 percent of deaths overall. The gap continues to grow between men and women, with nearly 45,000 more women than men dying of heart disease. However, more men than women are diagnosed with heart disease—fewer women have heart disease but are more likely to die from it when they have it.

Trends in Heart Disease Mortality Rates

Heart disease has been a health problem and a key cause of death, across cultures and to varying degrees, throughout documented history. Egyptian papyrus texts dating to 2000 B.C. reference medicinal preparations historians believe incorporated foxglove (the source of DIGITALIS, used for centuries

---

U.S. DEATHS FROM HEART DISEASE—2006

Form of Heart Disease	Percentage of Heart Disease Deaths
Coronary heart disease (coronary artery disease, ischemic heart disease)	51%
Cerebrovascular disease (transient ischemic attack, carotid stenosis, stroke)	17%
Other (rheumatic heart disease, congenital heart disease, valve disease, cardiomy opathy, arrhythmias)	14%
Heart failure	7%
Hypertension (high blood pressure)	7%
Vascular diseases (abdominal aortic aneurysm, atherosclerosis, arteriosclerosis, peripheral vascular disease, deep vein thrombosis)	7%

Source: U.S. Centers for Disease National Center for Health Statistics; American Heart Association

---

to treat ARRHYTHMIAS and HEART FAILURE) and belladonna (a natural source of ATROPINE, which stimulates heart contractions). Even though physicians knew little of the heart's function until English physician WILLIAM HARVEY published his landmark explanation of the cardiovascular system, *An Anatomical Treatise on the Motion of the Heart and Blood in Animals* in 1628, ancient healers knew the heart's beating was the quintessential hallmark of life and that abnormalities in its rhythm and force, which they could detect by feeling pulses, were indications of illness and often of impending death. Until the surge in knowledge and technology that took place during the 20th century, doctors had few means to diagnose or treat heart disease.

In the United States heart disease became the leading cause of death in 1900 with the rate of deaths due to heart disease peaking in 1950. In the second half of the 20th century, technological knowledge, comprehensive survey data, and growing understanding of the correlations between lifestyle (especially cigarette smoking) and heart disease converged to motivate concerted public health efforts to reduce the rate, severity, and mortality of heart disease. Each year since, the *rate* of deaths due to heart disease has declined. However, the *number* of deaths due to heart disease continued to climb until the mid-1980s, after which it began to edge downward. Epidemiologists (researchers who study trends in health and disease) postulate that if acquired (not congenital) heart disease were eliminated, average life expectancy would increase by seven years. However, at present heart disease remains a significant threat to both health and longevity. Based on current trends, epidemiologists project that a child born in 2000 has nearly a 50-50 chance of dying from heart disease as an adult.

Public Health Efforts to Reduce Heart Disease Mortality

With increased understanding of risk factors for heart disease, public health efforts to reduce risks proliferated. One of the earliest significant correlations was that between cigarette smoking and heart disease, which hit the public's attention with the first U.S. Surgeon General's report about it in 1964. Subsequent public health initiatives arose from the FRAMINGHAM HEART STUDY, the first large-scale study to definitively correlate risk factors such as high fat diet, sedentary lifestyle, and health conditions such as HYPERLIPIDEMIA (high blood CHOLESTEROL and TRIGLYCERIDES) and hypertension (high BLOOD PRESSURE) with coronary artery disease (CAD) and ischemic heart disease. Among these efforts have been:

- Healthy People 2000 and Healthy People 2010, which established goals for reducing risk factors and specific forms of heart disease
- numerous smoking cessation programs
- cholesterol-reduction programs such as widespread public cholesterol testing and the NATIONAL CHOLESTEROL EDUCATION PROGRAM (NCEP)
- programs to increase physical activity and reduce obesity
- efforts to increase awareness of health conditions that contribute to heart disease such as kidney disease, diabetes, and hypertension

Sources for Statistical Information

Key sources for statistical data, analysis, and other information related to heart disease prevalence (rate of frequency), morbidity (severity of disease), and mortality (deaths) are the U.S. Centers for Disease Control's National Center for Health Statistics (CDC-NCHS), the U.S. National Institutes of Health's National Heart, Lung, and Blood Institute (NIH-NHLBI), and the American Heart Association. Contact information for these organizations appears in Appendix I.

See also CARDIAC ARREST; HEART ATTACK; LIFESTYLE AND HEART HEALTH; PREVENTING HEART DISEASE; SUDDEN CARDIAC ARREST.

DeBakey, Michael E. (1908–2008) Pioneering American cardiovascular surgeon and researcher instrumental in developing numerous devices, instruments, and procedures now common in cardiovascular surgery. DeBakey started his career in medical research in 1932 while a medical student at Tulane University in New Orleans, Louisiana, when he designed the roller pump mechanism that became the foundation for the HEART-LUNG MACHINE. Highlights of his other contributions to medical science include:

- developed the concept and structure of mobile army surgical hospital (MASH) units following World War II
- developed the Veteran's Administration Medical Center system to provide care and treatment for military personnel wounded in war
- worked to develop and use prosthetic artery grafts made of Dacron and developed the techniques for using them to perform CORONARY ARTERY BYPASS GRAFT (CABG) surgery and replace other diseased arteries elsewhere in the body including CAROTID ENDARTERECTOMY and ABDOMINAL AORTIC ANEURYSM
- worked to develop early models of artificial hearts
- worked to establish the National Library of Medicine
- developed the classification system of CARDIOVASCULAR DISEASE (CVD) used to determine treatment options
- implanted the first partial artificial heart in 1966 and developed the first functional ventricular assist devices to serve as a "bridge" to support the heart of a person waiting for a heart transplant
- performed the first human HEART TRANSPLANT in the United States in 1968 and subsequently performed a total of 12 heart transplants

Credited with performing more than 60,000 cardiovascular operations during his career, DeBakey received international recognition and numerous awards, including the U.S. Presidential Medal of Freedom with Distinction (1969), the U.S. National Medal of Science (1987), and the United Nations Lifetime Achievement Award (1999). In 2001 DeBakey worked with NASA scientists to develop the DeBakey Ventricular Assist Device, which implemented technology used in the space shuttle program and earned NASA's Commercial Invention of the Year Award in 2002.

See also BARNARD, CHRISTIAAN; COOLEY, DENTON; DEVRIES, WILLIAM C.; JARVIK, ROBERT; LEFT VENTRICULAR ASSIST DEVICE (LVAD).

decongestants and blood pressure   See COLD/FLU MEDICATION AND HYPERTENSION.

deep vein thrombosis (DVT) The development of BLOOD clots (thrombi) in the inner veins, most commonly in the legs. These occur for various reasons arising from restricted blood flow through the veins, including CARDIOVASCULAR DISEASE (CVD), PERIPHERAL VASCULAR DISEASE (PVD; ATHEROSCLEROSIS that affects the veins in the extremities), injury that compresses a vein, and prolonged inactivity. The walls of veins are thinner and less muscular than the walls of arteries, making them vulnerable to damage and weakness. Veins have valves in them to keep blood from backflowing; when the wall of the vein weakens and stretches, or when there are plaque deposits in the veins, functioning of these valves becomes impaired.

Symptoms and Diagnostic Path

The primary symptoms of DVT are pain and swelling in the area of the clot. If a fragment of the clot breaks away it can lodge in the lungs, creating breathing difficulty. The main symptoms of this are a sudden cough without other cold or flu symptoms, chest pain, and shortness of breath. Clot fragments that lodge in the CORONARY ARTERIES can cause HEART ATTACK, and those that make it to the brain can cause STROKE.

Treatment Options and Outlook

Treatment typically includes a course of oral ANTICOAGULANT MEDICATION to prevent new clots from forming. Sometimes surgery is necessary to remove the blockage; a sonogram (ULTRASOUND) can help determine the size and location of the clot.

Risk Factors and Preventive Measures

Although anyone of any age can develop DVT, certain people have an increased risk. They include:

- Older people, because with aging the veins and their valves weaken, allowing blood to more easily pool.
- People who are overweight, because extra body bulk stresses the circulatory system overall and the veins in particular.
- People who travel by plane, because cramped seating arrangements prevent stretching the legs and inhibit easily getting up to walk around.

- People who smoke cigarettes, because nicotine and other chemicals in tobacco smoke cause the walls of blood vessels to stiffen.
- Women who are pregnant, because blood concentrations of clotting substances increases during pregnancy (especially in the third trimester).
- People who have DIABETES, because diabetes can damage peripheral blood vessels and impair peripheral blood circulation.
- People who are short enough that their feet do not touch the floor when they sit, because the increased pressure across the backs of the thighs can impair the flow of blood to and from the legs. Regular walking to maintain strong leg muscles helps to support function of the veins in the legs and to maintain good blood flow. Walking, or at least standing to stretch, every 20 minutes when seated for extended periods of time is important, especially on air flights. Sitting without crossing the legs is also important. Doctors may recommend low-dose aspirin as a mild anticoagulant, as a preventive measure for people at increased risk for DVT.

See also AGING, CARDIOVASCULAR CHANGES AS A RESULT OF; ARTERIOSCLEROSIS; CORONARY ARTERY DISEASE (CAD); SMOKING AND HEART DISEASE; TOBACCO USE; VENOGRAM.

defibrillation The administration of controlled electrical current to restore normal SINUS RHYTHM or HEART function during cardiac resuscitation. For defibrillation to be indicated, the heart must be beating in a pattern known as VENTRICULAR FIBRILLATION—rapid, erratic, and unsynchronized contractions of the myocardial fibers in the ventricles, the heart's primary pumping chambers—or PULSELESS VENTRICULAR tachycardia—contractions that are very rapid and rhythmic but ineffective and insufficient to generate a pulse although the type of electrical activity can be detected by ELECTROCARDIOGRAM (ECG). Neither pattern can sustain the heart's pumping functions but establishes that the heart still has electrical activity. If there is no heartbeat whatsoever, it is necessary to perform CPR (CARDIOPULMONARY RESUSCITATION) or administer drugs such as EPINEPHRINE and DOPAMINE in an attempt to stimulate electrical activity. Although defibrillation saves thousands of lives every year, it usually cannot start a heart that has no electrical activity of its own.

There are two kinds of defibrillation, manual and automated. Emergency medical professionals (such as doctors, nurses, paramedics) generally administer manual defibrillation, which requires interpretation of the ECG to determine whether the person is experiencing ventricular fibrillation or pulseless ventricular tachycardia. The medical professional must manually set the level of electrical current, apply the paddles with about 25 pounds of pressure when delivering the shock, and check the ECG to determine the defibrillation's effect. In situations of cardiac arrest, three discharges of current typically are administered in sequence.

Virtually anyone can use an AUTOMATED EXTERNAL DEFIBRILLATOR (AED) device in a cardiac emergency, and basic life support (BLS) training now includes AED use. The AED determines the person's cardiac rhythm and automatically delivers the appropriate level of electrical current. The user applies the defibrillator pads according to the instructions on the AED and activates the AED when the unit so instructs. It is not necessary to apply pressure with the defibrillator pads, which also send ECG readings back to the AED. The AED determines the current, frequency, and number of shocks to deliver.

For the person receiving defibrillation, the risks are slight relative to the benefit of restoring normal heart rhythm. Common adverse effects include skin and tissue burns, usually the consequence of improperly positioned paddles or inadequate conduction during manual defibrillation. The potential risks for the person administering defibrillation can be serious and include cardiac arrest due to electrical shock as well as burns from contact with the person receiving defibrillation (including clothing, equipment, and bed or gurney). All those rendering assistance during cardiac resuscitation must make sure they are not in contact to avoid accidental shock; hospitals and emergency response units have strict protocols for these procedures.

See also ARRHYTHMIA; CARDIOVERSION; DO NOT RESUSCITATE ORDERS; SUDDEN CARDIAC ARREST (SCA).

Demadex   See TORSEMIDE.

denial   A common reaction to a diagnosis of HEART DISEASE in which a person refuses to accept that the diagnosis is correct, or that it means making significant lifestyle changes. Denial is a normal, and the first, stage in the cycle of acceptance. Many health experts believe denial functions as a safety mechanism to let the mind come to grips with the significance of the information. For some people, a diagnosis of heart disease is so overwhelming that they stay in the denial phase for months or longer. Sometimes other people—family and friends— have difficulty accepting a loved one's diagnosis and what it means. It is frightening to recognize a loved one's vulnerability and mortality; heart disease forces confrontation with both.

Denial often manifests in ways that are not in the best health interests of the person with heart disease, such as refusing to make appropriate lifestyle changes (NUTRITION AND DIET, EXERCISE, smoking cessation). Others in the person's support network of family and friends can help to encourage positive changes. The most effective way to do this is to make similar changes themselves. Heart-healthy lifestyle choices benefit everyone and can help to delay or prevent adverse health consequences in people not yet at the disease stage. Many researchers believe that the foundation of heart disease starts early in life, in young adulthood or even childhood, progressing to a level of interference with health long before symptoms drive people to see their doctors. The body's amazing capacity to compensate makes it easy to ignore early warning signs for months, years, and even decades. When symptoms become obvious, or cause HEART ATTACK or STROKE, they often appear sudden even when clear or multiple RISK FACTORS FOR HEART DISEASE are present. At that point, it becomes as impossible to ignore the presence of heart disease as it is to accept it.

It is especially important for those diagnosed with heart disease to take any prescribed medications. If medications cause unpleasant side effects, doctors often can make substitutions to medications with fewer such problems. Some people find that it helps to talk about their concerns with others who have had similar experiences, such as through support groups. When denial persists beyond what is reasonable or begins to detrimentally affect the person's health, a therapist or psychologist might be able to help the person put concerns and worries in proper context and shift to a positive, supportive perspective. Denial that persists might be DEPRESSION, a potentially serious but treatable condition.

The earlier intervention begins, the more effective it can be in halting and sometimes even reversing the progression of heart disease.

See also CARDIAC REHABILITATION; LIFESTYLE AND HEART HEALTH; ORNISH PROGRAM.

dental procedures, prophylactic antibiotics for
See ANTIBIOTIC PROPHYLAXIS.

depression   A clinical condition in which profound sadness, unhappiness, and hopelessness interfere with the normal enjoyment of life. Depression appears to be a complex interplay between brain biochemistry and life experiences. In depression there is an imbalance of NEUROTRANSMITTERS in the brain, and in particular a low level of serotonin, a neurotransmitter that facilitates communication among nerve cells in regions of the brain that are responsible for mood and emotion. Researchers are not certain what causes such a biochemical environment.

Symptoms and Diagnostic Path

Symptoms of depression include:

- persistent sadness, helplessness, hopelessness, pessimism, worthlessness
- persistent lack of energy and interest in once pleasurable activities
- trouble concentrating and making decisions
- irritability
- SLEEP DISTURBANCES (trouble falling asleep, staying asleep, waking up)
- thoughts or expressions of suicide

People who have these symptoms for longer than two weeks should receive clinical evaluation.

Treatment Options and Outlook

Treatment for depression often includes ANTIDEPRESSANT MEDICATIONS, which help to restore the brain's biochemistry. Psychotherapy can help people with depression find ways to cope with their life circumstances. Physical activity and regular exercise are natural ways to boost brain chemicals related to mood as well as to improve cardiovascular health and overall well-being.

Risk Factors and Preventive Measures

Depression sometimes occurs as a side effect of certain medications, among them medications to treat HEART DISEASE. Depression is also common among people who are living with a chronic health condition such as heart disease. As well, there appears to be a correlation between depression and specific forms of heart disease including ANGINA and HYPERTENSION. Women are about twice as likely as men to have depression. Ongoing research suggests that depression can delay recovery from heart attack and may be a factor that contributes to the development of CARDIOVASCULAR DISEASE (CVD). Recognizing and treating the symptoms of depression early can prevent depression from becoming a significant general and cardiovascular health concern. Staying active and involved in favorite activities, walking daily, and eating nutritiously are effective lifestyle methods for improving mood and overall well-being.

See also DENIAL; EMOTIONS; LIVING WITH HEART DISEASE; MEDICATION SIDE EFFECTS.

DeVries, William C. (1943–)   The American cardiovascular surgeon best known for leading the surgical team that implanted the first permanent total artificial heart into retired Seattle dentist BARNEY CLARK in 1982. As a young physician, DeVries worked with the physician and researcher Willem Kolff, who had developed the first kidney dialysis machine and was testing an artificial heart in animals. Later in his career he developed a close working relationship with the researcher who developed the first permanent mechanical heart, ROBERT JARVIK. It was that design, the Jarvik-7, that DeVries implanted in Barney Clark. Clark's survival of 112 days spurred both hope and controversy. The mechanical heart's compressor was the size of a small freezer and kept Clark confined to his hospital bed and bedside chair. The details of Clark's successes and setbacks were in the media, and DeVries was in the spotlight daily for the duration of Clark's hospitalization.

The second patient into whom DeVries implanted a Jarvik-7, William Schroeder, lived the longest of the four of DeVries's patients who received mechanical hearts, 620 days. Although Schroeder suffered numerous STROKES and other complications following the implantation, he was able to live briefly outside the hospital in an apartment specially designed and equipped to accommodate the bulky compressor required to operate his mechanical heart. However, Schroeder's often difficult experiences were widely presented in the news, and the debate over whether the mechanical heart was morally and ethically right intensified.

During the time Schroeder lived with his mechanical heart, DeVries implanted a Jarvik-7 into two other patients, Murray Hayden and Jack Burcham, Sr., who also experienced numerous serious complications and setbacks. Hayden lived 488 days and Burcham only 10 days. Both public and professional opinion began to question whether the risks were worth what seemed to be little benefit. In the meantime, other surgeons had placed Jarvik-7 mechanical hearts as "bridge" devices to sustain life until DONOR HEARTS could be acquired and transplanted. This use of the mechanical heart was more successful, and Burcham was the last patient in whom DeVries implanted a permanent Jarvik-7.

In 2000 DeVries shifted from the private to the public arena, joining Walter Reed Army Medical Center's department of surgery as a consultant and becoming a lieutenant colonel in the U.S. Army reserve. At age 57, he was one of the oldest officers to complete basic officer's training and receive a commission. Military service fulfilled a longtime dream for DeVries, who had been prevented from joining the military as a young man because he was a sole surviving son.

See also BARNARD, CHRISTIAAN; COOLEY, DENTON; DEBAKEY, MICHAEL E.; HEART, ARTIFICIAL; HEART TRANSPLANT; LEFT VENTRICULAR ASSIST DEVICE (LVAD).

diabetes and heart disease   Diabetes mellitus is a health condition in which the body's insulin and glucose mechanisms function improperly or do not function at all. There are two kinds of diabetes, type 1 and type 2. Both significantly increase the risk for HEART DISEASE, particularly HYPERTENSION (high BLOOD PRESSURE) and CORONARY ARTERY DISEASE (CAD). Heart disease is the cause of death for two out of three people who have diabetes. Diabetes also is the leading cause of kidney disease and kidney failure, health conditions that affect the choices of medications and treatment options for heart disease. As well, there is growing evidence arising from research that points to dysfunction of the body's insulin/glucose mechanisms, particularly the insulin resistance of type 2 diabetes, as a common link between diabetes and CARDIOVASCULAR DISEASE (CVD).

Type 1 Diabetes

Type 1 diabetes occurs when the pancreas stops producing insulin, and generally comes on suddenly. Researchers believe it is an autoimmune disease in which the body produces antibodies that attack the pancreas and kill its insulin-producing islet cells, but they do not know what triggers this response although they suspect there might be a viral involvement. Based on current knowledge, there is no way to prevent type 1 diabetes, nor to predict who will develop it. There are no known risk factors for type 1 diabetes.

Type 1 diabetes usually develops during childhood, accounting for its former designation as juvenile diabetes. This is an inaccurate designation, however, as the condition continues throughout life. At present there is no cure for type 1 diabetes, although islet cell transplants and gene therapy hold great promise. Current treatment is insulin injections. About 1 million Americans have type 1 diabetes.

Type 2 Diabetes

Type 2 diabetes develops over time; some researchers believe over decades. The body's cells become resistant to the effects of insulin, requiring increasingly higher levels of insulin before they can accept glucose, their primary energy source. This causes BLOOD glucose levels to rise. Type 2 diabetes, sometimes called adult-onset diabetes as it was most common among people over age 50, is becoming increasingly common among younger people and even children. About 12 million Americans have been diagnosed as having type 2 diabetes and another 5 million have the condition but do not know it.

Some people with type 2 diabetes can control the disease through diet and EXERCISE, and others require oral anti-diabetes medications that improve cell sensitivity to insulin. About 40 percent of people with type 2 diabetes eventually need insulin injections to supplement or replace natural insulin. Although lifestyle changes often can reduce the need for medications to treat type 2 diabetes, there is no cure. Once type 2 diabetes develops, it does not go away. Health experts estimate that 80 to 90 percent of type 2 diabetes results from lifestyle factors—with OBESITY the leading cause—and could be prevented, like heart disease, through lifestyle change to incorporate nutritional eating habits, regular exercise, and WEIGHT MANAGEMENT.

Cardiovascular Changes in Diabetes

The metabolic imbalance that exists in diabetes causes numerous changes to take place in the structures of the CARDIOVASCULAR SYSTEM, particularly the arteries, arterioles, and capillaries. Insulin regulates the amount of glucose, the cell's primary energy source, that enters a cell. When cells become resistant to insulin, levels of glucose circulating in the bloodstream rise. The effect on cell metabolism—the processes by which cells use energy to carry out their functions—is analogous to throwing tinder on a campfire. Cell activity "flares," resulting in abnormal tissue growth particularly in the blood vessels. Doctors call these atherogenic changes, and their consequence is an acceleration of ATHEROSCLEROSIS (accumulations of arterial PLAQUE). The cascade of events that develops as a result includes hypertension, coronary artery disease, and increased risk of blood clots that can cause DEEP VEIN THROMBOSIS (DVT) and migrate to cause STROKE or HEART ATTACK.

Insulin Resistance: Common Ground

The INSULIN RESISTANCE that is the foundation of type 2 diabetes seems to be the common link between type 2 diabetes and heart disease; insulin resistance does not appear to be a factor in type 1 diabetes. Numerous research studies over the past decade have demonstrated that many people with hypertension and HYPERLIPIDEMIA also have insulin resistance, even when they do not have type 2 diabetes. Researchers estimate that one in four people who have insulin resistance will eventually develop type 2 diabetes. The most significant factor in that progression is obesity; insulin resistance is nearly always present in obesity, and obesity is a significant risk factor for both diabetes and heart disease.

Other Systemic Changes in Diabetes That Affect Cardiovascular Function

Diabetes causes numerous changes in the body beyond cardiovascular function, affecting every system. Critical changes take place in kidney function, which hypertension compounds by placing increased strain on the delicate blood vessels of the kidneys' inner structures. Elevated blood glucose levels can cause ANGIOGENESIS, a proliferation of tiny blood vessels. Peripheral neuropathy develops in response to changes in the nerve cells primarily in the feet and hands, creating impaired circulation that reduces blood supply.

Treatment Considerations

It is especially important to maintain as stable a balance between insulin and glucose as possible. This requires careful blood glucose monitoring, nutritious eating habits, regular exercise, and weight management. It also is important to keep blood lipid levels (cholesterol and triglycerides) low to slow the progression of atherosclerosis and coronary artery disease, and to keep blood pressure within normal limits. These efforts typically require medication in addition to lifestyle changes. People who have both diabetes and heart disease should see their doctors regularly and seek prompt medical attention for any new symptoms or changes in health status.

See also LIVING WITH HEART DISEASE; METABOLIC SYNDROME; NUTRITION AND DIET.

diaphragm   See PULMONARY SYSTEM.

diastolic blood pressure   See BLOOD PRESSURE.

diastolic dysfunction   An incomplete or abnormal relaxation of the ventricles (the HEART's lower, pumping chambers) during diastole. This makes it more difficult for BLOOD to flow into the ventricles from the atria (the heart's upper, collecting chambers). Diastole is the point during each CARDIAC CYCLE, or HEARTBEAT, at which the heart's ventricles are at rest between contractions; the second or bottom number in a BLOOD PRESSURE reading ends diastole. Diastolic blood pressure is an important indicator of resistance in the peripheral arteries, particularly the tiniest arterioles, and reflects the effort the heart must exert to move blood throughout the body.

Diastolic dysfunction, sometimes called diastolic heart failure, typically occurs with congestive HEART FAILURE; it can be primary (causing heart failure) or secondary (a result of heart failure). In either case, diastolic dysfunction causes pressure to build up and fluid to accumulate in the lungs (PULMONARY HYPERTENSION and PULMONARY CONGESTION), a consequence of the left ventricle's inability to accept all of the blood returning to it from the lungs, and in the body in general (diastolic HYPERTENSION and peripheral congestion, EDEMA, and ascites), a consequence of the right ventricle's inability to accept the blood that returns to the heart from the body. Diastolic dysfunction can affect only the right ventricle, only the left ventricle, or both ventricles. About 40 percent of people who have heart failure have diastolic dysfunction.

Symptoms and Diagnostic Path
The symptoms of diastolic dysfunction are those of heart failure: shortness of breath, weakness, and angina (particularly with exertion). Pulmonary congestion can cause coughing and difficulty breathing. An elevated right ventricle diastolic BLOOD PRESSURE suggests right diastolic dysfunction. Doctors use imaging technologies to diagnose left diastolic dysfunction. The most commonly used is ECHOCARDIOGRAM, a sonographic (ultrasound) procedure that allows real-time visualization of the heart's pumping action and flow of blood. From the echocardiogram, the cardiologist can calculate the LEFT VENTRICULAR EJECTION FRACTION (LVEF) a measure of the left ventricle's filling capacity and volume of blood pumped from the ventricle when the heart contracts. Occasionally the cardiologist also might use MAGNETIC RESONANCE IMAGING (MRI), if the echocardiogram is inconclusive or the cardiologist suspects other factors or conditions are also present.

Treatment Options and Outlook
Doctors most commonly prescribe BETA ANTAGONIST MEDICATIONS, ANGIOTENSIN-CONVERTING ENZYME (ACE) INHIBITOR MEDICATIONS, and CALCIUM CHANNEL ANTAGONIST MEDICATIONS to treat diastolic dysfunction; these medications help to relax myocardial muscle cells and reduce the heart's workload. Doctors might also prescribe DIGOXIN when systolic heart failure is the primary cause of the diastolic dysfunction. Most people are able to manage diastolic dysfunction with medications for quite a long time.

Risk Factors and Preventive Measures
Other cardiovascular diseases (CVD), including congestive heart failure, hypertrophic cardiomyopathy, aortic stenosis, ischemic heart disease (IHD), and untreated or poorly controlled chronic hypertension, are the primary risk factors for diastolic dysfunction. Diagnosing and appropriately treating these underlying conditions can improve cardiac function and slow, stop, or reverse diastolic dysfunction.

diet   See NUTRITION AND DIET.

diet, step   See NUTRITION AND DIET.

digitalis   A drug that strengthens the HEART's contractions and slows HEART RATE, taken to treat HEART FAILURE and ATRIAL FIBRILLATION. Chemically, digitalis is a cardiac glycoside that derives from the foxglove plant *(Digitalis purpurea)*. Ancient physicians recognized the effects of digitalis on the heart, even though they did not understand the mechanisms of heart function, and administered it in the form of tea brewed from foxglove leaves and stems. Today laboratories manufacture digitalis to precise pharmacological standards, and the term refers broadly to the group of medications, which includes DIGOXIN, DIGITOXIN, and related cardiac glycosides as the digitalis glycosides. Digitalis medications are the most widely prescribed MEDICATIONS TO TREAT HEART DISEASE.

The digitalis glycosides have two actions on the myocardium (heart muscle). One is to increase the amount of calcium within myocardial cells, causing them to contract more forcefully. The other is to inhibit the flow of electrical signals arising from the sinoatrial (SA) node (the heart's natural pacemaker), reducing the number of signals that trigger contractions and causing the heart rate to slow. Numerous medications interact with digitalis, with the potential to alter its effectiveness or toxicity level.

digitalis toxicity Digitalis toxicity is accumulation of digitalis glycosides in the body that can cause potentially life-threatening ARRHYTHMIAS (notably VENTRICULAR TACHYCARDIA and ventricular FIBRILLATION). Doctors carefully monitor digitalis levels in the BLOOD of people taking digitalis medications such as DIGOXIN or DIGITOXIN; these drugs have a narrow therapeutic index (NTI). They are effective at dosages that are just below the toxic, or harmful, level. Many factors influence this level. Symptoms of digitalis toxicity include nausea, loss of appetite, weakness, vision disturbances such as seeing double or seeing halos around objects, light-sensitivity, and irregular HEARTBEAT. Those taking digitalis medications who experience these symptoms should consult their doctors promptly. Treatment is to stop the digitalis medication temporarily until blood levels and heart rhythm return to safe points. Because the kidneys bear primary responsibility for filtering digitalis glycosides from the bloodstream, people with kidney disease or kidney failure have an increased risk for digitalis toxicity.

Young children who accidentally ingest the digitalis medications prescribed for adults such as grandparents can suffer rapid and potentially fatal poisoning. Older people who are not accustomed to having young children around the house sometimes keep their medications in daily dosage containers that do not have child-resistant closures. People taking digitalis medications should keep them in their originally dispensed containers, preferably with child-resistant caps, and store in a locked medicine cabinet. It is crucial to seek immediate emergency medical attention for any child suspected of accidentally ingesting a digitalis medication (such as digoxin or digitoxin). Even a small amount (a tablet or two) can cause serious or fatal heart arrhythmias.

digitoxin Digitoxin is a medication containing cardiac glycosides (digitalis glycosides) taken to treat heart failure or ATRIAL FIBRILLATION. Common brand names include Crystodigin. Derived, like other digitalis glycosides, from the foxglove plant, digitoxin has a longer half-life, or stays present in the body longer (five to seven days) than DIGOXIN (two days). This makes it easier to maintain a stable level of the drug in the bloodstream, although it also prolongs the effects of DIGITALIS TOXICITY should it occur. Digitoxin was the first pharmacological preparation of digitalis glycosides to become available for therapeutic use, but doctors do not commonly prescribe it because its lengthy half-life increases the risk for digitalis toxicity. Doctors sometimes prescribe digitoxin rather than digoxin for people who have kidney disease, as the kidneys are responsible for removing digitalis from the body, or who for other reasons have difficulty tolerating digoxin. Numerous medications interact with digitoxin, with the potential to alter its effectiveness or toxicity level. Among digitoxin's common side effects are ERECTILE DYSFUNCTION, gynecomastia (enlarged breasts in men), and cognitive disturbances.

digoxin Digoxin is a medication containing cardiac glycosides (DIGITALIS glycosides) taken to treat HEART FAILURE or ATRIAL FIBRILLATION. Common brand names include Lanoxin, Lanoxicaps, and Digitek. Digoxin is a commonly prescribed MEDICATION TO TREAT HEART DISEASE. Like other digitalis glycosides, digoxin derives from a species of the foxglove plant *(Digitalis lanata)*. Numerous medications interact with digoxin, with the potential to alter its effectiveness or toxicity level. In particular, POTASSIUM-depleting DIURETIC MEDICATIONS without potassium replacement increase the risk of DIGITALIS TOXICITY. Doctors typically request regular blood tests to monitor blood digoxin levels in people who are taking digoxin long-term.

digoxin immune fab　Digoxin immune fab is an antidote for severe DIGITALIS TOXICITY such as occurs with DIGOXIN overdose. Common brand names include Digibind and DigiFab. The preparation contains sterile, purified ovine antibodies (extracted from sheep) that bind with digitalis glycosides (cardiac glycosides) in the bloodstream. A fab is a fragment of immunoglobin prepared for specific antibody response. Digoxin immune fab is given by injection and works immediately. Some people experience fever or allergic reaction; severe allergic reaction is rare but can occur in someone who has an allergy to ovine proteins.

See also ANTIARRYTHMIA MEDICATIONS; MEDICATION SIDE EFFECTS.

diltiazem　A CALCIUM CHANNEL ANTAGONIST MEDICATION taken to treat HYPERTENSION (high BLOOD PRESSURE) and ANGINA (chest pain). Common brand names include Cardizem, Cardizem CD, Cardizem SR, Tiazac, Dilacor SR, and Cartia XT. Diltiazem comes in regular and extended release formulations. It works by relaxing the smooth muscle in the arteries. This decreases resistance to BLOOD flow, lowering blood pressure. It also allows a higher volume blood to move through the arteries, relieving angina by increasing the flow of blood to the myocardium (HEART muscle). Side effects are uncommon but can include ARRHYTHMIAS and BUNDLE BRANCH BLOCK, swelling of the legs (EDEMA), and CONSTIPATION. Cimetidine (Tagamet), a popular acid-reducing medication, increases the amount of diltiazem that enters the bloodstream and should not be taken with diltiazem.

See also ANTIARRHYTHMIA MEDICATIONS; DIURETIC MEDICATIONS; MEDICATION SIDE EFFECTS; MEDICATIONS TO TREAT HEART DISEASE.

Diovan　See VALSARTAN.

dipyridamole　An ANTICOAGULANT MEDICATION ("blood thinner") taken to treat or prevent BLOOD clots. Common brand names include Persantine and the combination product of dipyridamole and aspirin, Aggrenox. It works by slowing the tendency of platelets (blood cells responsible for initiating the clotting process) to clump together. Doctors often prescribe dipyridamole in combination with other anticoagulants such as WARFARIN or ASPIRIN to prevent blood clots in people who have had HEART valve replacement, CORONARY ARTERY BYPASS GRAFT (CABG), PERIPHERAL VASCULAR DISEASE (PVD), CAROTID STENOSIS, CAROTID ENDARTERECTOMY, DEEP VEIN THROMBOSIS (DVT), HEART ATTACK, or STROKE.

Common side effects include nausea, stomach irritation, headache, and DIZZINESS. These symptoms typically subside after the medication is taken for a few weeks. Dipyridamole also can cause ARRHYTHMIAS and fluctuations in BLOOD PRESSURE, which typically signal too high a dose. HERBAL REMEDIES including evening primrose oil, ginger, garlic, ginseng, and feverfew increase dipyridamole's inhibition of platelet aggregation and should not be taken when taking dipyridamole. Dipyridamole also interacts with various medications that can affect its actions, including BETA ANTAGONIST MEDICATIONS and some DIURETIC MEDICATIONS (notably loop diuretics such as FUROSEMIDE and thiazide diuretics such as CHLOROTHIAZIDE). When administered in large doses intravenously (by a cardiologist in a hospital or medical center setting), dipyridamole has a vasodilating effect on the CORONARY ARTERIES. This causes changes in heart function that simulate the effects of exercise.

See also COAGULATION; DIPYRIDAMOLE STRESS TEST; MEDICATION SIDE EFFECTS; MEDICATIONS TO TREAT HEART DISEASE; VALVE DISEASE; VALVE REPAIR AND REPLACEMENT.

dipyridamole stress test　The administration of intravenous DIPYRIDAMOLE to simulate the cardiovascular effects of EXERCISE. When given in larger doses than when using dipyridamole as an ANTI-

COAGULANT MEDICATION, dipyridamole causes the CORONARY ARTERIES to dilate. However, it does not affect peripheral arteries or cause any changes in BLOOD PRESSURE, HEART RATE, or myocardial (HEART muscle) oxygen needs, so the heart's actual workload remains unchanged. A cardiologist usually orders a dipyridamole stress test when it would be difficult for the person to do a conventional EXERCISE STRESS TEST, or when the results of an exercise stress test are inconclusive.

Procedure

A dipyridamole stress test takes about five or six hours to complete, with a four-hour wait between imagings for the heart's BLOOD flow to return to its pre-dipyridamole state. It begins with injecting dipyridamole and a small amount of a radionuclide (such as thallium or technitium) into a vein. Myocardial cells attract the radionuclide, and the dipyridamole initiates coronary vasodilation. A gamma camera records the patterns of low-level gamma radiation the radionuclides emit as the blood flow carries them throughout the heart muscle. A computer assembles these recordings into images of blood flow through the heart. This is done twice: first immediately after administering dipyridamole to capture the "exercise" phase, and repeated four hours later to capture the "rest" phase. The images show regions of strong and weak myocardial perfusion (blood distribution throughout the heart muscle), helping to identify any areas of inadequate blood supply during exercise (as the dipyridamole simulates) or at rest.

Risks and Complications

Some people find parts of the procedure uncomfortable. Starting the IV can cause minor, localized discomfort when the needle passes through the skin to enter the vein. The dipyridamole can cause flushing, nausea, headache, and ANGINA (CHEST PAIN due to the heart not getting enough oxygen). As well, it is necessary to lie still with the left arm upraised to allow the gamma camera to take pictures, which takes about 20 minutes. It is common to feel tired after a dipyridamole stress test. Although the dipyridamole stress test is an invasive procedure because it involves injecting substances into the body, the risks of any adverse reactions are very slight. The dipyridamole stress test, like other procedures that challenge the heart's capabilities, can initiate a myocardial infarction (HEART ATTACK), TRANSIENT ISCHEMIC ATTACK (TIA), or STROKE, although these are rare.

Outlook and Lifestyle Modifications

After resting at home for the remainder of the day, most people return to their regular activities.

See also ADENOSINE STRESS TEST; DOBUTAMINE STRESS TEST; RADIONUCLIDE SCAN.

disability due to heart disease Limitations on daily activities and job functions that result from various forms of HEART DISEASE. Heart disease is the leading cause of long-term disability in the United States. An estimated 60 million Americans live with heart disease, the majority of whom are able to maintain the lifestyles they desire (including work and leisure activities). About 10 percent of them—6 million—are not able to do so. STROKE alone disables one million Americans each year. CORONARY ARTERY DISEASE (CAD) and ISCHEMIC HEART DISEASE combined account for 20 percent of Social Security disability claims. Advances in diagnosing and treating heart disease have saved innumerable lives in the past two decades. Health-care experts stridently support shifting emphasis to prevention, which many believe could eliminate nearly all acquired heart disease (heart disease that is not congenital) and its corresponding disability. Such a result would add about seven years to average life expectancy and save billions of dollars in health-care expenses in the United States each year.

See also AMERICANS WITH DISABILITIES ACT (ADA); LIVING WITH HEART DISEASE.

disopyramide An ANTIARRHYTHMIC MEDICATION taken to treat potentially life-threatening irregular heartbeats, such as VENTRICULAR TACHYCARDIA, that do not respond to other medications. Common brand names available in the U.S. include Norpace and Norpace CR. Disopyramide works by altering various conductive processes among myocardial (HEART muscle) cells. Its actions are such that it can worsen moderate ARRHYTHMIAS, however, causing more serious or fatal irregularities in heart function. Taking disopyramide within two years of having a MYOCARDIAL INFARCTION (HEART ATTACK) significantly increases the risk of another. Disopyramide also can cause or worsen HEART FAILURE and cause HYPOTENSION. These potential risks limit disopyramide to people for whom other treatments have failed.

See also MEDICATION SIDE EFFECTS; MEDICATIONS TO TREAT HEART DISEASE.

Diuril See CHLOROTHIAZIDE.

diuretic medications A classification of medications prescribed to treat HYPERTENSION (high BLOOD PRESSURE) and to relieve EDEMA and ascites (swelling caused by fluid retention) as symptoms of HEART FAILURE. Diuretics work by drawing more water from the BLOOD. This reduces the volume of blood, lowering the resistance blood encounters as it flows through the arteries and reducing the amount of work the HEART must do to circulate blood through the body. These effects in turn lower blood pressure. The kidneys pass the excess water from the body in the urine, an action known clinically as diuresis, which is why diuretics have the nickname "water pills."

Diuretic medications typically are the first line of treatment for hypertension that persists after, or in addition to, lifestyle modifications (eating and EXERCISE habits). Many people can fully control mild to moderate hypertension with diuretics and lifestyle. Doctors often prescribe diuretics in combination with other MEDICATIONS TO TREAT HEART DISEASE. Frequent urination is common when first starting to take diuretics but usually goes away after a few weeks. Other possible side effects depend on the kind of diuretic. There are three primary kinds of diuretic medications, defined according to their actions in the body: loop diuretics, thiazide diuretics, and potassium-sparing diuretics.

Loop Diuretics

A loop diuretic gets its name from the action it has on a structure in the kidney called the loop of Henlé, which reabsorbs SODIUM from the urine as it passes through the kidney. The amount of sodium in the blood is a key regulator of the body's fluid/electrolyte (salt) balance. The amount of sodium (along with chloride) in the blood determines how much water the kidneys retain and return to circulation or pass in the urine to maintain this balance. When sodium in the blood decreases, the kidneys allow more water to leave the body in the urine. Loop diuretics significantly reduce sodium reabsorption, increasing the volume of water the kidneys pass from the body in the urine and lowering the volume of blood circulating in the body. Commonly prescribed loop diuretic medications are listed in the table.

Loop diuretics also cause the kidneys to pass more POTASSIUM in the urine. This can cause potassium depletion that can lead to ARRHYTHMIAS. Doctors generally recommend that people taking diuretics eat foods high in potassium such as bananas and raisins or might also prescribe a potassium supplement. Other common side

Loop Diuretic	Common Brand Names	Comments
Bumetanide	Bumex	possible cross-sensitivity in people with sulfa allergies
Ethacrynic acid, ethacry nate sodium	Edecrin	most potent of the loop diuretics but high potential for adverse side effects such as rapid dehydration and serious potassium depletion; typically prescribed when other loop diuretics are not as effective as desired
Furosemide	Lasix, Myrosemide	longest on the market; most frequently prescribed; can increase propanolol levels; possible cross-sensitivity in people with sulfa allergies
Torsemide	Demadex	possible cross-sensitivity in people with sulfa allergies; can cause ventricular tachycardia

effects include DIZZINESS, headache, dehydration, and increased risk for thromboembolism (blood clot) and HEART ATTACK. An infrequent but known side effect of loop diuretics is hearing loss, which often returns after lowering the medication dose or changing to a different kind of diuretic although the hearing loss can be permanent. Loop diuretics also can cause elevated blood glucose (sugar) in people with diabetes.

Thiazide Diuretics

Thiazide diuretics also act on the kidneys to block sodium reabsorption and increase water volume in the urine but are not quite as potent as loop diuretics. Thiazides inhibit the actions of certain proteins within nephrons (the primary filtering structures of the kidneys), blocking the ability of the proteins to transport sodium and chloride across cell membranes. Doctors might choose thiazide diuretics for people who also have calcium-based kidney stones, as these medications also reduce reabsorption of calcium (as well as magnesium and potassium).

There are numerous thiazide diuretics. Those commonly prescribed for heart conditions are comparably effective in their diuretic action and are listed on the table below.

Thiazides can increase the skin's sensitivity to sunlight, making it more susceptible to sunburn. Thiazides also can cause skin problems and hair loss. Chlorothiazide interacts with the LIPID-LOWERING MEDICATIONS, CHOLESTYRAMINE and COLESTIPOL; people taking both chlorothiazide and either of these medications should separate their doses by at least an hour.

Some medication products combine chlorothiazide with other drugs, providing a single medication to deliver common combinations of medications to treat heart disease. They are listed on the next page.

Possible side effects of combination products can include those for either or all drugs in the product. These medications work best for people who require multiple medications to control their hypertension and who are fairly stabilized on their medication regimens.

Potassium-Sparing Diuretics

Potassium-sparing diuretics, also called potassium-conserving diuretics, inhibit sodium and chloride reabsorption without affecting potassium reabsorption. They have the weakest effect of all the diuretics. Doctors often prescribe them in combination with other diuretics or with different antihypertensive medications when only a mild diuretic

Thiazide Diuretic	Common Brand Names	Comments
Bendroflumethiazide	Naturetin	
Chlorothiazide	Diuril, Diurigen	
Chlorthalidone	Hygroton, Thalitone	chemically related to thiazides but a different molecular structure; acts in the same ways
Hydrochlorothiazide (HCTZ)	Hydrochlor, HydroDiuril, Ezide, Esidrix, HydroPar, Microzide, Oretic	
Hydroflumethiazide	Diucardin, Saluron	
Methyclothiazide	Enduron, Aquatensen	
Metolazone	Diulo, Mykrox, Zaroxolyn	aspirin and NSAIDs can reduce effectiveness; Mykrox and Zaroxolyn are *not* metabolically equivalent and cannot be substituted for one another
Polythiazide	Renese	
Quinethazone	Hydromox	
Trichlormethiazide	Metahydrin, Trichlorex	

Thiazide Combination Diuretic	Common Brand Names	Comments
Amiloride with hydrochlorthiazide	Moduretic	potassium-sparing + thiazide
Chlorothiazide with reserpine	Diupress	thiazide diuretic + rauwolfia antihypertensive
Chlorthalidone with reserpine	Regroton	thiazide diuretic + rauwolfia antihypertensive
Hydrochlorothiazide with reserpine	Hydropres	thiazide diuretic + rauwolfia antihypertensive
Hydrochlorothiazide with reserpine and hydralazine	Ser-Ap-Es, Tri Hydroserp, UniSerp	thiazide diuretic + rauwolfia antihypertensive + vasodilator
Hydroflumethiazide with reserpine	Salutensin	thiazide diuretic + rauwolfia antihypertensive
Naldolol with bendroflumethiazide	Corzide	beta-blocker + thiazide diuretic
Triamterene with hydrochlorothiazide	Dyazide,	potassium-sparing + thiazide
Trichlormethiazide with reserpine	Metatensin	thiazide diuretic + rauwolfia antihypertensive

effect is necessary. Like loop and thiazide diuretics, potassium-sparing diuretics affect the functions of the kidneys but do so through different mechanisms. Sodium channel blocking diuretics act on a different area of the nephron than either loop or thiazide diuretics, one through which potassium reabsorption is limited. Spironolactone acts on the RENIN-ANGIOTENSIN-ALDOSTERONE (RAA) HORMONAL SYSTEM to block the actions of aldosterone, a hormone secreted by the adrenal glands. Aldosterone influences the amount of sodium the kidneys retain; blocking its action reduces sodium reabsorption.

Commonly prescribed potassium-sparing diuretics include:

Potassium-Sparing Diuretic	Common Brand Names	Comments
Amiloride	Midamor	can interact with ACE inhibitors
Triamterene	Dyrenium	
Spironolactone	Aldactone	blocks aldosterone binding; can cause erectile dysfunction and gynecomastia (enlarged breasts) in men and menstrual irregularities (including postmenopausal bleeding) in women

Potassium-sparing diuretics can allow excessive levels of potassium to build up in the bloodstream, particularly in people who have renal (kidney) disease. Elevated potassium can cause arrhythmias. Blood tests can be used to monitor potassium levels.

See also ANGIOTENSIN-CONVERTING ENZYME (ACE) INHIBITOR MEDICATIONS; ANTIHYPERTENSIVE MEDICATIONS; BETA ANTAGONIST MEDICATIONS; LIFESTYLE AND HEART HEALTH; MEDICATION SIDE EFFECTS; MEDICATIONS TO TREAT HEART DISEASE; RAUWOLFIA; VASODILATOR MEDICATIONS.

dizziness A sensation of LIGHT-HEADEDNESS and shakiness that most commonly results from reduced BLOOD flow to the brain such as occurs with a sudden drop in BLOOD PRESSURE. Dizziness is a key symptom of postural HYPOTENSION, a drop in blood pressure when moving from a lying or sitting position to standing. Postural hypotension is a common side effect of many MEDICATIONS TO TREAT HEART DISEASE and ANTIHYPERTENSIVE MEDICATIONS in particular (medications to treat high blood pressure). Dizziness also can signal TRANSIENT ISCHEMIC ATTACKS (TIAs), episodes of reduced blood flow to the brain resulting from blockages in the carotid arteries or "ministrokes" in which tiny blood clots lodge in the arterioles (tiny arteries) of the brain and stop the flow of blood through them. Occasional dizziness is benign. A doctor should evaluate persistent or frequent dizziness. If the cause is medication, the doctor might reduce the dose or prescribe a different formulation that will achieve the same result without the side effect of dizziness. Dizziness can cause loss of balance; when dizziness occurs, it is safest to sit or lie down until the sensation passes.

See also MEDICATION SIDE EFFECTS.

dobutamine stress test The administration of intravenous dobutamine, a medication that can cause changes in the HEART that simulate the cardiovascular effects of EXERCISE including increased myocardial (heart muscle) demand for oxygen. The cardiologist typically orders a dobutamine stress test when the person cannot easily complete an EXERCISE STRESS TEST (either because of cardiovascular disease or other health conditions that make physical activity difficult) or to obtain additional information when a conventional exercise stress test produces inconclusive results. Dobutamine causes the coronary arteries to dilate as they would under intense physical exercise, greatly and rapidly increasing blood flow to the myocardium (heart muscle).

Procedure

The test begins with an injection of a small amount of a radionuclide (such as thallium or technitium) into a vein in the arm, followed by an injection of dobutamine. The radionuclide is a tracer that has an affinity for myocardial cells. A special camera called a gamma camera takes pictures of the low-level radiation patterns the radionuclide emits as it travels through heart and attaches to myocardial cells. These patterns represent the heart's perfusion—how BLOOD flows through the myocardium and to myocardial cells. Areas of low or incomplete perfusion show damage to the myocardium. The cardiologist conducts the test twice, once with the dobutamine to view the heart at "exercise" and about four hours later when the effects of the dobutamine have worn off and the heart is "at rest."

Risks and Complications

Parts of the test, particularly inserting the IV into the vein, can be uncomfortable. It is common to experience flushing, nausea, headache, and ANGINA (CHEST PAIN) when the cardiologist injects the dobutamine, especially if there is significant CORONARY ARTERY DISEASE (CAD) or ISCHEMIC HEART DIS-

EASE. However, this discomfort is temporary. Some people feel extraordinarily tired when the test is finished. This is because even though they did not engage in any actual physical activity, their hearts functioned as though they did. Risks associated with a dobutamine stress test are similar to those associated with physical exercise or an exercise stress test and include HEART ATTACK (MYOCARDIAL INFARCTION), TRANSIENT ISCHEMIC ATTACK (TIA), or STROKE, as rare but potential consequences of the challenge to the heart's capabilities. Because of these risks, dobutamine stress tests are performed in hospitals or cardiac care facilities that are fully equipped and staffed to handle cardiovascular emergencies.

Outlook and Lifestyle Modifications

After resting, most people return to their normal activities by the following day.

See also ADENOSINE STRESS TEST; DIPYRIDAMOLE STRESS TEST; ECHOCARDIOGRAM; RADIONUCLIDE SCAN.

doctor visits The doctor's visit is the primary point of exchange between patient and physician. It is the opportunity for each to ask questions, evaluate the status of symptoms, and assess the effectiveness of treatment. Both doctors and patients know their time together is limited. There are many ways to make the most of that time. The doctor has clinical protocols that guide his or her interactions—reviewing test results, conducting a basic examination of heart and lung functions, and responding to findings. Most doctors, particularly specialists, are efficient in their methods for following these protocols. The typical patient, however, can find the experience unsettling, confusing, and even overwhelming, especially when an unexpected health crisis such as an ANGINA attack or HEART ATTACK has catapulted him or her into the midst of this strange and unfamiliar environment. Even people with long-standing heart conditions often find doctor visits disconcerting.

The leading complaint patients have about doctor visits is that there is not enough time for the doctor to explain or for questioning the doctor about procedures, diagnoses, and treatments. The leading concern doctors have about their visits with patients is that the patient did not mention or accurately represent symptoms, reactions to medications, and life circumstances that would have had significant bearing on clinical decisions. Although the factor of time is beyond the patient's (and usually the doctor's) control, there are ways to make sure doctor visits meet the needs of both doctor and patient. For each visit, regardless of its anticipated purpose and frequency, the patient should:

- Write a list of any questions in advance, take the list to the visit, and at the start of the visit let the doctor know there are questions.

- Write a list of all medications—prescription, over-the-counter, and herbal products—being taken. Write the name and strength of the product as this information appears on the label, the dose being taken, and how often. Also write any experiences that occur after taking the medication, such as feeling dizzy or nauseated. Take this list to every appointment and show it to the doctor.

- When explaining symptoms to the doctor, try to describe what happens, when it happens, how often it happens, and whether there are certain circumstances that cause the symptoms to occur, intensify, lessen, or go away. Write this information in advance, to help remember everything.

- Ask questions to clarify or understand what the doctor is saying. Do not leave the visit without knowing what the doctor has discovered, ordered, or decided, and why.

- When the doctor makes recommendations that are not feasible, practical, or possible, say so immediately. Often there are acceptable alternatives.

In the current health-care environment, continuity of care is also sometimes a concern. A person may not have a regular doctor at the time HEART DISEASE symptoms arise and may initially receive care through an emergency department and then from a cardiologist. Even when a person does have a regular doctor, communication gaps can develop when the cardiologist provides heart-related care and the regular doctor provides care for other health conditions. Some people have multiple health problems and see multiple specialists, further complicating coordination of care and communication. Also, it is increasingly common for a person to receive care through a health-care clinic or practice group in which appointments are made with the physicians who are available, so a person may go to the same location and see different doctors. Although notes about all care provided by any of the group's doctors go into the same medical record, the doctors may be unfamiliar with the person's health circumstances. These situations increase the importance of people being active participants in their health care—to keep their own notes and records of treatments, surgeries, and medications and to alert each doctor to the involvement of any other doctors or providers.

Ideally, the relationship between doctors and patient should be a partnership in which all work collaboratively toward improving the patient's health.

Initial Assessment Visit

The initial assessment visit can be 30 to 60 minutes long and generally centers around a comprehensive physical examination and health history. Before this visit, write a brief FAMILY HEALTH HISTORY that identifies blood relatives according to their relationship (father, mother, aunt, uncle, sibling, grandparent) who developed heart disease, suffered STROKES or HEART ATTACKS before age 60, or currently have heart disease. Answer questions about lifestyle—smoking, alcohol and drug use, eating habits, physical activity and exercise—honestly. This information is important to health status, not judgmental. At the end of this visit the doctor is likely to order tests or procedures. Make sure it is clear who needs to schedule them, within what time frame they should take place, and when to schedule the follow-up visit.

Diagnostic Visits

A diagnostic visit might involve procedures such as ELECTROCARDIOGRAM (ECG), ECHOCARDIOGRAM, DOPPLER ULTRASOUND, EXERCISE STRESS TEST, blood and urine tests, or various other procedures depending on the suspected diagnoses. These procedures might take place in a cardiac center, hospital, or clinic. Know what preparations each procedure requires, and follow them as instructed.

Routine or Follow-Up Visits

Routine or follow-up visits typically get short blocks of time on the doctor's schedule, sometimes just five or 10 minutes. Their purpose is for the doctor to ascertain that all is going as anticipated. It is essential to ask questions and describe any changes in symptoms. If the doctor prescribes new medications or changes medication doses, make sure he or she explains the reasons. Although the scheduled time for these visits is brief, both patient and doctor should feel comfortable taking the time necessary to address concerns. If this is not possible, ask the doctor to schedule a second, longer visit specifically for this purpose.

See DRUGS, FREE OR LOW-COST; LIVING WITH HEART DISEASE.

donor heart A human HEART surgically removed from a person who experiences death due to circumstances that leave the heart intact (such as brain injury) for transplant into a person whose own heart has damage too extensive to support life. A donor heart must be surgically removed within minutes of death, preserved on ice, and transplanted into the recipient within a few hours. The donor and recipient must share the same BLOOD type, and the donor cannot have any communicable diseases that the transplanted heart could transmit to the recipient. The identities of most donors remain unknown to the recipients.

Donor hearts are in short supply, with there being about four times as many people who need a HEART TRANSPLANT as there are donor hearts. The leading reason is that family members who must make the decision about organ donation often do not know of the person's wishes about donating organs. The death typically is sudden, and emotions are intense. Many states allow people to state their intentions in advance to donate their organs in the event of accidental or unexpected death. All adults should prepare ADVANCE DIRECTIVES, documents that state their desires and preferences about this and other matters related to end of life issues. When given to the physician, advance directives become part of the medical record.

The need to move the donor heart quickly from the donor to the recipient is another key factor in the shortage of donor hearts. There is a margin of several hours for donating other organs such as kidneys, corneas, and skin, but only minutes for hearts. Often doctors must use life support to keep the donor alive until a surgical team is available to harvest the heart, and not all hospitals have the appropriate facilities for such an extensive procedure. Two physicians not involved in the person's care must certify that brain death (cessation of brain activity) has occurred. Most hospitals have protocols that guide the process.

A surgical team, including at least one CARDIOVASCULAR SURGEON, removes the donor heart under sterile conditions in a hospital operating suite. When the team is ready, doctors discontinue any life support. The team must carefully cut the heart's great vessels to release the heart from the chest. After the heart is out, the surgeon closes the chest and there is no indication that the heart is not there. There is no charge to the donor's family for harvesting organs for donation.

See also UNITED NETWORK FOR ORGAN SHARING (UNOS).

dopamine An organic chemical the body naturally produces that functions as a HORMONE and as a NEUROTRANSMITTER to facilitate communication among cells and tissues throughout the body and brain. The brain produces its own supply of dopamine, which serves as a neurotransmitter to facilitate neuron communication related to movement as well as to perceptions of pleasure. Researchers believe addictive substances such as nicotine and narcotics activate dopamine receptors in the brain. Because the dopamine molecule is too large to pass across the blood-brain barrier (a membrane that protects the brain's blood supply from potentially harmful substances), the body produces its own supply of dopamine as well. A small structure in each carotid artery, called the carotid body, makes most of the body's dopamine. The adrenal medulla also makes some dopamine. Body, or peripheral, levels of dopamine are much lower than brain levels.

In the body, dopamine stimulates the rate and force of myocardial contractions, strengthening the HEARTBEAT and increasing the heart's output. The body primarily uses dopamine as a precursor from which it synthesizes EPINEPHRINE and NOREPINEPHRINE, hormones with much stronger actions on the CARDIOVASCULAR SYSTEM that are key to regulating HEART RATE and BLOOD PRESSURE. Doctors can administer dopamine as an injectable drug during cardiac crisis arising from HEART FAILURE, when the heart's pumping action has become ineffective. When given in such circumstances, dopamine has the added effect of increasing sodium reabsorption in the kidneys, which draws more water into the bloodstream and increases blood volume to raise blood pressure.

See also EMERGENCY CARDIOVASCULAR CARE.

Doppler ultrasound An imaging technique that uses high-frequency sound waves (ULTRASOUND) in combination with the Doppler effect to generate visual representations of BLOOD flow and moving structures within the body such as the HEART. In conventional diagnostic ultrasound, high-frequency sound waves travel through soft tissues— such as muscles and organs—and fluids until they encounter a solid object, such as bone, or gas, such as air in the lungs. The waves then bounce back or "echo," and the ultrasound machine records their lengths and presents them as a two-dimensional image.

The Doppler effect, first identified by the Austrian physicist Christian Doppler in 1842, is a phenomenon within physics in which the frequency of a sound appears to change as the object emitting the sound moves. A classic example of the Doppler effect occurs when listening to the sound of an approaching fire engine. Although the siren's signal remains at the same frequency, as the fire engine gets closer the signal's pitch seems to rise. As the fire engine then moves away, the pitch of its siren seems to drop. In actuality what happens is that the echoes of the sound signals shift in frequency as they bounce between the siren and the eardrum. These shifts then can be used to calculate the velocity of the object emitting the sound—in this example, the rate of speed the fire engine is traveling.

In Doppler ultrasound the ultrasound machine sends high-frequency sound waves toward a moving structure within the body, such as blood flowing through an artery or the heart. As the sound waves echo from the moving blood, their frequencies change. The ultrasound records these changes, from which the radiologist or cardiologist can calculate the rate of the blood's flow. Obstructions such as STENOSIS (narrowing) or arterial plaque accumulation in an artery change the rate, as do other heart problems such as diseased heart valves that cause the blood to swirl and pool. Depending on the method used and what the cardiologist wants to examine, the Doppler ultrasound can use color to highlight certain aspects of the blood flow (color Doppler ultrasound, amplitude Doppler ultrasound, or ultrasound angiography) or isolate a particular frequency range (pulsed Doppler ultrasound). Technicians also use Doppler ultrasound to check for air bubbles (which can act as clots in the body's blood vessels) in the blood returning from HEART-LUNG BYPASS MACHINES during OPEN-HEART SURGERY.

See also ANGIOGRAPHY; ECHOCARDIOGRAM; PLAQUE, ARTERIAL.

Down syndrome, heart malformations associated with Down syndrome, also called trisomy 21, is a chromosomal disorder in which cells contain a duplicate chromosome 21, giving them 47 instead of the normal 46 chromosomes. The syndrome produces characteristic facial features and diminished intellectual capability. Nearly half of those with Down syndrome have congenital HEART malformations. The most common, and characteristic, are abnormal openings between the heart's chambers:

- ATRIOVENTRICULAR (AV) CANAL DEFECT, in which the opening is between the atrium and the ventricle (the heart's upper and lower chambers); half of all babies born with this malformation have Down syndrome
- atrial SEPTAL DEFECT (ASD), in which the opening is between the right and left atria (the heart's upper chambers)
- VENTRICULAR SEPTAL DEFECT (VSD), in which the opening is between the right and left ventricles (the heart's lower, or pumping, chambers)

Often an operation can correct these malformations. However, when one malformation exists the probability of additional malformations existing increases. Malformed or incomplete valves commonly accompany canal and septal defects and require additional surgery. Complex malformations can be difficult to correct and account for the majority of deaths in infants with Down syndrome. Among the most common complex heart defects with Down syndrome are:

- PATENT DUCTUS ARTERIOSUS (PDA), in which a channel between the aorta and the pulmonary artery that is normal before birth fails to close following birth
- TETRALOGY OF FALLOT, a multiplicity of malformations that occur in a pattern
- HYPOPLASTIC LEFT HEART SYNDROME (HLHS), in which the left side of the heart fails to develop and cannot function

Congenital heart defects in Down syndrome can cause further heart disease including PULMONARY HYPERTENSION (increased pressure in the BLOOD vessels of the lungs) and HEART FAILURE (inability of the heart to effectively pump blood through the body). Conventional treatments, such as medications, generally are effective in managing these conditions after surgery has corrected their underlying causes.

See also HEART DISEASE; HEART DISEASE IN CHILDREN.

doxazosin An ALPHA ANTAGONIST MEDICATION taken to treat HYPERTENSION (high BLOOD PRESSURE). Common brand names include Cordura. Alpha blockers work by causing the muscles in the walls of the arteries to relax, widening the arteries so BLOOD flows through them with less resistance. Doxazosin is an alpha-1 adrenergic antagonist, which means it blocks activation of alpha-1 epinephrine receptors in smooth muscle cells. It has a vasodilation effect on the primary arteries and a vasoconstriction effect on the arterioles.

DIZZINESS and LIGHT-HEADEDNESS are common side effects that often lessen after taking the medication for several weeks. It is common for doctors to pre-

scribe doxazosin or another alpha blocker in combination with DIURETIC MEDICATIONS, BETA ANTAGONIST MEDICATIONS, or CALCIUM CHANNEL ANTAGONIST MEDICATIONS. Doctors sometimes prescribe doxazosin to treat benign prostatic hypertrophy (BPH) in men (noncancerous enlargement of the prostate gland), as the medication's alpha-1 antagonist action also relaxes smooth muscle in the genitourinary tract.

See also HYPOTENSION; MEDICATIONS TO TREAT HEART DISEASE; PRAZOSIN; TERAZOSIN.

driving Some forms of HEART DISEASE, or the medications taken to treat them, can cause impaired judgment or physical capability that limits driving. Driving is unsafe, no matter what health conditions exist, when there is the potential for loss of consciousness or of physical control, or when either has occurred within the previous three months. Such circumstances require investigation to determine the underlying causes and treatment if appropriate. Most people with heart disease are able to continue driving without limitations. Some states impose restrictions on the driver's licenses of people with certain medical conditions. Otherwise, health experts offer these general recommendations for driving with heart disease:

No Limitations or Restrictions Necessary
Coronary artery disease (CAD), ischemic heart disease, heart failure *without* ANGINA or other symptoms
Hypertension controlled through lifestyle or medication
Occasional ARRHYTHMIAS

Of course, it is imperative to follow the doctor's recommendations about driving regardless of these general guidelines. The capability to physically and mentally manage the many tasks of driving is highly individual. Most people who have been driving all of their adult lives do not have an accurate perception of what this capability entails. A person might feel fine, have no pain, and return to work following CORONARY ARTERY BYPASS GRAFT (CABG), yet it takes a minimum of six months for the sternum (breastbone) to fully heal after surgeons cut through it to gain access to the heart.

Should Not Drive	Length of Restriction
Coronary artery disease (CAD), ischemic heart disease, heart failure *with* other symptoms	Indefinite
Heart attack	Three to 12 months without further symptoms, stable on medications
Hypertension with dizziness, tiredness, weakness, or inability to maintain mental alertness	Three months of treatment without symptoms
Implantable defibrillator	Indefinite
Open-heart surgery (including coronary artery bypass graft and valve repair or replace- ment) or angioplasty	Three to 12 months without surgical or cardiovascular side effects
Pacemaker	Three months without symptoms or serious arrhythmias
Stroke and transient ischemic attacks (TIAs)	Variable according to degree of impairment; at least three months without further symptoms
Taking medications that cause dizziness, sleepiness, reduced alertness, or weakness	For the duration of these side effects and at least one month after they end or two weeks after stopping the medication
Unstable angina	Indefinite or until angina is stable for three months

As well, medication side effects sometimes are not noticeable to the person taking the medication yet significantly affect judgment and physical function. Although driving seems a routine and necessary activity, it involves considerable risk for the driver, passengers, and others when ability is impaired.

See also ACTIVITIES OF DAILY LIVING (ADLs); LIVING WITH HEART DISEASE.

drug abuse and heart disease Nearly any substance that enters the body can affect the HEART and CARDIOVASCULAR SYSTEM. This is the intended purpose of therapeutic drugs prescribed as medications to treat HEART DISEASE, and the unintended consequence of numerous medications taken to treat other health conditions as well as of drugs

taken for "recreational" purposes. Some illicit drugs, like cocaine and methamphetamine, can cause life-threatening ARRHYTHMIAS and SUDDEN CARDIAC ARREST even with first use. In most circumstances, cardiovascular damage is cumulative over time. In some situations the damage is reversible; in many cases it is permanent although often stops progressing when the drug is no longer being used.

Nicotine and Alcohol
Drugs can adversely affect the heart and cardiovascular system whether they are illicit, misused prescription medications, or nonpharmaceutical substances. Those that are most frequently abused and cause the greatest amount of cardiovascular disease are two that are so common that many people consider them social substances rather than drugs: NICOTINE (tobacco) and alcohol.

Heart disease is the most common health consequence of cigarette smoking, and cigarette smoking is one of the most significant causes of heart disease. Nicotine, the addictive chemical in tobacco, is a stimulant that has numerous effects on the cardiovascular system. It increases HEART RATE and BLOOD PRESSURE, causes the arteries to constrict, decreases "good" CHOLESTEROL (high-density lipoprotein or HDL), and increases platelet aggregation (clumping in the first stages of forming clots). As well, damage to the lungs from tar and other smoke residual diminishes the capability of the lungs to exchange oxygen, increasing the intensity with which the heart must work to meet the body's oxygenation needs.

Although some studies show that moderate alcohol consumption appears to have a protective effect with regard to heart disease, alcohol abuse (including alcoholism) causes changes in the cells of the heart that weaken their pumping effectiveness. Long-term alcohol abuse can cause nonischemic dilated hypertrophic CARDIOMYOPATHY, sometimes called alcoholic cardiomyopathy—an enlarged, poorly functioning heart. The walls of the heart may thicken and become stiff, further reducing their ability to contract to pump blood. Changes in myocardial cells interfere with their ability to convey electrical impulses, causing potentially fatal arrhythmias. Alcohol abuse causes myriad other changes in the body that affect cardiac function as well, including damage to the liver (affecting cholesterol mechanisms) and cells throughout the body.

Inhalants

Numerous common products are inhaled to produce a "high." Many of these products, such as paint and glue, are inherently toxic. Others that are aerosol-propelled, such as cooking oil sprays and hair sprays, introduce toxic propellants as well as damaging substances into the lungs. This severely limits the ability of the lungs to exchange oxygen and can easily cause immediate suffocation. Cardiovascularly, it sets in motion a crisis cascade of events intended to restore adequate oxygenation: accelerated pulse, elevated BLOOD PRESSURE, and intensified contractions of the heart. These events can cause sudden cardiovascular collapse.

Illicit Stimulants

Illicit stimulants such as methamphetamine, ecstasy, and other "designer" drugs that are amphetamine or methamphetamine derivatives have DOPAMINE-like actions that stimulate the central nervous system, causing euphoria and intensified alertness, and the cardiovascular system, causing rapid and irregular heartbeat, increased blood pressure, and changes in the walls of the arteries. Their use produces arrhythmias that can cause sudden cardiac arrest, particularly with large doses of the drugs, and rapid spikes in blood pressure that cause stroke. Sudden and significant vasoconstriction (narrowing of the arteries) can virtually close down the coronary arteries, causing HEART ATTACK. Over time, illicit stimulants appear to cause left ventricular dysfunction, cardiomyopathy, heart failure, and cerebrovascular damage (small hemorrhages in the arterioles in the brain).

Anabolic Steroids

Anabolic steroids (also called anabolic androgenic steroids) are taken to build muscle mass and do not produce any sort of "high." Although purported to increase cardiovascular capacity, their effect is in fact the opposite. Even with short-term use, anabolic steroids cause myocardial fibrosis—the growth of fibrous (scar) tissue within the walls of the heart. This weakens the heart, causing fairly rapid hypertrophy (enlargement) as the heart struggles to maintain normal function. Ischemic heart disease and heart failure are inevitable consequences if anabolic steroid use continues, and sometimes develop even after stopping the steroids. Compounding the actions of anabolic steroids on the myocardium are its vasoconstrictive actions on peripheral arteries, which elevates blood pressure, and on the coronary arteries, which can suddenly deprive the heart of oxygen. As well, anabolic steroids lower HDL, worsening the overall lipid profile and increasing the risk for atherosclerosis. Accelerated cardiovascular disease, heart attack, stroke, and sudden cardiac arrest are all consequences of continued anabolic steroid use.

Narcotics

When taken as prescribed, narcotics are effective pain relievers. When abused or illicit (such as heroin), they can cause a variety of cardiovascular disturbances including arrhythmias, bradycardia (slowed heart rate), HYPOTENSION (low blood pressure), and respiratory depression (slow or ineffective breathing). These effects can cause PULMONARY EDEMA and cardiovascular collapse. Injected narcotics further carry the risk of bacterial ENDOCARDITIS (infection of the heart walls or valves), which can create permanent damage to the heart and valves, making a valve replacement operation necessary, or the condition becomes life-threatening.

Cocaine

Cocaine's effects on the cardiovascular system are dramatic, rapid, and profound. Even with first use, there is significant potential for heart attack and sudden cardiac arrest as a result of severe arrhythmias or ISCHEMIA (lack of oxygen to the heart muscle). Cocaine increases the heart's force and rate of contractions while at the same time causing the coronary arteries to contract. This combination simultaneously increases the heart's demand for oxygen and shuts down the blood supply that brings it oxygen. Cocaine use causes the death of myocardial cells in much the same manner as a heart attack, and with similar consequences.

CARDIOVASCULAR EFFECTS OF ABUSED DRUGS

Drug	Cardiovascular Effects and Risks
Alcohol	arrhythmias, cardiomyopathy, heart failure, sudden cardiac arrest
Anabolic steroids	hypertrophic cardiomyopathy, ischemic heart disease, left ventricular dysfunction, heart failure; progression of heart disease even after stopping the drugs
Cocaine	myocardial cell death, ischemic heart disease, left ventricular dysfunction, heart attack, arrhythmias, sudden cardiac arrest; high risk of death with first use
Inhalants	suffocation, arrhythmias, hypertension, cardiovascular collapse
Methamphetamine and other stimulants	tachycardia, arrhythmias, hypertension and sudden spikes in blood pressure, left ventricular dysfunction, cardiomyopathy, heart failure, heart attack, stroke
Narcotics (prescription or illicit)	arrhythmias, bradycardia, hypotension, respiratory depression, bacterial
Nicotine (tobacco use)	atherosclerosis, arteriosclerosis, increased blood pressure, reduction of HDL ("good" cholesterol), increased platelet aggregation, narrowing of the coronary arteries, coronary artery disease, ischemic heart disease, heart failure

See also ALCOHOL CONSUMPTION AND HEART DISEASE; COCAINE AND HEART ATTACK; SMOKING AND HEART DISEASE; TOBACCO USE.

drug interactions, adverse   See MEDICATION SIDE EFFECTS.

drugs, free or low-cost   Medications to treat HEART DISEASE can be very expensive. Many health insurance plans provide little or no coverage for prescription drugs. For older people living on fixed incomes, these medications can be cost-prohibitive. The major pharmaceutical companies have programs through which they will provide certain medications free or low-cost to people who meet defined criteria (which usually are linked to income levels as well as other factors). Most programs require a physician's certification of the person's health status, financial need, and other circumstances. Doctors and pharmacists know what programs are available and can provide the contact information. For some programs, all that is necessary is for the doctor to complete the appropriate paperwork and submit it directly to the pharmaceutical company. The company then provides the medications to the doctor's office, which in turn provides them to the person who needs them.

Doctors also receive samples of medications from pharmaceutical companies, to give to patients at no cost to try out the medication. This is particularly helpful at the beginning of treatment, as there are numerous medications that could be effective but finding those that work best for each person is a process of trial and error. If the doctor does not offer samples when prescribing a new medication, ask if they are available. With numerous medications available in most classifications of drugs, prescribing them is a matter of physician choice. It is always appropriate to ask the doctor why he or she has selected particular medications. When paying for medications is a concern, let the doctor know this. Nearly always there are lower-cost options available that will have the same therapeutic effect.

See also LIVING WITH HEART DISEASE; MEDICATIONS TO TREAT HEART DISEASE.

dual chamber pacemaker   See PACEMAKER.

durable power of attorney for health care (DPHC)   See ADVANCE DIRECTIVES.

Dyazide   See DIURETIC MEDICATIONS.

DynaCirc   See ISRADIPINE.

dyslipidemia   See HYPERLIPIDEMIA.

dyspnea   Labored and sometimes painful breathing or shortness of breath that occurs when the body does not receive enough oxygenated BLOOD to meet its needs. Dyspnea is a symptom that can relate to numerous conditions involving the lungs and HEART, most commonly CHRONIC OBSTRUCTIVE PULMONARY DISEASE (COPD), EMPHYSEMA, PULMONARY CONGESTION/PULMONARY EDEMA, CORONARY ARTERY DISEASE (CAD), ISCHEMIC HEART DISEASE, and HEART FAILURE. Dyspnea also can occur following a HEART ATTACK (MYOCARDIAL INFARCTION) in which damage to the heart prevents it from pumping an adequate volume of blood into the body.

The way in which the dyspnea occurs is a key clue to its cause. Dyspnea that comes on suddenly and is accompanied by CHEST PAIN may suggest myocardial infarction, pulmonary embolism, PERICARDITIS, or pneumothorax (collapsed lung). Dyspnea that occurs at night points to congestive heart failure or chronic obstructive pulmonary disease (COPD). Dyspnea that appears to have no other symptoms and in which the person appears fine may indicate anxiety or panic attack. No matter its cause, however, dyspnea is a frightening experience. Oxygen administration sometimes relieves dyspnea in the short term. Long-term relief targets the underlying causes and improving LUNG CAPACITY.

See also EXERCISE STRESS TEST; ORTHOPNEA; INCENTIVE SPIROMETRY; SMOKING AND HEART DISEASE.

dysrhythmia   See ARRHYTHMIA.

early menopause and heart disease risk   During their childbearing years, women have a significantly lower risk for HEART DISEASE than men of the same age and comparable health status. Following menopause, a woman's risk rapidly increases to match that of a man's. A woman who experiences early menopause (before age 45) appears to have not only an earlier risk of heart disease but an increased risk for more severe forms of heart disease than women who go through menopause at age 50 or later and than men of the same age. It is not clear why this is, although researchers suspect genetic and lifestyle factors play significant roles.

For decades health experts believed that ESTROGEN gave women added protection against heart disease and this protection evaporated after menopause when estrogen levels plummet. In 1998 the HEART AND ESTROGEN/PROGESTIN REPLACEMENT STUDY (HERS) challenged this presumption, generating the first comprehensive data to compare the heart health of women after menopause taking HORMONE REPLACEMENT THERAPY (HRT) with those not taking it. HERS found that HRT afforded women after menopause no protection against heart disease.

Another study, the WOMEN'S HEALTH INITIATIVE (WHI), came to an early and abrupt close in 2002 when its more extensive data showed that women taking HRT (a combination of estrogen and progesterone) developed more heart disease than women not taking HRT. As well, they had more blood clots in the legs (DEEP VEIN THROMBOSIS) and developed more invasive breast cancers. Researchers did not expect such findings, and in response the National Heart, Lung, and Blood Institute (NHLBI), WHI's sponsor, ended the study early because the evidence was so compelling. In light of these findings, it becomes especially important for women to reduce as many RISK FACTORS FOR HEART DISEASE as possible before menopause.

See also LIFESTYLE AND HEART HEALTH; NUTRITION AND DIET; ORAL CONTRACEPTIVES; PREVENTING HEART DISEASE; SMOKING AND HEART DISEASE; TOBACCO USE; WOMEN AND HEART DISEASE.

eating disorders and heart disease   Anorexia nervosa, bulimia, and binge eating are eating disorders that affect the body and the HEART in numerous ways. The most significant cardiovascular risks are ARRHYTHMIAS that can cause SUDDEN CARDIAC ARREST, bradycardia, HYPOTENSION (low BLOOD PRESSURE), and HEART FAILURE. An estimated five to eight million Americans, 90 percent of them women who are in their teens to early adulthood, are diagnosed with eating disorders. Treatment for eating disorders involves a combination of medical support for physical symptoms (particularly with anorexia), which sometimes requires hospitalization, and psychological counseling to address the underlying issues.

Anorexia

Anorexia nervosa is a condition of distorted body image in which the person believes he or she is overweight, regardless of actual weight, and engages in actions to lose weight that typically include not eating and excessive exercise. The consequence is a state of perpetual starvation, with sufferers weighing 15 percent or less than healthy body weight. The effect of this is to engage the body's self-preservation mechanisms, which center around slowing the metabolism to conserve as much energy as possible. This results in slowed HEART RATE (bradycardia) and low BLOOD pressure (hypotension). The heart's workload inappropriately increases, however, as the heart works to maintain adequate circulation despite those circumstances. ANEMIA also is common. As anorexia persists over time, body systems become increasingly dysfunctional. Electrolyte imbalance develops as the body fails to replace calcium, magnesium, sodium, chloride, potassium, and other substances that it needs. This causes arrhythmias that can be life-threatening in combination with hypotension and bradycardia.

Damage to the cardiovascular system can be permanent, particularly heart failure, with increased risk of sudden cardiac arrest even after the disorder is under control and eating habits and weight return to normal. The death from anorexia-induced heart failure at age 32 of talented and popular singer and musician Karen Carpenter in 1983 brought eating disorders and their cardiovascular risks into the public eye, spurring numerous programs and facilities for treatment and support.

Bulimia

People with bulimia eat excessive amounts of food and then force themselves to throw up what they have eaten. It also is common for them to take laxatives and DIURETIC MEDICATIONS in an effort to remove as much food from their bodies as possible. The frequent vomiting has numerous gastrointestinal effects and also depletes the body's electrolytes. Diuretic medications that work by limiting the amounts of sodium and chloride the kidneys retain further alter the electrolyte balance and have the added consequence of reducing blood volume, which lowers blood pressure. The electrolyte imbalance causes various arrhythmias. Even in the presence of hypotension the less efficient heart (from arrhythmias) must work harder, leading to heart failure. The cardiovascular consequences of bulimia are not usually as severe as those associated with anorexia because the person is getting at least some nutrition so even though the body is underweight it is not in starvation mode. People with bulimia do have an increased risk of heart failure continuing after bringing the condition under control, as well as sudden cardiac arrest due to arrhythmias.

Binge Eating Disorder

People with binge eating disorder eat excessively and often secretly, without throwing up or purging themselves with laxatives and diuretics. Although the same body image issues exist, the consequence of binge eating disorder is more likely to be OBESITY than starvation. Heart disease that develops with this condition typically includes HYPERCHOLESTEROLEMIA (high blood cholesterol), early ATHEROSCLEROSIS, and HYPERTENSION. People with binge eating disorder are at high risk for developing type 2 diabetes as well, which further increases the risk for heart disease. Binge eating disorder tends to continue longer into adulthood than do anorexia and bulimia.

See also LIFESTYLE AND HEART HEALTH; NUTRITION AND DIET; OBESITY; WEIGHT MANAGEMENT.

Ebstein's anomaly A congenital heart condition in which the TRICUSPID VALVE separating the right atrium and the right ventricle (upper and lower chambers of the HEART) is displaced and malformed. A normal tricuspid valve has three uniform flaps, or leaflets, that open to allow BLOOD to flow from the right atrium into the right ventricle, and then close to prevent blood from returning to the atrium. In Ebstein's anomaly, two and sometimes all three of the tricuspid's leaflets develop low into the ventricle. This has two structural consequences: it allows blood to flow back into the atrium, and it distorts the sizes of each chamber so the atrium is larger than normal and the ventricle is smaller. Over time the structural distortion increases as the atrium further enlarges to accommodate the higher volume of blood it must contain. This constricts the function of the right ventricle, which pumps blood to the lungs for oxygenation. The right ventricle works harder but its diminished capacity makes the effort less efficient, increasing the heart's workload overall. This sets the stage for congestive HEART FAILURE as well as PULMONARY CONGESTION/PULMONARY EDEMA and PULMONARY HYPERTENSION.

Symptoms and Diagnostic Path

Symptoms vary in severity and the timing of their presentation and may include

- CYANOSIS
- abnormal heart sounds
- ARRHYTHMIAS

- difficulty breathing or shortness of breath (DYSPNEA)
- cough

When the anomaly is minor, symptoms may not develop until later in childhood or even adulthood. Significant malformations, especially when multiple anomalies are present, often produce symptoms shortly after birth. The diagnostic path begins with a general health assessment and procedures to assess the heart's structure and function. Such procedures commonly include ELECTROCARDIOGRAM (ECG), ECHOCARDIOGRAM, and chest X-ray.

Treatment Options and Outlook

Medications to manage symptoms such as heart failure and arrhythmias are generally the treatment approach when the anomalies are less severe. A significant Ebstein's anomaly requires surgical repair or replacement of the tricuspid valve and often occurs with other congenital defects, such as ATRIAL SEPTAL DEFECT (ASD), that require repair as well. Surgery is typically performed in childhood. A minor malformation can remain undetected well into adulthood and might come to light only incidentally during examination for other reasons. In adults, Ebstein's anomaly is a common cause of ATRIAL FIBRILLATION and WOLFF-PARKINSON-WHITE SYNDROME. People who have Ebstein's anomaly may need ANTIBIOTIC PROPHYLAXIS before dental and surgical procedures.

Risk Factors and Preventive Measures

Doctors are uncertain what causes Ebstein's anomaly, though suspect a combination of genetic and environmental factors. There is evidence to suggest that lithium, a medication to treat bipolar disorder, taken during pregnancy may cause this heart defect. A woman who is pregnant and taking lithium should discuss the potential risks with her physician. Otherwise, there are no known measures to prevent Ebstein's anomaly.

See also ACCESSORY PATHWAY; ARRHYTHMIA; ATRIOVENTRICULAR (AV) CANAL DEFECT; HEART DISEASE; HEART DISEASE IN CHILDREN; TETRALOGY OF FALLOT; VENTRICULAR SEPTAL DEFECT.

ECG See ELECTROCARDIOGRAM.

echocardiogram An imaging procedure that uses ULTRASOUND (high-frequency, inaudible sound waves) to generate images of the HEART; also called echocardiography. The procedure is painless and requires no preparation (other procedures done at the same time might require preparation). Doctors use echocardiogram to detect and evaluate structural problems with the heart, such as VALVE DISEASE and congenital malformations. In combination with other technologies, such as DOPPLER ULTRASOUND, echocardiogram can show the flow of BLOOD through the heart and coronary arteries as well.

Echocardiogram has become a standard first-line diagnostic procedure for most cardiovascular disease involving the heart. A typical echocardiogram takes about 60 to 90 minutes to conduct, and the results can be available to the cardiologist immediately. It is noninvasive, yet generates images that show the inner workings of the heart in great detail.

Procedure

During an echocardiogram, the technologist applies a thin layer of conductive gel to the surface of the chest, and then slides a transducer back and forth across the chest. The transducer emits and receives ultrasound signals. The returning signals are called echoes, which is what gives the procedure its name. A computer assembles the signals into images of the heart, and the cardiologist interprets them. Tissues and structures reflect the echoes in different ways, allowing the computer to generate images that have depth and dimension. Usually an electrocardiogram (ECG) is done at the same time as the echocardiogram, so the cardiologist can match the images with the heart's electrical activity.

A conventional echocardiogram is called transthoracic ("across the chest"). Sometimes the cardiologist wants a more precise recording, or the person has physical characteristics (such as barrel chest, infiltrative or obstructive lung disease, or OBESITY) that limit what a transthoracic echocardiogram can show. In such situations the cardiologist does a transesophageal echocardiogram instead. After giving a sedative for comfort and numbing the back of the throat, the technologist inserts a flexible tube with a very small but sensitive transducer at the end into the esophagus. This placement puts the transducer very close to the heart and produces extraordinarily clear images.

Risks and Complications

There are no risks or complications associated with undergoing standard echocardiogram. Echocardiogram may not show some kinds of heart problems and is often used to rule out certain issues to help guide further diagnostic testing decisions.

Outlook and Lifestyle Modifications

After completion of a standard echocardiogram, the person typically returns to usual activities.

See also COMPUTED TOMOGRAPHY (CT) SCAN; ELECTRON BEAM COMPUTED TOMOGRAPHY (EBCT) SCAN; MAGNETIC RESONANCE IMAGING (MRI); MULTI-UNIT GATED ACQUISITION SCAN; POSITRON EMISSION TOMOGRAPHY (PET) SCAN; RADIONUCLIDE SCAN; SINGLE PHOTON EMISSION COMPUTED TOMOGRAPHY (SPECT) SCAN.

ectopic beat An irregular contraction that appears to be an extra or skipped heartbeat; which depends on whether it immediately precedes or follows a normal beat. Ectopic means "out of place"; an ectopic HEARTBEAT occurs out of place in the heart's normal rhythm. In the normal CARDIAC CYCLE, each contraction originates when the SINO-ATRIAL (SA) NODE, the heart's natural pacemaker, discharges an electrical impulse. The impulse "fires" through the myocardium (HEART muscle) in a precise pattern, causing myocardial cells to contract in waves that collectively become the heartbeat. An ectopic heartbeat originates at another point along the pattern rather than within the SA node.

Ectopic heartbeats are common. Some people experience them as PALPITATIONS, although many people are unaware that they are having ectopic heartbeats until an ELECTROCARDIOGRAM (ECG) reveals them. Sometimes ectopic heartbeats signal ELECTROLYTE disturbances, but most often they are innocuous. Caffeine, tobacco, and alcohol use also are associated with ectopic heartbeats. Ectopic heartbeats do not themselves need treatment, although any underlying conditions causing them sometimes do.

See also ACCELERATED IDIOVENTRICULAR RHYTHM (AIVR); ARRHYTHMIA; CONDUCTION PATHWAY; PREMATURE VENTRICULAR CONTRACTION (PVC); SINUS RHYTHM; WOLFF-PARKINSON-WHITE SYNDROME.

edema Fluid that accumulates abnormally within body tissues, which can signal various health conditions including liver disease, lung disease, kidney disease, and HEART DISEASE. Fluid—water and the substances mixed with or suspended in it—comprises about 60 percent of the body by weight. In health, fluid moves between BLOOD and body tissues to maintain equilibrium, or a state of balance, between them. In edema, there is more fluid in body tissues than in the blood.

Edema can involve a specific part of the body (localized) or the entire body in general (systemic). Localized edema often suggests a narrowly focused problem such as DEEP VEIN THROMBOSIS (DVT). Systemic edema reflects a health condition that affects the entire body. A common presentation of edema in heart disease is swelling of the feet and ankles, and sometimes the wrists and hands. This is the result of the excess fluid following the pull of gravity—it naturally pools at the lowest point. Elevating the affected limbs to a level that places them above the HEART helps to ease the pressure and reduce the swelling. "Invisible" edema can affect the internal organs, most notably the lungs (PULMONARY EDEMA) or the brain (following STROKE or head injury). Rapid weight gain is an important sign of systemic edema. Doctors often ask people with heart failure and hypertension to weigh themselves at least daily.

Causes of Edema

Edema develops when the body attempts to restore fluid balance when there is excess volume or pressure within the blood vessels. The excess fluid in the blood seeps into the tissues surrounding the peripheral blood vessels, especially at the capillary level where the walls of the blood vessels are only a cell or two thick. Fluid gets pulled into the blood only when the balance shifts back again. The body's fluid balance becomes distorted for various reasons. Key among them in heart disease are electrolytes, BLOOD PRESSURE, and blood volume.

Electrolytes SODIUM and chloride, the electrolytes in greatest abundance in the body, draw fluid into the blood, which increases blood volume and causes BLOOD PRESSURE to rise. This is a give-and-take balance—when sodium and chloride levels drop, fluid leaves the blood. When blood electrolyte levels become chronically elevated, blood pressure and volume can remain elevated as well and edema develops.

Pressure High blood pressure also forces more fluid from the blood into the tissues, as fluid follows the flow of least resistance. When pressure is lower outside the blood vessels than within them, fluid leaves the blood vessels. This edema generally is systemic, although it might appear more prominently in the extremities.

Volume In HEART FAILURE the heart pumps harder but circulates less blood through the body, causing the volume of blood within the blood vessels to become excessive. This creates an environment of imbalance similar to that of HYPERTENSION, with the same result of edema. As well, edema can develop in the lungs (congestive heart failure). This causes PULMONARY CONGESTION, a chronic state of pulmonary edema that interferes with the ability of the lungs to exchange oxygen.

Consequences of Edema

Fluid-logged, or congested, cells cannot function properly, which has varying consequences depending on what tissues are involved. Peripheral edema involving the extremities can make it difficult to walk or engage in activities that require fine motor movements of the fingers. The edematous swelling acts to stiffen and restrict joints and tissues. If severe enough, such edema (particularly when chronic) can impair circulation in the affected limb, cutting off the flow of blood. Edematous extremities that are cold to the touch and appear dusky in color signal circulatory impairment that needs prompt medical attention.

Edema that affects primarily the abdominal cavity (called ascites) puts pressure on the organs and structures within the trunk. This can impair proper digestion as well as put pressure on the heart and lungs. This further reduces their effectiveness and causes the heart to work even harder. Doctors typically use injections of diuretic medications to relieve edema that reaches this level.

Symptoms and Diagnostic Path

The signs and symptoms of edema may include

- swelling that is often most noticeable in the hands, lower legs, and feet
- unexplained weight gain in which the weight appears most prominently around the midsection
- indentations in the skin that remain after pressing with the fingers
- a shiny, stretched appearance to the skin

Though mild to moderate edema is not usually painful, some people feel discomfort from rings, watches, and shoes that become too tight when swelling occurs. Severe edema can be painful because it creates substantial pressure on the affected tissues. The presence of edema is generally diagnosed by its appearance; the diagnostic challenge can be in determining its cause. Diagnostic procedures commonly include urine and blood tests, chest X-ray, and general physical examination. Further investigation depends on the direction these results suggest. When CARDIOVASCULAR DISEASE (CVD) already exists, it is still important to confirm that there are no other factors, such as kidney or liver dysfunction, that account for the edema.

Treatment Options and Outlook

Treatment of edema targets both the relief of symptoms and the underlying cause. Common approaches include DIURETIC MEDICATIONS to reduce fluid retention along with medications to treat the underlying condition. Compression garments (stockings, gloves, and sleeves) might also be helpful, though should only be used with the doctor's recommendation. Lifestyle measures that help reduce edema include limiting salt in the diet (salt draws fluid), elevating the edematous body parts several times a day, and regular physical activity (movement of the muscles helps keep fluid within the blood vessels). Sitting with the legs uncrossed and frequent walking help blood to return to the heart from the lower extremities.

Risk Factors and Preventive Measures

Edema typically arises as a consequence of chronic health conditions such as heart disease, liver disease, and kidney disease. Managing these conditions through appropriate medical treatment (such as medications) and healthy lifestyle practices helps to minimize edema.

See also CARDIAC OUTPUT; LIVING WITH HEART DISEASE.

edema, pulmonary See PULMONARY CONGESTION/PULMONARY EDEMA.

EDTA therapy See CHELATION THERAPY.

Einthoven, Willem (1860–1927) A Dutch physician whose combined interests and knowledge in medicine and physics led to his development of the multiple-lead ELECTROCARDIOGRAM (ECG), which has become the foundation of understanding and diagnosis of heart disease. He received the 1924 Nobel Prize in physiology or medicine for his work. Einthoven's research followed the trail that started with physicist Carlo Matteucci's discovery in 1842 that electrical impulses generate the HEARTBEAT and physiologist Augustus Waller's primitive recordings of those impulses in 1887. Einthoven designed a simplified electrometer (the machine that detects and records the heart's electrical impulses) that made such recordings practical and developed a new mathematical formula that standardized the electronic fluctuations inherent in the recording process. He also designated letter identifiers for the five primary wave deflections of the cardiac cycle—P, Q, R, S, and T—starting, as is the convention with mathematical formulas, with the second half of the alphabet given that his predecessors had used the first half of the alphabet in their formulas. These letter identifiers remain in use today.

See also ARRHYTHMIA; CORVISART, JEAN-NICHOLAS; HALES, STEPHEN; HEART BLOCK; PACEMAKER; LAËNNEC, RENÉ; SINUS RHYTHM; WOLFF-PARKINSON-WHITE SYNDROME.

Eisenmenger's syndrome A constellation of symptoms that develops as a consequence of form of CYANOTIC CONGENITAL HEART DISEASE.

Early in life, the underlying HEART defects allow unoxygenated and oxygenated BLOOD to mix through the opening between the ventricles. Because pressure is higher in the stronger, larger left ventricle (which pumps blood out to the body) than in the right ventricle (which pumps blood to the lungs), the blood flows from left to right. The initial effect of this is minimal and usually undetected unless there are other symptoms that instigate examination of cardiovascular function.

Over time pressure equalizes between the ventricles, which causes the right ventricle to pump blood into the lungs under greater pressure than normal. The arteries in the lungs stiffen in response, which establishes increased resistance. This resistance increases pressure within the right ventricle (PULMONARY HYPERTENSION). The flow of blood between the ventricles reverses to become right to left, and the left ventricle begins pumping unoxygenated blood out to the body.

Symptoms and Diagnostic Path

Symptoms of Eisenmenger's syndrome tend to arise between adolescence and early adulthood and appear in a characteristic constellation that includes

- CYANOSIS
- ARRHYTHMIAS
- difficulty breathing or shortness of breath (DYSPNEA)
- hemoptysis (coughing up blood)
- CHEST PAIN
- fatigue
- SYNCOPE (fainting) and dizziness
- extremely limited ability to engage in physical activity

The person may have had a HEART ATTACK or STROKE. Gout is also common (deposits of uric acid in the joints, causing painful swelling). The doctor's examination reveals further characteristic features of the consequential conditions that have developed, HEART FAILURE and pulmonary hypertension, which include clubbing of the fingers (an indication of chronic oxygen deprivation) and HEART MURMUR.

ECHOCARDIOGRAM and DOPPLER ULTRASOUND can detect the structural malformations and flow of blood in the HEART, confirming the diagnosis. Chest X-ray often provides the first incidental discovery of problems, showing the enlarged and sometimes displaced position of the heart and pulmonary artery.

Treatment Options and Outlook

If diagnosed in childhood or before permanent damage has become extensive, an operation to correct the septal defect can restore normal heart function. However, once pulmonary hypertension develops and pulmonary artery disease sets in, septal defect repair cannot correct or even offset the damage. Medications can relieve symptoms to some degree, but the pulmonary artery disease continues to progress. Some people with advanced Eisenmenger's syndrome benefit from HEART-LUNG TRANSPLANT, an extensive and high-risk treatment.

Risk Factors and Preventive Measures

The defects associated with Eisenmenger's syndrome include ATRIOVENTRICULAR (AV) CANAL DEFECT, VENTRICULAR SEPTAL DEFECT (VSD), PATENT DUCTUS ARTERIOSUS (PDA), TETRALOGY OF FALLOT, TRANSPOSITION OF THE GREAT ARTERIES (TGA), COARCTATION OF THE AORTA, EBSTEIN'S ANOMALY, TRUNCUS ARTERIOSUS, and TRICUSPID ATRESIA. Early diagnosis and surgical repair of congenital heart defects can prevent the development of Eisenmenger's syndrome. It is the more mild forms of heart defect that are most likely to escape early detection, and as yet there are few guidelines for screening newborns for congenital heart disease who have no symptoms.

See also CARDIOVASCULAR SYSTEM; DISABILITY DUE TO HEART DISEASE; HEART FAILURE; LIVING WITH HEART DISEASE; TETRALOGY OF FALLOT.

electrocardiogram (ECG) A procedure for detecting, recording, and interpreting the electrical activity of the HEART, sometimes abbreviated as EKG. A normal HEARTBEAT generates an ECG tracing with five predictable deviations from baseline, identified by the letters P, Q, R, S, and T, that track

the polarization (contraction) and repolarization (relaxation) of the myocardium.

- The SINOATRIAL (SA) NODE's release of the electrical impulse that initiates each cardiac cycle generates the first deviation, the P wave, which appears as a slight upward blip on the ECG tracing.

- The electrical impulse next travels through the complex of nerve structures (bundle of His, bundle branches, and PURKINJE NETWORK) in the heart to the first part of the ventricle. The ventricle's activation generates the next deviation, the Q wave, which appears as a slight downward blip.

- The main ventricular contraction produces the next ECG tracing, a sharp and prominent upward spike. This is the R wave.

- The remaining portions of the ventricles contract to produce the S wave, a slight downward spike on the ECG. Cardiologists typically refer to the three points representing ventricular contraction as the Q-R-S complex.

- The heart's return to relaxation generates the T wave, which on the ECG tracing rises slowly to baseline.

The ECG tracing changes in predictable patterns with various kinds of heart disease. Movement during the ECG can produce errant or artifact signals. A standard ECG uses 12 electrodes, although a monitoring ECG might use just three and some diagnostic ECGs use as many as 18. Their placements on the body occur in pairs that transect the heart, providing additional information about the heart's electrical activity. Generally six electrodes go on the chest and left side, and the remaining electrodes go on the arms and legs.

Procedure

A typical ECG takes place as the person rests quietly on an exam table. An ECG employs electrodes attached over the heart and at certain points on the arms and legs that transmit the heart's electrical signals to a machine that records them. There is no discomfort or risk with an ECG, and it usually requires no preparation (although sometimes it is necessary to shave the small area where the electrode goes, to make sure it has complete contact with the skin). Sometimes the cardiologist will want to examine the heart's electrical activity over an extended time, such as eight to 24 hours. This is called an ambulatory ECG or HOLTER MONITOR. The person wears electrodes and carries a small recording machine or a transmitting device that plugs into a telephone and sends signals to a recording machine in the doctor's office. For examination of the heart under more strenuous conditions, an ECG is done in conjunction with an EXERCISE STRESS TEST.

Risks and Complications

There are no risks or complications associated with undergoing a standard ECG. It is possible for a person to have an ARRHYTHMIA that is not detected on the ECG. When symptoms or concerns persist, the cardiologist may request specialized testing that enhances the ECG signal.

Outlook and Lifestyle Modifications

After completion of a standard electrocardiogram, the person typically may return to his or her usual activities.

See also ECHOCARDIOGRAM; EINTHOVEN, WILLEM; HEART BLOCK.

electrolyte An ionized (electrically charged) chemical in the BLOOD. The most common ones are SODIUM (Na), chloride (Cl), POTASSIUM (K), MAGNESIUM (Ma), phosphate (P), and calcium (Ca). Electrolytes have many functions in the body and are especially important to conducting the electrical impulses that regulate the HEARTBEAT. Imbalances among the body's electrolytes can cause HEART conditions such as ARRHYTHMIAS and increased or decreased BLOOD PRESSURE, as well as EDEMA. The kidneys primarily regulate electrolyte concentrations in the blood.

Electrolytes and Blood Pressure

Electrolytes are part of the body's mechanism for regulating blood volume and blood pressure. Sensitive structures within the inner parts of the kidneys detect the levels of electrolytes in the blood, par-

ticularly sodium and chloride. When blood electrolyte levels drop, the kidneys reduce the amounts of them excreted into the urine. This draws water into the blood as well, which increases both blood volume and blood pressure. DIURETIC MEDICATIONS taken to treat mild to moderate hypertension and edema act on the kidneys to interfere with this process.

Electrolytes and Heart Contractions

Electrolytes carry electrical signals among the cells of the myocardium (heart muscle), and the sodium/calcium exchange within myocardial cells stimulates them to contract. Many of the medications taken to treat heart failure act on these functions to slow and strengthen the contraction of the cells, causing the heart to pump more efficiently. When the myocardium's blood supply becomes restricted, such as from CAD or with ischemic heart disease, the altered contractions of the myocardial cells cause shifts in the blood electrolyte balance. Blood tests show this, which is one indicator of myocardial distress including heart failure from heart attack.

Electrolyte Imbalance

Electrolyte imbalance occurs when there is too much or too little of a particular electrolyte in the blood. It can occur as a consequence of HEART DISEASE and the medications to treat it and also from other circumstances such as intense EXERCISE, stress, vomiting, diarrhea, dehydration, and health conditions other than heart disease (notably diabetes, pulmonary disease, liver disease, and kidney disease) and the medications to treat them. Electrolyte imbalance can affect heart function, causing PREMATURE VENTRICULAR CONTRACTIONS (PVCs) and other arrhythmias. Electrolyte imbalance that affects heart function most commonly involves sodium and potassium, and less commonly magnesium.

- **Hypokalemia** (low blood potassium) nearly always results from the body excreting too much potassium in the urine, which most commonly occurs with thiazide and loop diuretics taken to treat hypertension and congestive heart failure. Blood levels of potassium may also drop in significant edema. Increasing dietary potassium intake is often effective for mild hypokalemia. Foods that are high in potassium include bananas, baked potato with skin, figs, raisins, and milk (lowfat or nonfat). Switching to a potassium-sparing diuretic or oral potassium supplementation might also be necessary.

- **Hyperkalemia** (high blood potassium) most often develops when using salt substitute products that contain potassium chloride and when increasing dietary potassium when taking a potassium-sparing diuretic (such as spironolactone and triamterene). Other causes of hyperkalemia include ANGIOTENSIN-CONVERTING ENZYME (ACE) INHIBITOR MEDICATIONS, BETA ANTAGONIST MEDICATIONS, DIGOXIN TOXICITY, fluctuating insulin levels such as occur in type 1 diabetes (insulin regulates potassium movement in and out of cells), kidney disease, liver disease, and RHABDOMYOLYSIS. It is also possible for a blood test to present a false hyperkalemia result, called pseudohyperkalemia. This happens when blood cells in the blood sample rupture. Repeating the blood test can determine whether this is the case. The doctor may also request an ECG because true hyperkalemia produces arrhythmias.

- **Hyponatremia** (low blood sodium) may occur with HEART FAILURE, rhabdomyolysis, liver disease, kidney disease, and thiazide diuretics. It may also develop following surgery, with severe emotional stress, and as a consequence of excessive water consumption. Treatment depends on the cause and may be as simple as changing to a different diuretic medication or reducing water intake.

- **Hypernatremia** (high blood sodium) typically results from significant dehydration such as may occur with excessive sweating without appropriate fluid replacement or prolonged vomiting or diarrhea. Diuretic medications, notably loop diuretics, also can cause hypernatremia. Endocrine disorders such as diabetes insipidus and adrenal gland tumors can also cause hypernatremia, as can hyperglycemia in diabetes. An early symptom of hypernatremia is excessive thirst. Treatment depends on the cause and may include increasing water consumption, changing to a different diuretic, and stabilizing blood glucose levels.

- **Hypomagnesemia** (low blood magnesium) can occur with loop and thiazide diuretic medications. It is less common than other electrolyte imbalances resulting from diuretic therapy, though sometimes accompanies hypokalemia. Magnesium deficiency may also develop in people who undergo gastric bypass surgery as treatment for significant OBESITY, because the portion of the small intestine that is bypassed is where most magnesium absorption takes place. Changing to another diuretic, increasing dietary magnesium, or magnesium supplement therapy may be necessary to restore magnesium blood levels to normal.

Routine blood tests to check electrolyte levels can detect imbalances before they have health consequences. When electrolyte imbalances are detected, the doctor may request an electrocardiogram (ECG) to check for arrhythmias.

See also BLOOD TESTS TO DETECT HEART ATTACK; CALCIUM CYCLE; EATING DISORDERS AND HEART DISEASE.

electron beam computed tomography (EBCT) scan A sophisticated imaging procedure that uses a focused beam of electron particles to intensify X-rays. It also is called ultrafast CT scan or "heart scan." EBCT produces detailed images of the heart and coronary arteries that can be useful in early diagnosis of CORONARY ARTERY DISEASE (CAD).

Procedure

Conventional COMPUTED TOMOGRAPHY (CT) SCAN uses X-rays to take images, like snapshots, that are cross-sectional slices of internal structures and organs. A computer then collates these slices into two-dimensional images that display the organ. The speed with which the X-rays can be discharged determines the thickness of each slice; the thickness of the slice determines the detail the completed image can show. EBCT is up to 10 times faster than a conventional CT scan, generating much thinner slices. The rate is fast enough to "freeze-frame" the heart without blurring. When the computer collates the EBCT slices, it uses additional calculations to integrate digital signals into three dimensional images that show the heart's structures in great detail.

Risks and Complications

Among the most significant information EBCT can reveal is the amount of calcium contained in the arterial plaque within the CORONARY ARTERIES. Researchers know there is a strong correlation between the calcium and the likelihood of CAD advanced enough to be a risk for HEART ATTACK. Controversy exists among researchers and physicians, however, over how effective EBCT is as a predictor of potentially life-threatening coronary artery occlusion. This is because arterial calcium deposits appear to occur with aging, making it difficult to determine whether their presence is normal or a sign of advanced CAD. Generally, heavy calcium presence in the coronary arteries of a person under age 60 indicates significant CAD.

Although some researchers advocate for EBCT scanning to become part of normal health screenings for all adults, others express concern that the correlation between calcified deposits in the coronary arteries and heart attack is inconsistent. Further studies are under way. At present, heart experts recommend that people at risk for CAD or who show early signs of CAD receive an EBCT scan as a routine diagnostic procedure.

The radiation exposure with EBCT is about the same as occurs with mammogram. Because health risk associated with radiation exposure correlates to cumulative exposure, the radiation risk of EBCT by itself is very low. People who have recently had other exposure to radiation (such as through X-rays, mammogram, chest CT scan, ANGIOGRAPHY) should let the cardiologist and radiologist know. As well, some people may have hypersensitivity reactions to the dye that is injected intravenously during the procedure.

Outlook and Lifestyle Modifications

Unless there are underlying health concerns that restrict activities, most people return to their normal routine after the EBCT is completed.

See also INFLAMMATION AND HEART DISEASE; LIVING WITH HEART DISEASE; MAGNETIC RESONANCE IMAGING (MRI); PLAQUE, ARTERIAL; POSITRON EMISSION TOMOGRAPHY (PET) SCAN; SINGLE PHOTON EMISSION COMPUTED TOMOGRAPHY (SPECT) SCAN.

embolism A circumstance in which debris in the bloodstream, called an embolus, causes blockage of an artery that impedes or stops the flow of BLOOD. The most common source of this debris is a thrombus, or blood clot. When a thrombus migrates from its original location to another site in the body and blocks flow, it is called a thromboembolus and the condition it causes is called thromboembolism. Other sources of emboli include clumps of cells or bacteria, fragments of arterial plaque or fatty tissue, and air bubbles.

Thrombi (blood clots) can form when circulation is poor, when there is significant ATHEROSCLEROSIS (accumulated fatty particles and arterial plaque along the inner walls of the arteries), or following surgical procedures.

Symptoms and Diagnostic Path

Symptoms of embolism vary depending on the composition and location of the embolus. An embolus may cause pain and swelling at its location, such as with DEEP VEIN THROMBOSIS (DVT) in which blood clots form in the legs. A PULMONARY EMBOLISM may cause CHEST PAIN and difficulty breathing (DYSPNEA). An embolism that blocks a coronary artery often causes symptoms of HEART ATTACK. The diagnostic path may include COMPUTED TOMOGRAPHY (CT) scan, chest X-ray, ANGIOGRAPHY, and other imaging procedures depending on the suspected location of the embolus. The doctor will ask questions about recent surgeries, injuries, CARDIAC EVENTS such as MYOCARDIAL INFARCTION (MI), and existing CARDIOVASCULAR DISEASE (CVD) such as CORONARY ARTERY DISEASE (CAD) and PERIPHERAL ARTERY DISEASE (PAD).

Treatment Options and Outlook

Treatment depends on the type and location of the embolism. THROMBOLYTIC MEDICATIONS may be administered if the cause is suspected to be a blood clot; however, use of these medications must begin within a few hours of the clot's development to be effective. Emboli that occur in the coronary arteries, arteries in the lungs, and arteries in the brain can be life-threatening. Sometime surgery is required to remove an embolus. Treatment for air embolism is hyperbaric OXYGENATION, in which the person enters a sealed chamber to receive pressurized oxygen. This increases the oxygen level in the blood and helps to get oxygen to tissues deprived of it by the air bubble and also to shrink the air bubble's size. Eventually the air will be absorbed into the body; the important part of this treatment is to get oxygen to the tissues beyond the point of the blockage. The outlook for recovery also depends on the type and location of the embolism and the effectiveness of treatment. When oxygenation beyond the embolism can be quickly restored, damage is usually minimal. However, sometimes the damage is permanent, such as when brain embolism results in STROKE.

Risk Factors and Preventive Measures

ATHEROSCLEROSIS, CAD, PAD, DVT, ATRIAL FIBRILLATION, VALVE DISEASE, MITRAL VALVE PROLAPSE (MVP), and impaired blood circulation create increased risk for embolism. People who have prosthetic heart valves or have had CORONARY ARTERY BYPASS GRAFT (CABG) are at high risk for embolism as well. Having HYPERTENSION (high BLOOD PRESSURE) intensifies the risk because it can cause arterial plaque deposits to break free and enter the blood circulation. Significant injury, surgery, long airplane flights, and extended immobility may also increase the risk for embolism. Doctors typically prescribe prophylactic ANTICOAGULATION MEDICATIONS for people who are at high risk for embolism.

An air bubble can enter the bloodstream during operations or when a needle punctures an artery to draw blood for arterial BLOOD GASES. HEART-LUNG BYPASS MACHINES contain special filters to eliminate air bubbles from the blood before returning it to the body. An air embolus also can develop following rapid decompression after diving. Rarely, an air bubble can enter the circulation when receiving intravenous fluids, although IV tubing contains filters to prevent this from occurring.

See also PLAQUE, ARTERIAL; THROMBOLYSIS; THROMBOSIS.

emergency cardiovascular care (ECC) A structure of multilevel education, prevention, and resuscitation methods to reduce the number of lives lost to CARDIOVASCULAR DISEASE (CVD), HEART ATTACK, and STROKE. It encompasses training and education in basic cardiac life support (BCLS), advanced cardiac life support (ACLS), CPR (cardiopulmonary resuscitation), and AUTOMATED EXTERNAL DEFIBRILLATORS (AED). The American Heart Association (AHA) publishes comprehensive guidelines for emergency cardiovascular response. The guidelines come from a panel of international experts who review procedures and outcomes to determine the most effective methods for the public and for health-care professionals to employ. ECC targets reviving those who suffer CARDIAC ARREST and getting them to hospitals that can administer advanced care. Statistics show that fewer than 5 percent of people who go into cardiac arrest live long enough to receive hospital treatment; current ECC procedures aim to improve that percentage. The AHA updates ECC guidelines as new information becomes available.

See also CHAIN OF SURVIVAL.

emotions and heart disease There are two dimensions to the role of emotions in HEART DISEASE: emotions as contributing to the causes and development of heart disease, and emotions in the context of learning to cope with having (or living with a loved one who has) heart disease.

Emotions as They Contribute to Heart Health and Heart Disease

Through the last several decades, there has been considerable research into the relationship between emotions and health, with strong correlations emerging between emotions and both disease and recovery. In the 1980s researchers made the first definitive connections between biochemical activity in the brain and emotions such as fear and joy. Though clinical evidence remains inconclusive, it appears that people with a bright outlook who can find joy in everyday life are not only happier but live longer and with fewer symptoms than people whose emotional outlook is dark and negative.

For many years, doctors observed correlations between certain modes of emotional expression and the likelihood of heart disease. People, particularly men, who were outwardly expressive with their anger and aggression, the "type A" personality, had higher rates of HYPERTENSION (high BLOOD PRESSURE) and CORONARY ARTERY DISEASE (CAD) than did those with a "type B" personality whose emotional expressions were less volatile. Recent studies of people with IMPLANTABLE CARDIOVERTER DEFIBRILLATORS, which deliver a shock to the heart when ARRHYTHMIAS threaten the HEARTBEAT, showed that there is a correlation between the expression of anger and arrhythmia. Scientists have long known that strong fear activates the body's "FIGHT-OR-FLIGHT" response, which raises blood pressure, increases the heart's pumping force, and increases HEART RATE. Continuous stress has the same effect. Although there is no clear evidence that emotions cause heart disease, it does seem certain that they contribute to it at least in subtle ways.

Emotions and Living with Heart Disease

The diagnosis of heart disease brings varied emotional responses for the person with heart disease as well as family members and friends. Sometimes people feel they cannot express their emotions for fear of hurting the feelings of others. Yet withholding emotional expression increases frustration and stress. It is important for those whose lives are affected by heart disease to share their emotions with one another. Fear, anger, and DENIAL are common. So, too, are joy and happiness. Many hospitals and community organizations have support groups for people with heart disease or who have had heart surgery, and for their loved ones. Such support groups provide opportunities to express feelings and share concerns with others who are having similar experiences.

See also LIFESTYLE AND HEART HEALTH; LIVING WITH HEART DISEASE; ORNISH PROGRAM; PERSONALITY TYPES; STRESS AND HEART DISEASE; STRESS REDUCTION TECHNIQUES.

enalapril An ANGIOTENSIN-CONVERTING ENZYME (ACE) INHIBITOR MEDICATION taken to treat HYPERTENSION (high BLOOD PRESSURE) and HEART FAILURE. Common brand names include Vasotec. Doctors sometimes prescribe enalapril in combination with a DIURETIC MEDICATION to treat hypertension, or as

ADJUNCT THERAPY with a digitalis medication such as digoxin to treat HEART failure. As with other ACE inhibitors, enalapril works by interfering with the action of angiotensin-converting enzyme (ACE) to convert angiotensinogen (angiotensin I) into angiotensin II, a powerful vasoconstrictor that acts on the arterioles, the body's smallest arteries. ACE is an integral component of the RENIN-ANGIOTENSIN-ALDOSTERONE (RAA) HORMONAL SYSTEM, the body's primary mechanism for regulating blood pressure. Enalapril, like other ACE inhibitors, has numerous potential side effects. Among the most common are headache, DIZZINESS, weakness, skin irritation, and a persistent cough.

See also ANGIOTENSIN II RECEPTOR ANTAGONIST MEDICATIONS; ANTIHYPERTENSIVE MEDICATIONS; BENAZEPRIL; CAPTOPRIL; FOSINOPRIL; LISINOPRIL; MEDICATIONS TO TREAT HEART DISEASE; MOEXIPRIL; RAMIPRIL; TRANDOLAPRIL.

endarterectomy An operation to open an artery to remove an occlusion and restore normal blood flow. The most commonly performed variation is CAROTID ENDARTERECTOMY to treat CAROTID STENOSIS, a narrowing of the carotid artery in the neck usually resulting from an accumulation of arterial plaque. Endarterectomy of arteries in the legs and arms can relieve occlusions resulting from peripheral vascular disease, opening the arteries and restoring free circulation. ANGIOGRAPHY helps to isolate the area of occlusion.

Procedure

The surgeon then makes an incision near the area to expose and then cut into the artery. The procedure includes removing the inner layer of the artery's wall at the location of the occlusion. A new inner layer grows in a few weeks, providing a smooth, clean surface that resists the adherence of arterial plaque and other deposits.

Risks and Complications

Endarterectomy carries a substantial risk of thromboembolism that can result in HEART ATTACK or STROKE. Tiny fragments of debris can break away into the bloodstream, lodging in the small arteries in the HEART or brain. Other risks include infection that can quickly become systemic as bacteria have rapid entry into the bloodstream.

Outlook and Lifestyle Modifications

The procedure generally requires several days of hospitalization for recovery and two or three weeks of recuperation at home. The area of artery cleared by the endarterectomy typically stays free from arterial plaque accumulation, although other areas and arteries often develop occlusions. ATHEROSCLEROSIS tends to be a systemic rather than localized disease, so when it involves one artery, it generally affects all arteries to some extent.

See also ATHERECTOMY; CORONARY ARTERY DISEASE (CAD); PLAQUE, ARTERIAL; STENT; SURGERY TO TREAT CARDIOVASCULAR DISEASE.

endocarditis   Inflammation or infection of the interior of the HEART, often involving the valves. The infective agent can be viral or bacterial, although most commonly is bacterial. Occasionally a medical procedure such as CARDIAC CATHETERIZATION, ANGIOGRAPHY, or ANGIOPLASTY can traumatize heart valves or myocardial tissue as the catheter passes through the heart, creating susceptibility to infection or introducing the bacteria that cause an infection.

Symptoms and Diagnostic Path

The symptoms of endocarditis often are generalized, making diagnosis difficult. The person may experience fever, chills, shortness of breath, chest tightness, night sweats, and occasionally angina-like CHEST PAIN. Some people develop HEART MURMURS, which indicate the heart's valves are not functioning properly. (Heart murmur alone is fairly common and is not by itself a symptom of endocarditis.) Endocarditis can smolder for months; often there are few symptoms until the infection significantly impairs cardiac function and has spread to other parts of the body. Meningitis (infection of the membranes surrounding the brain) and septicemia (infection involving multiple body systems) are common and serious consequences of untreated bacterial endocarditis, as blood passing through the heart picks up the bacteria and circulates it throughout the body. ECHOCARDIOGRAM and blood cultures to test for bacterial growth are important but not conclusive diagnostic tools.

Treatment Options and Outlook

Treatment for bacterial endocarditis requires intravenous antibiotics, usually given for four to six weeks depending on the bacteria and the severity of symptoms. This can take place on an outpatient basis once it is clear the infection is responding. Occasionally surgery is necessary to remove any diseased and damaged valves and clean out the remaining areas of infection. Sometimes the infection causes scarring when tissues and especially valves heal, requiring surgery to repair or replace valves that no longer function properly.

Viral endocarditis is less common. Because they travel in the bloodstream, viruses can infect virtually any organ system or structure of the body. Treatment is primarily supportive while the virus runs its course. Another uncommon form of endocarditis is sterile endocarditis, in which the heart and valves become inflamed but there is no infection. Sterile endocarditis generally develops in people who have other chronic diseases, including metastatic cancer and systemic lupus erythematosus (an autoimmune disorder affecting the connective tissue). Treatment in such situations targets the underlying causes or is primarily supportive.

Risk Factors and Preventive Measures

Known risks for bacterial endocarditis include:

- recent heart operation
- recent dental procedures or gum infection
- recent bacterial throat infection (particularly streptococcus or "strep throat")
- prosthetic heart valves
- intravenous drug use or extended intravenous therapy
- AIDS

Some people have increased susceptibility to endocarditis, which means they are more likely to develop endocarditis with bacterial exposure and should take prophylactic antibiotics before dental procedures, endoscopic procedures, and any non-sterile operative procedures (such as podiatric). As well, certain heart conditions increase susceptibility to endocarditis. Among them are:

- CYANOTIC CONGENITAL HEART DISEASE
- congenital heart malformations (even if surgically repaired)
- clinically significant MITRAL VALVE PROLAPSE (MVP)
- hypertrophic CARDIOMYOPATHY (enlarged heart)
- acquired valve disease
- history of RHEUMATIC HEART DISEASE
- previous endocarditis or PERICARDITIS (inflammation or infection of the membranes surrounding the heart)

Antibiotic prophylaxis is the most effective means of preventing endocarditis in people who have increased susceptibility. As well, it is important to appropriately treat bacterial infections elsewhere in the body, such as the throat.

See also ANTIBIOTIC PROPHYLAXIS; VALVE REPAIR AND REPLACEMENT.

endorphins and enkephalins Substances the brain produces that act like natural pain-relievers. Classified as neuropeptides, endorphins and enkephalins are closely related amino acid structures that function as neurotransmitters to facilitate signals related to pain and pleasure in the brain. They interact with opioid receptors in the brain in the same manner as do narcotics such as morphine. Various stimuli cause the brain to release endorphins and enkephalins, although researchers are investigating the mechanisms of release. Enzymes that brain cells release at the same time quickly neutralize the endorphins and enkephalins, so their natural time of effectiveness is limited. Some studies suggest that ACUPUNCTURE stimulates the release of endorphins and enkephalins, accounting for its effectiveness in relieving pain.

Researchers discovered endorphins and enkephalins in the 1970s, and research has continued since that time to find ways to synthesize them for use as pain medications. Although scientists have been successful in replicating the chemical struc-

tures of these neuropeptides, the brain barrier prevents them from ᴦ blood to the brain.

endovascular abdominal aortic aneurysm repair
See ABDOMINAL AORTIC ANEURYSM.

enhanced external counterpulsation (EECP) A treatment for congestive HEART FAILURE that uses pressure alternatingly applied and released to the legs and arms to support the heart's efforts to circulate blood. A computer synchronizes the counterpulsation with the CARDIAC CYCLE.

Procedure

For EECP, pressure cuffs similar to large blood pressure cuffs go around the lower extremities, buttocks, and arms. When the heart contracts (SYSTOLE), the cuffs sequentially deflate from the arms downward. When the heart relaxes (DIASTOLE), the cuffs sequentially inflate from the lower legs upward. This pattern augments the heart's pumping action, helping to ease the peripheral resistance against which the heart pumps and the heart's (particularly the left ventricle's) workload.

For a typical treatment regimen, the person goes to a cardiology clinic or hospital location for EECP treatment for one hour five days a week for seven weeks, a total of 35 treatments.

Risks and Complications

Some people may find the alternating pressurization to be mildly uncomfortable. People who have ATRIAL FIBRILLATION, poorly controlled HYPERTENSION (high BLOOD PRESSURE), DEEP VEIN THROMBOSIS (DVT), significant PERIPHERAL ARTERY DISEASE (PAD), or congestive heart failure should not undergo EECP.

Outlook and Lifestyle Modifications

Most people feel immediate improvement when each EECP session begins and feel progressive improvement as the treatments continue.

The effect of EECP are long-term for most people, lasting up to three years after a treatment period. Many people who have symptomatic coronary artery disease (CAD) and undergo EECP experience significant or complete relief of ANGINA and are able to return to normal activities, whereas before EECP treatment their angina even with medication was limiting. Exercise stress tests show that EECP significantly improves myocardial perfusion—that is, the flow of blood through the myocardium (heart muscle).

Researchers have understood the principle of external counterpulsation since the 1950s. Early applications used alternating but nonsequential counterpulsation as a treatment for cardiovascular shock. It became a practical treatment for heart failure in the 1990s when computer technology allowed sequential counterpulsation synchronized with the cardiac cycle.

See also LIVING WITH HEART DISEASE; MEDICATIONS TO TREAT HEART DISEASE.

enlarged heart   See CARDIOMYOPATHY.

enzyme   A protein structure that regulates the interactions of other proteins, HORMONES, and chemicals in the body. There are thousands of enzymes that have roles in nearly every chemical interaction that takes place. Body tissues release enzymes in response to actions taking place within them, such as when the myocardium (heart muscle) releases CTNI (CARDIAC TROPONIN I), CTNT (CARDIAC TROPONIN T), CREATINE KINASE (CK), and CREATINE KINASE MB (CK-MB) following HEART ATTACK (MYOCARDIAL INFARCTION). The predictable rise and fall of the levels of these enzymes in the blood helps doctors to determine the severity and timeline of a heart attack. Enzymes also have therapeutic application. Doctors administer the enzymes STREPTOKINASE and TISSUE PLASMINOGEN ACTIVATOR (TPA) following STROKE or HEART ATTACK, if treatment can begin quickly enough, to help dissolve blood clots blocking the arteries and minimize or prevent permanent damage.

See also BLOOD TESTS TO DETECT HEART ATTACK; CARDIAC ENZYMES.

ephedra   A stimulant chemically related to amphetamine found in some over-the-counter appetite suppressants, diet aids, and products claiming to enhance athletic performance. Its use is associated with HYPERTENSION (high BLOOD PRESSURE) and deaths due to cardiac ARRHYTHMIAS, HEART ATTACK, and STROKE. Ephedra comes from the Chinese herb ma huang which was once a common ingredient in many over-the-counter nutritional supplements though is now banned in the United States. Ephedra's active ingredient is ephedrine, a substance once common in decongestant products but now prohibited in over-the-counter medications in the United States.

Ephedra works by stimulating, in similar fashion to EPINEPHRINE, the body's mechanisms that increase blood pressure, HEART RATE, the force of the HEARTBEAT, and respirations (breathing rate). It also intensifies mental alertness. This is the body's "call to action" response, and it has the corresponding consequence of diminishing functions nonessential to physical activity such as appetite. Numerous athletic organizations—among them the International Olympics Committee (IOC), the National Football League (NFL), the National Collegiate Athletic Association (NCAA), and all high school athletic associations—ban athletes from using products containing ephedra or ephedrine. Strenuous exercise also elevates blood pressure, heart rate, and respirations. When this is in addition to the elevations that ephedra already has activated, the body can quickly reach the level beyond which it cannot cope. Blood pressure and pulse can skyrocket, sending the body into a state of shock. The Food and Drug Administration (FDA) has documented more than 100 deaths and several thousand reports of adverse reactions among athletes taking ephedra products.

Ephedra seems to be especially hazardous for the HEART when taken in combination with caffeine, which also is a stimulant. This increases the stress on the heart during exercise. Because nutritional supplements are not subject to FDA regulations that require labels to list ingredients, many products do not identify ephedra or its variations as an ingredient. Ma huang, Chinese ephedra, botanical ephedrine, and epitonin are all forms of ephedra.

See also COLD/FLU MEDICATION AND HYPERTENSION; EXERCISE; NUTRITION AND DIET; PSEUDOEPHEDRINE; SUDDEN CARDIAC ARREST; WEIGHT MANAGEMENT.

epinephrine A chemical the body naturally produces that has numerous effects on the nervous and cardiovascular systems; sometimes called adrenaline (more common outside the United States). It is primarily a cardiovascular stimulant that increases HEART RATE, the force of the HEARTBEAT, and, by causing peripheral arteries to constrict, BLOOD PRESSURE. It also increases respiratory rate (breathing). It is at the center of the body's "FIGHT-OR-FLIGHT" stress response. Epinephrine belongs to the chemical family catecholamines, as do NOREPINEPHRINE and DOPAMINE. The adrenal medulla, the inner portion of the adrenal gland and a structure of the autonomic nervous system, produces epinephrine (as well as norepinephrine and dopamine). Doctors inject epinephrine directly into the heart (intracardiac) or intravenously in a CARDIAC ARREST to "jump-start" the heart. BETA ANTAGONIST MEDICATIONS taken to treat HYPERTENSION (high blood pressure) block the actions of epinephrine on the HEART and BLOOD vessels.

Because epinephrine causes blood vessels to constrict, local anesthetics (numbing medications) injected for dental procedures and minor medical procedures sometimes include it. Several studies have shown that people who have had HEART TRANSPLANTS have intensified sensitivity to some of the systemic effects of epinephrine, notably that it increases heart rate shortly after being injected into the tissues. Whether this is clinically important is unclear; there is not the corresponding increase in blood pressure that epinephrine typically also initiates. People who have transplanted hearts should let their dentists and doctors know of this before receiving any local anesthetic injection.

See also ALPHA ANTAGONIST MEDICATIONS; HORMONE; NEUROTRANSMITTER; PHEOCHROMOCYTOMA.

erectile dysfunction The inability of a man's penis to become or remain erect enough for sexual intercourse. Erectile dysfunction can develop as a consequence of ATHEROSCLEROSIS (deposits within the arteries that narrow the channel for the flow of BLOOD) and other CARDIOVASCULAR DISEASE (CVD) that impairs circulation. For an erection to occur, the spongy channels within the penis (the corpora cavernosa) must fill with enough blood to engorge them and stiffen the penis. The arteries that supply the penis are narrower than arteries in other parts of the body and often are among the first to be affected by arterial plaque and atherosclerotic deposits. This can slow or even cut off the flow of blood into the penis, preventing blood from completely filling the corpora cavernosa. A man who has CVD is four times more likely to have erectile dysfunction than a man who does not have HEART DISEASE, although overall the likelihood of erectile dysfunction increases with a man's age.

Erectile dysfunction also can occur as a side effect of MEDICATIONS TO TREAT HEART DISEASE, particularly ANTIHYPERTENSIVE MEDICATIONS such as BETA ANTAGONIST MEDICATIONS that act to relax smooth muscle tissue of the walls of the arteries throughout the body including the penis. Changing to a different antihypertensive medication often reduces or ends this interference. Treatments that reduce arterial plaque accumulations, such as exercise and LIPID-LOWERING MEDICATIONS, can improve blood flow to the penis as well as throughout the body.

Psychological factors can influence erectile dysfunction as well. When recovering from HEART ATTACK, STROKE, or operations such as ANGIOPLASTY or CORONARY ARTERY BYPASS GRAFT (CABG), it is normal and natural for men to feel worry and even fear about resuming sexual activity. This can inhibit sexual arousal and further concerns about not only sexual performance but also whether the activity will exacerbate the heart problems. If the cardiologist gives the okay to resume sex, then it is not likely to affect heart function any more than walking up three or four flights of stairs.

One of the most promising treatments for erectile dysfunction are the nitrate compound medications that inhibit phosphodiesterase (PDE5), the ENZYME that cause an erection to subside. This makes it easier for a man to obtain and keep an erection. About 60 to 70 percent of men who have erectile dysfunction benefit from PDE5 inhibitors (such as sildenafil, commonly known by its brand name Viagra). Men who take nitrate-based medications such as nitroglycerin or amyl nitrate for ANGINA should not take PDE5 inhibitors.

For men who cannot take, or do not receive benefit from, sildenafil, there are other options to treat erectile dysfunction including alprostadil urethral suppositories or injections, penile implants, and medications such as papaverine and phentolamine that the man injects directly into the side of his penis. It is especially important for couples to be open and loving toward each other and about erectile dysfunction, and to maintain an intimate relationship that includes close physical contact even when intercourse does not occur. Men need to let their doctors know if they are experiencing erectile dysfunction, as often there are treatments that can help.

See also PLAQUE, ARTERIAL; SEXUAL ACTIVITY AND HEART DISEASE; SEXUAL DYSFUNCTION.

erythrocyte   See BLOOD.

erythropoietin (EPO)   A HORMONE the kidneys produce that stimulates stem cells in the bone marrow to produce red blood cells (erythrocytes). The kidneys release EPO when oxygen levels in the BLOOD drop; red blood cells transport oxygen. EPO also is given, by injection, as a treatment for severe anemia (particularly the anemia accompanying chemotherapy) and for people on renal dialysis for kidney failure.

When taken as a performance-enhancing substance, which is illegal, EPO use is called "blood doping." It artificially increases the number and percentage of red cells in the blood, increasing the blood's capacity to carry oxygen. This inherently increases AEROBIC CAPACITY. Such use of EPO is illegal in all forms of international and national competition. Blood tests can measure the amount of EPO in the bloodstream. EPO use can cause or worsen HYPERTENSION (high BLOOD PRESSURE).

See also DRUG ABUSE AND HEART DISEASE; EXERCISE; HEMOGLOBIN.

estrogen   The collective name for the HORMONES that regulate female fertility. Estrogen levels rise at puberty, remain cyclic but elevated through a woman's 20s, 30s, and 40s, and diminish as fertility draws to an end, for most women, in the early 50s. In addition to its role in secondary sex characteristics, ovulation, conception, and pregnancy, estrogen has numerous other effects in a woman's body. One of the most important, although not yet fully understood, is its involvement in cholesterol metabolism.

Women in their fertile years when estrogen levels are high have more high-density lipoprotein (HDL), the "good" cholesterol, and less low-density lipoprotein (LDL), the "bad" cholesterol. This relationship slips in the other direction after menopause, with LDL rising and HDL dropping. As it is LDL that is linked with ATHEROSCLEROSIS and CORONARY ARTERY DISEASE (CAD), this is a disturbing switch. Estrogen supplementation after menopause (hormone replacement therapy, or HRT), was once common and seemed to halt and even restore the cholesterol ratio to near premenopausal levels. This appeared to give estrogen, taken via HRT, a protective effect against HEART DISEASE.

Studies in the late 1990s and early 2000s refuted this premise, providing startling yet clear evidence that this was not the case. Whatever protective effect estrogen has with regard to heart disease, attempting to maintain its levels in the body after menopause does not restore it. In fact, women taking HRT were at greater risk for early heart disease. Research continues to search for explanations. One line of scientific exploration looks at the interplay between genetics and estrogen. Others undertake to investigate the roles of lifestyle factors such as WEIGHT MANAGEMENT, EXERCISE, and eating habits.

See also CHOLESTEROL, BLOOD; EARLY MENOPAUSE AND HEART DISEASE RISK; LIFESTYLE AND HEART HEALTH; NUTRITION AND DIET; WOMEN AND HEART DISEASE, WOMEN'S HEALTH INITIATIVE (WHI).

estrogen replacement therapy (ERT)   See HORMONE REPLACEMENT THERAPY (HRT).

exercise   Physical activity of moderate to strenuous effort that increases cardiovascular functions. Although many people think of exercise as dedicated to "working out" or establishing and maintaining fitness, it can be any physical activity a person performs for 15 to 60 minutes. Exercise is a cornerstone of lifestyle efforts to support HEART health. There are two main kinds of exercise, aerobic and anaerobic (resistance). Both are important for optimal health and fitness; aerobic exercise is essential for cardiovascular fitness.

Aerobic Exercise

The word *aerobic* means "with air." Aerobic activities increase the body's need for oxygen. During aerobic exercise, the heart beats faster and harder, the breathing accelerates, the BLOOD PRESSURE goes up. The CARDIOVASCULAR SYSTEM needs aerobic activity to maintain optimal efficiency in exchanging and delivering oxygen. Regular aerobic exercise causes new capillaries to grow, improving oxygen exchange at the tissue level. It also causes mitochondria within cells, the structures that generate energy, to increase.

People of nearly any age and fitness level can engage in aerobic activity that will improve cardiovascular efficiency. Walking is an ideal aerobic exercise because it requires no special equipment (except comfortable clothing and sturdy, well-fitted shoes). Increasing aerobic fitness requires aerobic activity at a sustained level that elevates HEART RATE for a minimum of 15 minutes at a time. The longer and more intense the exercise, the more stamina and strength the cardiovascular system develops. Athletes in training and people striving for optimal aerobic fitness monitor their heart rates to keep them at target heart rate, a percentage of maximum heart rate (which varies with age). With higher levels of aerobic fitness, resting heart rate is lower. A normal resting heart rate is 80 to 100 beats per minute. The resting heart rate of a person in excellent aerobic condition can be 60 beats per minute or lower. This reduces the heart's workload.

Although people tend to think of activities such as running, swimming, and bicycling when they think of aerobic exercise, YOGA and TAI CHI can both provide cardiovascular workouts if performed to do so. These activities also emphasize breath control, which is essential for aerobic fitness. No matter what the aerobic activity, it is important to start at a level of moderate exertion and work up to more intense exercise. Cardiac rehabilitation programs and organizations such as the YMCA can provide structured, progressive programs that accommodate any special needs made necessary by existing

Aerobic Activity	Light	Moderate	Strenuous
basketball		X	X
bicycling	X	X	X
jogging/running		X	X
step aerobics	X	X	X
swimming	X	X	X
tai chi	X	X	
tennis		X	X
volleyball		X	X
walking	X	X	
yoga	X	X	

heart disease or by physical impairments. These are some common aerobic activities:

Anaerobic (Resistance) Exercise

Anaerobic exercise builds muscle bulk by working muscle fibers against resistance. This causes them to thicken and elongate, giving them increased strength. The most common form of anaerobic exercise is weight lifting or resistance training. Increased muscle strength and bulk make the muscles more efficient, so they use less oxygen to accomplish their activities. This benefits the heart by lessening the force and rate with which it must contract. An added benefit of anaerobic exercise is a toned physical appearance. Regular resistance activities give shape and form to muscle groups.

Most people should begin resistance exercise through structured programs, such as through health clubs, to learn proper movement, breathing, and lifting techniques. It is easy to become injured by trying to lift, push, or pull too much resistance or weight. Some workout routines support overall muscle strengthening and toning, and others can support specific aerobic activities. The most effective approach to exercise blends aerobic and anaerobic activities that complement one another.

Weight Management

Excess body fat (OBESITY) is a significant risk factor for HEART DISEASE. Regular exercise that combines aerobic and anaerobic activities increases the body's metabolism (rate at which the body uses energy). When coupled with nutritious eating habits, this helps people to lose excess body fat and weight, and to maintain healthy body fat and weight. This also lowers the risk for type 2 diabetes, another significant RISK FACTOR FOR HEART DISEASE.

See also AEROBIC CAPACITY; LIFESTYLE AND HEART HEALTH; NUTRITION AND DIET.

exercise stress test A diagnostic procedure to evaluate the heart's function and performance during strenuous physical activity, which increases the demand on the HEART. A cardiologist might request an EXERCISE stress test as part of an overall cardiology examination, or to look at specific symptoms such as ANGINA (CHEST PAIN arising from restricted blood flow to the heart muscle) or ARRHYTHMIAS (irregular heartbeat) that occur primarily or exclusively during exercise. An exercise stress test also helps the cardiologist to evaluate the degree of occlusion present in CORONARY ARTERY DISEASE (CAD) by challenging the ability of the CORONARY ARTERIES to meet the heart's OXYGENATION needs during activity. A standard exercise stress test employs ELECTROCARDIOGRAM (ECG) readings before, during, and after directed and monitored exercise such as walking/running on a treadmill or riding a stationary bicycle.

For an exercise stress test, the technologist applies ECG electrodes to the person's torso and extremities and first records a resting ECG and also takes BLOOD PRESSURE readings. Then the person exercises for a defined period of time and repeats the ECG and blood pressure. Sometimes the test also includes an evaluation of lung capacity and oxygen exchange, in which case the person blows into a tube when instructed during the test. A standard exercise stress test takes 60 to 90 minutes. There is a slight risk that an exercise stress test can initiate a cardiac event such as angina, arrhythmia, and even HEART ATTACK or STROKE. This is uncommon, however, and the cardiac testing center has the equipment and staff to respond immediately to any cardiac emergency.

Sometimes cardiologists combine the exercise stress test with a RADIONUCLIDE SCAN to get a more clear picture of the heart's activity. When this is the case, the technologist injects a small amount of a gamma-radiation emitting "tag" that migrates to myocardial cells. A gamma camera records the radiation emissions (which are harmless), and a computer assembles their patterns into images that show the heart, its circulation, and the flow of BLOOD through the heart. The procedure is done at rest, during physical activity, and sometimes again at rest following exercise. This captures a comprehensive picture of any constraints HEART DISEASE places on the heart's function.

See also ADENOSINE STRESS TEST; DIPYRIDAMOLE STRESS TEST; DOBUTAMINE STRESS TEST.

experimental drugs See INVESTIGATIONAL NEW DRUGS (INDs).

external counterpulsation See ENHANCED EXTERNAL COUNTERPULSATION (EECP).

extrasystole See PREMATURE VENTRICULAR CONTRACTION (PVC).

fad diets   See NUTRITION AND DIET.

family health history   A compilation of significant health information about immediate BLOOD relatives, living or deceased, focusing on parents, siblings, grandparents, aunts, uncles, and adult children. A family health history should include information about major health factors in general as well as detailed information about health conditions for each relative that reflect possible risk for heart disease, such as:

- Causes and ages of death. Premature deaths—deaths that occur before the person reaches the age of average life expectancy for his or her generation—are particularly important. Death certificates typically list the primary cause of death, although this sometimes is general and might not reflect the health circumstances leading to the cause of death.
- Cardiovascular disease, current or past, particularly before age 50 in men and age 60 in women as early onset of HEART DISEASE suggests hereditary or familial connections. This includes ATHEROSCLEROSIS, ARTERIOSCLEROSIS ("hardening of the arteries"), aneurysm, HEART ATTACK, STROKE, HYPERTENSION (high blood pressure), CORONARY ARTERY DISEASE (CAD), HEART FAILURE, ANGINA, ARRHYTHMIAS, and congenital heart malformations.
- Cardiovascular surgeries such as ANGIOPLASTY, CORONARY ARTERY BYPASS GRAFT (CABG), valve repair or replacement, repair of congenital heart defects, aneurysm repair, arterioplasty or venoplasty, heart transplant.
- Blood or bleeding disorders such as hemophilia or clotting disorders.

- Cancer, particularly breast, endometrial (uterine), and colorectal.
- Metabolic disorders such as thyroid disease (HYPOTHYROIDISM, HYPERTHYROIDISM) and diabetes.
- Kidney disease, kidney surgery (including transplant), kidney dialysis.
- Surgeries involving the HEART, blood vessels, gastrointestinal tract (including liver and stomach), and brain and nervous system.

Viewed in combination with personal health status and history, family health history helps to identify added risks for health problems, particularly with regard to heart disease. Knowing what these risk factors are makes it possible to implement strategies to delay or prevent the health problems from developing.

See also HEREDITY AND HEART DISEASE; LIFESTYLE AND HEART HEALTH.

fascicular block   See HEART BLOCK.

fat, dietary   See NUTRITION AND DIET.

fat, limiting in diet   See NUTRITION AND DIET.

fatigue   A state of feeling tired and without energy. Fatigue most often occurs in HEART DISEASE when the body's tissues are unable to receive enough BLOOD and oxygen to support their activities. This can happen because the HEART itself does not get enough oxygen, as in CORONARY ARTERY DISEASE (CAD) and ISCHEMIC HEART DISEASE. This limits the heart's capacity to pump blood through the body. Fatigue also can happen when the blood getting out to the body lacks adequate oxygen, as with CYANOTIC CONGENITAL HEART DISEASE. Fatigue is a key symptom of HEART FAILURE and CARDIOMYOPATHY, in which damage limits the heart's pumping efficiency.

Some people with heart disease experience fatigue only when stressing their bodies, as during moderate to strenuous physical activity or EXERCISE. This is more common with moderate CAD or ischemic heart disease. Others feel fatigued even when at rest, as is typical with heart failure. It is important to heed signals from the body that it needs adequate rest. People who have trouble sleeping are more likely to experience fatigue regardless of heart disease. Regular exercise helps to improve cardiovascular fitness, improving the efficiency with which cells use oxygen. This reduces their overall oxygen needs, helping them to do more with the same level of oxygen.

Some medications cause or increase fatigue, or cause drowsiness that contributes to feelings of fatigue. When fatigue follows a new medication, check with a pharmacist about the medication's possible side effects. Often, such side effects wear off after taking the medication for three to four weeks. If symptoms appear related to the timing of the medication and continue beyond this time, the doctor might be able to prescribe a different drug with the same therapeutic results but not the side effects.

See also MEDICATION SIDE EFFECTS; SLEEP DISTURBANCES.

felodipine A CALCIUM CHANNEL ANTAGONIST MEDICATION taken to treat moderate HYPERTENSION (high BLOOD PRESSURE), usually as a second-line treatment when other medications do not provide adequate control. It works by relaxing the smooth muscle in the walls of the arteries, which lowers the resistance BLOOD encounters as it flows through them. Common brand names include Plendil. Doctors sometimes prescribe felodipine in combination with other ANTIHYPERTENSIVE MEDICATIONS such as DIURETIC MEDICATIONS and BETA ANTAGONIST MEDICATIONS, and sometimes to treat HEART FAILURE. As

with other calcium channel blockers, GRAPEFRUIT JUICE consumed within two to four hours of taking felodipine causes higher than expected levels of the drug in the bloodstream. Common side effects include HYPOTENSION, ARRHYTHMIAS, headache, light-headedness, CONSTIPATION, peripheral EDEMA (swelling of the lower part of the legs and hands), and cough. Women who are pregnant or breast-feeding should not take felodipine.

See also CALCIUM CYCLE; MEDICATION SIDE EFFECTS; MEDICATIONS TO TREAT HEART DISEASE; SODIUM CHANNEL BLOCKING MEDICATIONS.

fenfluramine A medication prescribed to suppress appetite as a treatment for OBESITY. Common brand names include Pondimin. Fenfluramine is no longer available in the United States. Following reports of an unusually high rate of heart valve disease among people taking the medication, the U.S. Food and Drug Administration (FDA) requested that the manufacturer remove fenfluramine, along with the closely related medication dexfenfluramine, from the U.S. market in September 1997. Although the highest rate was among those taking fenfluramine in combination with phentermine, popularly known as Fen-Phen, assessment of available data pointed to fenfluramine (and dexfenfluramine) as the primary connection. PULMONARY HYPERTENSION, high pressure in the arteries within the lungs that increases the workload of the heart's efforts to pump blood to the lungs, also appears linked to fenfluramine.

Health experts advise anyone who previously took any of these medications to obtain comprehensive cardiovascular examinations, including echocardiogram to detect any valve disease. Complications such as these appear to be most common in people who took fenfluramine (or dexfenfluramine) for longer than four weeks. Adverse health problems such as valve disease primarily manifest within the first year after taking the medication. People who took fenfluramine or Fen-Phen and have not had follow-up cardiovascular examinations should talk with their doctors about whether this is necessary.

See also NUTRITION AND DIET; WEIGHT MANAGEMENT.

fenofibrate   A LIPID-LOWERING MEDICATION taken to treat HYPERLIPIDEMIA and HYPERTRIGLYCERIDEMIA. Common brand names include Tricor. Doctors prescribe fenofibrate when low-density lipoprotein (LDL), very low-density lipoprotein (VLDL), and TRIGLYCERIDES BLOOD levels remain higher than desired with other therapies. Fenofibrate works by blocking the body's production of triglycerides and by accelerating the metabolism of triglycerides already in circulation. Common side effects include nausea and gastrointestinal upset. Rare but serious side effects include RHABDOMYOLYSIS (abnormal destruction of muscle tissue) and kidney failure. People taking fenofibrate should report any signs of muscle weakness or paralysis to their doctors without delay.

See also EXERCISE; GEMFIBROZIL; HYPERLIPIDEMIA; LIFESTYLE AND HEART HEALTH; MEDICATIONS TO TREAT HEART DISEASE; NUTRITION AND DIET.

fiber, dietary   See NUTRITION AND DIET.

fibrillation   A pattern of ARRHYTHMIA (irregular HEARTBEAT) in which the heart's contractions are rapid, uncoordinated, and ineffective and occur when electrical impulses originate within individual myocardial fibers rather than from the SINOATRIAL (SA) NODE that normally paces the heart's electrical activity. Fibrillation can involve the atria (the heart's upper chambers) or the ventricles (the heart's lower chambers).

ATRIAL FIBRILLATION is common with many forms of HEART DISEASE such as CORONARY ARTERY DISEASE (CAD) and HEART FAILURE, particularly when the atria have become enlarged, and can reach rates of 300 to 500 beats per minute (the heart's normal rate is 60 to 100 beats per minute). Because the initiating electrical signals originate in the atria, most of them do not affect the ventricles. However, the discordant atrial contractions stimulate the ventricles, causing them to contract irregularly. Many people feel atrial fibrillation as PALPITATIONS (the sensation that the HEART "leaps" in the chest). Treatment targets the underlying HEART DISEASE to the extent possible. As well, ANTIARRHYTHMIA MEDICATIONS such as BETA ANTAG-ONIST MEDICATIONS or DIGOXIN often are effective in restoring normal atrial rhythm. Atrial fibrillation is not itself life-threatening. Doctors sometimes treat persistent atrial fibrillation with CARDIOVERSION, a procedure that delivers controlled electrical shock to the heart to synchronize its electrical activity.

VENTRICULAR FIBRILLATION is life-threatening and must receive immediate emergency treatment. The ventricles pump BLOOD out of the heart, and when their contractions are ineffectual in doing so, body tissues do not receive oxygen. Ventricular fibrillation sometimes occurs with HEART ATTACK (MYOCARDIAL INFARCTION). Treatment is defibrillation, delivering a series of measured electrical shocks to the heart through paddles or electrodes placed on the outside of the chest.

See also AUTOMATED EXTERNAL DEFIBRILLATOR (AED); COCAINE AND HEART ATTACK; COMMOTIO CORDIS; SUDDEN CARDIAC ARREST.

fibrinogen   A protein present in the BLOOD that participates in initiating the actions of clotting. An elevated fibrinogen level signals an increased risk for HEART ATTACK and STROKE for people who have CORONARY ARTERY DISEASE (CAD) and ISCHEMIC HEART DISEASE. There is some evidence that elevated fibrinogen might be an early indicator of the tendency to develop CAD, much in the same way as elevated blood lipids (cholesterol and TRIGLYCERIDES). Although the blood fibrinogen level cannot be lowered, ANTICOAGULANT MEDICATIONS can slow the formation of clots. Regular EXERCISE tones BLOOD vessels and the tissues supporting them, helping to keep blood flowing. This also reduces the potential for clots to form.

Recent research into inflammation and heart disease suggests that the combination of elevated fibrinogen and elevated C-REACTIVE PROTEIN blood levels signals a significantly increased risk for MYOCARDIAL INFARCTION (MI). However, it remains unclear why this is so. It also remains unclear whether the risk for MI diminishes with treatment, such as with antiinflammatory medications or HMG CoA REDUCTASE INHIBITOR MEDICATIONS. At present, most experts believe there is little value in looking to fibrinogen levels as potential avenues for evaluating heart disease risk except to support anticoagulation therapy decisions.

See also ATHEROSCLEROSIS; CHOLESTEROL, BLOOD; RISK FACTORS FOR HEART DISEASE.

fibroelastoma A nonmalignant tumor that usually develops on a HEART valve. Tumors of any kind involving the heart are rare. Fibroelastomas, sometimes called papillary fibroelastomas, are made of fibrous tissue that adheres to the heart valve in a small patchlike structure. Although they usually are small, fibroelastomas alter the flow of BLOOD through the valve, causing turbulence. The fibrous tissue attracts platelets, which form tiny clots on the tumor's surface. When these clots break away, they can lodge in the brain, causing STROKE; in the heart, causing HEART ATTACK; or in the lung, causing pulmonary EMBOLISM. Most fibroelastomas are detected incidentally, when ECHOCARDIOGRAM performed for other reasons detects their presence. Sometimes fibroelastomas do cause symptoms, which might include ANGINA (CHEST PAIN) or shortness of breath when the tumor significantly impedes the flow of blood. Treatment is surgical removal of the tumor. Because fibroelastomas tend to distort the valve's structure, most of the time it is necessary to also replace the valve, usually with a prosthetic valve.

See also CANCER OF THE HEART; MYXOMA; VALVE DISEASE; VALVE REPAIR AND REPLACEMENT.

fibromuscular dysplasia (FMD) A condition in which cells in the walls of the arteries grow abnormally (dysplasia), forming thickened areas similar to scar tissue. These formations, called lesions, characteristically resemble a string of beads in imaging studies such as ANGIOGRAPHY. The lesions cause irregular narrowing and stiffening of the arterial wall, which creates turbulence in the flow of BLOOD through the affected arteries. This turbulence allows blood to pool, which in turn allows clots to form. The swirling movement of the blood then dislodges the clots. These circumstances present a high risk for HYPERTENSION (high BLOOD PRESSURE), STROKE, ANEURYSM, and MYOCARDIAL INFARCTION (MI). FMD most commonly affects the renal arteries in the kidneys, the carotid arteries in the neck, and the mesenteric arteries that carry blood to the abdominal organs. However, FMD can affect any artery in the body, and in more than a fourth of those who have the condition affects multiple arteries.

Symptoms and Diagnostic Path

For many people who have FMD, the first indication of the condition is a STROKE or HEART ATTACK. When earlier symptoms are present, they typically correlate to the body region where there are lesions in the arteries. FMD affecting the renal arteries commonly causes abnormal kidney function, which doctors detect through routine blood tests. FMD affecting the carotid arteries may cause symptoms such as headache, DIZZINESS, and vertigo (sensation that the room is spinning). FMD affecting the mesenteric arteries may cause abdominal pain, digestive difficulties, and abnormal liver function. When arteries in the legs are involved, symptoms are similar to those of INTERMITTENT CLAUDICATION: pain and cramping in the legs, difficulty walking, numbness, coldness, and the sensation of pins and needles.

The diagnostic path begins with a general physical examination with special focus on any areas of symptoms. Routine blood tests can reveal abnormal kidney or liver function. Because FMD appears to run in families, the doctor will also take a comprehensive health history, asking questions about family members who might have similar symptoms or who have been diagnosed with FMD. An angiography, in which the cardiologist injects dye into the bloodstream and observes its movement through the blood vessels via X-rays, provides the conclusive clinical evidence for the diagnosis. Other diagnostic procedures used sometimes include ULTRASOUND, COMPUTED TOMOGRAPHY (CT) SCAN, and MAGNETIC RESONANCE IMAGING (MRI).

Treatment Options and Outlook

The preferred treatment for occlusive FMD—FMD that severely restricts the flow of blood—is ANGIOPLASTY, a procedure to compress the lesions and restore the patency of the artery. Often the cardiologist may choose to do angioplasty at the same time as the angiography. Open surgery may also be necessary to repair a dissecting aneurysm (weakened arterial wall that is beginning to tear). Medical therapies include ANTIHYPERTENSIVE MEDICATIONS to treat high blood pressure, ANTICOAGULANT MEDICATIONS or ANTIPLATELET MEDICATIONS to reduce the risk for blood clots, and lifestyle modifications such as smoking cessation.

Most people are able to return to their usual and normal activities once they are recovered from any procedures and the FMD is stabilized. Angioplasty typically offers long-term, although not permanent, relief. Many people experience recurrence of the lesions as well as the development of lesions in other arteries. Medications to control clot formation can significantly lower the risk for complications such as stroke or heart attack. The greatest challenge in treating FMD is that many people are not diagnosed until after a catastrophic event, such as heart attack or stroke, has occurred. Treatment options and outlook for recovery in such situations depend on the medical event and any complications.

Risk Factors and Preventive Measures

FMD affects women between ages 20 and 50 far more frequently than it affects men, although the condition can affect anyone at any age (including children). FMD does appear to have a genetic correlation; having family members with FMD is the most significant risk factor. However, it is not yet clear the extent to which environmental factors come into play although it is certain that lifestyle exerts some influence. Among people who have no apparent family history of FMD, cigarette smoking appears to increase the risk for FMD.

Until recently, doctors believed FMD was rare. However, routine screening of living kidney donors revealed that FMD appears to affect 4 to 5 percent of the American population. Increased awareness of this condition, coupled with advances in diagnostic imaging, is making earlier diagnosis more frequent. People who have relatives in whom FMD has been diagnosed should make sure to tell their doctors; when a strong family history exists, the doctor may choose to use noninvasive imaging methods such as ultrasound or MRI to screen for FMD even when there are no obvious symptoms. Aside from smoking cessation, there do not appear to be any measures, lifestyle or interventional, to prevent FMD.

See also FAMILY HEALTH HISTORY; HEREDITY AND HEART DISEASE; LIVING WITH HEART DISEASE; SMOKING AND HEART DISEASE.

"fight-or-flight" response Autonomic nervous system reactions to perceived threats that set into motion a series of physiological events giving the body the ability to save itself. The response is a primal survival mechanism that activates the release of the hormones EPINEPHRINE and NOREPINEPHRINE to raise BLOOD PRESSURE, HEART RATE, and breathing rate. At the same time, these chemicals cause peripheral blood vessels to constrict, sending more blood to the body's core organ systems and to the muscles. Quite literally, the body is ready to either fight or flee. When the perception of threat subsides, epinephrine and norepinephrine levels return to normal, allowing the body's systems to do the same.

Stressful situations not related to survival activate the "fight-or-flight" response as well. Health experts believe continued such activations contribute to numerous health problems, particularly involving systems and structures the response activates—contributing to HEART conditions such as HYPERTENSION (high blood pressure), for example. The premise is that the body becomes so accustomed to always being on "high alert" status that it gradually readjusts to that level of function as its standard. Blood pressure, pulse rate, and respirations remain elevated even when the threat, or in most cases the stressful situation, abates, contributing to health problems such as hypertension (high blood pressure). The body is not designed to maintain itself at this level, which creates physical stress and eventual damage to cells, tissues, and organs.

See also STRESS AND HEART DISEASE; STRESS REDUCTION TECHNIQUES.

first degree AV block See HEART BLOCK.

fish and fish oil See OMEGA FATTY ACIDS.

fitness level The degree to which a person's physical condition allows physical activity. Fitness level represents the body's strength, endurance, and efficiency—how much the body can do for how long and how quickly. There are various scales that attach numeric or descriptive qualifiers to fitness level, although there is no single standard. Fitness level improves with regular physical activity, both aerobic ("air"; improves cardiovascular function) and anaerobic (builds more muscle). The higher the fitness level, the more efficiently cells throughout the body function, reducing the amounts of oxygen and glucose (their two primary fuel sources) they require. This lowers the demand on the HEART. People with higher fitness levels generally have lower BLOOD PRESSURE and slower, stronger heart rates at rest and at exercise than people with lower fitness levels. Regardless of current fitness level, working toward improvement benefits health overall. Fitness level is one of the most important controllable factors in reducing the risks for HEART DISEASE.

See also AEROBIC CAPACITY; EXERCISE; FUNCTIONAL CAPACITY; LIFESTYLE AND HEART HEALTH; NUTRITION AND DIET.

flavonoids Substances found naturally in fruits, vegetables, grains, and legumes (such as soy) that appear to have protective abilities. Flavonoids are ANTIOXIDANTS, chemicals that reduce the amounts of free radicals (waste particles remaining after metabolism) in the body. Scientists believe that many degenerative diseases such as HEART DISEASE develop as a result of oxidation, or the creation of free radicals. Flavonoids and other antioxidants interfere with this process. Flavonoids also appear to have an effect on the clotting process, reducing platelet aggregation. Foods that contain high concentrations of flavonoids include teas, especially green teas, and red wines.

Gaining attention for its dual role as an antioxidant and an antiinflammatory is the flavonoid quercetin. Some studies show quercetin has a beneficial effect in protecting the arteries from damage due to low-density lipoprotein (LDL) CHOLESTEROL—the "bad" cholesterol. It seems to do so by reducing inflammation within the arterial walls and lessen-

ing the ability for LDL and other substances to stick to the walls of the arteries (ATHEROSCLEROSIS). Red wines contain an abundance of quercetin. Quercetin is also available as a dietary supplement.

See also HERBAL REMEDIES; NUTRITION AND DIET.

fluoroscopy A radiology procedure that uses continuous X-rays to create real-time dynamic images viewed on a television screen monitor. Cardiologists use fluoroscopy during CARDIAC CATHETERIZATION to visualize and guide the catheter through the body's BLOOD vessels and into the HEART and CORONARY ARTERIES. The cardiologist also might inject dye into the blood vessels to improve visualization of the blood flow through the coronary arteries, revealing the extent of occlusion and STENOSIS (narrowing), and through the chambers of the HEART. Even though the X-ray beam is continuous, X-ray exposure is minimal.

For fluoroscopy in conjunction with cardiac catheterization, preparation is minimal (usually restricting food and drink the night before). An IV is started before the procedure begins, which can cause some discomfort. The cardiologist then administers a sedative to help the person feel comfortable. Some people feel a sensation of warmth if the cardiologist injects dye during the fluoroscopy.

See also ANGIOGRAPHY; COMPUTED TOMOGRAPHY (CT) SCAN; ELECTRON BEAM COMPUTED TOMOGRAPHY (EBCT) SCAN; MAGNETIC RESONANCE IMAGING (MRI); POSITRON EMISSION TOMOGRAPHY (PET) SCAN; SINGLE PHOTON EMISSION COMPUTERIZED TOMOGRAPHY (SPECT) SCAN.

fluvastatin A LIPID-LOWERING MEDICATION taken to treat HYPERCHOLESTEROLEMIA. Common brand names include Lescol. Fluvastatin is a HMG CoA REDUCTASE INHIBITOR MEDICATION, commonly called a statin drug, that works by slowing the liver's ability to produce cholesterol to replace the cholesterol the body uses that is already in circulation. This causes overall blood cholesterol levels to drop, as replacement decreases with use of statins. Doctors prescribe fluvastatin for people who have mild to moderate ATHEROSCLEROSIS (accumulations of fatty deposits along the insides of the arteries) or high levels of blood cholesterol to limit or help prevent CORONARY ARTERY DISEASE (CAD). Common side effects of fluvastatin include nausea, gastrointestinal distress, headache, and cough.

See also CHOLESTEROL, BLOOD; EXERCISE; FAMILIAL HYPERLIPIDEMIA; LIFESTYLE AND HEART HEALTH; MEDICATIONS TO TREAT HEART DISEASE; NUTRITION AND DIET.

folic acid A B-complex vitamin that occurs naturally in dark green, leafy vegetables such as spinach; also called folate (depending on its form). Folic acid also is available as a nutritional supplement, both alone and as a common ingredient in multiple vitamin formulas. It is vital to many body functions including cell growth, new tissue development, and healing. Folic acid and other B-vitamins are important for neurological processes, and for the proper development of the spine and nervous system in the fetus. Because of its importance, folic acid is added in the United States, along with other B-vitamins, to many wheat-based foods such as breads and cereals; labels identify these products as "fortified."

Some studies show a correlation between increased folic acid intake and lower levels of HOMOCYSTEINE, an amino acid in the blood that appears linked to CARDIOVASCULAR DISEASE (CVD). People with CVD—particularly ATHEROSCLEROSIS (deposits of lipids that collect along the inside walls of the arteries), CORONARY ARTERY DISEASE (CAD), and ischemic heart disease—typically have elevated homocysteine levels, and some research suggests that homocysteine plays a role in the body's lipid management processes. Folic acid breaks down homocysteine.

Many people take B-vitamin and folic acid supplements to help prevent HEART DISEASE. Health experts caution that although this likely has no adverse effects for most people, it is not a substitute for healthy lifestyle habits, including eating and EXERCISE.

See also LIFESTYLE AND HEART HEALTH; NUTRITION AND DIET.

Fontan procedure The final in a series of surgical procedures to repair the congenital HEART malformation SINGLE VENTRICLE. The normal heart has two atria, the upper chambers, and two ventricles, the lower chambers. The right atrium receives unoxygenated BLOOD from the body and passes it to the right ventricle, which pumps it from the heart to the lungs via the pulmonary artery. The left atrium receives the oxygenated blood returning from the lungs and passes it to the left ventricle, which pumps it out to the body. In single ventricle malformations, one ventricle does all the pumping so blood going out to the body is a mix of unoxygenated and oxygenated blood.

The Fontan procedure creates a channel (also called a baffle) through the heart that connects the inferior vena cava, which returns blood from the lower body to the heart, with the pulmonary artery so the blood returning from the body to the heart goes directly to the lungs via the pulmonary artery, bypassing the heart. Typically, previous surgeries already have connected the superior vena cava, which returns blood from the head and upper body, to the pulmonary artery. The final result, with the Fontan procedure, is that the heart uses its single ventricle to pump out only oxygenated blood.

Risks and Complications

The risks and complications of the Fontan procedure include those of OPEN-HEART SURGERY, anesthesia, and cardiopulmonary bypass as well as those related to the procedure. Postoperative infection, bleeding, blood clots, and pneumonia are also concerns. There is also the possibility that the procedure fails to improve cardiac function as intended, which requires additional surgery or HEART TRANSPLANT. The risk of death in the first five years is high, about 15 percent. Late failure of the procedure occurs gradually in about 20 percent of those who survive beyond 10 years, causing progressively severe ARRHYTHMIAS.

Although the Fontan procedure gives the single-ventricle heart the ability to deliver adequate oxygenated blood throughout the body, it does not produce a normally structured heart. With one ventricle to do the work of two, heart failure is inevitable, and most survivors begin to experience this complication after about 20 years following the operation. It is unlikely that a single-ventricle can sustain a normal life span; heart transplant likely looms in the future of most survivors. Thromboembolism and DEEP VEIN THROMBOSIS (DVT) are also significant and chronic risks throughout life.

Outlook and Lifestyle Modifications

The series of corrective operations generally takes place in the child's first two or three years. Although the repaired heart is not normal, it typically can support the body's cardiovascular functions fairly well. However, limitations on physical activity due to exercise intolerance are mild to moderate throughout life. About 85 percent of children who undergo Fontan procedure survive 20 years. They require ongoing treatment with medications to prevent thrombosis (anticoagulation therapy), manage arrhythmias, and otherwise support cardiovascular function. Nonetheless, the Fontan procedure has greatly extended life expectancy for those born with very severe heart defects, and most survivors are able to enjoy a satisfactory QUALITY OF LIFE.

See also BIDIRECTIONAL GLENN PROCEDURE; BLALOCK-TAUSSIG PROCEDURE; HEART DISEASE IN CHILDREN; NORWOOD PROCEDURE; PALLIATION, STAGED.

foramen ovale   See HEART DISEASE IN CHILDREN.

fosinopril   An ANGIOTENSIN-CONVERTING ENZYME (ACE) INHIBITOR MEDICATION taken to treat HYPERTENSION (high BLOOD PRESSURE). Common brand names include Monopril. Fosinopril works by preventing the body from forming angiotensin II, a potent substance that causes BLOOD vessels to constrict. This is part of the body's mechanism to raise blood pressure. Doctors sometimes prescribe fosinopril in combination with DIURETIC MEDICATIONS. Common side effects include nausea, headache, and persistent cough. Women who are pregnant should not take fosinopril, and women who become pregnant when taking it should talk with their doctors immediately about changing to another medication. Like other ACE inhibitors, fosinopril can cause damage and death of the unborn baby in the second and third trimesters of pregnancy.

See also ANGIOTENSIN-CONVERTING ENZYME (ACE); ANTIHYPERTENSIVE MEDICATIONS; MEDICATION SIDE EFFECTS; MEDICATIONS TO TREAT HEART DISEASE.

foxglove   A family of plants that are the natural source for DIGITALIS, DIGOXIN, and DIGITOXIN. Foxglove contains chemicals called cardiac glycosides or digitalis glycosides that affect the ways myocardial cells in the HEART contract. Taken therapeutically in the form of digoxin or digitoxin, cardiac glycosides strengthen and slow the HEART RATE, allowing the heart to pump more efficiently. Accidentally ingested, the plant is highly toxic and can cause serious ARRHYTHMIAS (irregular HEARTBEAT) and bradycardia (slow heart rate). Ancient physicians brewed tea from the leaves and chopped stems of foxglove plants, administering it to treat "weakness of the heart."

Different foxglove species supply the cardiac glycosides that become medications. *Digitalis purpurea,* which has a purple flower, is the source for digitoxin. *Digitalis lanata,* which has a white bloom, is the source for digoxin. The chemical formulations of these cardiac glycosides are very similar, differing primarily in how rapidly they reach peak effect in the body. There are numerous species of foxglove that grow naturally in many regions of the United States. Gardeners often cultivate them for their tall, spired stalks of bell-shaped flowers, which come in many colors and can reach five feet or more in height. Accidental poisoning can occur when plant sap gets on the skin and then is ingested. Thorough hand-washing after handling foxglove plants and flowers prevents this.

See also DIGOXIN IMMUNE FAB.

Framingham Heart Study   The longest-running epidemiological study of cardiovascular health in the United States. The Framingham Heart Study started with 5,209 men and women between the ages of 30 and 62 in the town of Framingham, Massachusetts. Participants agreed to undergo extensive physical examinations at the start of the study, and to return for follow-up examinations every two years. The study's conceptual objective was simple: to learn about how HEART DISEASE affects people's lives, and what lifestyle factors influence the development of heart disease. What was then the National Heart Institute, now the National Heart, Lung, and Blood Institute (NHLBI), designed and funded the study.

Over the next two and a half decades, researchers correlated the development of heart disease to risk factors such as cigarette smoking, dietary habits, and EXERCISE patterns. They identified the relationships between eating a diet high in fat and high blood cholesterol levels, and between high blood cholesterol levels and ATHEROSCLEROSIS, CORONARY ARTERY DISEASE (CAD), HEART ATTACK, and STROKE. They followed family patterns in heart disease, distinguishing between those that appeared hereditary and those that appeared lifestyle. They then integrated these epidemiological observations with emerging clinical data about the mechanisms of heart disease.

The result was the first comprehensive identification of lifestyle factors that increased the risk of cardiovascular disease (CVD), with emphasis on HYPERTENSION (high BLOOD PRESSURE), CAD, and ISCHEMIC HEART DISEASE: smoking, high-fat diet, lack of exercise (sedentary lifestyle), and clinical findings such as high blood cholesterol levels, OBESITY, and diabetes. Researchers also determined that changing these risk factors could delay, minimize, or prevent the onset of CVD. Health organizations such as the American Heart Association developed recommendations for modifying these risk factors, and health-care providers throughout the United States embarked on the journey of preventive care for heart disease.

In 1971 the study expanded to include 5,124 children (and their spouses) of the original study participants, known as the Offspring Cohort. This added a second generation to the study, giving researchers the first extensive opportunity to look at links between lifestyle and heart disease across generations. By this time CLINICAL RESEARCH STUDIES had produced significant new understandings about how heart disease develops from a physiological perspective. New medications and treatments, including heart surgery and, by the end of the 1970s, HEART TRANSPLANTS, reshaped perceptions of and approaches to treating heart disease. In 2001 the Framingham Heart Study expanded

again, this time to include more than 4,000 children (and their spouses) of the second generation participants—grandchildren of the original participants. This group is called the Generation Three Cohort, or Gen III for short.

This next phase of the study hopes to gain understanding of newly identified risk factors such as homocysteine and FIBRINOGEN levels, and to further explore the consequences of changes in lifestyle (eating habits and exercise) to determine whether there are optimal points in the development of heart disease at which such changes have the most significant effects. Researchers also intend to explore the value of new imaging procedures such as ELECTRON BEAM COMPUTED TOMOGRAPHY (EBCT) SCANS for detecting CAD in its earliest stages, when preventive measures are most likely to be effective. They also hope to learn more about the role of heredity and genetics in how heart disease develops as well as in preventing it.

Through the decades, Framingham Heart Study researchers have frozen blood samples collected from study participants. Recent advances in technology are being applied to study those samples through the SABRe in CVD Initiative (Systems Approach to Biomarker Research in Cardiovascular Disease). This gives researchers an amazing window back in time to examine various aspects of heart health and heart disease over multiple generations. The Framingham Heart Study also studies neurological health and disorders. Its Brain Tissue Donation Program uses brains and brain tissues donated at death (post-mortem) to analyze the aging process and examine healthy brains as a means for improved understanding of diseases related to aging such as Alzheimer's disease and Parkinson's disease. The NHLBI continues to fund, support, and oversee the Framingham Heart Study.

See also CHOLESTEROL, BLOOD; DEATHS FROM HEART DISEASE; LIFESTYLE AND HEART HEALTH; LIVING WITH HEART DISEASE.

free radicals Molecular particles that are the waste by-products of metabolism. They are released when cells use oxygen for energy, in a process called oxidation. Free radicals are molecularly unattached. They bind with other molecules that will receive them, forming nonfunctional structures that have no purpose in the body. Scientists believe that over time, free radicals are damaging to cells and that many diseases, including heart disease develop as the damage accumulates. ANTIOXIDANTS are natural chemicals that bind with free radicals and alter their molecular structures so the body can process them as waste and remove them.

Recent research implicates oxidative stress, which results from free radical binding, as a significant factor in the development of inflammatory heart diseases such as ATHEROSCLEROSIS and CORONARY ARTERY DISEASE (CAD). However, recent clinical studies have also demonstrated that the use of antioxidants such as vitamin E are not effective in lowering LDL CHOLESTEROL, reducing inflammation that leads to atherosclerosis, or improving CAD. Additional studies are under way to gain better understanding of the relationship between free radicals, oxidative stress, and heart disease.

See also FLAVONOIDS; INFLAMMATION AND HEART DISEASE; NUTRITION AND DIET.

free-standing cardiac catheterization facility A CARDIAC CATHETERIZATION facility that is not part of a hospital. Generally a cardiologist or group of cardiologists owns and operates a free-standing cardiac catheterization facility, which is staffed and equipped to perform a range of procedures to diagnose heart conditions, including ELECTROCARDIOGRAM (ECG), ECHOCARDIOGRAM, EXERCISE STRESS TEST, and ANGIOGRAPHY. The facility has surgical suites for sterile procedures, radiology and imaging equipment, recovery rooms, laboratory, and other appropriate patient services for outpatient care. All cardiac catheterization facilities should be staffed and equipped to handle any level of cardiovascular emergency. Such a facility's environment generally is less intimidating for patients than is that of a hospital setting, and the facility is more cost-effective to operate.

See also SURGERY TO TREAT CARDIOVASCULAR DISEASE.

functional capacity The level of physical activity a person with HEART DISEASE, particularly HEART FAILURE, is capable of doing. It integrates the NEW YORK HEALTH ASSOCIATION (NYHA) CLASSIFICATION SYSTEM, the standard for clinical grading of heart failure, with the cardiologist's subjective and objective findings about the person's health status and life situation. Functional capacity assessment often determines a person's disability determination for job- and insurance-related matters. It also helps to quantify the effect heart disease is having on the person's QUALITY OF LIFE. Functional capacity assessment typically combines evaluation of symptoms such as ANGINA (CHEST PAIN) and shortness of breath with the limitations they impose on the person's regular daily activities. Functional capacity changes with treatment and with the progression of disease. It is sometimes one of the criteria used for determining whether certain treatment options are viable, such as CORONARY ARTERY BYPASS SURGERY (CABG), VALVE REPLACEMENT, and HEART TRANSPLANT.

See also ACTIVITIES OF DAILY LIVING (ADLs); LIVING WITH HEART DISEASE.

furosemide A DIURETIC MEDICATION taken to relieve the body of excess fluid, usually to treat HYPERTENSION (high BLOOD PRESSURE) and congestive HEART FAILURE. Common brand names include Lasix and Myrosemide. Furosemide is a loop diuretic, a reference to its actions on a structure of the kidney called the loop of Henlé. This structure regulates the amounts of sodium, chloride, and other ELECTROLYTES that either remain in the bloodstream or pass from the body in the urine. When the loop of Henlé retains electrolytes, it pulls water into the bloodstream. This increases BLOOD volume and, correspondingly, BLOOD PRESSURE. Furosemide's effect is to inhibit SODIUM and chloride retention, helping to lower blood volume and, correspondingly, blood pressure. This action also helps to relieve peripheral EDEMA (swelling due to fluid retention) that results from heart failure.

Furosemide is one of the oldest loop diuretic formulations on the market, and the most commonly prescribed. Because it does prevent POTASSIUM, along with other electrolytes, from being drawn back into the bloodstream, people taking furosemide often need to ingest additional potassium either through diet (foods such as bananas and raisins) or potassium supplements. Potassium depletion is the most common side effect of furosemide. Frequent urination, which people taking furosemide often view as an undesired side effect, is an expected action of furosemide as its purpose is to remove excess fluid from the body. Doctors often prescribe furosemide in combination with other medications taken to treat HYPERTENSION, heart failure, and other cardiovascular conditions. Furosemide never should be taken with the diuretic medication ethacrynic acid, as the combination can cause severe potassium depletion leading to potentially life-threatening ARRHYTHMIAS.

See also MEDICATIONS TO TREAT HEART DISEASE; MEDICATION SIDE EFFECTS.

Galen (A.D. 129–199)   The ancient Greek physician whose theories and teachings about the structure and function of the human body guided the practice of medicine for 14 centuries. He rightly determined that the arteries carried BLOOD, not air as was the common belief of his time. Although the laws and religious beliefs of Galen's time prohibited human vivisection and autopsy, Galen used the knowledge he acquired from dissecting animals such as pigs and monkeys to postulate about human anatomy and physiology. He established a rudimentary understanding of blood and the circulatory system, the relationship between the pulse and the HEART, and the premise that the body continuously produced blood.

In his efforts to make connections between structures and functions without actually observing them within the body, Galen also established numerous false premises that medical teachings perpetuated until well into the 17th century. His view of the circulatory system, for example, rightly had the arteries arising from the heart but wrongly attributed the liver as the source of the veins. Ingested food, Galen believed, went to the liver, which used it to produce blood that went out to nourish the rest of the body via the veins. Galen accurately described the chambers and pumping action of the heart but presented a confused process for how blood moved through the heart. Despite its flaws, the Galenic view of cardiovascular function remained the mainstay of medical understanding until English physician William Harvey conclusively refuted it in 1628.

See also CORVISART, JEAN-NICHOLAS; EINTHOVEN, WILLEM; HALES, STEPHEN; HARVEY, WILLIAM; LAËNNEC, RENÉ.

garlic and garlic oil   An alternative therapy approach for lowering BLOOD cholesterol levels and BLOOD PRESSURE. CLINICAL RESEARCH STUDIES suggest that garlic, particularly in its natural (food) form, helps the body to metabolize cholesterol and other lipids. There is less supportive evidence for any affect on BLOOD PRESSURE. Garlic contains allium compounds that decrease the body's production of cholesterol overall, lowering total blood cholesterol levels, and particularly low-density lipoprotein (LDL) or "bad" cholesterol, which has a greater tendency to form arterial plaque that adheres to the inside walls of the arteries. Allium compounds also appear to have mild vasodilation effects, helping arteries to relax, and mild anticoagulant properties, slowing the blood clotting process. Allium compounds might help to lower HOMOCYSTEINE levels as well.

Because of garlic's distinctive odor, many people who want to benefit from garlic's possible effects choose to use supplements that are odorless. In studies that have looked at this, there seems to be little difference between how they and natural garlic act in the body. Although garlic has been a medicinal remedy in many cultures for centuries, relatively few clinical research studies have explored its actions and effects. Most doctors feel it does no harm to use garlic, especially in its food form. Excessive amounts of garlic, usually from supplements, can cause unpleasant symptoms such as gastrointestinal upset and skin rash. People who take ANTICOAGULANT MEDICATIONS should first consult their doctors or pharmacists before using garlic at medicinal levels (beyond ordinary seasoning in foods); dosages for anticoagulant medications ("blood thinners") are sensitive and even a very mild added anticoagulant effect can increase the risk for excessive bleeding. Onions also contain allium compounds.

See also CHOLESTEROL, BLOOD; COMPLEMENTARY THERAPIES; FLAVONOIDS.

gemfibrozil A LIPID-LOWERING MEDICATION taken to treat HYPERLIPIDEMIA and HYPERCHOLESTEROLEMIA for people who are not able to bring their BLOOD lipid levels down through diet and EXERCISE. Common brand names include Lopid and Gemcor. Gemfibrozil lowers very low-density lipoprotein (VLDL) and TRIGLYCERIDES, and raises high-density lipoprotein (HDL). The most common side effects are gastrointestinal upset and increased risk for gallbladder disease, particularly gallstones. Doctors sometimes prescribe multiple medications to treat severely elevated blood lipids that do not respond as desired to treatment efforts. However, taking gemfibrozil with a statin lipid-lowering medication (HMG, CoA REDUCTASE INHIBITOR MEDICATIONS) increases the risk for a rare but serious complication, RHABDOMYOLYSIS, in which chemical processes within the body destroy muscle tissue.

See also CHOLESTEROL, BLOOD; NUTRITION AND DIET; MEDICATIONS TO TREAT HEART DISEASE.

generic drug The basic chemical formulation of a medication. When new medications first become available, their manufacturers market nearly all of them as brand-name products. Under the United States patent system, this allows exclusive production of the medication for a certain period of time. The premise of this system is to encourage pharmaceutical companies to put their resources into new drug development. The "reward" is that only the company holding the patent (or companies which the patent holder authorizes) has the right to earn money from selling the drug for the time the patent is in effect. Today most medications come to market under patent for three to seven years. Once the patent expires, other manufacturers can use the generic formula to make their own versions of the medication. At this point pricing becomes competitive, with generic products significantly less expensive than brand-name products. Generic products often also have brand names, but the medication is not under patent.

Medical experts disagree about whether generic medications have comparable bioavailability—that is, the same actions and effects in the body. Although the chemical formula of the active ingredients is the same, the substances used as "filler" (the nonactive ingredients) can affect how the body absorbs the medication. This is more of a concern with oral medications (taken by mouth) because many factors influence their absorption from the gastrointestinal system including foods consumed at the same time. For medications with a NARROW THERAPEUTIC INDEX (NTI), such as certain ANTICOAGULANT MEDICATIONS or DIGOXIN, doctors and pharmacists generally recommend staying with the same brand (whether generic or the original patent product) to avoid any possible problems due to variations across products.

The costs of prescription medications for treating the various forms of HEART DISEASE are significant. Many health plans that cover prescription drugs require pharmacists to dispense generic medications when they are available, as a cost-control measure. Most often, this is a benefit for the consumer, who typically has to pay at least a portion of the prescription costs. Many health plans do not pay for prescription drugs because of the costs. Most states allow generic substitution unless the prescribing physician specifically prohibits it. It is important to ask the doctor when he or she writes the prescription if the medication can be dispensed as a generic product.

See also DRUGS, FREE OR LOW-COST.

gene therapy Treatment approaches that focus on the particular actions (or lack of actions) within specific cells or cellular components. Scientists know that many disease processes originate with changes that take place at the cellular level when the cell's genetic code governing its behavior becomes distorted. Sometimes this distortion results from inherent gene mutations, or inborn flaws in the cell's genetic code. Scientists believe this is what happens in familial disorders (when diseases "run in the family"). Gene therapy might someday enable doctors to inject genetic material that replaces defective genetic code, restoring normal function of the cells.

More often, researchers believe, the mutations take place over time as genetic material becomes damaged during replication. This allows other damage to take place, such as ATHEROSCLEROSIS (accumulations of PLAQUE in the arteries) and

ARTERIOSCLEROSIS (stiffening of the arterial walls). Therapies that target the cellular changes which allow such damage seem promising as preventive measures with regard to HEART DISEASE, as most heart conditions develop over time.

At present gene therapy for heart disease is primarily experimental. Scientists hope that in the near future gene therapy will present the opportunity to heal heart damage such as that which occurs in HEART FAILURE, replacing injured cells with healthy ones. Gene therapy also holds promise for treating some kinds of HYPERTENSION (high blood pressure) by replacing damaged peripheral artery cells and restoring artery contraction and dilation to normal. Some scientists believe it eventually will be possible to target nearly every form of heart disease through gene therapy.

See also ANGIOGENESIS; GENETICALLY ENGINEERED CELLS; INVESTIGATIONAL TREATMENTS.

genetically engineered cells   Cells in which scientists manipulate genetic code (DNA) to cause the cells to grow or act in a certain way. One of the earliest and most commonly used applications of genetically engineered cells is laboratory production of human insulin. Genetic engineering also is the foundation of cloning technology, in which cells can be directed to grow as specific tissues. Although this technology is in its infancy, researchers believe that eventually it will be possible to use genetic engineering to "grow" replacement tissues from a person's own cells. Applications of this technology in HEART DISEASE could mean replacing diseased coronary arteries or heart valves with new ones of the person's own tissue, for example.

Genetic engineering shows particular promise in ANGIOGENESIS, where researchers have been able to use certain growth factors to stimulate new blood vessels to grow around areas of damaged heart tissue following heart attack. Laboratory manipulation of stem cells also holds promise for growing specific kinds of cells, such as those that produce the heart's electrical activity. Such an advance would be a great boon for people who rely on electronic PACEMAKERS because natural cells have the ability to respond to changes in the heart's needs such as with EXERCISE. Yet another aspect of genetic engineering is that of manipulating food-source animals such as cattle to produce meats with inherently lower saturated fats, the idea being to preserve the beneficial qualities of eating meat while diminishing the risks to cardiovascular health.

Genetically engineered cells might also be introduced into the body in such a way as to avert disease development in the first place, for example altering the cells of the lining of the arteries so they are more resistant to plaque accumulations.

See also CLONING RESEARCH.

genetic predisposition   See HEREDITY AND HEART DISEASE.

ginkgo biloba   An extract from the Chinese ginkgo tree that has mild anticoagulant and vasodilator effects. This has a relaxing effect on smooth muscle tissue such as in the walls of the arteries. It also limits platelet aggregation, an early stage in the blood clotting sequence in which platelets start sticking together. Some CLINICAL RESEARCH STUDIES show ginkgo biloba can relieve the symptoms of mild to moderate peripheral vascular disease (PVD) and INTERMITTENT CLAUDICATION, conditions of impaired circulation in the legs. Ginkgo biloba also acts as an ANTIOXIDANT, limiting the accumulation of FREE RADICALS in the body. Many researchers believe free radicals, molecular fragments that remain as the waste by-products of cell metabolism, cause many diseases that develop over time. Gingko biloba is reputed to aid dementia, Alzheimer's disease, sexual dysfunction, DEPRESSION, and asthma, and to boost energy. Its medicinal uses in traditional practices trace back several thousand years.

Because of ginkgo biloba's popularity as an herbal remedy for a wide range of health conditions, the National Institutes of Health's National Center for Complementary and Alternative Medicine (NCCAM) is supporting a number of studies into its actions and effects. Ginkgo biloba comes in numerous NUTRITIONAL SUPPLEMENTS and related products. Because the U.S. Drug and Food Administration (FDA) does not regulate such products, it is important to read labels to determine how much ginkgo biloba extract, sometimes abbreviated as GBE, the product contains although not all products include this information. Ginkgo biloba can interact with or alter the effects of numerous medications, among them ANTICOAGULANT MEDICATIONS ("blood thinners") such as WARFARIN and CLOPIDOGREL. People who want to take ginkgo biloba should first talk with their doctors or pharmacists.

See also COMPLEMENTARY THERAPIES; FLAVONOIDS; GARLIC AND GARLIC OIL; NUTRITION AND DIET.

good cholesterol   See CHOLESTEROL, BLOOD.

grapefruit and grapefruit juice   Grapefruit and grapefruit juice affect the way the liver metabolizes many heart medications, particularly anticoagulant medications and calcium channel blocking medications, allowing higher levels of the medications to enter the bloodstream and to stay longer. This lowers the toxicity threshold for these medications, sometimes significantly. This affect does not occur with other citrus fruits. Generally the effect is minimal when more than two hours separates the medication and consuming grapefruit or grapefruit juice, but some medications are sensitive enough that the grapefruit should be avoided altogether. People who take medications to treat heart disease should ask the pharmacist about grapefruit. There is a fad diet for WEIGHT MANAGEMENT, the grapefruit diet, that incorporates high consumption of grapefruit. This could be particularly risky for someone taking heart medications; the most effective approach for weight loss and weight management is a nutritional diet combined with regular EXERCISE.

See also MEDICATION SIDE EFFECTS; NUTRITION AND DIET.

guanabenz   A medication taken to treat moderate HYPERTENSION (high BLOOD PRESSURE). Common brand names include Wytensin. Doctors commonly prescribe guanabenz in combination with thiazide diuretics. Guanabenz is an ALPHA ANTAGONIST MEDICATION; it acts by blocking signals from the autonomic nervous system to prevent them from activating the release of EPINEPHRINE. This causes

the arteries to dilate, lowering the resistance BLOOD encounters as it flows through them. It also slows HEART RATE. Common side effects include headache, dry mouth, and SEXUAL DYSFUNCTION.

See also ANTIHYPERTENSIVE MEDICATIONS; BETA ANTAGONIST MEDICATIONS; DIURETIC MEDICATIONS; GUANADREL; GUANETHIDINE; GUANFACINE; MEDICATIONS TO TREAT HEART DISEASE.

guanadrel   A medication taken to treat moderate HYPERTENSION (high BLOOD PRESSURE). Common brand names include Hylorel. Guanadrel is an ALPHA ANTAGONIST MEDICATION that acts on the peripheral nervous system to inhibit NOREPINEPHRINE release. This prevents BLOOD pressure from rising and helps to dilate peripheral arteries, lowering resistance to blood flow during DIASTOLE (the resting phase of the CARDIAC CYCLE). Common side effects include headache, fatigue, urinary frequency, and SEXUAL DYSFUNCTION. Guanadrel interacts with tricyclic ANTIDEPRESSANT MEDICATIONS, can worsen asthma or cause asthma attacks, and should not be taken in combination with BETA ANTAGONIST MEDICATIONS.

See also ANTIHYPERTENSIVE MEDICATIONS; GUANABENZ; GUANETHIDINE; GUANFACINE; MEDICATION SIDE EFFECTS; MEDICATIONS TO TREAT HEART DISEASE.

guanethidine   A medication taken to treat moderate to severe HYPERTENSION (high BLOOD PRESSURE). Common brand names include Ismelin. Doctors often prescribe guanethidine in combination with DIURETIC MEDICATIONS as part of a multilevel approach to treating BLOOD pressure that remains elevated with other ANTIHYPERTENSIVE MEDICATIONS or to treat hypertension in which both systolic and diastolic pressures are elevated. Guanethidine is an ALPHA ANTAGONIST MEDICATION that acts on the peripheral nervous system to inhibit NOREPINEPHRINE release. This relaxes the arteries, particularly during DIASTOLE (the resting phase of the CARDIAC CYCLE), and reduces resistance to blood flow. Guanethidine also inhibits norepinephrine action on myocardial (HEART muscle) cells, slowing heart rate. Side effects can include DIZZINESS, peripheral EDEMA (swelling of the ankles, feet, wrists, and hands), and SEXUAL DYSFUNCTION). Guanedrine also can cause bradycardia (slow HEART RATE) and postural HYPOTENSION (sudden drop in blood pressure upon rising to a standing position).

See also GUANABENZ; GUANADREL; GUANFACINE; MEDICATION SIDE EFFECTS; MEDICATIONS TO TREAT HEART DISEASE.

guanfacine　A medication taken to treat moderate to severe HYPERTENSION (high BLOOD PRESSURE). Common brand names include Tenex. Guanfacine is an ALPHA ANTAGONIST MEDICATION that acts on the central nervous system to interrupt the nerve signals that increase the release of EPINEPHRINE. This prevents vasoconstriction, helping to keep the arteries relaxed and reducing resistance to BLOOD flow. Doctors often prescribe guanfacine in combination with DIURETIC MEDICATIONS to further reduce blood pressure and prevent peripheral edema (swelling of the limbs due to excess fluid). Common side effects include drowsiness, dizziness, headache, dry mouth, and SEXUAL DYSFUNCTION.

See also ANTIHYPERTENSIVE MEDICATIONS; BETA ANTAGONIST MEDICATIONS; GUANABENZ; GUANADREL; GUANETHIDINE; MEDICATION SIDE EFFECTS; MEDICATIONS TO TREAT HEART DISEASE.

guar gum fat replacer　See NUTRITION AND DIET.

guided imagery　A method of relaxation and stress relief. Guided imagery is a conscious effort to create a sense of calm and perspective by focusing the mind on specific images. Some people use guided imagery to create a "place" that they can go to in their minds, such as a peaceful garden. Others use guided imagery to generate an inner vision of healing and health, such as when recovering from HEART ATTACK, STROKE, or surgery, or in preparation for an operation. Guided imagery experiences can be brief interludes during a busy day, such as a five-minute break at work. Or they can become a transition from the stress of the day to restful relaxation and rest at night. Guided imagery taps into the powerful mind-body connection and can result in lowering BLOOD PRESSURE and HEART RATE to diminish strain on the HEART AND CARDIOVASCULAR SYSTEM.

See also BIOFEEDBACK; LIFESTYLE AND HEART HEALTH; LIVING WITH HEART DISEASE; MEDITATION; MINDFULNESS; ORNISH PROGRAM; QUALITY OF LIFE; STRESS AND HEART DISEASE; STRESS REDUCTION TECHNIQUES.

habits, eating See NUTRITION AND DIET.

Hales, Stephen (1677–1761)   English scientist who was the first to measure BLOOD PRESSURE and to determine that the pressure of BLOOD in the arteries and veins differed. Hales, an ordained minister, had a keen interest in understanding the mechanics of the natural world. He researched and wrote extensively about plant physiology. He was the first to thoroughly demonstrate and detail the way plants draw in and use water, absorb nutrients, and circulate sap. His success in this area inspired him to investigate the circulation of blood, about which little had been learned since WILLIAM HARVEY's determination a century earlier that blood did in fact circulate within the body. Hales used wax castings to measure the size of blood vessels in various animals after their deaths and inserted a glass catheter into major arteries and veins of three living horses to measure the pressure and volume of blood. Hales's research established that the pressure of blood differed between arteries and veins. He published his findings in 1733 in the monograph *Haemostaticks.* It would be 150 years later when other scientists finally developed noninvasive methods for measuring blood pressure.

See also CORVISART, JEAN-NICHOLAS; EINTHOVEN, WILLEM; LAËNNEC, RENÉ; SPHYGMOMANOMETER; STETHOSCOPE.

hardening of the arteries See ARTERIOSCLEROSIS; ATHEROSCLEROSIS.

Harvey, William (1578–1657)   English physician who determined that the HEART pumps BLOOD in circulation throughout the body. Still popular in Harvey's time were GALEN's interpretations of the heart and circulation, at the cornerstone of which was the premise that venous blood and arterial blood coursed through the body in separate systems. Arterial blood originated in the heart and contained "pneuma," which gave the body life. Venous blood originated in the liver and nourished the body, which consumed it. In the Galen model, the arteries pulsed because of the pneuma in the blood they carried, and the heart was a passive structure.

By the time he was 40 years old, Harvey was a prominent physician and lecturer in anatomy at the Royal College of Physicians. He used living frogs to demonstrate the function of the heart in moving blood through the body and the volumes of blood the heart pumped each minute. He dissected other animals to demonstrate the muscular, chambered structure of the heart and to further elaborate the function of the circulatory system. By tying a band around a volunteer's arm and selectively tightening and loosening it, Harvey also proved that blood flowed into the arm via arteries and returned via veins. Lastly, Harvey demonstrated, through dissection of various animals, that veins had one-way valves that regulated the flow of blood within them to move toward the heart. Harvey published his findings in 1628 in the manuscript *Exercitatio anatomica de motu cordis et sanguinis in animalibus* (An anatomical treatise on the movement of the heart and the blood in animals). Harvey's views made him somewhat of an eccentric among his peers, who still held to the Galen model. However, by the time Harvey died at age 79, his model of cardiovascular structure and function had become widely accepted.

See also CORVISART, JEAN-NICHOLAS; EINTHOVEN, WILLEM; HALES, STEPHEN; LAËNNEC, RENÉ.

heart The heart powers the CARDIOVASCULAR SYSTEM. This muscular, four-chambered organ is about the size of a man's closed fist and weighs 10 to 12 ounces. Placed slightly left of center in the chest, the heart nestles between the organs with which it has the most intimate relationship, the lungs. The ribs encircle the chest to provide a protective cage around these vital structures, with the flat, broad sternum (breastbone) shielding the exposed, vulnerable front of the chest and the spine giving a rail of added protection down the back. The heart's job, which it carries out with precise efficiency, is to collect deoxygenated blood from the body and pump it to the lungs and to receive oxygenated blood from the lungs and pump it to the body.

A fluid-filled membranous sac called the pericardium surrounds and envelops the heart; it protects the heart from contact with other structures in the chest and provides lubrication to minimize friction as the heart beats. A thin membrane, the endocardium, lines the inside walls of the heart's chambers, providing a smooth surface that keeps blood from sticking to the insides of the heart.

The heart has four chambers:

Right atrium The right atrium receives deoxygenated BLOOD returning from the body through two large veins, the superior (upper) vena cava and the inferior (lower) vena cava. In timed sequence with the heart's rhythm, the right atrium contracts to pass its volume of blood through the tricuspid valve into the right ventricle. Each contraction of the right atrium dispenses about 2 1/2 ounces (80 ml) of blood and initiates a cardiac cycle.

Right ventricle The right ventricle receives the deoxygenated blood from the right atrium. When the right ventricle contracts, it sends the blood through the pulmonary valve into the pulmonary artery, which carries the blood to the lungs to become oxygenated.

Left atrium Oxygenated blood from the lungs returns to the heart via the pulmonary veins into the left atrium. The left atrium pumps the oxygenated blood through the mitral valve into the left ventricle.

Left ventricle The left ventricle is the workhorse of the heart. Its walls are thicker and stronger than the walls of the other heart chambers to support its efforts to pump against the high arterial BLOOD PRESSURE (tremendous resistance) to push blood through the body. The left ventricle pumps blood into the aorta, the body's largest artery. Each contraction of the left ventricle concludes a CARDIAC CYCLE.

The muscular, thick wall of the heart is the myocardium. The right side of the heart—right atrium and right ventricle—is responsible for receiving blood and getting blood to the lungs for OXYGENATION. The left side of the heart—the left atrium and left ventricle—is responsible for delivering the oxygenated blood to the body. A thick wall, the septum, runs the length of the heart, separating the right and left sides.

One-way valves keep blood flowing through the heart in the proper direction, and prevent it from backflowing into a chamber following the chamber's contraction.

Pulmonary valve The pulmonary valve regulates the flow of deoxygenated blood from the right ventricle into the pulmonary arteries, which carry the blood to the lungs. It has three cusps and opens into the right ventricle at the peak of the ventricle's contraction (systole). The pulmonary valve closes when the right ventricle's contraction is complete. The pulmonary valve's opening coordinates with the tricuspid valve's closing.

Aortic valve The aortic valve regulates the flow of oxygenated blood from the left ventricle into the aorta, the artery that carries the blood out to the body. It has three flaps, called cusps, that open into the aorta at the peak of the left ventricle's contraction (systole). The aortic valve closes when the left ventricle's contraction is complete. The opening of the aortic valve coordinates with the closing of the mitral valve.

Tricuspid valve The tricuspid valve regulates the flow of blood between the right atrium and the right ventricle. It has three cusps and opens into the right ventricle when the ventricle relaxes (diastole). The opening of the tricuspid valve coordinates with the closing of the pulmonary valve.

Mitral valve The mitral valve regulates the flow of oxygenated blood between the left atrium and the left ventricle. It has two cusps and opens into the left ventricle when the ventricle relaxes (diastole) and the aortic valve closes, allowing oxygenated blood newly arrived to the left atrium from the lungs to flow into the left ventricle. The mitral valve's opening coordinates with the closing of the aortic valve.

The coronary arteries supply blood to the heart itself. They encircle the heart like a crown; "coronary" means crownlike. The arteries and veins through which blood enters and leaves the heart are collectively called the great vessels. They are the largest blood vessels in the body:

Superior and inferior vena cavae The superior vena cava and the inferior vena cava are the veins that bring deoxygenated blood back to the heart from the upper body and lower body, respectively. The superior vena cava enters the right atrium from the top and the inferior vena cave enters the right atrium from the lower side, just above the tricuspid valve.

Aorta The aorta leaves the heart from the inner top of the left aorta, tucking beneath the pulmonary artery. This enormous artery, an inch in diameter along most of its structure, arches over the top of the heart and then curves downward to drop behind the heart. From the heart to the top of the aortic arch is the ascending aorta; from the aortic arch to the central abdomen is the descending aorta.

Pulmonary artery The pulmonary artery leaves the heart from the top of the right ventricle and is the blood's route to the lungs. It comes to a T at the aortic arch, where it separates into the right pulmonary artery and the left pulmonary artery, which go to the right and left lungs, respectively. The pulmonary arteries are the only arteries in the body that carry deoxygenated blood.

Pulmonary veins The two pairs of pulmonary veins, one pair from the right lung and one pair from the left lung, enter the sides of the left atrium to bring oxygenated blood to the heart.

The heart's four chambers contract and relax in a synchronized pattern, regulated by the heart's conduction system. The electrical impulse that initiates each cardiac cycle originates in a cluster of specialized cells at the top of the right atrium, the sinoatrial (SA) node. The impulse electrifies the myocardial cells of the atria in a wavelike pattern that causes them to contract. A second cluster of specialized cells in the septum at the base of the atria, the atrioventricular (AV) node, serves as a circuit breaker of sorts, interrupting the flow of the electrical impulse. The AV node refocuses the impulse and then releases it into the His-Purkinje network, which carries the impulse like a beam to the apex of the ventricles. The beam then splits and spreads out to electrify the myocardial cells of the ventricles, causing them to contract.

A contraction increases the tension of the valves and forces the mitral and tricuspid valves closed. The force of the blood pushes the aortic and pulmonary valves open. When the heart chamber relaxes, tension decreases and allows the mitral and tricuspid valves to open; the higher pulmonary artery and aortic pressure forces the pulmonary and aortic valves to close. Fibrous cords help to anchor the mitral and tricuspid valves, limiting their movement to prevent overdistention during contraction when tension is increased.

heart, artificial A mechanical pumping device to replace a badly diseased or damaged natural HEART. An American heart surgeon, MICHAEL DEBAKEY, implanted the first artificial heart in 1963 as an emergency measure to save the life of a man who, while awaiting surgery to replace a faulty aortic valve, had a CARDIAC ARREST. The bulky, compressor-driven device sustained the man's life for four days—not enough to carry him through to the operation that could have prolonged his life by decades, but long enough to raise the hope that an artificial heart could become a viable treatment option for those whose own hearts fail. Thirty years would pass before an artificial heart design was developed that had the potential to fulfill that hope.

Early Efforts: The Heart-Lung Bypass Machine

In the 1930s the American physician John Gibbon began a lifetime's work of research to develop a machine that could temporarily take over the functions of the heart and lungs, primarily to allow surgery on the heart. His efforts culminated in the first successful OPEN-HEART SURGERY in 1953 by rerouting the patient's BLOOD supply and cardiovascular functions (circulation and oxygenation) through a prototype HEART-LUNG BYPASS MACHINE. The enormous piece of equipment featured membrane oxygenation in which blood was pumped past a permeable membrane that allowed oxygen and CARBON

DIOXIDE exchange. Large cannulas diverted blood flow from the heart's great vessels to the machine, which then returned the blood to the aorta for distribution to the body. The heart-lung bypass machine was the 20th century's most significant breakthrough in cardiovascular medicine, and it fueled the enthusiasm of researchers who believed building a replacement heart was possible.

The Jarvik 7

The cardiovascular researcher ROBERT JARVIK was in the forefront of scientific enthusiasm in artificial heart research. The American physician devoted his career to designing a functional, total replacement artificial heart. In 1982 he received approval from the U.S. Food and Drug Administration (FDA), the agency responsible for overseeing the development and use of medical devices, to implant his latest model of artificial heart, the Jarvik 7, and the first artificial heart to make it to human testing, into human volunteers. As is typical for such devices, the FDA restricted the pool of volunteers to those in complete heart failure who had no other treatment options available to them and who were expected to die within a month.

The first eligible volunteer was BARNEY CLARK, a retired dentist who was in end-stage heart failure. In December 1982 heart surgeon William DeVries implanted the Jarvik 7 into Clark's chest after cutting away the badly diseased and damaged left ventricles (the pumping chambers) of Clark's natural heart. Though the Jarvik 7 itself fit into Clark's chest cavity, the compressor required to operate it was the size of a console television. Seven feet of tubing connected Clark's artificial heart to the compressor, defining Clark's range of mobility. Clark suffered numerous medical setbacks during the 112 days he survived with the mechanical pump circulating blood through his body; he died in March 1983.

Over the next few years about 70 people received pumping assistance from implanted Jarvik 7 artificial hearts, most of whom were awaiting heart transplants. The exception was William Schroeder, who lived 620 days with a Jarvik 7. It was clear, however, that a viable replacement heart would have to be not only small enough to fit inside the chest cavity but also fully self-contained to permit adequate QUALITY OF LIFE. As well, other research began to suggest that supporting, rather than replacing, a diseased heart could allow the heart to heal enough to return to function. Researchers turned their efforts to pursue these directions.

Ventricular Assist Devices

The development of the axial flow pump in the late 1980s represented another breakthrough in artificial heart design that allowed surgeons to implant a small pump to augment, rather than replace, the natural heart. The axial flow pump, less than an inch long and about the diameter of a pencil, features a screw-style continuous flow pumping design. Researchers recognized that the heart pauses between beats to give the myocardium (heart muscle) a brief rest and the ability to recharge (repolarize) between contractions. With a mechanical device that is not susceptible to physiological fatigue, this pausing is unnecessary. A continuous flow pump has far fewer moving parts and accomplishes the heart's primary function, which is to move oxygenated blood through the body.

Similar in concept to screw-drive propulsion systems on boat motors, the tiny axial flow pump fits inside the heart's ventricle to boost the flow of blood and relieve the ventricle's workload. Ventricular assist devices often are called pulseless pumps as the continuous flow mechanism does not generate a pulse. Different designs accommodate placement in the left ventricle (LEFT VENTRICULAR ASSIST DEVICE [LVAD]), right ventricle (right ventricular assist device or RVAD), or both ventricles (biventricular assist device or BVAD). The most common placement is in the left ventricle, as this is the primary pumping chamber of the heart and the ventricle most severely damaged in heart failure. In 2002 the FDA approved the LVAD for use in people who have end-stage heart failure and for whom there are no other treatment options. Among the models in use is the Jarvik 2000.

The Total Artificial Heart (TAH)

Research with ventricular assist devices and continuous flow pumps led to the development in the late 1990s of the total artificial heart, a self-contained device implanted to replace the natural heart. There are various designs and models, most of which are dual chamber pumps that use continuous flow technology and compensation microsensors to adjust the flow of blood between the ventricles (the left ventricle pumps a greater volume of blood, and at greater force, than the right ventricle) as well as to accommodate changes in activity level and oxygen needs. The first recipient of the TAH, 59-year-old Robert Tools, received an AbioCor model in July 2001 and lived for five months with the device. Though plagued by problems with blood clots and bleeding, Tools was able to go home with his artificial heart. Other recipients of the TAH have survived for longer periods of time, though researchers remain uncertain whether the TAH will become a viable permanent solution for severely damaged hearts or serve as a bridge device for those awaiting HEART TRANSPLANT.

Implantable Artificial Heart (IAH)

Technology took leaps in 2004 with the FDA's approval of the first fully implantable temporary artificial heart and in 2006 when the first fully implantable permanent artificial heart received FDA approval. Both devices are permitted for people who have irreversible, end-stage failure of both ventricles. The temporary IAH serves as a bridge pump to augment cardiac function until a DONOR HEART becomes available for heart transplant. The permanent IAH is for people who do not meet the criteria for heart transplant. Both types have rechargeable internal batteries that can hold a short charge and external battery packs and power sources that operate the IAH as well as recharge the internal batteries. These systems use coils that transmit energy through the skin without direct contact; there are no exposed wires, tubes, or other components. Such designs eliminate the risk of infection and allow more freedom for people who have them.

The Challenges of Mechanical Circulation

The human heart is an amazing design of engineering efficiency, the functioning of which is nearly impossible to replicate. Initial efforts to develop an artificial heart focused on doing just that by designing valves and pumping mechanisms as close to the human model as mechanical engineering could make possible. The efforts were abysmally inef-

fective; researchers could not generate adequate pumping force and the valve mechanisms were prone to both failure and accumulating blood clots. Testing on such models did not make it past the stage of experimental surgeries on dogs. There also was the challenge of powering the device, which, until the explosive growth of microtechnology in the 1990s, required external sources such as compressed air or hydraulics. The size of mechanical devices such as LVADS and TAHs remains a factor in their widespread use; even as small as some models are, they are too large to be implanted in smaller adults.

A persistent challenge of mechanical circulation remains the formation of blood clots around the device's synthetic components. This is the same challenge of artificial heart valves; despite the sophistication of synthetic materials available for constructing mechanical devices for implantation in the body, the materials are not as effective as natural body tissues at shedding blood cells that make contact with them. Stroke is a particularly grave risk with implanted pumping devices, and people who have them must take fairly high doses of ANTICOAGULANT MEDICATIONS to help prevent blood clots from forming. The therapeutic index of such medications is extremely narrow, however, and the balance between adequate anticoagulation and excessive bleeding is intricate and precarious.

See also COOLEY, DENTON; MECHANICAL CIRCULATORY SUPPORT.

Heart and Estrogen/Progestin Replacement Study (HERS) A landmark clinical research study that evaluated the effectiveness of HORMONE REPLACEMENT THERAPY (HRT) in reducing a postmenopausal woman's risk for CARDIOVASCULAR DISEASE (CVD). The study enrolled nearly 2,800 women, average age 67, who had CORONARY ARTERY DISEASE (CAD) or ISCHEMIC HEART DISEASE, and randomly assigned half of them to take HRT (combination estrogen/progesterone) and the other half of them to take a placebo (inactive substance). The study ran for four years and reported its findings in 1998.

HERS was the first comprehensive study to evaluate the perceived cardiovascular benefits of HRT in a clinical, rather than observational, context, and its findings shocked researchers, physicians, and women alike. HRT was found to significantly increase the risk of BLOOD clots causing pulmonary embolism and deep vein thrombosis (DVT). As well, there was no evidence that HRT improved the women's cardiovascular status, and the suggestion emerged that taking HRT might instead increase a woman's risk for HEART ATTACK and death resulting from CVD during the first two years of taking HRT, when the woman already has CVD.

A later and larger study, the WOMEN'S HEALTH INITIATIVE (WHI), provided even more striking evidence that HRT provided no cardiovascular benefit for postmenopausal women and increased the risk of HEART attack and death (and also that HRT significantly increased a woman's risk for endometrial cancer and some breast cancers). The National Heart, Lung, and Blood Institute (NHLBI), WHI's sponsor, stopped the study ahead of schedule in 2002 and issued a warning about the potential risks of HRT.

CLINICAL RESEARCH STUDIES continue to investigate the role of estrogen, progesterone, and other HORMONES in heart disease and other forms of CVD. Most doctors recommend that women who are considering HRT do so only to relieve significant symptoms related to menopause and take the lowest dose possible for the shortest period of time. It is important for a woman to discuss with her doctor the full range of possible benefits and potential risks relative to her personal health situation before she makes a decision about HRT.

See also EARLY MENOPAUSE AND HEART DISEASE RISK; LIFESTYLE AND HEART HEALTH; WOMEN AND HEART DISEASE.

heart attack   The death of myocardial (HEART muscle) tissue and interruption of the heart's functions. Heart attack occurs when the heart's blood supply, and hence oxygen supply, is interrupted; it is also called myocardial infarction, which means "death of heart muscle." The myocardium uses two to three times as much oxygen as other tissues in the body. Myocardial cells begin to die within two minutes of oxygen depletion, and the heart has very limited ability to replace the dead cells. When the area of infarction is minimal the surrounding cells often can compensate with little consequence to overall heart function. Heart attack may result in full CARDIAC ARREST (stoppage of the heart) or present no symptoms, depending on the extent of damage and what areas of the heart the damage affects.

More than 1 million Americans have heart attacks each year; just under half of them die. Among those who die of heart attacks, half do so during the first hour following the heart attack and before reaching a hospital. Immediate emergency medical attention is crucial when heart attack occurs or is suspected. Treatment is most effective when received within one hour of a heart attack's onset. Yet among those who have heart attacks, only one in five seeks medical attention within the first hour; most wait two hours or longer. Women are more likely than men to have severe first heart attacks and to die from first heart attacks; the reasons for this are unclear but likely involve multiple factors.

Symptoms and Diagnostic Path

The classic image of heart attack presenting as crushing CHEST PAIN is familiar to many people. Only about half of heart attacks present in this way, however. Women in particular are less likely to experience classic symptoms. Early signs of heart attack often are vague, and many people do not clearly recognize them as cardiac. Doctors call these early warning signs prodromal signs. They include:

- sensation of pressure or squeezing in the center of the chest that lasts longer than a few minutes or that comes and goes over a period of time
- nagging discomfort, ranging from dull and achy to sharp and stabbing, in the back under the shoulder blade, in the shoulder, along the collarbone, or in the jaw (usually on the left side but can occur on either side or both sides of the body)
- breaking out in a cold sweat
- feeling short of breath when at rest
- nausea and upset stomach
- episodes of DIZZINESS, wooziness, or LIGHT-HEADEDNESS

- vague uneasiness or feeling that something is wrong
- unusual or persistent fatigue

Inasmuch as people fear mistaking gastrointestinal distress for heart attack, the symptoms can be quite similar. Equally as many people err in the other direction, believing they are experiencing gastrointestinal distress (or sometimes cold symptoms) when they are in the early stages of heart attack. All too many people delay seeking medical attention because they are waiting to be sure; such delay can be fatal. Discomfort that persists beyond 20 minutes or that develops in a person who has diagnosed heart disease of any kind (or family history of early heart disease) requires immediate medical evaluation.

Treatment Options and Outlook

When there is any suspicion that a person is having a heart attack, whether oneself or someone else, call 911 to summon emergency medical aid, then sit quietly to limit the heart's workload. Rapid treatment is essential to maintain adequate circulation and contain damage to the heart. Intravenous or intracardiac ANTIARRHYTHMIA MEDICATIONS and ionotropic drugs such as EPINEPHRINE and DOPAMINE, as well as DEFIBRILLATION (controlled electrical shock) might be necessary when the heart's rhythm is erratic. Efforts such as administering THROMBOLYTIC MEDICATIONS ("clot-busters" that dissolve blood clots blocking the coronary arteries) or emergency ANGIOPLASTY (removing the occlusion using a catheter threaded through the blood vessels and into the blocked coronary artery) can halt the heart attack, stop the spread of damage, and even allow the heart to begin to recover. The window of opportunity for these treatment options to have such effect is narrow, however, typically two to four hours after the heart attack begins. Sometimes heart attack "stuns" myocardial cells, sending them into a state of suspended function that cardiologists refer to as hibernation. With timely and appropriate treatment to restore blood flow to the cells, sometimes the damaged area of heart muscle tissue can recover and return to full function. This recovery process can take a few days to several weeks.

When treatment is not received so rapidly, the situation becomes one of repairing rather than preventing damage. This might include angioplasty or CORONARY ARTERY BYPASS GRAFT (CABG) to remove the occlusion and repair (or, with CABG, replace) the obstructed coronary artery; often it is necessary to wait for the heart muscle to stabilize before performing either of these operations, as the damaged tissue can lose its firmness. Nearly all hospital emergency departments have thrombolytic medications; not all hospitals are staffed and equipped to perform angioplasties or bypass procedures. When the damage is extensive, doctors can place an INTRA-AORTIC BALLOON PUMP (IABP), a tiny device placed via CARDIAC CATHETERIZATION into the aorta as it leaves the heart, to help move blood out of the heart and relieve the effort the heart must exert when pumping. About a third of people who have heart attacks recover completely, and about 90 percent of those under age 65 at the time of their heart attacks are able to return to work and many other activities that were part of their lives before their heart attacks. However, one in five men and one in two women who have heart attacks end up having permanent limiting or disabling heart failure as a result. The risk for subsequent heart attack is highest among those who are under age 65 when they have their first heart attacks. Medical treatment and lifestyle modification help to moderate, although cannot eliminate, this increased risk.

Risk Factors and Preventive Measures

Any event that interrupts the flow of blood to the myocardium can cause heart attack. The primary causes of heart attack are CORONARY ARTERY DISEASE (CAD), in which accumulations of arterial plaque collect along the inside walls of the coronary arteries and reduce the flow of blood, and ISCHEMIC HEART DISEASE, in which the myocardium's blood supply (and oxygenation) is chronically deficient, usually as a consequence of CAD. Arterial plaque accumulations narrow the passageway for blood, and the irregular surfaces that form inside the arteries attract debris and clots that can occlude, or block, the artery entirely. The occlusion prevents blood from flowing through the artery, and myocardial tissue on the other side of the blockage no longer receives the oxygen it needs. CORONARY ARTERY SPASM also can interrupt blood flow long enough to cause heart attack, as can arrhythmias such as ventricular tachycardia or ventricular fibrillation that disrupt the heart's ability to pump blood.

There are several methods researchers believe reasonably predict the likelihood that a person will have a heart attack within a certain framework of time, provided the person makes no lifestyle changes. The value of such predictive ability is to alert people at high risk so they can take appropriate actions to reduce their risks. Some methods are invasive or technical; others are simple.

- **Waist circumference** greater than 35 inches in women and greater than 40 inches in men strongly correlates with high abdominal adiposity ("spare tire" body fat distribution pattern or apple body shape) and probable heart attack.

- **WAIST-TO-HIP RATIO** greater than 0.8 in men and 1.0 in women also strongly correlates with high abdominal adiposity and heart attack.

- **BODY MASS INDEX (BMI)** greater than 35 (men or women) indicates more than 20 percent excess body fat, which greatly increases the risk of conditions such as HYPERLIPIDEMIA, HYPERTENSION (high blood pressure), and DIABETES—all leading causes of heart attack.

- **Elevated C-reactive protein** levels in the blood suggest unstable arterial plaque accumulations in the arteries.

- **ELECTRON BEAM COMPUTED TOMOGRAPHY (EBCT) scan** measures the level of calcium in arterial plaque; the higher the concentration of calcium, the more unstable the plaque.

As well, anyone who has had one heart attack has an eightfold increase in risk for a second heart attack. The National Heart, Lung, and Blood Institute (NHLBI) reports that within six years, 18 percent of men and 35 percent of women will have second heart attacks.

Preventing CVD is the most effective way to prevent heart attack; rarely does heart attack occur in a person who does not have some form of CVD. Key preventive actions include smoking cessation, eating nutritiously (with fewer than 30 percent of calories from fat), getting regular physical exercise (minimum 30 minutes, four times a week), maintaining healthy weight, and managing other health conditions such as diabetes that contribute to heart disease. Rapid treatment at the earliest signs of heart attack can mitigate damage to the heart.

See also CHAIN OF SURVIVAL; CPR LIFESTYLE AND HEART HEALTH; PLAQUE, ARTERIAL; WEIGHT MANAGEMENT; WOMEN AND HEART DISEASE.

heartbeat The completion of a CARDIAC CYCLE in which the heart pumps blood to the lungs and to the body. The heartbeat can be felt as the pulse, at points where the arteries come near the surface of the skin such as at the wrists, crook of the elbows, sides of the neck, groin, back of the knees, and tops of the feet. It is used to obtain BLOOD PRESSURE readings (the force with which blood moves through the arteries) and measure the HEART RATE (the pace at which the heart contracts). Detecting heartbeat is the classic indicator of life.

See also AUSCULTATION; SPHYGMOMANOMETER.

heart block A disorder of the heart's electrical system. The SINOATRIAL (SA) NODE, a small cluster of nerve fibers at the apex of the right atrium, releases the electrical impulse that begins the CARDIAC CYCLE. The impulse moves in a wave across the atria, causing them to contract. In a healthy HEART the ATRIOVENTRICULAR (AV) NODE, a cluster of nerve fibers on the septum at the top of the ventricles, receives the impulse and retransmits it through the bundle of His to the right and left bundle branches, the network of nerves that cause and coordinate ventricular contraction. In heart block, when the impulse reaches the AV node it slows or stops. The consequence is slowed contraction of the ventricles and asynchronous contraction of the heart. The more severe the heart block, the greater the lack of synchronization between atrial contractions and ventricular contractions. In severe heart block there might not be enough electrical stimulation to contract the ventricles, which can result in SUDDEN CARDIAC ARREST.

Sometimes heart block can be a drug reaction; DIGITALIS medications taken to control ARRHYTHMIAS or to strengthen the heart in HEART FAILURE, can cause heart block. Occasionally there is accidental damage to the bundle of His or the bundle branches during heart surgery. Heart block also can be congenital (present at birth) or accompany a MYOCARDIAL INFARCTION (HEART ATTACK). However, most of the time doctors do not know what causes heart block. Heart block also is called AV block, as the impairment takes place at or after the AV node.

Symptoms and Diagnostic Path

Symptoms, if there are any, might include LIGHTHEADEDNESS, DIZZINESS, fainting, and shortness of breath not related to exertion. Doctors diagnose heart block using ELECTROCARDIOGRAM (ECG) to examine the electrical patterns of the heartbeat and sometimes ECHOCARDIOGRAM to visualize the heart's pumping action.

Treatment Options and Outlook

There are three classifications of heart block: first degree, second degree, and third degree. Treatment depends on the type of heart block.

First degree heart block First degree heart block is the most mild form of heart block. It generally does not produce symptoms, and doctors find it coincidentally on ECG done for other reasons. The ECG indicates it is taking longer for the electrical impulse to travel through the AV node than the normal two-tenths of a second; this travel time is called the PR interval. Other causes of first degree heart block can include heavy alcohol use, substance abuse, and certain medications taken for legitimate therapeutic purposes. Digitalis medications often cause first degree heart block, for example. The heart's rate and rhythm generally are normal in most people who have first degree heart block, so body tissues receive the blood and oxygen they need despite the short delay in signal transmission. First degree heart block typically does not require treatment beyond monitoring to identify whether it worsens over time; for many people first degree heart block remains relatively stable for years.

Second degree heart block In second degree heart block, some SA node impulses make it through the AV node and some do not. These are called dropped beats. There are two forms of

second degree heart block, type 1 and type 2. In type 1 second degree heart block, which is the more common, the dropped beats gradually slide out of synchronization such that the PR interval becomes longer with each beat until eventually the heart skips a beat. This effect sometimes causes the person to feel momentarily light-headed or to perceive the skipped heart. Generally there is no loss of pumping efficiency or cardiovascular risk with type 1 second degree heart block, and no treatment is necessary. In type 2 second degree heart block dropped beats may be frequent and the ventricular contraction often is delayed and weakened. When the signal does make it through, the ventricular contraction is normal. The erratic contractions can cause unstable blood pressure; often type 2 second degree heart block requires treatment with ANTIARRHYTHMIA MEDICATIONS or an implanted pacemaker.

Third degree heart block Third degree heart block is the most serious form of heart block. Untreated it is life-threatening, as the AV node cannot itself generate a fast enough electrical impulse to maintain adequate ventricular contractions. People with third degree heart block often have symptoms of heart failure including a slow and/or erratic pulse and unstable blood pressure, although sometimes the only sign of third degree heart failure is an abnormal ECG. Third degree heart block requires an implanted PACEMAKER to artificially maintain a normal heart rhythm.

Risk Factors and Preventive Measures

Most heart block develops as a consequence of other CARDIOVASCULAR DISEASE (CVD) that causes damage to myocardial tissues, including nerve paths. CORONARY ARTERY DISEASE (CAD), ISCHEMIC HEART DISEASE, HEART ATTACK (MYOCARDIAL INFARCTION), CARDIOMYOPATHY, heart failure, and congenital heart malformations (even after surgical repair) are the most common risk factors for heart block. Heart block, like most CVD, is more prevalent with age. Preventive efforts are the same as for CVD in general, with emphasis on lifestyle factors such as nutritious eating habits, regular physical EXERCISE, WEIGHT MANAGEMENT, and no smoking.

See also HEART DISEASE; HEREDITY AND HEART DISEASE; NUTRITION AND DIET; TILT TABLE TEST.

heart disease A collective term for the health conditions that affect the heart. Heart disease is a dimension of CARDIOVASCULAR DISEASE (CVD). Diseases of the heart generally include disorders of conduction and rhythm, the myocardium (heart muscle), and structure, although the heart's structure and function are closely integrated and often there are overlaps.

Disorders of Conduction and Rhythm

Disorders of conduction and rhythm involve the heart's electrical system. ARRHYTHMIAS in which the heart rate is too slow, too fast, or irregular can affect one atrium, both atria, one ventricle, both ventricles, or the entire heart. Often arrhythmias result from other diseases of the heart or cardiovascular disease such as HYPERTENSION (high BLOOD PRESSURE). Conductive disorders such as heart block, in which electrical impulses do not travel through the heart's electrical system as they should, can be functional or structural in origin. Electrocardiogram (ECG), which amplifies and transmits the heart's electrical activity into patterns printed on paper, is the primary diagnostic tool for disorders of conduction and rhythm. Treatment for disorders of conduction and rhythm is ANTIARRHYTHMIA MEDICATIONS and, if necessary, interventions such as CARDIOVERSION, DEFIBRILLATION, and PACEMAKERS. Disorders of conduction and rhythm often improve and sometimes go away when they result from underlying CVD that resolves with treatment, such as CORONARY ARTERY BYPASS GRAFT (CABG) to replace occluded CORONARY ARTERIES or hypertension controlled with ANTIHYPERTENSIVE MEDICATIONS or lifestyle modifications. Independently occurring conductive disorders and arrhythmias often

become permanent conditions that require ongoing medical monitoring and treatment. Preventive measures are as for CVD in general.

Disorders of the Myocardium

The most common disorders of the myocardium, or heart muscle, are CORONARY ARTERY DISEASE (CAD), CARDIOMYOPATHY, ISCHEMIC HEART DISEASE, and HEART FAILURE. These conditions are most often the consequences of lifestyle factors and progress slowly over decades of life. In this regard, they are often preventable through lifestyle modification to incorporate nutritious eating habits, regular physical EXERCISE, WEIGHT MANAGEMENT, and no smoking. ANGIOPLASTY and CABG can partially correct disorders from CAD and restore the heart's circulation to normal or near-normal, though CAD is likely to return without changes in lifestyle.

Some forms of cardiomyopathy arise from unpreventable causes. Arrhythmogenic right ventricular cardiomyopathy (ARVC) develops when fibrous tissue and fat infiltrate the myocardium, weakening it. Hypertrophic cardiomyopathy is genetic in origin. Cardiomyopathy also can arise from congenital malformations of the heart (disorders of structure) as well as from other diseases such as HEMOCHROMATOSIS (a metabolic disorder in which iron deposits accumulate in organs including the heart) and amyloidosis (protein deposits in the heart). Treatment depends on the cause and on any underlying or coexisting CVD. In general, cardiomyopathy cannot be cured, although medications and lifestyle can help to manage and moderate its symptoms.

Myocarditis (inflammation or infection of the heart muscle), can cause temporary or permanent

DISEASES OF THE HEART		
Disorders of Conduction and Rhythm	**Disorders of the Myocardium**	**Disorders of Structure**
Arrhythmias; bradycardia, tachycardia, fibrillation, ectopic beats, premature ventricular contractions	Ischemic heart disease	Congenital malformations
	Coronary artery disease (CAD)	Valve disease
Heart block	Cardiomyopathy	
	Heart failure	
	Tumors	
	Myocarditis	

damage to the myocardium. Early treatment, usually with anti-inflammatory medications and antibiotics, can halt myocarditis before it does extensive damage. Tumors of the myocardium, also considered diseases of the heart, are rare but do occur. Benign (noncancerous) tumors include MYXOMA, fibromas, and rhabdomyomas. Primary cancer of the heart (malignant tumors that originate in the heart) are even more rare than benign tumors; the two most likely to arise are rhabdomyosarcomas (cancers of muscle connective tissue) or cardiac angiosarcomas (cancers of the blood vessels of the heart). Secondary, or metastatic, cancerous tumors occur somewhat more commonly than primary cardiac malignancies but still are rare. Treatment is surgery to remove a benign or primary malignant tumor; for metastases, treatment targets the original cancer.

Disorders of Structure

Congenital malformations of the heart account for most disorders of structure involving the heart, and range in complexity from easily repairable openings in the septum (septal defects) to multiple operations that literally rebuild the heart. There are almost always lifelong consequences with complex congenital malformations, even after they have been surgically repaired or reconstructed. VALVE DISEASE is an acquired disorder of structure in which the shape and hence function of the valve become altered. Valve disease usually is corrected with valve replacement surgery. Often the replaced valve restores the heart's normal function and there is little or no residual damage to the heart.

Symptoms and Diagnostic Path

Many people are unaware they have heart disease until a crisis such as HEART ATTACK or STROKE occurs. When symptoms of heart disease are present, they commonly include

- CHEST PAIN (ANGINA pectoris), tightness, or pressure
- shortness of breath or difficulty breathing
- sensation of racing, fluttering, or "skipping" HEARTBEAT (PALPITATIONS)
- SYNCOPE (fainting), LIGHT-HEADEDNESS, or DIZZINESS

- coughing (especially with HEART FAILURE)
- inability to engage in physical exertion

Symptoms may develop so slowly and over such a long period of time that a person unknowingly adjusts and accommodates for them, such as limiting activities like climbing the stairs or walking distances. In such situations, and also when no symptoms are present, the doctor may detect conditions such as hypertension (high blood pressure), arrhythmias, and valve disorders (HEART MURMUR) upon routine physical examination.

The diagnostic path typically begins with a personal and family health history, which provides a base for an individual's risk for heart disease. The stronger the family history, the more likely a person is to develop heart disease. The health history should include questions or discussion about:

- all significant medical concerns that are causing symptoms or for which the person is receiving treatment
- recent operations
- all medications currently being taken, including prescription, over the counter, and herbal or naturopathic
- alcohol, drug, and TOBACCO USE (past and present)
- family history of early heart disease (typically before age 50 in men and age 60 in women)
- general eating habits
- current level of physical activity

The physical examination may be comprehensive or focus specifically on cardiovascular symptoms. At minimum, the examination should include height, weight, blood pressure, and pulse taken at several locations (neck, wrists, and feet are most common). The doctor also should look at the fingers and nail beds, which can indicate the presence of CYANOSIS or other markers that point to heart disease. Many doctors will also do a baseline electrocardiogram (ECG). What, if any, additional diagnostic procedures are necessary depends on the base findings. Further testing might include ECHO-CARDIOGRAM, imaging procedures, sophisticated conduction studies to evaluate arrhythmias, blood and urine tests, and X-rays.

Treatment Options and Outlook

Treatments and outlook vary depending on the diagnosis and may include medical, surgical, and lifestyle components. Millions of Americans live with heart disease; current treatments increase both longevity and QUALITY OF LIFE. Because lifestyle is such a significant factor and because nearly all heart disease (except congenital) develops over decades, there is intense focus on preventive measures to reduce and eliminate modifiable risk factors. However, despite the extent to which health researchers believe heart disease is preventable, it remains the leading cause of death among adults over age 40 in the United States.

Risk Factors and Preventive Measures

Researchers consider two classifications of risk factors—significant and contributing—that affect the likelihood for an individual to develop heart disease. Significant risk factors are known to cause heart disease and their mechanisms are fairly well understood. Contributing risk factors are suspected of involvement in the development of heart disease though the ways in and extent to which they do so are not clear. Some risk factors, such as gender and age, are fixed: they cannot be altered or reduced. Most risk factors for heart disease are mutable: they are matters of lifestyle that are within the ability of individuals to influence and reduce.

Significant Risk Factors

Among the significant, or major, risk factors for heart disease are three that are fixed:

- **Age.** The risk for heart disease increases with age; the majority of people who have heart disease are age 65 or older. By age 85, nearly everyone has some form or degree of heart disease.

- **Gender.** Men are at higher risk for heart disease than women until about age 80, when the risk of heart disease for women increases to be comparable to that for men. The reasons for this are not entirely clear though likely are related to the influence of testosterone on cellular functions in

a man's body and perhaps a protective influence of estrogen on cellular functions in a woman's body.

- **Genes.** An individual's heredity may establish predisposition for certain kinds of heart disease such as coronary artery disease (CAD) or hypertension (high blood pressure). It also may direct the development of heart disease related to gene mutations, such as MARFAN SYNDROME, LONG QT SYNDROME, and hypertrophic CARDIOMYOPATHY. Hereditary influence may be familial or racial.

That these risk factors are fixed does not mean that having one or more of them makes heart disease inevitable (with the exception of heart disease resulting from gene mutations). Rather, having one or more of these risk factors increases the importance of modulating significant and contributing risk factors that are within individual influence to lower one's cumulative risk profile.

Other health conditions can become major risk factors for heart disease as well. Key among them are:

- **Diabetes.** The elevated and erratic blood glucose levels characteristic of DIABETES are devastatingly damaging to nerve structures and blood vessels. As well, increased insulin levels alter the body's lipid management systems, contributing to high blood CHOLESTEROL and high blood TRIGLYCERIDES. Many forms of heart disease are associated with diabetes, including peripheral vascular disease (PVD), CAD, hypertension, heart attack, and STROKE.

- **Obesity.** OBESITY is a complex medical condition with multiple cardiovascular implications. Hypertension, INSULIN RESISTANCE, diabetes, cardiomyopathy, and HEART FAILURE all are associated with excess body mass. Doctors now consider obesity as much of a risk factor for heart disease as cigarette smoking.

- **Kidney disease.** Kidney disease may result from hypertension, diabetes, obesity, or other causes. As well, it can cause hypertension, as the body's key blood pressure regulation mechanisms are based in the filtering structures (the glomeruli) of the kidneys, giving the kidneys a complex and multifaceted role in maintaining appropriate blood pressure.

- **Hypertension.** Though a form of heart disease in its own right, hypertension also contributes to the development of other forms of heart disease including heart failure, cardiomyopathy, heart attack, and stroke.

- **Hyperlipidemia, hypercholesterolemia, and hypertriglyceridemia.** Elevated blood lipid levels suggest atherosclerotic processes are at work. ATHEROSCLEROSIS, the accumulation of fatty acids and arterial PLAQUE along the inner walls of the arteries, contributes to hypertension, PVD, and CAD.

For most people who have any of these conditions there are significant lifestyle components, that, when modified even after the conditions develop can improve cardiovascular status.

Lifestyle Risk Factors

Health experts believe that lifestyle modifications in four key areas could eliminate nearly all acquired heart disease. These areas are:

- **Physical activity.** Only about 20 percent of Americans engage in the minimum level of physical activity necessary to maintain cardiovascular health: 30 to 45 minutes of moderately intense EXERCISE four to five days a week and 60 minutes of aerobically intense exercise two to three days a week. Physical activity has multiple cardiovascular benefits, improves the efficiency of metabolism, and helps maintain healthy body weight.

- **Nutrition and diet.** A diet high in saturated fats and carbohydrates contributes to excess body weight and also provides the body with the ingredients to manufacture cholesterol and other fatty acids. As there is never "enough" of these substances from the body's perspective, the body continues to produce them as long as the ingredients to do so are available. Excess becomes stored in ways that are detrimental to cardiovascular health and that contribute to conditions such as atherosclerosis and CAD.

- **Weight management.** Only about 35 percent of Americans are of healthy body weight. Excess

body mass increases the workload of the heart and contributes to other health conditions (such as diabetes) that are risk factors for heart disease. About 80 percent of people who are obese—have a BODY MASS INDEX over 35—have hypertension.

- **Tobacco use.** The leading health consequence of cigarette smoking is not lung cancer, as many people believe, but rather heart disease. NICOTINE, the primary chemical ingredient of tobacco, is a potent vasoconstrictor that has immediate as well as long-lasting effects on the walls of the blood vessels. Over time, nicotine alters the structure of cells in the blood vessels, accelerating the development of atherosclerosis (accumulations of arterial plaque along the inner walls of the arteries) and ARTERIOSCLEROSIS (stiffening and loss of flexibility of the arteries). As well, tobacco smoke contains hundreds of chemicals of varying toxicity, and the smoke itself damages the delicate alveoli in the lungs. These consequences limit the ability of the lungs to deliver oxygen to the blood.

Contributing or Other Risk Factors

Contributing risk factors are those that doctors believe play roles in the development of heart disease though there is little evidence for how they might do so. Among them are:

- **Stress.** Stress activates physiological responses in the body that raise blood pressure and increase the rate and force of the heartbeat. These responses are known to produce changes in cellular metabolism and structure; the extent to which and the mechanisms through which they do so remain largely unknown.

- **Oral contraceptives.** Women who are over age 35 or who smoke face increased risk for heart disease when they take ORAL CONTRACEPTIVES. Doctors are unsure why this is though they suspect interrelationships between the extra hormones in the oral contraceptives and functions within the body, perhaps interference with the natural protectiveness estrogen seems to provide.

- **Excessive alcohol consumption.** Despite studies that show moderate alcohol consumption may have cardio-protective benefits, alcohol is a toxin from the body's perspective. Excessive alcohol consumption (more than one drink daily) damages the cells of the heart and blood vessels and damages nerve endings, which can result in hypertension, cardiomyopathy, and heart failure.

Nearly all forms of heart disease have associated lifestyle factors that if eliminated, researchers at the U.S. Centers for Disease Control and Prevention (CDC) hypothesize, would eradicate as much as 90 percent of heart disease and add seven years to life expectancy. As presently 62 million Americans live with some form of heart disease, the personal, societal, and economic implications of preventing heart disease are staggering. Two Americans die from heart disease every minute—nearly a million people every year. Ninety percent of Americans between the ages of 55 and 65 have or will develop HYPERTENSION (high blood pressure). Direct health-care expenses related to medical care for heart disease exceed $350 billion.

Organized prevention efforts combine education and intervention; numerous government and private organizations sponsor structured programs for specific cardiovascular concerns such as the National Cholesterol Education Program (NCEP), an initiative of the National Heart, Lung, and Blood Institute (NHLBI), which encourages people to have their blood cholesterol levels checked and to maintain diet and exercise habits to keep those levels under control to prevent coronary artery disease (CAD). The American Heart Association (AHA) and the American Stroke Association sponsor similar education efforts that target the public at large as well as specific high-risk populations (notably those who have diabetes, are obese, or are African American) to detect, treat, and prevent hypertension.

The national health promotion and disease prevention initiative Healthy People 2010 has as one of its objectives achieved longevity and a good QUALITY OF LIFE for all Americans. To accomplish this ambitious undertaking, the initiative has established both broad and focused goals for public health efforts, seeking to integrate the participation of hundreds of health organizations throughout the United States. Among the initiative's 28 focus areas are four major categories that target reducing cardiovascular disease (CVD):

- **Heart disease and stroke.** This focus area targets efforts to prevent CAD, ANGINA, and ISCHEMIC HEART DISEASE (IHD), known collectively as CORONARY HEART DISEASE (CHD), and cerebrovascular disease (STROKE and TRANSIENT ISCHEMIC ATTACKS [TIAs]) by reducing blood cholesterol and blood pressure.

- **Nutrition and overweight.** This focus area aims to educate people about dietary and nutritional choices and their consequences for heart health or heart disease, with emphasis on OBESITY and portion sizes.

- **Physical activity and fitness.** This focus area aims to improve muscle strength and endurance, flexibility, and AEROBIC CAPACITY by encouraging people to participate in physical activities and by encouraging communities to support services to make facilities and organized activities available to their citizens.

- **Tobacco use.** This focus area targets reducing direct tobacco use, particularly cigarette smoking, as well as exposure to environmental (secondhand) smoke.

Many private health-care centers and community organizations sponsor a broad spectrum of preventive efforts as well, from local heart walks to free blood cholesterol and blood pressure clinics. In most communities there are numerous opportunities for free blood pressure readings. State, county, and city public health departments also provide certain preventive services at no charge. Appendix I contains contact information for numerous specific programs and organizations that participate in prevention efforts.

See also AFRICAN AMERICANS AND HEART DISEASE; CARDIORENAL SYNDROME; DIABETES AND HEART DISEASE; WEIGHT MANAGEMENT; WOMEN AND HEART DISEASE.

heart disease in children Though there is a broad public perception that HEART DISEASE is a health concern for older people, CARDIOVASCULAR DISEASE (CVD) is the second-leading cause of death in children age 15 and under. More than 40,000 infants are born with heart malformations or disorders of heart function in the United States each year. Much congenital heart disease remains of health concern in adulthood as even with surgical correction there is altered structure and function of the heart. As well, children can acquire nearly any form of heart disease that adults can develop including HYPERTENSION (high BLOOD PRESSURE), CORONARY ARTERY DISEASE (CAD), CARDIOMYOPATHY, HEART FAILURE, and STROKE (cerebrovascular disease). Lifestyle factors such as high-fat diet, lack of physical activity, OBESITY, and cigarette smoking contribute to these forms of CVD in youth just as they do in adults.

Congenital Heart Malformations

Most congenital heart malformations occur spontaneously; there is no known reason for them. Other heart malformations are strongly linked with genetic conditions such as Down syndrome. Among the more common congenital malformations are:

- ATRIOVENTRICULAR (AV) CANAL DEFECT, an opening in the heart wall between the atrium and the ventricle that allows BLOOD to pass between the two chambers.

- BICUSPID AORTIC VALVE, in which the valve between the left ventricle and the aorta has two instead of the normal three leaflets, weakening its ability to prevent blood from backflowing into the left ventricle.

- COARCTATION OF THE AORTA, a narrowing of the aorta as it leaves the left ventricle that limits the volume of blood the heart can pump out to the body.

- EBSTEIN'S ANOMALY, a malformation of the tricuspid valve.

- EISENMENGER'S SYNDROME, a complex that includes one or more forms of septal defect in combination with PULMONARY HYPERTENSION.

- Hypoplastic left heart syndrome (HLHS), in which the left ventricle is too small to be functional.

- PATENT DUCTUS ARTERIOSUS (PDA), in which the ductus arteriosus, a natural opening between the

pulmonary artery and the aorta in the fetus, fails to close after birth.

- Pulmonary or tricuspid atresia, in which the pulmonary valve or the tricuspid valve fails to form and there is no opening between the pulmonary artery and the right ventricle or the right atrium and the right ventricle.

- SINGLE VENTRICLE, in which the heart has just one ventricle instead of the normal two; nearly always there are other malformations as well.

- TETRALOGY OF FALLOT, a complex of four concurrently occurring malformations involving the valves and structure of the heart.

- TRANSPOSITION OF THE GREAT ARTERIES (TGA) in which the aorta arises from the right ventricle and the pulmonary artery arises from the left ventricle, a reversal that sends unoxygenated blood into circulation in the body and oxygenated blood back to the heart.

- VENTRICULAR SEPTAL DEFECT (VSD), an opening in the septum or wall separating the right and left ventricles that allows unoxygenated and oxygenated blood to mix.

Surgery successfully repairs most simple congenital heart malformations, such as septal defects and patent ductus arteriosus, with few residual effects. Complex malformations require multiple operations that may provide limited to complete restoration of heart function depending on various factors. Complex malformations typically require lifelong follow-up and may result in heart disease in adulthood. Anyone born with a congenital heart malformation, even when successfully corrected, should receive annual physical examinations that include cardiac assessment and should take ANTIBIOTIC PROPHYLAXIS before most medical or dental procedures.

Kawasaki Disease

This uncommon childhood disease, also known as mucocutaneous lymph node syndrome, mostly afflicts children under age five and twice as many boys than girls for reasons researchers do not understand. Researchers suspect an infectious agent, likely a virus, causes Kawasaki disease but so far have not identified it. The initial course of disease consists of high fever and swollen lymph glands in the neck with accompanying inflammation and redness in and around the mouth, the whites of the eyes, the palms of the hands, and the soles of the feet. Four in five children recover fully and uneventfully in about three weeks. One in five develops serious cardiovascular complications resulting from inflammation that spreads to the arteries throughout the body, including the CORONARY ARTERIES that supply the heart. This inflammation can weaken the arteries, making them susceptible to ANEURYSM (ballooning and possible rupture of the arterial wall). Aneurysm requires rapid medical attention, typically surgery to repair the damaged portion of the artery.

The Japanese physician Tomisaku Kawasaki first reported the disease that bears his name and its cardiovascular complications in 1967; today its diagnosis is 100 times more prevalent among Japanese than American children. There are no preventive measures for Kawasaki disease; it is possible for the same child to have the disease twice but very rare for more than one child in a family to get it. Treatment is primarily supportive, though high doses of immunoglobulin administered early in the disease seem able to avert cardiovascular complications and shorten the course of the disease. As yet researchers do not know whether childhood infection with Kawasaki disease increases the risk for coronary artery disease (CAD) and peripheral vascular disease (PVD) in adulthood.

See also BIDIRECTIONAL GLENN PROCEDURE; BLALOCK-TAUSSIG PROCEDURE; CYANOTIC CONGENITAL HEART DISEASE; DAMUS-KAYE-STANSEL PROCEDURE; FONTAN PROCEDURE; HEART DISEASE; NORWOOD PROCEDURE; SURGERY TO TREAT CARDIOVASCULAR DISEASE.

heart failure   The inability of the HEART to pump enough BLOOD to meet the body's needs. Heart failure can occur as a gradual loss of function independent of other HEART DISEASE, such as through the changes that take place in the body with aging, though it most commonly develops as a consequence of other heart conditions, notably CORONARY ARTERY DISEASE (CAD), HYPERTENSION (high BLOOD PRESSURE), CARDIOMYOPATHY, HEART ATTACK (MYOCARDIAL INFARCTION), and congenital heart disease. Heart failure results when the heart no longer can adjust, physically or functionally, to compensate for damage or dysfunction. Heart failure can affect the right heart, left heart, or entire heart. When heart failure causes fluid to accumulate in the lungs it is called congestive heart failure. Heart failure is systolic when the heart becomes enlarged and weakened; it is diastolic when the myocardium (heart muscle) becomes stiff.

Heart failure is one of the most common forms of CARDIOVASCULAR DISEASE (CVD), affecting five million Americans. Though heart failure can occur at any age, it is most common in people over age 65 and is the leading cause of hospitalization for people over age 65. OBESITY is a particularly significant risk factor for heart failure, irrespective of the presence of other heart conditions, as excess body fat

NYHA HEART FAILURE CLASSIFICATIONS

NYHA Classification	Symptoms	Functional Capacity Limitations
Category I	Few or none	none
Category II	Mild edema; shortness of breath and tiredness with strenuous activity No symptoms at rest	strenuous physical activity
Category III	Moderate edema; shortness of breath with mild activity; fatigue Rest relieves symptoms	cannot engage in physical activities that require exertion
Category IV	Significant edema; shortness of breath; fatigue; gastrointestinal distress; mild to moderate cognitive dysfunction (intermittent) Symptoms present at rest	cannot engage in any level of physical activity; may require continuous oxygen therapy; fully disabled

increases the oxygen demand as well as the resistance blood encounters at the level of the arterioles (the tiniest arteries that permeate body tissues). This increased resistance forces the heart to pump harder to meet the body's circulatory needs.

Treatment for heart failure aims to manage symptoms and limit disease progression; for most people with heart failure there is no cure, though many people experience measurable to significant improvement with treatment. Treatment typically consists of medications to strengthen the contractions of the heart to make them more efficient, as well as to manage related, underlying, or coexisting cardiovascular conditions. In certain situations such as heart failure that originates as cardiomyopathy due to structural defects in the heart, HEART TRANSPLANT or, if pulmonary damage also is extensive as a consequence of long-term PULMONARY HYPERTENSION as can occur with severe congestive heart failure, HEART-LUNG TRANSPLANT is a treatment option. Prevention efforts target reducing or eliminating overall risk for heart disease as well as managing other diagnosed CVD to help safeguard the heart and control the progression of damage.

Symptoms and Diagnostic Path

Heart failure can develop gradually or come on suddenly. The typical symptoms are rather general and many people do not correlate them with potential heart problems until a doctor makes the diagnosis. Common symptoms of heart failure include:

- shortness of breath (DYSPNEA), especially when lying down and with exertion
- persistent coughing and wheezing with no indication of viral infection (cold or flu)
- fatigue and lack of energy when doing common tasks such as grocery shopping
- loss of appetite and nausea after eating
- cognitive difficulties (impaired thought processes and memory)
- fluid retention and unexplained weight gain
- rapid pulse

AUSCULTATION typically reveals characteristic abnormal heart sounds. Chest X-ray or ECHOCAR-DIOGRAM (ultrasound examination of the heart) often shows an enlarged heart, and echocardiogram also may reveal physical changes to the structure of the heart such as thickening or thinning of the ventricular walls. Electrocardiogram (ECG) may show mild to moderate ARRHYTHMIAS (disturbances of the heart's normal electrical patterns), either as underlying disease or compensatory changes the heart makes as it attempts to maintain pumping effectiveness. Further diagnostic procedures, if necessary, may include RADIONUCLIDE SCAN, LEFT VENTRICULAR EJECTION FRACTION (LVEF), cardiac MAGNETIC RESONANCE IMAGING (MRI), and MULTI-UNIT GATED ACQUISITION (MUGA) SCAN to assess the heart's function and capacity. Diagnosis indicates whether heart failure affects the right, left, or both sides of the heart; this determines treatment options and prognosis (outlook). When heart failure results in fluid retention, it is generally referred to as congestive heart failure.

Left heart failure The left side of the heart pumps blood to the body; left heart failure develops when the left ventricle cannot contract with enough force to push blood out of the heart and into the body. This can be the consequence of damage to the ventricle such as from congenital malformation, heart attack, certain arrhythmias, hypertension, coronary artery disease, RHEUMATIC HEART DISEASE that damages the myocardium or the heart valves, heart valve disease, and cardiomyopathy. Left heart failure can cause fluid to accumulate in the lungs, resulting in PULMONARY CONGESTION/PULMONARY EDEMA.

Right heart failure Right heart failure generally develops as a consequence of left heart failure, although it can exist independently as a consequence of congenital heart malformations, or rarely because of myocardial tumors. The right side of the heart pumps blood to the lungs; right heart failure means the heart cannot pump adequate volumes of blood to the lungs for oxygenation. Right heart failure also can develop when resistance to blood flow is high in the arteries of the lungs, such as with CHRONIC OBSTRUCTIVE PULMONARY DISEASE (COPD), emphysema, and PULMONARY HYPERTENSION. In its late stages right heart failure can cause abdominal swelling (ascites) and swelling throughout the body (systemic EDEMA).

Total heart failure   Generally the progression of either left or right heart failure is such that both sides of the heart ultimately experience failure. This is called total heart failure or sometimes biventricular heart failure. Total heart failure is considered end-stage heart disease.

Congestive heart failure   When heart failure causes peripheral or pulmonary edema (fluid accumulation in body tissues or in the lungs), it is considered congestive heart failure. Nearly all heart failure eventually progresses to congestive heart failure as the heart's inability to pump efficiently becomes increasingly compromised. Congestive heart failure affects lung function as well as cardiovascular function. People who have congestive heart failure may experience rapid weight gain with fluid accumulation.

Restrictive heart failure   Restrictive heart failure is uncommon and develops when there are physical factors that constrict the heart's movement. Such factors might include PERICARDITIS (inflammation of the sac surrounding the heart), restrictive cardiomyopathy (in which changes take place in the walls of the heart that make them rigid and inflexible), and conditions such as HEMOCHROMATOSIS and amyloidosis in which iron or protein deposits respectively cause the myocardium to stiffen. Depending on the causes, other health conditions, and the person's age, heart transplant is sometimes a treatment option for severe restrictive heart failure.

NYHA Heart Failure Classification System

The New York Heart Association (NYHA) classification system for heart failure has become the standard measure of determining the severity of heart failure and its affect on daily living. The NYHA classification is a key factor when determining disability status for employment or insurance purposes.

Treatment Options and Outlook

Treatment for heart failure consists of lifestyle modifications and a medication regimen to minimize fluid retention, strengthen the heart's contractions, and dilate peripheral blood vessels to reduce the resistance of blood flow and decrease the effort the heart must expend to move blood throughout the body.

- DIURETIC MEDICATIONS ("water pills") cause the kidneys to extract more salt and fluid from the blood.
- DIGITALIS medications (DIGOXIN, DIGITOXIN) strengthen the contraction effort of heart muscle cells.
- ANGIOTENSIN-CONVERTING ENZYME (ACE) INHIBITOR MEDICATIONS cause peripheral blood vessels to dilate, lowering blood pressure and decreasing resistance.
- BETA ANTAGONIST MEDICATIONS slow the heart rate and stabilize the heart's rhythm.
- ANTIARRHYTHMIA MEDICATIONS correct dysfunctions in the heart's rhythm such as HEART BLOCK and ATRIAL FIBRILLATION.

Lifestyle modifications are as important as medications for effectively managing heart failure and cardiovascular health overall. Doctors recommend that people with heart failure:

- restrict SODIUM (salt) intake to help control fluid retention
- eat a nutritious, low-fat diet
- get daily physical EXERCISE to the extent possible
- monitor body weight daily to watch for rapid weight gain that can signal fluid retention
- lose weight if necessary to maintain a healthy body weight
- avoid TOBACCO USE, ALCOHOL, and CAFFEINE

Surgical treatment options for heart failure are appropriate only in limited circumstances. Surgical correction of underlying cardiovascular disease, such as CORONARY ARTERY BYPASS GRAFT (CABG) to treat coronary artery disease, can improve the underlying condition and thus the heart failure. Heart transplant and LEFT VENTRICULAR ASSIST DEVICE (LVAD) implant are options for some people. Procedures called ventricular remodeling, such as the BATISTA HEART FAILURE PROCEDURE, remove segments of myocardial tissue from the affected ventricle to reduce the size of the heart and strengthen its ability to contract. Cardiovascular surgeons are experimenting with other procedures to accomplish long-term improvement, though at present the long-term results of surgery for heart failure are unpredictable.

Risk Factors and Preventive Measures

Heart failure typically develops secondary to other forms of heart disease or conditions affecting the body's ability to regulate fluid volume such as chronic and significant liver disease or kidney disease. Preventing or minimizing the risks for underlying health conditions, cardiovascular and other, also helps prevent heart failure.

See also ACTIVITIES OF DAILY LIVING (ADLs); CARDIOMYOPLASTY; CARDIORENAL SYNDROME; DIASTOLIC DYSFUNCTION; SEXUAL ACTIVITY AND HEART DISEASE; SYSTOLIC DYSFUNCTION; WEIGHT MANAGEMENT; WOMEN AND HEART DISEASE.

heart-lung bypass machine A machine that takes over the basic functions of the HEART—oxygen—carbon dioxide exchange and circulation during OPEN-HEART SURGERY. The machine's functions often are referred to as cardiopulmonary bypass, extracorporeal ("out of the body") perfusion, or pump oxygenation. The surgeons connect large tubes (cannulas) to the BLOOD vessels carrying blood to and from the heart (the superior and inferior vena cava entering the right atrium and the aorta leaving the left ventricle) to reroute the body's blood supply from the heart to the bypass machine. The machine oxygenates the blood and pumps it to the body at the aorta, bypassing the heart and lungs to allow surgeons to stop the heart to perform operations. Generally the heart-lung bypass machine also cools the blood, which slows the body's metabolism and thus its oxygen needs.

Research to develop a heart-lung bypass machine began in the 1930s with the work of physician John H. Gibbon, Jr. (1903–73), credited as the inventor of the technology that 20 years later would redraw the boundaries of cardiovascular surgery. On May 6, 1953, Gibbon's device made it possible for surgeons to repair the congenital heart defect of 18-year-old Pennsylvania college student Cecelia Bavolek. In 1960 Gibbon's heart-lung bypass machine, with modifications and improvements from other researchers, was approved for use in open-heart surgeries and made possible

what has become one of the most commonly performed operations today, CORONARY BYPASS ARTERY GRAFT (CABG). Early heart-lung machines were large and cumbersome pieces of equipment that took considerable space; the modern heart-lung bypass machine is about the size of an office desk and is wheeled into the operating room when the surgeons are ready to use it.

Inherent in the heart-lung bypass machine's design and function is the tendency for microemboli, tiny fragments of blood clots and other arterial debris, to become dislodged from the blood vessels. Though the heart-lung bypass machine contains filters to capture these microscopic particles, some are small enough to slip through and make their way to the arterioles in the brain where they become lodged and cut off the blood flow. The resulting damage is minimal but sometimes apparent as confusion, memory loss, and cognitive dysfunction after surgery. Often these disturbances are temporary, but in some people they are permanent. Cardiovascular surgeons and researchers are working on new technologies and surgical techniques that permit open-heart surgery without use of the heart-lung bypass machine; at present about 20 percent of the U.S. cardiovascular surgeons who perform open-heart surgery offer "off-pump" options to selected patients (typically those whose surgical needs are minimal and nonemergency).

See also CARDIOVASCULAR SYSTEM; MINIMALLY INVASIVE CARDIAC SURGERY.

heart-lung transplant An operation in which a person whose own heart and lungs are damaged beyond the ability to sustain life receives the heart and lungs from a donor who dies of causes that leave these organs healthy. Surgeons at Stanford University in California performed the first heart-lung transplant in 1981. Heart-lung transplant presently is a treatment of final option for people with end-stage heart and lung disease, partly because donor organs are difficult to acquire and partly because the surgery is complex, the recovery uncertain, and the prognosis limited. Currently fewer than 100 people undergo heart-lung transplant in the United States each year.

Complex congenital heart malformations with complications such as EISENMENGER'S SYNDROME account for nearly half the heart-lung transplants performed. Other reasons for heart-lung transplant are primary PULMONARY HYPERTENSION, cystic fibrosis, and acquired lung diseases such as emphysema, pulmonary fibrosis, pulmonary sarcoidosis, and pulmonary asbestosis (conditions that cause extensive scarring of lung tissue, rendering it ineffective for oxygen–carbon dioxide exchange). Matching the donor and the recipient requires the usual blood and tissue type compatibility necessary for any organ transplant and also must take into consideration the physical size of donor and recipient. The lungs grow to fill the chest cavity. The lungs of a donor who is six-feet two-inches tall will not fit in the chest of a person who is five-feet two-inches tall.

Procedure

Heart-lung transplant is a complex operation in which transplant surgeons remove the diseased organs and replace them with the donor organs. The donor organs must be transplanted within about six hours of being removed from the donor. A typical heart-lung transplant operation takes eight to 12 hours, though this varies according to individual circumstance. After the person is anesthetized and on CARDIOPULMONARY BYPASS, the surgeon removes the diseased lungs at the main bronchi and blood vessels and cuts away the diseased heart except for the backs of the atria which remain attached to the chest wall. The donor organs are then prepared for transplant, which includes matching the bronchus size and alignment and cutting away the backs of the DONOR HEART atria. Often only one lung is transplanted and remains attached to the donor heart. The surgeon first attaches the donor lung, then aligns the DONOR HEART atria to the backs of the original heart and sutures them in place. After the donor organs are in place, the surgeon stops the cardiopulmonary bypass and allows blood to flow through the body and the new heart. Often the heart begins beating on its own; if it does not, the surgeon administers an electrical shock to start it beating.

Risks and Complications

When recovery is routine, the person stays in the intensive care unit for a few days and 10 to 14 days total in the hospital. The immediate risks are of bleeding, failure of the donor heart or lung to function properly, rejection of the donor organs, and infection. Long-term complications arising from heart-lung transplant include development of bronchiolitis obliterans, an obstructive pulmonary disease that affects the bronchioles (small airways), and CAD. Although the donor heart beats normally and generates a pulse, there is no connection between the donor heart and the person's nervous system. Because of this, the person will not feel cardiac pain such as ANGINA. As well, sometimes a PACEMAKER is necessary to maintain an appropriate rhythm because the donor heart does not receive signals from the nervous system that would cause it to accelerate or decelerate. Immunosuppresive medications are highly effective in minimizing the risk for rejection, though raise the risk for infection because they block immune system function. They also increase the likelihood of developing lymphoma (cancer of the lymphatic structures).

Outlook and Lifestyle Modifications

The follow-up care required after heart-lung transplant is both costly and time-consuming. Myocardial tissue biopsies, done via cardiac catheterization to look for signs of rejection, are necessary frequently during the first year and at least once a year for life. Some people are able to return to jobs and activities that were part of their lives before the diseases that destroyed their hearts and lungs, though most must make modifications to accommodate their ongoing medical needs.

The rate of organ rejection is much higher than with other transplanted organs, as is the overall complication rate. At present the five-year survival rate for heart-lung transplant is about 50 percent. A person who has a heart-lung transplant must take immunosuppressive drugs for the remainder of his or her life to reduce the risk of organ rejection. This immunosuppressive therapy creates vulnerability to infection, which is the leading cause of death among those who receive heart-lung transplants. As well, the person's long-standing cardiopulmonary disease results in compensatory changes in the cardiovascular system that the body sometimes cannot overcome. It is common for conditions such as hypertension to continue, worsen, or develop after heart-lung transplant.

See also ALLOGRAFT; ALLOGRAFT FAILURE; CYCLO-SPORINE; HEART TRANSPLANT.

heart murmur   A soft, distinctive sound a physician can detect when listening to the HEART through a STETHOSCOPE if one or more of the heart's four valves does not open or close properly. It is called a murmur because of the whisperlike quality of its sound compared to other heart sounds. Heart murmurs are common and often transient; it is common for a valve occasionally to open or close incompletely. Persistent heart murmur can signal VALVE DISEASE or damage, most commonly insufficiency or stenosis of the aortic or mitral valves. An ECHOCARDIOGRAM (ultrasound examination of the heart) often can confirm whether there is valve disease. CARDIAC CATHETERIZATION allows the cardiologist to visualize the functioning of the heart valves to determine the extent of damage and consider appropriate treatment options. Certain valve problems respond to treatment with medication, while others require that the valve be surgically repaired or replaced.

See also AUSCULTATION; RHEUMATIC HEART DISEASE; VALVE REPAIR AND REPLACEMENT.

heart rate   The pace, measured in beats per minute, at which the HEART contracts. A normal heart rate for an adult at rest is 60 to 100 beats per minute (usually 60 to 80); during strenuous exercise the heart rate can jump to three times its resting rate. The higher a person's level of AEROBIC CAPACITY (the efficiency with which the body uses oxygen), the lower the resting heart rate and the less work the heart is doing to meet the body's oxygen needs, which is why aerobic conditioning is so important to cardiovascular health. An athlete in peak condition might have a resting heart rate of 45 to 50 beats per minute; a person whose lifestyle is sedentary (physically inactive) might have a resting rate of 80 to 100 beats per minute. Heart rate increases with physical activity, in response to intense emotion such as fear and anger, and when the heart's pumping efficiency drops, such as in disease conditions.

Heart Rate and Cardiovascular Health

Heart rate reflects the efficiency with which the heart pumps blood through the body and becomes altered in various forms of CARDIOVASCULAR DISEASE (CVD) such as HEART FAILURE. In cardiovascular health the heart gets maximum value from each cardiac cycle, contracting with appropriate force to move blood into the body. When the heart's pumping efficiency becomes compromised, as in heart failure, the autonomic nervous system that regulates heartbeat and blood pressure sends signals to the heart to pick up its pace. Accordingly, the heart beats faster although not necessarily with improved efficiency. Over time the increased workload this places on the heart can result in cardiomyopathy and heart failure; increased heart rate also is a sign of these conditions. Heart rate does not directly reflect the heart's rhythm.

Heart Rate and Aerobic Conditioning

Doctors and exercise physiologists look at resting heart rate, maximum heart rate, and target heart rate when determining an appropriate level of physical activity for aerobic conditioning. Resting heart rate is the heart's pumping pace at minimal effort; the object of aerobic conditioning is to establish a level of fitness that supports a resting heart rate around 60 beats per minute. Maximum heart rate is the hypothetical upper limit at which the heart can safely maintain a pumping rhythm. For decades, the rule of thumb has been that one's maximum heart rate is 220 minus one's age. A 20-year-old's maximum heart rate is around 200 beats per minute; a 60-year-old's maximum heart rate is 160.

Aerobic conditioning is most effective when the heart functions at target heart rate, which is 60 to 75 percent of maximum heart rate, for 15 to 60 minutes at a time. This, according to prevailing philosophy regarding aerobic conditioning, is the optimal balance between pushing the heart to work hard and avoiding overload. Not all exercise experts agree with this approach, however, and many recommend that people simply focus on pushing themselves to the extent that they still enjoy what they are doing, rather than focusing on hypothetical numbers.

See also EXERCISE; LIFESTYLE AND HEART HEALTH; NUTRITION AND DIET.

heart sounds   See AUSCULTATION.

heart's regenerative ability   The extent to which the heart can repair itself after damage due to ISCHEMIC HEART DISEASE, HEART FAILURE, or HEART ATTACK (myocardial infarction). Researchers and doctors long have believed that the heart's ability to regenerate is extremely limited, as heart muscle cells, called cardiomyocytes, do not replicate as do cells in other parts of the body, such as in skeletal muscle. New directions of exploration made possible by technological advances in the early 2000s have shed new light on myocardial regeneration and suggest that cardiomyocytes do replicate, albeit slowly, to replace cells lost to damage.

Researchers are investigating new methods, such as GENE THERAPY, to stimulate cardiomyocyte replication. As well, the heart's ability to establish collateral circulation—develop new networks of coronary arterioles—to bypass areas of atherosclerotic and other damage to native blood vessels demonstrates at least minimal capacity for self-repair. When these mechanisms unfold naturally they are slow and often do not produce results adequate to overcome the effects of cardiovascular disease. Scientists are hopeful that new technologies will lead to treatments that can accelerate these mechanisms, stimulating the heart to repair itself.

See also COLLATERAL CIRCULATION.

heart transplant   A surgical operation to remove a badly diseased or damaged HEART and replace it with a healthy heart harvested from a donor who died of causes that left the heart intact and undamaged. South African heart surgeon Dr. CHRISTIAAN BARNARD performed the first heart transplant on December 3, 1967, in Cape Town, South Africa. Donor DENISE DARVALL suffered unsurvivable injuries in an automobile accident; Barnard's team transplanted the 25-year-old's heart into 53-year-old LOUIS WASHKANSKY, a dentist in severe HEART FAILURE brought on by DIABETES. Although Washkansky died of pneumonia after just 18 days with his new heart, his surgery established heart transplant as a viable treatment option for people with end-stage heart disease, typically HEART FAILURE. Today there are about 2,200 heart transplants performed in the United States every year and 130 U.S. hospitals that perform heart transplantation.

Generally the recipient must be no older than 64 years and in good health other than his or her diseased heart. The DONOR HEART must match the blood type of the recipient and must be transplanted into the recipient within six hours or so. Healthy adult hearts are in general about the same physical size in men and women; gender is not a relevant factor with heart transplant alone although it becomes so with HEART-LUNG TRANSPLANT. There are about half as many donor hearts available as there are people waiting to receive them. This is largely because the donor must be sustained on life support until there is a match with a recipient so the heart can be removed just before transplant. As well, many people do not make their organ donor preferences known to family members who often must make the decision. Many states offer the option of including this information on the driver's license, which health experts encourage people to do.

Procedure

Heart transplant is a complex operation, although it has become standardized over the more than 40 years it has been performed. The surgeon first removes the diseased heart and then replaces it with the donor heart. A donor heart must be transplanted within about six hours of being removed from the donor. A typical heart transplant operation takes four to eight hours, depending on the condition of the diseased heart. A badly damaged or previously operated on heart often has extensive scar tissue and other challenges that make its removal more difficult.

After the person is anesthetized and placed on CARDIOPULMONARY BYPASS, the surgeon cuts away the diseased heart. There are several approaches to this; the most common is called orthotopic and involves leaving the backs of the atria attached to the chest wall (although sometimes only the left atrium is left attached). The backs of the donor heart's atria are cut away to match, and the new heart and its blood vessels are aligned and sutured into place. After the donor heart is in place, the surgeon stops the cardiopulmonary bypass and allows blood to flow through the body and the new heart. Often the heart begins beating on its own; if it does not, the surgeon administers an electrical shock to start it beating.

Risks and Complications

When recovery is routine, the person stays in the intensive care unit for one to three days and seven to 10 days total in the hospital. The immediate risks are of bleeding, failure of the donor heart to function properly, rejection of the donor heart, and infection. A significant long-term complication of heart transplant is the development of cardiac allograft vasculopathy (CAV), a chronic condition in which the coronary arteries thicken and harden. This diminishes blood flow to the heart and can cause ARRHYTHMIAS, heart failure, and SUDDEN CARDIAC ARREST. Although the donor heart beats normally and generates a pulse, there is no connection between the donor heart and the person's nervous system. Because of this, the person cannot feel cardiac pain such as ANGINA. As well, sometimes a PACEMAKER is necessary to maintain an appropriate rhythm because the donor heart does not receive signals from the nervous system that would cause it to accelerate or decelerate. Immunosuppressive medications are highly effective in minimizing the risk for rejection, though raise the risk for infection because they block immune system function. They also increase the likelihood of developing cancer, notably lymphoma (cancer of the lymphatic structures).

Outlook and Lifestyle Modifications

Heart transplant requires significant lifelong medical follow-up. Myocardial tissue biopsies, done via cardiac catheterization to look for signs of rejection, are necessary frequently during the first year and at least once a year for life. Some people are able to return to previous jobs and activities, but most must make modifications to accommodate their ongoing medical needs.

At present the five-year survival rate for heart transplant is 72 percent for men and and 67 percent for women; heart transplant has become a fairly mainstream treatment option for people whose hearts are severely damaged by CARDIOMYOPATHY, congenital malformations, and heart failure. One in four heart transplant recipients are under age 35. Heart transplant recipients must take IMMUNO-SUPPRESSIVE MEDICATIONS, such as CYCLOSPORINE, for the remainder of their lives to protect against organ rejection (the immune system perceiving the donor heart to be an "invader" and attacking it). Many heart transplant recipients who recover fully from the surgery are able to enjoy productive, full lives without restriction.

See also HEART, ARTIFICIAL; LEFT VENTRICULAR ASSIST DEVICE (LVAD); LIVING WITH HEART DISEASE; SURGERY TO TREAT CARDIOVASCULAR DISEASE.

heart valve   See HEART.

Heimlich maneuver   A procedure to dislodge an obstruction, often a piece of food, from the upper airway. The maneuver involves delivering a quick upward thrust to the area of the solar plexus (between the navel and the base of the rib cage) while standing behind the person who is choking. A variation of the Heimlich maneuver can be self-performed as well, by placing a fist in the area of the solar plexus and using the other hand to thrust the fist upward. Physician Henry J. Heimlich, M.D., developed the method, then called subdiaphragmatic pressure, in 1974. It quickly replaced the "back slap" method of dislodging obstructions, which has the disadvantage of forcing the obstruction deeper into the windpipe, and in 1985 the Heimlich maneuver became the U.S. surgeon general's recommended method for aiding choking victims.

See also CPR.

Helsinki Heart Study   One of the first primary prevention trials, conducted over five years in the 1980s, to conclusively demonstrate the benefit of taking the HMG CoA REDUCTASE INHIBITOR MEDICATION (statin) GEMFIBROZIL to raise high-density lipoprotein (HDL) and lower low-density lipoprotein (LDL) levels to reduce the risk of HEART ATTACK.

Researchers at the University of Helsinki in Finland involved 4,000 men who had HYPERLIPIDEMIA but no symptoms of HEART DISEASE in the study. Half of the men took the statin medication gemfibrozil (Lopid) and half of the men took a placebo (inactive substance). At the study's conclusion, those taking gemfibrozil experienced 34 percent fewer diagnoses of heart disease than those taking placebo. Other studies corroborate these findings and form the basis of support for the current clinical practice of prescribing statin medications not only to lower blood lipid levels but also as a preventive measure following heart attack.

See also CHOLESTEROL, BLOOD; CLINICAL RESEARCH STUDIES; FRAMINGHAM HEART STUDY; NURSES' HEALTH STUDY; LYON DIET HEART STUDY; TRIGLYCERIDES.

hemochromatosis A disorder of iron absorption in which abnormally high levels of iron accumulate in the body. Hemochromatosis is primarily hereditary and involves at least two identified mutations, called C282Y and H63D, of the HFE gene responsible for how the body absorbs iron. Other mutations are also likely. Doctors once considered hemochromatosis rare but now believe as many as one in 200 Americans, about 1 million people, have the disorder. Though hemochromatosis causes abnormal iron absorption from birth, the accumulation is slow, and symptoms generally do not become apparent until midlife. Early symptoms are vague and nonspecific and might include fatigue, joint pain, erectile dysfunction, and amenorrhea (lack of menstrual periods), or early menopause. Later symptoms relate to the organs that are affected, most commonly the liver (liver dysfunction, failure, and cancer), pancreas (DIABETES), and HEART (ARRHYTHMIA, CARDIOMYOPATHY, and HEART FAILURE).

Laboratory tests that measure the iron levels of BLOOD and tissue samples can confirm a diagnosis of hemochromatosis. The most commonly used tests are serum ferritin and transferrin saturation, blood tests that measure proteins in the blood that are involved in iron transport. These tests are not conclusive, however, because there is not yet a clear correlation established between ferritin and transferrin levels and conditions such as hemo-chromatosis. A liver biopsy is sometimes necessary to provide a definitive diagnosis if questions remain, as the liver stores the greatest amount of iron in the body.

Treatment for hemochromatosis is phlebotomy; removing blood through a process similar to blood donation. (However, most blood banks will not accept blood from people who have hemochromatosis.) Phlebotomy removes blood one unit (pint) at a time until blood iron levels return to normal; the frequency depends on the extent of iron accumulation and can be as often as twice weekly at the onset of treatment. Regular phlebotomy, the frequency again depending on blood iron levels, is necessary to maintain normal iron levels. Any damage already done to organs can constitute permanent health conditions, however, and must be treated as is appropriate for those conditions. Returning blood iron levels to normal prevents further damage as a result of the hemochromatosis, although the particular condition, such as heart failure, may continue progressing. In its later stages untreated hemochromatosis can cause the skin to turn a characteristic bronze color, which sometimes is the first sign of the disorder and is what gives the disorder its name. Though hemochromatosis affects men and women equally, men are more likely to show symptoms earlier in their lives. Doctors believe this is because the bleeding of menstruation serves to remove iron from women's bodies, so women do not develop symptoms until after menopause.

At present there are no recommendations for routine screening for hemochromatosis, even though some health experts believe as many as one in 10 Americans are carriers of the mutated genes. This is largely due to the imprecision of blood tests and an incomplete understanding of the prevalence of hemochromatosis, as well as the expense and complexity of genetic testing. The U.S. Centers for Disease Control and Prevention (CDC) currently recommends that people whose parents or siblings are diagnosed with hemochromatosis undergo testing, as there is a 25 percent chance that they also have the disorder. A rare form of hemochromatosis, juvenile hemochromatosis, which does not appear to result from mutations of the HFE gene, causes liver disease and heart disease in children and adolescents. Its symptoms manifest early in childhood and are pronounced, although by the time diagnosis occurs the organ damage is usually significant. Diagnosis and treatment for juvenile hemochromatosis are the same as for hereditary hemochromatosis.

See also ANEMIA; BLOOD; HEMOGLOBIN.

hemoglobin A protein molecule in red BLOOD cells that binds with oxygen. Hemoglobin contains iron, which gives it (and red blood cells) a red pigmentation. Inadequate levels of hemoglobin (often the consequence of depleted red blood cells) result in ANEMIA, a condition in which the blood cannot carry enough oxygen to body tissues. Inadequate oxygenation triggers the body's mechanisms to increase the heart's workload and output. When these increases continue over an extended time, the heart enlarges in an effort to maintain the extra capacity (just as any muscle enlarges with continued use). The eventual consequence often is HEART FAILURE. Low hemoglobin generally is easy to treat with iron supplements or drugs called hematopoesis stimulators that cause the bone marrow to increase red blood cell production.

See also HEMOCHROMATOSIS.

hemorrhage Uncontrolled bleeding. Hemorrhage that involves an artery, major vein, or blood-rich organ such as the liver or spleen is dangerous and can cause death in a matter of minutes. Hemorrhage in the brain causes a form of STROKE (hemorrhagic stroke). Hemorrhage can occur from a wound to a blood vessel, from an aneurysm, or as a consequence of a bleeding or clotting disorder, and it can be profuse or seeping. People taking ANTICOAGULANT MEDICATIONS (including ASPIRIN) have increased risk for hemorrhage. Internal hemorrhage can be difficult to detect; signs and symptoms might include unexplained weakness, fatigue, DIZZINESS, disorientation, pallor, erratic or weak pulse, and swelling and sometimes pain in the location of the hemorrhage.

External hemorrhage is apparent as heavy or steady bleeding. Bleeding from a vein is typically steady and the BLOOD is dark; bleeding from an artery often spurts and the blood is bright red. Arterial hemorrhage can be especially difficult to control because blood travels through the arteries under considerable pressure; as the loss of blood becomes significant enough to affect BLOOD PRESSURE, the body's mechanisms increase heart rate to attempt to restore blood pressure, exacerbating the blood loss. Hemorrhage from a major artery such as the femoral artery in the upper thigh can cause death within minutes. For any external hemorrhage the first response must be to apply pressure to the bleeding area to attempt to slow or stop the flow of blood. Hemorrhage that involves a limb might require a tourniquet (a band of cloth or a belt placed tightly between the wound and the heart) to slow or stop bleeding until emergency medical attention is available. Immediate emergency medical care is essential for any obvious or suspected hemorrhage.

See also COAGULATION.

hemorrhagic stroke See STROKE.

heparin A chemical that inhibits COAGULATION (blood clotting). Heparin forms naturally in the body, synthesized primarily by the liver and intestines. It also is available as an injectable drug that can be given intravenously (into a vein) or deep subcutaneously (into the fatty tissue under the skin) in anticoagulant therapy. Intravenous heparin is fast-acting, with peak effect within 30 minutes. Subcutaneous heparin has more sustained release, providing a longer action.

Heparin works by inactivating BLOOD factors essential for the formation of fibrin, a sticky, threadlike substance that forms the structure familiar as a blood clot (thrombus). Heparin cannot dissolve clots that already are formed. Doctors commonly use heparin therapy to prevent clots from forming after cardiovascular surgery, STROKE, HEART ATTACK, pulmonary EMBOLISM, and DEEP VEIN THROMBOSIS (DVT). Heparin is also often an adjunct therapy to THROMBOLYTIC MEDICATIONS. DIGITALIS medications, NICOTINE (tobacco), and certain antibiotics can interfere with heparin's actions. Heparin is prepared from porcine (pig) sources and can cause hypersensitivity reactions.

See also ANTICOAGULANT MEDICATIONS; ASPIRIN; TOBACCO USE; WARFARIN.

herbal remedies Products manufactured from botanicals, sold in the United States as over-the-counter nutritional supplements that do not require a physician's prescription. A number of these products are marketed as preventives and remedies for heart problems. Perhaps the best known is garlic to lower blood cholesterol levels; clinical studies have affirmed that garlic has a mild effect, and millions of Americans eat garlic or take garlic supplements for this purpose. Small studies suggest that tea—black and green but not herbal—contains chemicals called catechins that counter oxidation in the body. Most herbal remedies taken for heart health have their foundations in folk or traditional medicine and have not undergone clinical research trials, the standard by which Western medicine assesses a treatment's effectiveness and potential harm. Accordingly, it is not possible to say whether most herbal remedies have any effect on heart health or HEART DISEASE.

Herbal remedies may produce mild effects not likely to provide the level of intervention necessary when heart disease exists, and perhaps not a level necessary for prevention. Hence conventional treatments remain the recommendation for treating all forms of heart disease. It is important first to consult a physician or pharmacist before taking any herbal preparations, as herbs can interact with prescribed and over-the-counter medications. Most doctors encourage lifestyle modification—notably SMOKING CESSATION, low-fat diet, and regular EXERCISE—because it is clearly demonstrated to provide at least the same level of benefit as commonly and anecdotally attributed to many herbal remedies and has no adverse consequences. People with diagnosed heart disease, particularly HYPERTENSION, should avoid licorice, EPHEDRA (ma huang), and ginseng, as these substances raise BLOOD PRESSURE. Researchers continue to explore the effectiveness of hawthorn (berries, tea, and extract forms) as a treatment for HEART FAILURE, as this herb appears to affect the heart's rhythm and force of contractions. Hawthorn contains high concentrations of procyanidins (also called procyanidolic oligomers), which are FLAVONOIDS also found in lower concen-

POPULAR HERBAL REMEDIES FOR CARDIOVASCULAR HEALTH

Herbal Remedy	Probable Active Ingredients	Possible Effects	Potential Side Effects
Garlic (raw, extract)	Allium compounds, ajoene	Mild to moderate lipid-lowering effect; mild anticoagulant; antioxidant	Gastrointestinal upset
Ginkgo biloba	Flavone glycosides	Mild anticoagulant; antioxidant	Interaction with prescription anticoagulants; delayed blood clotting
Grape seed extract	Procyanidins, flavonoids	Mild antihypertensive	Gastrointestinal upset
Hawthorn (berries, tea, extract)	Procyanidins, flavonoids	Mild antiarrhythmic; mild antihypertensive; mild effect on force of myocardial cell contractions	Arrhythmias, hypotension, gastrointestinal upset
Onion	Adenosine compounds, allium compounds	Mild lipid-lowering effect; mild anticoagulant; antioxidant	Gastrointestinal upset
Soy	Soy isoflavones	Mild to moderate lipid-lowering effect	
Tea (green and black, not herbal)	Catechins; flavonoids	Mild anticoagulant; lower LDL cholesterol	
Willow bark	Salicylic compounds	Mild anticoagulant	Interaction with prescription anticoagulants; cross sensitivity in aspirin allergy

trations in grapes and grape seeds (including grape seed extract), wine, blueberries, and cranberries. People who have diagnosed heart failure should not take hawthorn in any form unless their physicians give the go-ahead to do so.

It is important to remember that even though herbal remedies are sold as nutritional supplements, they contain numerous chemicals that act as drugs in the body and can interact with medications. Many "heart health" products contain a blend of herbs and organic substances, so it also is important to read the label's list of ingredients. People taking medications for any form of heart disease should first talk with a physician or pharmacist before beginning any herbal products and should let their doctors know of any herbal products they already are taking.

See also COMPLEMENTARY THERAPIES; MEDICATION SIDE EFFECTS; VITAMIN AND MINERAL SUPPLEMENTS.

heredity and heart disease The correlations between genetic risk factors and the development of HEART DISEASE. Researchers have identified a number of genes and gene mutations that influence a person's tendency to develop certain forms of CARDIOVASCULAR DISEASE (CVD) such as familial HYPERLIPIDEMIA, hypertrophic CARDIOMYOPATHY, LONG QT SYNDROME, and MARFAN SYNDROME. Other genetic correlations are less specific. People speak of them in the context of heart disease that "runs in the family." Such conditions include HYPERTENSION (high BLOOD PRESSURE), familial HYPERCHOLESTEROLEMIA, familial hyperlipidemia, familial HYPERTRIGLYCERIDEMIA, ATHEROSCLEROSIS, CORONARY ARTERY DISEASE (CAD), early HEART ATTACK (MYOCARDIAL INFARCTION), some ARRHYTHMIAS, and STROKE.

Identified Gene Mutations

Thanks in large part to the ambitious international undertaking to map the human genome (which was completed in 2003), researchers have identified numerous genes and their responsibilities in the body, and correspondingly their mutations and consequences of them. Many such mutations affect the ways the body synthesizes and uses proteins, the basic structures that direct the myriad functions that take place within the cells. Gene muta-

tions can cause subtle or dramatic changes; most that establish predispositions toward heart disease engender subtle (and often cumulative) changes. Forms of heart disease for which there are identified gene mutations include:

- hypertrophic cardiomyopathy, traced to mutations of genes on chromosome 1 (affecting cardiac troponin T [cTnT]; chromosome 19 (affecting cardiac troponin I [cTnI]); and chromosomes 11, 14, and 15 (affecting cardiac myosins)
- long QT syndrome, traced to mutations of genes on chromosomes 3, 7, 11, and 21 that affect the heart's ion channels
- Marfan syndrome, traced to the mutation of a gene on chromosome 15 that directs the formation of fibrin proteins
- familial lipid disorders (hypercholesterolemia, hyperlipidemia, hypertriglyceridemia), traced to numerous gene mutations on various chromosomes including apolipoprotein B100 (apo B) and other low-density lipoprotein (LDL) receptor genes

Researchers hope that by identifying gene mutations responsible for various forms of cardiovascular disease, they also can develop therapies that target either the genes or correct their misdirections, essentially "turning off" their abilities to contribute to disease development. Such therapies remain highly speculative.

Familial Tendencies

Various forms of heart disease have familial tendencies in which researchers have not identified specific gene mutations. These nonspecific hereditary correlations likely reflect the involvement of numerous genes as well as interactions with environmental factors such as oxidation and mitochondrial damage—factors that affect the functions of individual cells. When such factors cumulatively come to affect enough cells, they may contribute to cardiovascular conditions such as atherosclerosis, coronary artery disease, and hypertension. Family history of heart disease becomes an important aspect for early monitoring and intervention efforts, although control of lifestyle factors such as diet,

EXERCISE, and smoking likely is more significant in terms of reducing the risk for heart disease.

The Importance of Lifestyle Factors

With the exception of genetic disorders such as Turner's syndrome or Down syndrome, in which malformations of the heart are common, researchers believe genetic factors establish predisposition for, but do not necessarily cause, cardiovascular disease. It appears that environmental, or lifestyle, factors influence nearly all CVD. Seldom does a single risk factor result in heart disease; rather, it is a cumulative effect of multiple risk factors that converge to cause certain disease states to develop. The presence of any hereditary tendencies toward CVD underscores the importance of managing modifiable lifestyle risk factors for heart disease to the best extent possible. Such management includes:

- nutritious eating habits
- regular exercise
- no TOBACCO USE
- WEIGHT MANAGEMENT

These efforts greatly mitigate most lifestyle risk factors. Though it probably is not possible to entirely prevent heart disease in someone who has significant hereditary predisposition, health experts believe it is possible to minimize through lifestyle management (and medical intervention as appropriate) the course of any CVD that does develop.

Congenital Heart Disease

Most congenital heart disease occurs randomly; there are no consistent gene mutations responsible for them. However, parents who have one child with serious heart malformations such as TETRALOGY OF FALLOT, HYPOPLASTIC LEFT HEART SYNDROME (HLHS), or TRANSPOSITION OF THE GREAT ARTERIES (TGA) have as high as a 10 percent likelihood of having a second child with serious heart malformations. More common and less serious malformations such as SEPTAL DEFECTS (atrial septal defect [ASD]), ATRIOVENTRICULAR [AV] CANAL DEFECT, VENTRICULAR SEPTAL DEFECT [VSD]), and PATENT DUCTUS ARTERIOSUS do not seem to have familial tendencies.

See also AFRICAN AMERICANS AND CARDIOVASCULAR DISEASE; DOWN SYNDROME, HEART MALFORMATIONS ASSOCIATED WITH; FRAMINGHAM HEART STUDY.

high blood pressure   See HYPERTENSION.

high-density lipoprotein (HDL)   See CHOLESTEROL, BLOOD.

HIV/AIDS and heart disease   See AIDS AND HEART DISEASE.

HMG CoA reductase inhibitor medications   A family of LIPID-LOWERING MEDICATIONS, commonly called statins, that block the action of 3-hydroxy-3-methyl-glutaryl coenzyme-A reductase (HMG CoA), an enzyme necessary in the early stages of cholesterol synthesis. Doctors prescribe these medications to lower blood cholesterol and blood TRIGLYCERIDES levels as well as to reduce the risk of subsequent HEART ATTACK (MYOCARDIAL INFARCTION) following a first HEART ATTACK. These medications also have an anti-inflammatory effect on the walls of the arteries, helping to minimize the damage arterial plaque causes to the arterial walls. Commonly prescribed HMG CoA reductase inhibitors include:

- atorvastatin (Lipitor)
- fluvastatin (Lescol)
- lovastatin (Mevacor)
- pravastatin (Pravachol)
- simvastatin (Zocor)

Gastrointestinal side effects such as nausea, dyspepsia (upset stomach), diarrhea, flatulence (gas), and CONSTIPATION are common when first starting treatment with HMG CoA reductase inhibitors; these side effects typically ease after six to eight weeks of taking the medication. A rare but potentially life-threatening side effect of the statins is RHABDOMYOLYSIS, a condition in which muscle tissue rapidly breaks down and floods the kidneys with protein, which can cause kidney failure. Statin drugs interact with numerous other medications including the post-transplant immunosuppressive drug CYCLOSPORINE; the antibiotic erythromycin; the lipid-lowering medications gemfibrizol, clofibrate, and fenofibrate; DIGOXIN; and ORAL CONTRACEPTIVES (birth control pills). Specific HMG CoA reductase inhibitors may have additional interactions. Women who are pregnant should not take these medications, as cholesterol is essential for normal cell reproduction and the lack of cholesterol can cause birth defects in the developing fetus.

See also CHOLESTEROL, BLOOD; EXERCISE; LIFESTYLE AND HEART HEALTH; NUTRITION AND DIET.

Holter monitor A device that records the HEART'S electrical activity over an extended period, commonly 24 hours. Small, adhesive-backed electrodes placed on the outside of the chest are connected by wires to a small recorder worn around the neck or in a pocket. The Holter monitor provides a continuous ELECTROCARDIOGRAM (ECG) recording, and while wearing it the person keeps a 24-hour log or diary of symptoms. At the end of the monitoring period the cardiologist evaluates the ECG in comparison with the symptom diary to correlate symptoms with any electrical anomalies. The extended monitoring helps to detect and diagnose transient cardiac events and episodic ARRHYTHMIAS such as atrial flutter; symptoms such as ANGINA or shortness of breath that may be associated with ATRIAL FIBRILLATION, atrial multifocal tachycardia, paroxysmal supraventricular tachycardia, PALPITATIONS; and unexplained SYNCOPE (DIZZINESS and fainting).

See also CARDIOVASCULAR SYSTEM; HEART BLOCK.

home health care Professional nursing services such as wound care, BLOOD PRESSURE and DIABETES checks, and intravenous medications provided in the home for people recovering from surgery and illness, typically following discharge from the hospital. Home health care agencies provide a defined number of visits according to the doctor's order and the person's medical condition and health needs.

Home health care nurses also work with individuals and caregivers to teach care techniques and provide education about LIVING WITH HEART DISEASE, including related health matters such as diabetes, WEIGHT MANAGEMENT, and NUTRITION AND DIET. The goal is to increase a person's ability to independently manage his or her medical conditions to maintain health to the best extent possible. Many medical insurance plans and Medicare pay for certain home health care services, though often these services require preauthorization. Home health care should be part of discharge planning when a person is leaving the hospital.

See also HOSPICE.

homeostasis The body's natural efforts to maintain balance among its organ systems and their functions. The HEART and CARDIOVASCULAR SYSTEM continually adjust functions such as BLOOD PRESSURE and heart rate to ensure there is adequate blood flow at all times to meet the body's needs. The HYPOTHALAMUS, a structure within the brain toward the front of the brain stem, coordinates the numerous interactions necessary to maintain cardiovascular homeostasis through a perpetual flow of neurological and biochemical signals to and from the body's organs and systems. CARDIOVASCULAR DISEASE (CVD) is one representation of a point at which the body reaches the limits of homeostasis and an adjusted (and dysfunctional) state becomes the norm, as with HYPERTENSION (high blood pressure) or HEART FAILURE.

homocysteine An amino acid normally present in the BLOOD. The body uses homocysteine to form other amino acid structures. Researchers have discovered that about 20 percent of people with CORONARY ARTERY DISEASE (CAD) have higher blood levels of homocysteine than people who do not have CAD and suspect that when present in excess homocysteine causes irritation and inflammation of the walls of the arteries. However, scientific evidence to support such a causal relationship remains scant. As yet there is no established "normal" level of homocysteine, which makes it difficult to determine at what point homocysteine levels might become harmful to health.

Vitamins B_6, B_{12}, and folic acid (folate) work naturally in the body to break down homocysteine, leading to a belief that taking supplements of these substances will increase homocysteine metabolism and reduce the potential harmful actions of excess homocysteine. This correlation has led many people to take, and some doctors to recommend, vitamin B and folic acid supplementation as homocysteine-lowering therapies. However, recent research suggests this approach may increase, rather than decrease, the risk for further HEART DISEASE in people who have already had MYOCARDIAL INFARCTION (MI).

One large randomized study, the Norwegian Vitamin Trial (NORVIT), followed 3,749 men and women in Norway, all of whom had MIs within seven days of the study's start, from 1998 to 2004. Study participants who took only B_6 and those who took B_{12} plus folic acid had no different rate of further heart disease than those who took placebo (an inert substance). Those who took a combination of B_6, B_{12}, and folic acid (a common therapeutic regimen) had a statistically significant higher rate of further heart disease, including SUDDEN CARDIAC ARREST. On the basis of these findings, the NORVIT researchers recommend against using vitamin B and folic acid supplements as homocysteine-lowering therapies. However, health experts do continue to recommend making nutritious food choices including those high in B vitamins (such as fortified grains, breads, and cereals) because such foods and nutrients are essential for good health overall.

See also C-REACTIVE PROTEIN; LIFESTYLE AND HEART HEALTH; NUTRITION AND DIET.

hormone A chemical the body produces that acts as a messenger to initiate or end functions among cells within the body. Hormones regulate many of the body's activities, from METABOLISM to sexual characteristics. Most hormones have a direct or indirect effect on the CARDIOVASCULAR SYSTEM. Those having a direct effect include EPINEPHRINE, NOREPINEPHRINE, renin, aldosterone, antidiuretic hormone (ADH), cortisol, calcitonin, and parathy-

roid hormone; these hormones regulate functions related to HEART RATE, BLOOD PRESSURE, and cardiovascular HOMEOSTASIS. The RENIN-ANGIOTENSIN-

HORMONES AND THEIR CARDIOVASCULAR EFFECTS

Hormone	Actions	Produced by
Adrenocorticotropic hormone (ACTH)	Stimulates adrenal glands to release cortisol	Pituitary gland
Aldosterone	Regulates excretion or reabsorption of sodium and potassium in the kidneys; reabsorbs to raise blood pressure and excretes to lower blood pressure	Adrenal glands
Antidiuretic hormone (ADH)	Limits urine production by the kidneys to increase blood volume	Pituitary gland
Calcitonin	Prevents bones from releasing calcium and increases calcium excretion by kidneys to lower blood calcium levels	Thyroid gland
Cortisol	Increases blood pressure, heart rate, and respiration rate	Adrenal glands
Epinephrine	Increases heart rate and force of the heart's contractions; constricts peripheral arteries	Adrenal glands
Erythropoietin	Stimulates bone marrow to produce red blood cells	Kidneys
Norepinephrine	Constricts peripheral arteries to raise blood pressure	Adrenal glands
Parathyroid hormone	Causes bones to release calcium and decreases calcium excretion by kidneys to raise blood calcium levels	Parathyroid glands
Renin	Initiates the sequence of events that raise blood pressure	Kidneys
Thyroid hormone (thyroxine)	Regulates metabolism	Thyroid gland

ALDOSTERONE (RAA) HORMONAL SYSTEM is the body's key mechanism for regulating blood pressure; many ANTIHYPERTENSIVE MEDICATIONS target various functions of the RAA hormonal system. Key hormones that exert indirect effects on the cardiovascular system include adrenocorticotropic hormone (ACTH), thyroid hormone, and ERYTHROPOIETIN. The endocrine glands, which include the thyroid, pituitary, adrenal, pancreas, and parathyroid glands, as well as the ovaries in women and the testicles in men, produce most of the body's hormones. The kidneys, gastrointestinal system, and brain also produce hormones.

See also CALCIUM CYCLE; CARDIAC CYCLE; ESTROGEN; METABOLIC SYNDROME.

hormone replacement therapy (HRT)

The practice of giving women ESTROGEN and progesterone supplements during and after menopause, primarily to relieve the discomforts of this hormonal transition. For many years doctors believed HRT also afforded a woman an extra measure of protection against HEART DISEASE, a conclusion drawn from the apparent protective effects of estrogen against heart disease. Before menopause a woman's risk for CARDIOVASCULAR DISEASE (CVD) is substantially lower than the risk for a man of comparable age and health status. This has lead to the conclusion that estrogen, a hormone in high supply during a woman's fertile years, safeguards a woman's body from many of the processes that cause CVD.

Extensive research conducted in the late 1990s and early 2000s demonstrated that there is no such protective effect from estrogen taken as a perimenopausal or postmenopausal supplement. Further, these studies provided clear evidence that women who do take HRT after menopause are at increased risk for early heart disease, which tends to be of more rapid onset and more severe consequence. In 2002 health officials changed their recommendations regarding HRT to advise against long-term HRT and suggest short-term HRT (two years or less) only to relieve menopausal symptoms, only under the close supervision of a physician who can monitor the woman for cardiovascular changes and early CVD, and only in women who have no personal or family history of endometrial (uterine) or breast cancer.

See also EARLY MENOPAUSE AND HEART DISEASE; HEART AND ESTROGEN/PROGESTIN REPLACEMENT STUDY (HERS); WOMEN AND HEART DISEASE; WOMEN'S HEALTH INITIATIVE.

hospice Care and services provided in the home or in a special unit of a hospital for people who are terminally ill, typically with a survival prognosis of six months or less. Hospice services include nursing and personal assistance care as well as respite care for family members who are caregivers. People with HEART FAILURE who are assessed as New York Heart Association (NYHA) category IV, the widely accepted classification system for HEART FAILURE, generally are considered terminal. Other diagnosed HEART DISEASE or CARDIOVASCULAR DISEASE (CVD) factors, such as ARRHYTHMIAS and residual damage following HEART ATTACK (MYOCARDIAL INFARCTION) also may qualify, depending on the responsiveness to treatment, the person's age, and other health conditions (such as HIV/AIDS) that may exist. A doctor must certify a person's terminal status for Medicare, Medicaid, and most private medical and long-term care insurance plans to pay for hospice services.

See also AIDS AND HEART DISEASE; HOME HEALTH CARE.

hot tubs and high blood pressure See HYPERTENSION.

hydralazine An ANTIHYPERTENSIVE MEDICATION taken to lower BLOOD PRESSURE. Doctors also prescribe hydralazine (Apresoline) to treat some forms of congestive HEART FAILURE. Hydralazine is a VASODILATOR MEDICATION; it acts directly on the smooth muscle tissue in the walls of the arteries to relax and dilate the arteries, increasing the flow of BLOOD and decreasing its resistance. These actions in turn lessen the heart's workload and reduce blood pressure. Doctors often prescribe hydralazine in combination with other antihypertensive medications for increased effectiveness. Hydralazine can cause

HYPOTENSION, especially orthostatic hypotension (a drop in blood pressure upon rising), ARRHYTHMIAS, headache, nausea, diarrhea, and symptoms that resemble those of systemic lupus erythematosus (SLE) though hydralazine does not cause this AUTOIMMUNE DISORDER.

See also ANTIARRHYTHMIA MEDICATIONS; MEDICATIONS TO TREAT HEART DISEASE.

hydrochlorothiazide (HCTZ) A DIURETIC MEDICATION taken to reduce fluid accumulations in the body and to help lower blood pressure by reducing BLOOD volume. Hydrochlorothiazide (HCTZ) belongs to the family of drugs known for their actions on the proximal portion of the distal tubules of the kidneys. HCTZ works by preventing the kidneys from reabsorbing SODIUM, which in turn decreases the amount of fluid (water) the kidneys return to the bloodstream. Less fluid results in lowering the volume of blood, which reduces the amount of pressure needed to circulate the blood through the body. Doctors commonly prescribe HCTZ in combination with other ANTIHYPERTENSIVE MEDICATIONS that have different mechanisms of action on BLOOD PRESSURE.

HCTZ, like other thiazide diuretics, also prevents the kidneys from reabsorbing POTASSIUM. Because potassium is less abundant in the diet, the increased excretion of potassium in the urine can result in potassium depletion in the blood (hypokalemia). People taking HCTZ typically have regular blood tests to monitor blood potassium levels. Eating foods high in potassium may be enough to keep blood potassium levels normal. Such foods include bananas, baked potato with skin, raisins, figs, cantaloupe, and tomatoes. Salt substitute products typically contain potassium chloride, although should be used sparingly if at all. Sometimes it is not possible to maintain normal blood potassium levels through diet alone, in which case the doctor may prescribe a potassium supplement or switch to a potassium-sparing diuretic such as triamterene (which is available in a combination product with HCTZ). Thiazide diuretics also can cause the kidneys to allow more potassium to pass in the urine, which can cause potassium depletion. People who take HCTZ should consult their doctors about maintaining adequate blood potassium levels.

See also ANTIHYPERTENSIVE MEDICATIONS; MEDICATION SIDE EFFECTS; MEDICATIONS TO TREAT HEART DISEASE.

Hydrodiuril See DIURETIC MEDICATIONS.

hydrogenated fat See NUTRITION AND DIET.

hypercholesterolemia A condition in which BLOOD levels of total CHOLESTEROL, low-density lipoprotein (LDL) cholesterol, and very low-density lipoprotein (VLDL) cholesterol are elevated. Hypercholesterolemia can be familial (have genetic components) or nonfamilial, and it may or may not be part of a larger picture of HYPERLIPIDEMIA that includes elevated levels of TRIGLYCERIDES and other lipids (fatty acids in the bloodstream). Hypercholesterolemia increases the risk of developing ATHEROSCLEROSIS, an accumulation of arterial PLAQUE along the inside walls of the arteries that causes the arteries to narrow and stiffen. Atherosclerosis is a harbinger of CARDIOVASCULAR DISEASE (CVD), such as CORONARY ARTERY DISEASE (CAD) and PERIPHERAL VASCULAR DISEASE (PVD), and carotid artery disease raises the risk for STROKE. A desirable blood cholesterol level is less than 200 milligrams (mg) per deciliter (dL) of blood; hypercholesterolemia exists when the level reaches or exceeds 240 mg/dL.

Symptoms and Diagnostic Path
Hypercholesterolemia has no symptoms, although people with extremely high blood cholesterol levels (greater than 600 mg/dL) such as occur with familial hypercholesterolemia may have deposits of cholesterol that collect beneath the skin called XANTHOMAS. Hypercholesterolemia is detected by a blood test that measures the amount of cholesterol in the bloodstream. It is important to fast (nothing to eat or drink except water) for 12 hours before blood is drawn for a cholesterol test.

Treatment Options and Outlook
Typically treatment for either familial or nonfamilial hypercholesterolemia first targets lifestyle modification. This is the most effective treatment for

nonfamilial hypercholesterolemia, and for people with mild to moderate cholesterol elevations it is often adequate for lowering blood cholesterol levels to healthy ranges. When lifestyle modifications alone do not adequately lower blood cholesterol levels, when blood cholesterol levels are extremely high and there are other risks for heart disease, or when doctors suspect familial hypercholesterolemia, treatment includes LIPID-LOWERING MEDICATIONS. The medications prescribed depend on the person's health situation and health history. Familial hypercholesterolemia may not respond well to treatment, making control of other modifiable risk factors for heart disease especially important.

Risk Factors and Preventive Measures
Health experts estimate that familial hypercholesterolemia affects about seven in 1,000 Americans, men and women equally. At present there are two gene mutations identified with these forms of hypercholesterolemia; inheriting one or both establishes a predisposition for the condition. Genetic testing to confirm hypercholesterolemia is limited and expensive, and not necessary from a clinical perspective because treatment is the same as for nonfamilial forms of hypercholesterolemia. The main advantage of knowing whether there are genetic factors at play is early intervention.

The most common forms of hypercholesterolemia are nonfamilial; that is, they result primarily from lifestyle factors such as a diet high in saturated fats and carbohydrates and lack of physical activity and exercise. Often obesity and type 2 diabetes are present as well; high levels of insulin such as exist with insulin resistance and diabetes interfere with LDL and VLDL synthesis and metabolism.

Many health organizations provide free screenings for elevated blood cholesterol. As well, blood tests to measure cholesterol levels are part of routine physical examinations. When detected and treated early, hypercholesterolemia can be reversed in most people to reduce the risk for CVD.

See also HEREDITY AND HEART DISEASE; NUTRITION AND DIET.

hyperglycemia A circumstance in which the level of glucose (sugar) in the BLOOD is elevated.

Hyperglycemia is a hallmark sign of INSULIN RESISTANCE and DIABETES. Excessive thirst, hunger, and urination are the classic indicators of hyperglycemia; rapid weight loss sometimes accompanies them. Glucose is one of the primary fuel sources for cells throughout the body. When it is present in higher than normal amounts, glucose causes cell metabolism to accelerate. This has numerous and varied adverse consequences including permanent damage to nerves and blood vessels throughout the body. In the 1990s researchers began to conclusively correlate hyperglycemia and HYPERLIPIDEMIA (high levels of fatty acids in the blood), particularly elevated very low-density lipoprotein (VLDL) levels, with an increased risk for ATHEROSCLEROSIS and CORONARY ARTERY DISEASE (CAD). Hyperglycemia causes changes in the structure of cells lining the inner walls of the arteries, making the arteries more susceptible to accumulations of arterial plaque. Hyperglycemia also appears to accelerate many forms of CARDIOVASCULAR DISEASE (CVD) including peripheral vascular disease (PVD).

See also CHOLESTEROL, BLOOD; PLAQUE, ARTERIAL.

hyperkalemia See ELECTROLYTE.

hyperlipidemia A collective term for conditions in which BLOOD levels of LIPIDS (fatty acids) such as cholesterol and TRIGLYCERIDES are elevated, creating increased risk for CARDIOVASCULAR DISEASE (CVD) and HEART ATTACK. More than 40 million Americans have some form of hyperlipidemia, which includes HYPERCHOLESTEROLEMIA (elevated blood levels of cholesterol) and HYPERTRIGLYCERIDEMIA (elevated blood levels of triglycerides). Hyperlipidemia appears to accelerate ATHEROSCLEROSIS (accumulations of arterial plaque within the walls of the arteries) and may have other involvement in the development of CVD.

Symptoms and Diagnostic Path
Hyperlipidemia has no symptoms and is detected by blood tests that measure the levels of cholesterol, triglycerides, and other lipids in the blood. It is necessary to fast (nothing to eat or drink except

water) for 12 hours before blood is drawn for a lipids test.

Treatment Options and Outlook

Treatment targets lowering blood lipid levels to healthy ranges and begins with lifestyle modifications that emphasize nutritious (and usually low-fat) eating habits, daily physical EXERCISE, and WEIGHT MANAGEMENT (weight loss if appropriate). Doctors often prescribe LIPID-LOWERING MEDICATIONS as well, especially when there is a family history of hyperlipidemia.

Risk Factors and Preventive Measures

Key factors contributing to hyperlipidemia are primarily lifestyle in origin and include a diet high in fat and carbohydrate and a low level of physical activity. Health conditions that contribute to hyperlipidemia include OBESITY, INSULIN RESISTANCE, and DIABETES; these conditions often coexist.

One form of hyperlipidemia that is inherited is familial combined hyperlipidemia, in which family members have elevated blood levels of triglycerides, total cholesterol, low-density lipoprotein (LDL) cholesterol, and very low-density lipoprotein (VLDL) cholesterol irrespective of lifestyle factors, although diet and exercise influence the severity of the hyperlipidemia. Low blood levels of high-density lipoprotein (HDL) might also be present. Diagnosis and treatment are the same as for nonfamilial forms of hyperlipidemia, though results may not be as pronounced. Familial combined hyperlipidemia is associated with early CVD, especially CORONARY ARTERY DISEASE (CAD), and early heart attack.

See also CHOLESTEROL, BLOOD; PLAQUE, ARTERIAL; INFLAMMATION AND HEART DISEASE.

hypertension A health condition of chronically elevated BLOOD PRESSURE, also called high blood pressure. The body's mechanisms for regulating blood pressure are complex, and there are numerous reasons that blood pressure can become elevated. Hypertension is the leading cause of STROKE and contributes to HEART FAILURE and HEART ATTACK.

As many as 50 million Americans have hypertension though only about half of them know it and only about a third have their blood pressure controlled. Hypertension is more common among people who are overweight, older, African American or Hispanic; have a family history of high blood pressure or CARDIOVASCULAR DISEASE (CVD); and are physically inactive. Hypertension also is more common in people who have INSULIN RESISTANCE, DIABETES, kidney disease, or other forms of HEART DISEASE.

Symptoms and Diagnostic Path

Most people with hypertension have no symptoms until they experience a catastrophic cardiovascular event, which is why health experts recommend routine blood pressure screening for all adults beginning at age 21 and why blood pressure measurement is a routine element of nearly every visit to the doctor regardless of the reason for the visit. Health-care providers use a device called a SPHYGMOMANOMETER, consisting of an inflatable cuff that goes around the arm above the elbow and a gauge that represents blood pressure in terms of millimeters of mercury (mm Hg), to measure blood pressure. Some sphygmomanometers are electronic and provide digital readouts.

A blood pressure reading consists of obtaining two measurements, the pressure at systole (the peak of the heart's contraction) and the pressure at diastole (the relaxation phase of the CARDIAC CYCLE). The health-care provider places the sphygmomanometer cuff around the upper arm, puts a STETHOSCOPE against the PULSE point at the bend in the arm on the inside of the elbow, and inflates the cuff until it is no longer possible to hear the heart beat. The health-care provider then slowly deflates the cuff while listening for the heart beat. The first beat heard is the systolic measurement and the last beat heard is the diastolic measurement. The reading generally is written as a fraction presenting systolic/diastolic, for example 118/68. Systolic, diastolic, or both measurements can be elevated.

Hypertension is diagnosed after there are a minimum of two elevated readings on separate visits to the doctor. This is because many variables influence blood pressure, including anxiety about going to the doctor (sometimes called "white coat" hypertension). Often if an initial blood pressure reading is high the doctor will repeat it at the end of

HYPERTENSION

Systolic Measurement	Diastolic Measurement	Diagnostic Category	Treatment
119 mm Hg or lower	79 mm Hg or lower	Normal	Maintain healthy lifestyle habits; weight management
120 to 139 mm Hg	80 to 89 mm Hg	Prehypertension	Lifestyle modifications to include daily physical exercise, low sodium diet, and weight loss
140 to 159 mm Hg	90 to 99 mm Hg	Stage 1	Lifestyle modifications plus antihypertensive medication such as a diuretic or beta-blocker
160 mm Hg or higher	100 mm Hg or higher	Stage 2	Lifestyle modifications plus multiple antihypertensive

Source: Guidelines of the Seventh Report of the Joint National Committee on Prevention, Detection, Evaluation and Treatment of High Blood Pressure issued May 2003

the visit to see if there is a difference. Other factors the doctor also considers when making a diagnosis of hypertension are general health status, weight, age, race, family history, and lifestyle. When blood pressure readings are inconsistent or borderline the doctor might suggest a period of watchful waiting, often in combination with lifestyle modifications to support cardiovascular health.

The doctor or other health-care provider may take readings in both arms to see if they are the same. Differences can suggest specific health conditions that bear further investigation, such as AORTIC STENOSIS or COARCTATION OF THE AORTA (narrowing of the aorta), AORTIC REGURGITATION (malfunctions or malformations of the aortic valve), or structural anomalies of the aorta or heart. Blood pressure measurements should be taken when sitting at rest. Caffeine, cold and flu preparations containing decongestants, and herbal energy drinks or products can cause elevated blood pressure.

Risk Factors and Preventive Measures

Hypertension can exist as a primary condition (independent of other causes) or as a secondary condition (caused by other health conditions or circumstances). About 95 percent of people who have hypertension have primary hypertension, sometimes called essential hypertension, which exists independently of other health conditions known to increase blood pressure (though may coexist with other forms of cardiovascular disease). Typi-

cally there are no symptoms; the doctor detects the elevated blood pressure during a routine examination or at a visit for other health concerns. Though doctors understand the hemodynamic mechanisms that result in hypertension, the precise reasons hypertension develops remain elusive.

Secondary hypertension exists as a consequence of another health condition or circumstance such as a medication side effect. A kidney condition due to renal artery stenosis (narrowing of the main artery to the kidney) is the most common causes of secondary hypertension. This activates one of the body's mechanisms for regulating blood pressure, initiating increases in the rate and force of the HEARTBEAT. The kidneys are the center of action for the body's primary blood pressure regulatory mechanism, the RENIN-ANGIOTENSIN-ALDOSTERONE (RAA) HORMONAL SYSTEM, and also control the body's fluid volume, another mechanism of blood pressure control. Any changes in kidney function affect these mechanisms.

Paroxysmal hypertension consists of episodes of sudden severe spikes in blood pressure that produce symptoms such as headache, DIZZINESS, PALPITATIONS, and nausea. These episodes are usually stress induced, although the reason for the stress can be quite removed from the timing of the episode (delayed traumatic stress syndrome). When this is the case, it can be difficult for both the person having the episodes and the doctor evaluating them to make the correlation. Paroxysmal hypertension can also result from pheochromocytoma, a tumor of the adrenal gland that causes excessive EPINEPHRINE production.

Other health conditions that cause hypertension include Cushing's syndrome (a disorder in which the adrenal glands oversecrete cortisol), adrenal tumors such as pheochromocytoma and adenoma, aldosteronism (a disorder, often familial, in which the adrenal glands oversecrete aldosterone), HYPERTHYROIDISM (overactive thyroid gland), HYPOTHYROIDISM (underactive thyroid gland), and sleep apnea (periods of delayed breathing during sleep).

Certain medications can raise blood pressure as a side effect. These include:

- decongestants (pseudoephedrine, neosynephrine nose spray or drops)
- appetite suppressants prescribed to treat obesity (phentermine, sibutramine)
- nonsteroidal anti-inflammatory medications (ibuprofen, naproxen, ketoprofen)
- thyroid hormone supplements (levothyroxine, thyroid extract)
- prescription corticosteroid anti-inflammatory medications (hydrocortisone, prednisone) and steroid supplements such as human growth hormone (HGH)
- tricyclic antidepressants (amitriptyline, imipramine, doxepin)

In many situations, treating the underlying health condition restores blood pressure to normal. However, the longer blood pressure remains elevated, the more likely it is to stay so even when contributory conditions are resolved. Diabetes damages peripheral arteries and arterioles, increasing the resistance blood encounters as it moves through these blood vessels. Hypertension associated with diabetes is nearly always permanent because the damage done to the peripheral blood vessels is permanent.

Treatment Options and Outlook

Lifestyle modification often is adequate for controlling prehypertension; lifestyle modification in combination with ANTIHYPERTENSIVE MEDICATIONS is the standard approach for managing stage 1 and stage 2 hypertension. Doctors commonly prescribe antihypertensives in combination with one another, particularly when other cardiovascular disease is present. As well, it is important to manage any coexisting or underlying health conditions that influence blood pressure such as other forms of heart disease (such as atherosclerosis, coronary artery disease, peripheral vascular disease, heart failure), diabetes, and kidney disease. WEIGHT MANAGEMENT and regular EXERCISE are particularly important; weight loss alone can reduce blood pressure and physical activity maintains overall cardiovascular health. Health experts recommend a low-SODIUM diet (2 grams or less of sodium daily) for people with stage 2 hypertension, and that all people cut back on sodium consumption. Processed foods and fast-food items are especially high in sodium. People who have hypertension should avoid hot tubs and saunas, as the sudden dilation of peripheral blood vessels in response to the heat while taking vasodilating medications for high blood pressure can cause blood pressure to decrease too much.

Untreated hypertension is deadly. High blood pressure is the leading cause of stroke and a key cause of kidney disease and kidney failure. Hypertension also causes ANEURYSM and contributes to emboli (blood clots) in the blood that cause heart attack (MYOCARDIAL INFARCTION). It also causes arteries to stiffen, which worsens the situation by further increasing the heart load (high resistance and low compliance) blood encounters as it flows through them, and causes the heart to enlarge (cardiomyopathy) and ultimately weaken (heart failure). Because the cardiovascular system is a closed system, there is no way for the body to release excess pressure. Extremely high blood pressure can result in hypertensive crisis, a condition of medical emergency in which organ systems begin to shut down as a protective mechanism. The damage that has occurred to cells, tissues, and organs as a result of hypertension often remains even after blood pressure is brought under control. Health experts recommend all adults have routine blood pressure checks every year to screen for hypertension.

See also ALPHA ANTAGONIST MEDICATIONS; ANGIOTENSIN-CONVERTING ENZYME (ACE) INHIBITOR MEDICATIONS; ANGIOTENSIN II RECEPTOR ANTAGONIST MEDICATIONS; BETA ANTAGONIST MEDICATIONS; CALCIUM

CHANNEL ANTAGONIST; DIURETIC MEDICATIONS; HYPOTENSION; HALE STEPHEN; LIVING WITH HEART DISEASE; MEDICATIONS TO TREAT HEART DISEASE; NUTRITION AND DIET.

hypertension, pulmonary See PULMONARY HYPERTENSION.

hypertension, white coat See HYPERTENSION.

hypertensive crisis See HYPERTENSION.

hyperthyroidism A medical condition in which the thyroid gland secretes too much thyroid HORMONE, causing a variety of symptoms including accelerated HEART RATE, ARRHYTHMIAS (notably ATRIAL FIBRILLATION), and HYPERTENSION (high BLOOD PRESSURE).

Most cells in the body, including those of the myocardium (HEART muscle), are receptive to thyroid hormone, which influences metabolism (the rate at which cells consume energy). In the cells of the heart (cardiomyocytes), excessive thyroid hormone intensifies CONTRACTILITY and accelerates calcium transport to increase the force and rate of heart contractions. Thyroid hormone also acts on the smooth muscle cells that form the walls of the peripheral arteries, causing them to relax, and influences the body's primary blood pressure regulatory mechanism, the RENIN-ANGIOTENSIN-ALDOSTERONE (RAA) HORMONAL SYSTEM; these two circumstances cause blood pressure to rise. The combination of all of these effects dramatically increases the heart's output and workload such that in a short time the heart can experience atrial or ventricular enlargement.

Symptoms and Diagnostic Path

Hyperthyroidism causes numerous noncardiovascular symptoms, including rapid weight loss, generalized weakness and fatigue, irritability, and disturbances of the menstrual cycle in women. Cardiovascular symptoms include tachycardia (rapid pulse), PALPITATIONS, shortness of breath with EXERCISE or exertion (DYSPNEA), elevated systolic blood pressure, and HEART MURMURS. Laboratory tests to measure the levels of thyroid hormone in the blood can diagnose hyperthyroidism.

Treatment Options and Outlook

Treatment for hyperthyroidism depends on the cause and may include surgery to remove growths on the thyroid gland or radioactive iodine therapy to destroy hyperactive thyroid tissue. Untreated, the effects of hyperthyroidism can result in fatal arrhythmias, permanent damage to the heart, and HEART FAILURE. Treatment of the hyperthyroidism halts the progression of cardiovascular symptoms and often resolves arrhythmias, though conditions such as hypertension and heart failure may continue and require treatment independent of the hyperthyroidism. It is important to consider both the hyperthyroidism and the manifestations of cardiovascular disease (CVD) with regard to treatment, as many medications taken to treat heart disease affect the balance of thyroid hormone in the body.

Risk Factors and Preventive Measures

Though the risk overall for developing hyperthyroidism increases with age, women of all ages have up to 10 times greater likelihood of developing the condition than do men. Health experts recommend annual blood tests to check thyroid levels after age 35. People who take the ANTIARRHYTHMIA MEDICATION amiodarone, which may be prescribed to treat certain types of serious ventricular arrhythmias, should have thyroid levels checked regularly because amiodarone contains a high level of iodine and iodine causes the thyroid gland to make thyroid hormone. The most common causes of hyperthyroidism are Graves' disease and thyroiditis, both of which are autoimmune disorders. There are no measures to prevent these causes of hyperthyroidism.

See also HYPOTHYROIDISM.

hypertriglyceridemia A condition of elevated blood TRIGLYCERIDES (a form of fatty acid) levels that is a significant but modifiable risk factor for HEART DISEASE. Health experts estimate that as many as one in 300 Americans have hypertriglyceridemia. There are two general forms of hypertriglyceridemia, familial (genetic) and nonfamilial.

Symptoms and Diagnostic Path

Hypertriglyceridemia has no symptoms. A blood test can measure the level of triglycerides in the blood. It is necessary to fast (nothing to eat or drink except water) for 12 hours before blood is drawn for a triglycerides test. Diagnosis is made by laboratory tests to measure the concentration of triglycerides in the blood; 150 mg/dL or lower is considered normal; 200 mg/dL or higher is considered clinical hypertriglyceridemia.

Treatment Options and Outlook

Treatment targets lowering blood triglycerides levels to healthy ranges, typically through a combination of lifestyle measures (nutritious and low-fat eating habits, daily physical EXERCISE, and WEIGHT MANAGEMENT or weight loss if OBESITY is a factor) and LIPID-LOWERING MEDICATIONS such as GEMFIBROZIL (Lopid), OMEGA-3 FATTY ACID supplements, and NIACIN. People with nonfamilial hypertriglyceridemia are usually able to bring their blood triglycerides levels down significantly within a few months after starting treatment; people who have familial hypertriglycerides may drop their blood triglycerides levels though still be very high.

Risk Factors and Preventive Measures

Researchers have identified a number of gene mutations affiliated with hypertriglyceridemia, most of which create predisposition or susceptibility toward developing elevated triglycerides but do not necessarily cause a disease state. There appear to be numerous interactions among several gene mutations as well as lifestyle influences that result in elevated blood triglycerides levels. Key factors that point to a hereditary connection include:

- elevated blood levels of triglycerides that remain high despite reasonable lifestyle modification efforts (dietary and exercise changes) and initial treatment with lipid-lowering medications
- elevated blood levels of triglycerides and normal blood levels of other lipids

- evidence of early CARDIOVASCULAR DISEASE (CVD) such as ATHEROSCLEROSIS or CORONARY ARTERY DISEASE (CAD)
- family history of elevated blood triglycerides levels

Familial hypertriglyceridemia typically involves dysfunctions of the enzymes involved in lipid synthesis and METABOLISM. These dysfunctions allow more fatty acids, particularly triglycerides, to enter and remain in circulation in the bloodstream. In some rare genetic mutations, triglycerides levels can rise well above 2000 mg/dL, more than 100 times the upper limit of the healthy concentration and the point at which symptoms such as pain develops and may be mistaken for ANGINA or HEART ATTACK. Treatment focuses on getting and keeping triglycerides levels below 1000 mg/dL and lower if possible, primarily with the aid of lipid-lowering medications such as GEMFIBROZIL (Lopid), OMEGA-3 FATTY ACID supplement, and niacin. Regular physical activity and a nutritious diet also help. Various factors contribute to nonfamilial hypertriglyceridemia, in which there are no apparent hereditary connections. These factors include:

- diet in which 60 percent or more of calories come from carbohydrates
- lack of physical activity and exercise (sedentary lifestyle)
- INSULIN RESISTANCE or DIABETES
- medications that interfere with lipid synthesis and metabolism to cause hypertriglyceridemia as a side effect
- obesity

Treatment focuses on lifestyle modifications, including nutritious diet and regular physical exercise (30 to 60 minutes of aerobic exercise daily), with a goal of weight loss if obesity is a factor. Lipid-lowering medications such as gemfibrozil and niacin also may be necessary.

See also HYPERCHOLESTEROLEMIA; HYPERLIPIDEMIA; NUTRITION AND DIET; XANTHOMA.

hypertrophic cardiomyopathy (HCM)   See CARDIOMYOPATHY.

hypertrophic obstructive cardiomyopathy (HOCM)
See CARDIOMYOPATHY.

hyperventilation A pattern of rapid, deep breathing. An adult at rest typically breathes at a rate of 10 to 16 breaths per minute; during hyperventilation this rate can double or triple, which causes DIZZINESS and a feeling of not getting enough air. However, during hyperventilation the body's CARBON DIOXIDE level, not oxygen level, drops. This can rapidly alter the acid-alkaline balance of the blood, which can have serious consequences if it continues.

Most hyperventilation is stress- or panic-related; closing the mouth and holding one nostril closed to breathe just through the open nostril forces a slowed respiration rate and can restore normal breathing within a few minutes. (Although doctors once recommended breathing into a paper bag, health experts have determined that this can raise the level of carbon dioxide too high and no longer recommend the method.) Panic or stress hyperventilation can be a frightening experience, especially the first time, but it usually has no long-term effects. People who are prone to hyperventilation episodes can learn to identify their early indications and take measures, such as visualization or meditation, to head them off.

Less commonly, hyperventilation can develop in lung conditions such as CHRONIC OBSTRUCTIVE PULMONARY DISEASE (COPD) and pulmonary EMBOLISM (blood clot in the lung) as well as in late-stage HEART FAILURE. These are circumstances that require immediate medical intervention as they indicate that the body is not receiving adequate oxygenation. Generally treatment targets the underlying disease and the hyperventilation goes away with its relief.

See also HYPOXIA; STRESS AND HEART DISEASE; STRESS REDUCTION TECHNIQUES.

hypoglycemia A circumstance in which the level of glucose (sugar) in the BLOOD is below normal. Hypoglycemia typically occurs in people with DIABETES who take oral antidiabetes medications or insulin and reflects an imbalance between glucose and insulin in the body, though it can develop with strenuous physical EXERCISE and inadequate carbohydrate intake in someone who does not have diabetes. Because glucose is a primary fuel source for cell activity, the body attempts to compensate for low glucose levels by boosting HEART RATE to increase circulation, which a person may feel as PALPITATIONS. Other indications of hypoglycemia include diaphoresis (profuse sweating), headache, confusion, and possibly loss of consciousness. Ingesting simple carbohydrates, such as orange juice or even a candy bar, can quickly bring the glucose level up.

See also HYPERGLYCEMIA.

hypokalemia See ELECTROLYTE.

hyponatremia See ELECTROLYTE.

hypoplastic left heart syndrome (HLHS) A life-threatening congenital HEART malformation in which the heart's left ventricle fails to develop fully and is too small to be functional at the time of birth. The right side of the heart often is dilated (enlarged) in compensation, although this does not improve the heart's ability to function. Other malformations are also present, commonly aortic and mitral valve STENOSIS or atresia (narrow or closed passage from the left ventricle to the aorta, the artery carrying BLOOD from the heart to the body, and the mitral valve between the left atrium and left ventricle).

The unborn baby is able to grow and develop because while in the womb its circulatory system bypasses the lungs. Oxygen in the baby's blood instead comes from the mother, transferred across the placenta from the mother's blood to the baby's blood (though there is no mixing of blood between mother and baby). Temporary structures exist in the baby's heart and blood vessels to accommodate this circulatory pattern, and both ventricles pump oxygenated blood. A key temporary structure is the ductus arteriosus, a passage between the aorta and the pulmonary artery. At birth, pressure changes and other processes cause these temporary structures to begin closing and the regular structures to begin taking over. The ductus arteriosus begins closing around three days after birth and is completely closed by the time the baby is 10 to 12 days old, except in the condition of PATENT DUCTUS ARTERIOSUS (PDA), in which the ductus arteriosus fails to close.

Symptoms and Diagnostic Path

Before birth, there are no signs or symptoms that the baby has HLHS. In about half of babies who have HLHS, the diagnosis is made incidentally on prenatal ULTRASOUND. When the diagnosis does not occur until after birth, the signs and symptoms are those of a classic "blue" baby: CYANOSIS, rapid breathing, and rapid HEART RATE. The baby's skin may feel cool and moist. Typically the doctor examining the baby at birth detects a heart MURMUR. ECHOCARDIOGRAM shows the malformations and confirms the diagnosis. The pediatric cardiologist may also do an ELECTROCARDIOGRAM (ECG) to assess the heart's electrical patterns.

Treatment Options and Outlook

Surgery to reconstruct the heart or heart transplant are the only treatment options for survival and generally must be done within a week of birth. Reconstructive surgery is done in three stages over the course of the child's first three years and results in a two-chamber heart (one atrium and one ventricle) rather than the normal four-chamber heart (two atria and two ventricles). When diagnosis is made before or at birth, doctors can initiate therapy with prostaglandin E2 (PGE2), which maintains a patent (open) ductus arteriosus. The PDA allows arterial and venous blood to mingle, which permits partially oxygenated blood to circulate through the body. This therapy is effective only when it starts before the ductus arteriosus begins to close, and its purpose is to delay the necessary surgery to begin repairing the heart until the baby is a little older and stronger.

Risk Factors and Preventive Measures

Although doctors do not know what causes HLHS, congenital heart malformations involving the left heart tend to run in families, which leads researchers to believe there are genetic factors at play. These factors remain unidentified. About 1,000 babies with HLHS are born in the United States each year, a rate of about one in 5,000 births. Among families who have babies with HLHS, there is about a 10 percent chance that a second baby will also have a left heart malformation.

As viable treatments for HLHS have been available only since the mid-1980s, doctors are uncertain about long-term effects though they know there are lifelong consequences. The present five-year survival rate is about 75 percent overall. Infants who undergo reconstructive surgery generally have compromised cardiovascular capacity because the two chambers of their reconstructed hearts must conduct the functions a normal heart carries out with four chambers, though the extent to which this limits life activities and QUALITY OF LIFE as adults remains to be seen.

Infants who RECEIVE HEART TRANSPLANTS must take immunosuppressive drugs for the rest of their lives to prevent their bodies from rejecting their transplanted hearts; immunosuppressive therapy increases susceptibility to infection. As well, doctors do not know how long a transplanted heart will function; like most surgical replacements, there is a high probability that the organ itself has a life expectancy. Immunosuppressive therapy cannot totally prevent rejection over the long term, so this eventually becomes a problem. The longest an adult has lived with the same transplanted heart is 25 years; the average is about 10 years.

See also BIDIRECTIONAL GLENN PROCEDURE; BLALOCK-TAUSSIG PROCEDURE; FONTAN PROCEDURE; NORWOOD PROCEDURE; SINGLE VENTRICLE.

hypotension LOW BLOOD PRESSURE. Hypotension results in inadequate BLOOD flow to all organ systems in the body, including the brain and the HEART. Hypotension can result from taking too high a dose of an ANTIHYPERTENSIVE MEDICATION (to treat hypertension or high blood pressure) or as a side effect of various medications. It also can develop as a condition related to damage to the systems that regulate blood pressure or because of severe blood loss.

Secondary hypotension Hypotension can develop secondary to other health conditions such as DIABETES, HEART FAILURE, and ARRHYTHMIAS. Hypotension in diabetes results when there is damage to the nerves that affects mechanisms regulating blood pressure. Heart failure and arrhythmias can affect the heart's ability to pump enough blood to maintain adequate blood pressure. Hypotension also is common following STROKE if there is damage to the centers of the brain that regulate functions such as HEART RATE and blood pressure, or HEART ATTACK (myocardial infarction) when the heart's pumping ability is impaired.

Orthostatic hypotension Orthostatic hypotension, sometimes called postural hypotension, is a sudden drop in blood pressure upon rising, usually from lying down to sitting or standing. It most often occurs as a medication side effect, although can result from arrhythmias and heart failure. In health, the body compensates for the added physical stress of changing position by initiating a brief and minor increase in blood pressure. This mechanism does not function properly in orthostatic hypotension, for various reasons.

Symptoms and Diagnostic Path

The most common symptoms of hypotension are LIGHT-HEADEDNESS, DIZZINESS, and SYNCOPE. The diagnostic path typically includes several blood pressure measurements, blood tests, an ELECTROCARDIOGRAM (ECG), and a review of medications being taken. The diagnosis is confirmed when blood pressure readings are consistently low and other possible causes, such as arrhythmia, are ruled out.

Treatment Options and Outlook

In most situations, an episode of hypotension either resolves itself or can be resolved by sitting or by lying with the feet higher than the heart. Treatment targets the underlying condition or circumstance and may consist of changing the timing or doses of medications or switching to different medications. Increased fluid consumption eliminates dehydration-related hypotension. Most of the time, hypotension can be corrected.

Risk Factors and Preventive Measures

The risk for hypotension is greatest among young children and older adults. Dehydration is a common cause among younger people, so ensuring adequate fluid consumption is an effective preventive measure. Rising from a prone or sitting position more slowly, bending and moving the legs when standing for prolonged periods of time, and wearing support hose are also ways to prevent hypotension. Orthostatic hypotension is common in Parkinson's disease.

See also CARDIOVASCULAR SYSTEM; HYPERTENSION.

hypothalamus A small structure within the brain that plays a key role in regulating BLOOD PRESSURE and HEART RATE as well as other functions of the AUTONOMIC NERVOUS SYSTEM, including the body's stress response. The primary function of the hypothalamus is to maintain the body's HOMEOSTASIS (balance). It continually sends and receives messages through nerve signals and hormones, using both the nervous system and the endocrine system as its channels of access to either initiate or inhibit actions. Clusters of nerves that serve as message centers, called baroreceptors, are located in the carotid arteries and the aortic arch. These baroreceptors provide most of the information the hypothalamus receives about blood pressure. The baroreceptors register the slightest change in blood pressure, which causes the hypothalamus to activate the appropriate response. The hypothalamus operates without conscious awareness or participation from the conscious mind; it is one of the brain's most primitive structures, solely concerned with the body's physical survival.

See also HORMONE.

hypovolemia A loss of BLOOD volume such as can occur with a serious wound, during surgery, or with severe dehydration. Hypovolemia sometimes develops after open-heart operations or when diuretic doses are too high. Hypovolemia can result in either HYPOTENSION (low BLOOD PRESSURE) and bradycardia (slowed HEART RATE) if there is not enough blood to support adequate blood pressure or HYPERTENSION (high BLOOD PRESSURE) and tachycardia (rapid HEART RATE) as the body attempts to compensate for the reduced BLOOD volume. Conditions such as HEART FAILURE also can produce hypovolemia when the heart is unable to pump blood through the body.

Diagnosis may involve blood tests to look at the concentrations of blood cells compared to plasma, imaging technologies to investigate the possibility of internal bleeding such as from an ANEURYSM, or invasive measures such as pulmonary artery catheterization in which the doctor inserts a catheter (thin, flexible, long tube) into a large blood vessel near the surface of the skin and passes it through the vessel into the HEART and the pulmonary artery. Treatment depends on the underlying cause, and for some situations it is as simple as administering intravenous fluids to restore the diminished volume. For other situations, such as heart failure, treatment would focus on strengthening the heart's ability to pump.

hypoxia Inadequate OXYGENATION of body tissues. Hypoxia can affect a single organ or structure, such as a STROKE that deprives the brain of oxygen, or the entire body, such as following CARDIAC ARREST (stopping of the HEART) or a pulmonary EMBOLISM that stops the flow of BLOOD to a portion of the lung. ANGINA (CHEST PAIN emanating from the heart) reflects hypoxia involving the myocardium (heart muscle). Hypoxia can be a sign that the heart cannot circulate enough oxygenated blood to meet the body's needs, as with HEART FAILURE, in which case there is a general lack of oxygen throughout the body. Systemic hypoxia might also develop as a result of strenuous physical activity that exceeds the ability of the lungs and heart to adequately oxygenate and circulate blood, in a person whose AEROBIC CAPACITY is low or whose cardiovascular capacity is compromised by disease.

See also ISCHEMIC HEART DISEASE (IHD).

Hytrin See TERAZOSIN.

idiopathic hypertrophic subaortic stenosis (IHSS)
See CARDIOMYOPATHY.

idiopathic ventricular tachycardia (VT) See
TACHYCARDIA.

Imdur See ISOSORBIDE.

immunosuppressive medications Drugs taken to
subdue the response of the immune system to
prevent rejection following organ transplant. A
common therapeutic combination is CYCLOSPORINE,
prednisone, and azathioprine. A new immunosuppressive agent that shows promise is mycopheno-
late mofetil. A person with a transplanted organ
must take immunosuppressive medications for the
rest of his or her life. The effect on the HEART AND
CARDIOVASCULAR SYSTEM can be direct, as in HEART
TRANSPLANT or HEART-LUNG TRANSPLANT, or indirect when the transplanted organ is a kidney or
the liver. In either situation, immunosuppressive
medications have substantial side effects (notably
reduced resistance to infection, HYPERTENSION, and
EDEMA) and interactions with other medications
including those commonly prescribed to treat
HEART DISEASE.

Medical management for a person taking immunosuppressive medications is a delicate balance
between preventing organ rejection and rendering
the body's defense mechanisms impotent. Exposure to common viruses such as chicken pox and
measles, and to opportunistic infections such as
herpes simplex and cytomegalovirus (CMV), present particular challenges. The person who is taking
immunosuppressive therapy must learn to identify
early signs of difficulty, and health-care providers
must respond quickly to treat situations before
they become complications. The potential for drug
interactions increases the difficulty of managing
coexisting conditions such as hypertension. The
doctor monitors the effectiveness of immunosuppressive therapy with regular biopsies of the transplanted organ, looking for signs of rejection.

See also ALLOGRAFT.

implantable cardioverter defibrillator (ICD) A
device surgically placed in the body that has a PULSE
generator and electrodes that attach to the HEART,
also called automatic implantable cardioverter defibrillator (AICD). The electrodes transmit signals
from the heart to the pulse generator. When the
HEART RATE exceeds a preset limit, the pulse generator discharges an electrical shock that realigns
the electrical impulses moving through the myocardium (heart muscle) to slow them and restore
them to synchronized contractions. Cardiologists
use ICDs to treat ventricular ARRHYTHMIAS (ventricular FIBRILLATION and VENTRICULAR TACHYCARDIA)
that do not respond to treatment with ANTIAR-
RHYTHMIA MEDICATIONS or other treatments such as
ABLATION. Ventricular arrhythmias are the leading
cause of SUDDEN CARDIAC ARREST (SCA).

As with a pacemaker, an ICD can control the
heart rate by delivering small (imperceptible) electrical impulses to the heart muscle. In addition,
an ICD is able to rapidly recognize and diagnose
life-threatening rhythm abnormalities. If such a
rhythm persists beyond a few seconds, the ICD
delivers a powerful shock to restore a normal heart
rhythm. Although such a DEFIBRILLATION shock is
painful to the person with the ICD, it may also be
life-saving. Contrary to widespread belief, the ICD

shock cannot be felt by another person, even if that person is touching the person with the ICD when the shock is delivered. A long-lasting battery powers the ICD; it may need to be replaced every five years or so.

Although most electronic equipment and home appliances are unlikely to interfere with ICDs or PACEMAKERS, some devices with electromagnetic motors can cause problems. These devices include car engine alternators, home generators, and such. Despite rumors to the contrary, use of microwave ovens, cell phones, and other handheld devices are not major concerns, although doctors do advise to avoid putting electronic devices in the shirt pocket overlying the implanted ICD or pacemaker.

Most people can resume their normal activities once the ICD stabilizes their arrhythmias. Some states may restrict driving privileges depending on the diagnosis and potential for loss of consciousness episodes such as SYNCOPE. It is important to recognize that even though the ICD maintains a relatively stable heart rate, the risk still exists for syncope and SCA. These risks should be carefully considered when returning to occupations in which such events could present hazards. Many kinds of diagnosed arrhythmias, especially ventricular arrhythmias, preclude commercial driver's licenses or pilot's licenses, regardless of treatment.

See also BRUGADA SYNDROME; CARDIOMYOPATHY; HEART FAILURE; LONG QT SYNDROME.

implantable loop recorder (ILR)   A small device surgically placed within a pocket of tissue on the upper chest to detect and record the HEARTBEAT during episodes of SYNCOPE (fainting). An ILR can help to diagnose ARRHYTHMIAS when other monitoring methods, such as HOLTER MONITOR, have not produced useful information. There are no leads into the HEART; the ILR picks up electrical signals through the chest wall when there is a CARDIAC EVENT and stores them electronically. The person may press a button on an activator to turn on the recording when he or she feels an episode coming on, or the ILR can be set to turn on automatically. The cardiologist can download recorded data. An ILR can stay in place for about two years; the car-

diologist will remove it sooner if it provides enough data to be diagnostic.

See also PACEMAKER.

indapamide   A DIURETIC MEDICATION taken to treat HYPERTENSION and edema that develops as a consequence of congestive HEART FAILURE. Indapamide (Lozol) is similar in chemical composition and action to the thiazide diuretics, though it is not a thiazide. It can cause potassium depletion; doctors often recommend eating foods high in potassium such as bananas and raisins, or may prescribe low-dose potassium supplementation. Indapamide may be one of several medications prescribed to treat hypertension; it is common to use a diuretic in combination with other kinds of ANTIHYPERTENSIVE MEDICATIONS for maximum BLOOD PRESSURE control. Indapamide should not be taken with other diuretics. People who have allergies to sulfonamides (such as sulfa antibiotics) may have cross-sensitivity to indapamide. Headache, DIZZINESS, and nausea are the most common side effects and usually resolve after taking indapamide for several weeks.

See also ANTIHYPERTENSIVE MEDICATIONS; BETA ANTAGONIST MEDICATIONS; ANGIOTENSIN-CONVERTING ENZYME (ACE) INHIBITOR MEDICATIONS; ANGIOTENSIN II RECEPTOR ANTAGONIST MEDICATIONS; MEDICATIONS TO TREAT HEART DISEASE.

Inderal   See PROPRANOLOL.

inferior vena cava   See HEART.

inflammation and heart disease   The correlations between inflammation in the arteries, the development of CARDIOVASCULAR DISEASE (CVD), and the likelihood for MYOCARDIAL INFARCTION (MI). Inflammation is part of the body's normal immune response to injury. In some people this response goes awry, causing the body to perceive injury where it does not exist (autoimmune disorder). In most people, inflammation becomes a problem over time as the body continually responds to microinjuries. When this process affects the joints, for example, the result is arthritis. Rheumatoid arthritis is an example of arthritis that results from dysfunctions in the immune response; osteoarthritis is an example of arthritis that results from continual damage.

In the CARDIOVASCULAR SYSTEM, inflammatory damage develops within the walls of the arteries. Fragments of fatty acids (blood lipids), calcium, and other substances are able to collect along inflamed cells. These collections can eventually form hardened deposits that stiffen the arterial walls and narrow the passage through which BLOOD flows. Doctors believe this inflammation plays a key role not only in the development of CORONARY ARTERY DISEASE (CAD) and PERIPHERAL ARTERY DISEASE (PAD) but also in raising the risk for HEART ATTACK and STROKE. They also believe it helps to explain why people who have normal blood levels of cholesterol and TRIGLYCERIDES still develop CVD.

The primary diagnostic tool for heightened inflammatory response with cardiovascular risk is a blood test that measures the level of a substance called C-REACTIVE PROTEIN, which rises when there is active inflammation in the body. When coupled with the presence of other risk factors for heart disease, the C-reactive protein level helps to identify people in whom prophylactic anti-inflammatory therapy, such as ASPIRIN or ANTICOAGULANT MEDICATIONS, can lower the risk for heart attack or stroke. People with high blood lipid levels (cholesterol and triglycerides) also benefit from lipid-lowering medications. Lifestyle modifications, primarily weight loss/WEIGHT MANAGEMENT and daily EXERCISE, are also effective in reducing inflammation. It is also important to control other health conditions such as diabetes and HYPERTENSION (high BLOOD PRESSURE) and to stop smoking.

See also ARTERIOSCLEROSIS; CHOLESTEROL, BLOOD; DIABETES AND HEART DISEASE; LIFESTYLE AND HEART HEALTH; METABOLIC SYNDROME.

informed consent A formal process of fully disclosing and explaining to the person who is the patient, in language the person understands, the possible benefits and potential risks of a particular treatment. Generally informed consent applies to invasive (such as surgery) or investigational therapies, or when a person chooses to decline treatment. Depending on the circumstances, the person may be asked to sign a document affirming the explanations and his or her understanding and acceptance of them. Informed consent safeguards the legal rights of patients and providers.

Health-care providers (physicians and facilities) should have clear and explicit policies dealing with informed consent. Especially when the procedure is urgent, it is easy to feel that the informed consent documents are simply more paperwork. However, it is important to question information that seems vague or complications that were not previously presented. It is also valuable to ask providers what measures they take to reduce the likelihood of the identified risks and complications. Such discussions can sometimes lead to other approaches that might have greater benefit and/or less risk.

See also ADVANCE DIRECTIVES; CLINICAL RESEARCH STUDIES; INVESTIGATIONAL NEW DRUGS (INDs); INVESTIGATIONAL TREATMENTS; SURGERY TO TREAT CARDIOVASCULAR DISEASE.

innocent heart murmur See HEART MURMUR.

insulin A HORMONE the pancreas produces that regulates the amount of glucose available to cells and is essential for numerous functions within the body related to energy production and storage (METABOLISM). Insulin is also available as a hormone supplement medication for insulin replacement therapy in people who have insulin-dependent DIABETES (all people with type 1 diabetes and about 40 percent of people who have type 2 diabetes). Insulin significantly affects cardiovascular health and the development of CARDIOVASCULAR DISEASE (CVD).

Insulin-Glucose Balance
The body maintains an intricate balance between insulin and glucose. Glucose is one of the body's two primary fuel sources (the other being oxygen). Most cells in the body require insulin to allow them to use glucose; the notable exceptions are cells in

the brain and the liver. During digestion, the body converts carbohydrates to glucose, a form of sugar that passes easily into the bloodstream from the small intestine. Glucose molecules bind with specialized protein molecules in the blood that serve as glucose transporters.

The pancreas, a glandular organ located in the upper left abdomen behind the stomach, releases insulin when glucose levels in the bloodstream rise. Insulin allows the glucose transporters to pick up (bind with) glucose molecules. Insulin molecules also bind with insulin receptors in cells, "unlocking" access for glucose molecules to enter the cell and regulating their passage. These binding processes lower both glucose and insulin levels in the blood, which in turn slows additional binding to "lock" cellular access to glucose. The balance is such that, in health, cells receive the amount of glucose they need to function efficiently and effectively. When this balance becomes disturbed, cells receive either too little or too much glucose (energy).

Insulin also stimulates the liver to convert glucose into an intermediate storage form of energy, glycogen. The body stores glycogen in the liver as well as in fat cells throughout the body. The pancreas produces another hormone, glucagon, that converts glycogen back to glucose when the body's glucose levels fall too low. Cells that require high and continual glucose supplies, such as those of the nervous system and brain, can draw directly from glycogen stores. Though this process is inefficient for long-term energy needs, it allows such cells to continue vital functions in the short term when the body's normal insulin-glucose balance becomes disturbed.

Insulin and Lipids

Lipids, or fatty acids, are the body's long-term energy storage forms. Glucose that enters the bloodstream goes first to meet the immediate energy needs of cells, then to the liver for conversion into glycogen. When the body reaches its limit for glycogen stores, the liver switches from manufacturing glycogen to increasing lipid production. The body has virtually an endless capacity to store lipids, which comprise the bulk of adipose (fat) tissue throughout the body. Adipose cells can swell to more than 100 times their normal size to accommodate fatty acid deposits and can infiltrate most tissue structures within the body including the heart.

Insulin has two roles in lipid production and storage. First, it activates the enzymes in the liver that synthesize lipoproteins, the carriers for fatty acid molecules (including cholesterol, which the liver also manufactures). This puts more lipoproteins, especially low-density lipoprotein (LDL) and very low-density lipoprotein (VLDL), into circulation in the bloodstream. Second, insulin blocks the action of enzymes that allow fat cells to release lipids, which prevents the body from "burning" fat as an energy source.

Insulin's Roles in Cardiovascular Health and Disease

As the gatekeeper for cellular metabolism, insulin influences the health and function of most cells in the body. The cells of the cardiovascular system have a narrow margin of tolerance; their functions are precise. Through its actions to regulate glucose levels, insulin maintains appropriate cellular metabolism. Persistent elevated levels of glucose in the bloodstream, such as in INSULIN RESISTANCE and diabetes, allow cellular metabolism to increase, ultimately resulting in damage to cells throughout the body and particularly those that comprise the inner walls of the arteries.

Because the arterioles and peripheral arteries are so small, damage to their walls can cause them to rupture and impair peripheral circulation. One of the body's mechanisms for regulating blood pressure relies on declines or rises in peripheral resistance (how hard the heart must work to get blood to the most distant arteries) as a signal to lower or raise blood pressure. When it becomes widespread, damage to these distant arteries and arterioles causes this mechanism to perceive increased peripheral resistance and initiates the sequence of events that raise blood pressure. Over time this contributes to HYPERTENSION (high BLOOD PRESSURE).

The inner walls of the large arteries experience damage as well, becoming fragile and vulnerable to tears. The blood clots that form to heal these tears attract fatty acid molecules, especially VLDL and LDL, accelerating arterial PLAQUE accumulations. The fragile state of the arterial walls makes it more likely that these plaque accumulations will rupture, sending fragments into the bloodstream where they become a significant risk for HEART ATTACK and STROKE. Its roles in lipid manufacture and storage make insulin a significant factor in the development of OBESITY and also contribute to cardiovascular diseases resulting from accumulations of arterial plaque such as ATHEROSCLEROSIS and CORONARY ARTERY DISEASE (CAD).

See also CHOLESTEROL, BLOOD; LIFESTYLE AND HEART HEALTH; NUTRITION AND DIET.

insulin resistance A condition in which cells become desensitized to the presence of INSULIN and require higher insulin levels before they respond. Insulin is instrumental in metabolism with one of its key roles being "gatekeeper" for entry of glucose (sugar), the body's primary source of energy, into the cells. When cells become resistant to insulin's action, higher levels of glucose remain in circulation in the bloodstream.

Symptoms and Diagnostic Path
Diagnosis of insulin resistance considers the coexistence of several features:

- elevated blood levels of TRIGLYCERIDES
- reduced blood levels of high-density lipoprotein (HDL), the "good" cholesterol
- elevated blood glucose level (fasting)
- OBESITY
- polycystic ovary disease in women

Researchers do not know whether these features generate the circumstance of insulin resistance or whether insulin resistance causes these features to develop. They do know that lifestyle factors can prevent, halt, and even reverse insulin resistance in most people.

Treatment Options and Outlook
Lifestyle modifications can reverse insulin resistance in some people and delay its progression in nearly everyone who has it. EXERCISE is particularly effective in increasing insulin sensitivity as well as boosting HDL and lowering triglycerides. Reducing

dietary carbohydrates (sugars) to no more than 60 percent of calories consumed and fats to no more than 30 percent (10 percent or less saturated fats) also is important. The doctor may prescribe a lipid-lowering medication to bring down blood triglycerides levels. Otherwise there are no medical interventions for insulin resistance; medical treatment options enter the picture only when insulin resistance progresses to type 2 diabetes.

Risk Factors and Preventive Measures
Insulin resistance is the first stage of type 2 diabetes and sometimes is called prediabetes. About half of those who have insulin resistance will develop type 2 diabetes. Health experts estimate that about one in four adults has insulin resistance. People with insulin resistance often have some degree of CARDIOVASCULAR DISEASE (CVD) as well, commonly ATHEROSCLEROSIS, CORONARY ARTERY DISEASE (CAD), and HYPERTENSION (high BLOOD PRESSURE). Insulin resistance appears to be the foundation for a complex of metabolic disorders collectively referred to as the metabolic SYNDROME.

See also CHOLESTEROL, BLOOD; DIABETES AND HEART DISEASE.

intermittent claudication See CLAUDICATION.

intra-aortic balloon pump (IABP) counterpulsation An interim treatment for relieving the heart's workload following HEART ATTACK or in severe HEART FAILURE that uses alternating inflation and deflation of a small balloon to generate somewhat of a wavelike motion of BLOOD from the left ventricle into the aorta. The waves, or counterpulsations, help to pull blood from the ventricle, easing by as much as 40 percent the effort the ventricle must exert to pump the blood out.

Procedure
The cardiologist inserts the intra-aortic balloon pump (IABP) through a catheter that enters the body through an incision in the femoral artery in the groin. Using FLUOROSCOPY (moving X-rays) to guide the catheter, the cardiologist threads the balloon pump through the arteries and HEART until it rests

in the aorta just before the left subclavian artery branches off. Once the balloon pump is in place the cardiologist uses helium to inflate a small outer cuff that holds it against the walls of the aorta.

A computerized control unit receives electrical signals from the heart and times the inflation and deflation of the inner ring, or lumen, of the balloon with the electrical impulses of the person's CARDIAC CYCLE such that the balloon inflates during DIASTOLE and deflates at the start of left ventricular ejection (the point at which the filled left ventricle begins to push blood through the aortic valve into the aorta). This pattern lowers the pressure in the aorta during SYSTOLE, which facilitates the flow of blood from the heart and reduces ventricular afterload (the "clenching" type of pressure the left ventricle must hold immediately following peak contraction to keep the aortic valve open and prevent blood from flowing back into the ventricle during the last phase of systole).

Cardiologists often use IABP counterpulsation to stabilize a heart that has sustained significant damage during myocardial infarction (heart attack). Allowing the heart to recover enough to undergo CORONARY ARTERY BYPASS GRAFT (CABG), or in other circumstances in which the heart's pumping ability has failed, such as end-stage cardiomyopathy while awaiting HEART TRANSPLANT, or traumatic injury to the heart. IABP counterpulsation also might be used to treat SHOCK of cardiovascular origin (cardiogenic shock) to restore circulation throughout the body. Once the person's heart and cardiovascular functions are stabilized, the cardiologist removes the IABP.

Risks and Complications

The potential risks of this treatment include infection and perforation of the aorta or any of the arteries along the insertion path; these are uncommon events.

Outlook and Lifestyle Modifications

IABP counterpulsation is highly effective in decreasing the heart's workload and improving OXYGENATION of the blood. The procedure also makes it possible for many people who are awaiting donor hearts for transplant to survive until a suitable DONOR HEART is obtained. People who undergo this procedure have significant and sometimes end-stage heart disease, however, which affects the ultimate outlook.

See also CARDIAC CATHETERIZATION; CARDIOVASCULAR SYSTEM; ENHANCED EXTERNAL COUNTERPULSATION; SURGERY TO TREAT CARDIOVASCULAR DISEASE.

intraventricular conduction defect   An ARRHYTHMIA condition identified by an irregularity in the ELECTROCARDIOGRAM (ECG) that shows a widened QRS complex (pattern of electrical activity). This means that the electrical signals that cause the myocardium (heart muscle) to contract become delayed as they pass through the left ventricle, prolonging the contraction and diminishing the heart's pumping efficiency. An intraventricular conduction defect often is associated with CARDIOMYOPATHY and HEART FAILURE or may follow heart surgery such as CORONARY ARTERY BYPASS GRAFT (CABG). Diagnosis is by ECG; treatment with ANTI-ARRHYTHMIA MEDICATIONS is sometimes effective, though often an implanted PACEMAKER that uses electrical impulses to regulate heart rate is required.

See also BUNDLE BRANCH BLOCK; HEART BLOCK.

investigational new drug (IND)   A classification for drugs that have not yet received full approval for use from the U.S. Food and Drug Administration (FDA) that permits limited use of the drug under specified circumstances as well as its transportation across state lines. Typically an investigational new drug (IND) is in the final stage of CLINICAL RESEARCH STUDIES and has demonstrated its efficacy and relative safety within established parameters of use. Approval of IND status allows the drug to be used in multicenter studies as well as in emergency circumstances when it would clearly benefit a person for whom conventional treatments have not been successful. For example, an IND immunosuppressive agent might be used to treat a person with a transplanted heart who is facing organ rejection because currently available IMMUNOSUPPRESSIVE MEDICATIONS are no longer effective. Numerous requirements and controls apply to INDs, including the settings in which they are used and who administers them.

See also INFORMED CONSENT; INVESTIGATIONAL TREATMENTS.

investigational treatments Therapies (medications and devices) that show promise for treatment but have not yet received full approval for use from the U.S. Food and Drug Administration (FDA). Some investigational treatments involve approved medications or devices being applied to different clinical circumstances than their original approvals, and others are new products. Typically an investigational treatment has been successful in early (phase I) clinical research but its full benefits and risks remain undetermined.

At any given time there are hundreds of CLINICAL RESEARCH STUDIES soliciting volunteers to participate in the next levels of testing, which involves using the product in its intended therapeutic approach in people who have the health condition the treatment is intended to benefit. Doctors sometimes suggest investigational treatments for people who are not receiving benefit from conventional treatments and whose conditions will continue to decline without intervention. It is crucial to understand the ramifications, to the extent possible, of choosing an investigational treatment, especially with regard to how ongoing and future medical care will be provided.

See also INFORMED CONSENT; INVESTIGATIONAL NEW DRUG (IND).

irbesartan A medication taken to treat HYPERTENSION (high BLOOD PRESSURE). Irbesartan (Avapro) is an ANGIOTENSIN II RECEPTOR ANTAGONIST MEDICATION that doctors often prescribe in combination with HYDROCHLOROTHIAZIDE, a thiazide DIURETIC MEDICATION, for more effective BLOOD pressure control. Like other ANGIOTENSIN II RECEPTOR antagonists, irbesartan works by preventing the enzyme angiotensin II from binding with its receptors in the walls of the arterioles. Angiotensin II is a powerful vasoconstrictor that causes the arterioles to contract, signaling the body to raise blood pressure. Blocking the action of angiotensin II stops this process. Irbesartan's side effects generally are mild and may include headache, gastrointestinal distress,

and dizziness. Women who are pregnant should not take irbesartan or other angiotensin II receptor antagonists, as these medications are known to cause birth defects.

See also ANGIOTENSIN-CONVERTING ENZYME (ACE) INHIBITOR MEDICATIONS; ANTIHYPERTENSIVE MEDICATIONS; MEDICATIONS TO TREAT HEART DISEASE.

iron A mineral that has many vital uses in the human body. One of the most important from a cardiovascular perspective is its ability to bind with oxygen molecules and transport them through the BLOOD to cells throughout the body. Red blood cells contain hemoglobin, which carries the iron. Low levels of iron in the blood cause iron-deficiency ANEMIA, a condition in which the blood cannot carry enough oxygen to meet the body's needs. Anemia increases the workload of the heart, typically increasing HEART RATE and BLOOD PRESSURE as the HEART attempts to move larger volumes of blood as a means of accommodating the low oxygen load. Sometimes doctors administer blood transfusions after heart attacks in people who are anemic to boost the blood's ability to transport oxygen and relieve some of the heart's workload.

Excesses of iron can result in deposits within tissues that cause damage, especially to the heart and liver. Because iron transports oxygen and thus facilitates oxidation processes within cells as a function of metabolism, some researchers have raised questions whether borderline high levels of iron in the blood contribute to oxidation damage through the formation of FREE RADICALS (unstable molecular particles implicated in numerous diseases including cardiovascular disease).

Iron comes primarily from dietary sources. Foods that are high in iron include dark green leafy vegetables such as spinach and kale, meats, and fortified grain products such as cereals and pastas. People who are iron-deficient might require iron supplements; a doctor should make this determination as too much iron is toxic and because chronic iron deficiency can signal other health problems such as internal bleeding (as from gastrointestinal ulcers) or metabolic disorders.

See also HEMOCHROMATOSIS; NUTRITION AND DIET; THROMBOCYTHEMIA.

ischemia Oxygen deprivation resulting from impaired BLOOD flow to an organ or tissue. The word means "to hold back blood." Ischemia results when there is a restriction or an OCCLUSION to the blood supply, such as the narrowing of arterial channels that occurs with ATHEROSCLEROSIS (accumulations of arterial plaque along the inner walls of the arteries) or when a clot blocks blood flow through an artery. Ischemia can have especially serious health consequences when it affects the brain, kidneys, or HEART. Generally the occlusion is partial so there is some blood flow; the deprivation might become apparent only when the tissue or organ comes under the stress of increased functional demand. With the heart, for example, this may be with increased physical exertion or exercise.

See also CORONARY ARTERY DISEASE (CAD); EDEMA; HEART ATTACK; ISCHEMIC HEART DISEASE (IHD); PLAQUE, ARTERIAL; STROKE; TRANSIENT ISCHEMIC ATTACK (TIA).

ischemic heart disease (IHD) Damage to the myocardium (HEART muscle) that results from continued temporary oxygen deprivation. The most common cause of ischemic HEART DISEASE is CORONARY ARTERY DISEASE (CAD), narrowing and occlusion of the CORONARY ARTERIES resulting from ATHEROSCLEROSIS (accumulations of arterial plaque along the inner walls of the arteries). CORONARY ARTERY SPASM also can cause ischemic attacks. Ischemic heart disease often becomes apparent through ANGINA, CHEST PAIN that originates in the HEART, though it can be present without symptoms (called silent ischemic heart disease). About 14 million Americans have IHD.

Ischemic heart disease and coronary artery disease sometimes are collectively referred to as coronary heart disease (CHD); their disease processes and symptoms are so intertwined that it is difficult to separate them. Seldom does one exist without the other. A prolonged ischemic attack can become a myocardial infarction (HEART ATTACK), a loss of oxygenation substantial enough to cause permanent damage to the myocardium. Ischemic heart disease affects both the mechanical and electrical functions of the heart and can cause potentially life-threatening ARRHYTHMIAS (irregularities in the heartbeat).

Symptoms and Diagnostic Path

Abnormalities detected on routine ELECTROCARDIOGRAM (ECG) may be the first indication of ischemic heart disease in the absence of symptoms such as angina, though often when there are no symptoms myocardial infarction is the first sign that ischemic heart disease (and typically coronary artery disease as well) is present. Angina, especially with exercise, exertion, or stress, is a key symptom of ischemic heart disease.

Cardiologists typically identify ischemic heart disease according to the layers of heart tissues the ischemia penetrates:

- Transmural ischemia affects the full depth of the myocardium.
- Subendocardial ischemia affects the endocardium, the inner layer of the myocardium.
- Subepicardial ischemia affects the epicardium, the outer layer of the myocardium.

Diagnosis of ischemic heart disease generally is by ECG, with CARDIAC CATHETERIZATION or ANGIOGRAPHY if necessary to determine the extent of coronary artery disease that is present.

Treatment Options and Outlook

Treatment may consist of medications to relieve angina symptoms, if present, and to strengthen and slow the HEARTBEAT to reduce the heart's workload. When appropriate, the cardiologist may recommend ANGIOPLASTY or CORONARY ARTERY BYPASS GRAFT (CABG) to remedy the underlying cardiovascular disease causing ischemic attacks.

Risk Factors and Preventive Measures

CAD is the leading risk factor for IHD; the narrowed and stiffened coronary arteries become unable to respond to the heart's changing needs for oxygen. Other forms of heart disease, such as hypertension and having previously had a heart attack, are also factors that contribute to risk. Measures to prevent, diagnose, and treat these conditions reduces the risk for IHD. Smoking cessation and efforts to lower blood lipid levels (cholesterol and TRIGLYCERIDES) are also beneficial.

See also AFRICAN AMERICANS AND CARDIOVASCULAR DISEASE; CARDIOVASCULAR DISEASE; ISCHEMIA; LIVING WITH HEART DISEASE; PLAQUE, ARTERIAL; WOMEN AND HEART DISEASE.

isoptin See VERAPAMIL.

isosorbide A NITRATE MEDICATION taken to prevent ANGINA (CHEST PAIN) due to ISCHEMIC HEART DISEASE (IHD) or CORONARY ARTERY DISEASE (CAD). Isosorbide comes in two forms, dinitrate and mononitrate. Common brand names of isosorbide dinitrate available in the United States, include Isordil, Sorbitrate, and Dilatrate SR; isosorbide mononitrate is available as the brand-name product Imdur. Isosorbide works by causing the arteries and the veins throughout the body to relax and dilate. This reduces arterial resistance for BLOOD flowing from the HEART and slows the rate of venous blood returning to the heart; in combination these actions reduce the heart's workload and thus oxygen requirements, preventing angina.

It is essential to take isosorbide on the schedule prescribed, as the body develops a tolerance to its effects and doses are spaced to minimize this. A "nitrate headache" is common at the start of isosorbide therapy, a consequence of the systemic vasodilation the nitrate causes. For most people this goes away after a few weeks of taking the medication. Nitrate medications interact with numerous other medications; it is important to follow label directions precisely and to discuss all other medications with the doctor or pharmacist when isosorbide is first prescribed.

See also MEDICATION MANAGEMENT; MEDICATIONS TO TREAT HEART DISEASE; PDES INHIBITOR MEDICATIONS.

isradipine A medication taken to treat HYPERTENSION (high BLOOD PRESSURE). Isradipine, available as the brand-name products DynaCirc and DynaCirc CR, is a CALCIUM CHANNEL ANTAGONIST MEDICATION. Doctors often prescribe isradipine in combination with a thiazide DIURETIC MEDICATION such as HYDROCHLOROTHIAZIDE for more effective blood pressure regulation. Like other calcium channel blockers, isradipine works by slowing the flow of calcium into myocardial (HEART muscle) cells. This in turn slows the rate and force with which the cells contract, reducing the heart's workload and lowering blood pressure. Generally isradipine becomes a therapeutic choice when other medications fail to adequately control blood pressure. Side effects include gastrointestinal upset (nausea, diarrhea, and constipation), PALPITATIONS, edema, and occasionally ARRHYTHMIAS such as ATRIAL FIBRILLATION. There has been some concern that calcium channel blockers increase the risk for HEART ATTACK (myocardial infarction) and SUDDEN CARDIAC ARREST in people with moderate to severe HEART FAILURE or HEART BLOCK; however, recent large-scale research studies have resolved or at least diminished this concern, as no evidence of increased heart attack or sudden cardiac arrest was observed in these studies.

See also ANGIOTENSIN II RECEPTOR ANTAGONIST MEDICATIONS; ANGIOTENSIN-CONVERTING ENZYME (ACE) INHIBITOR MEDICATIONS; CALCIUM CYCLE; MEDICATIONS TO TREAT HEART DISEASE; SODIUM CHANNEL BLOCKING MEDICATIONS.

J

Jantene procedure See ARTERIAL SWITCH PROCEDURE.

Jarvik, Robert (1946–) The physician and biomedical engineer who designed the first permanent implantable artificial heart, the Jarvik-7. Jarvik and his artificial heart made history in 1982 when a team of cardiovascular surgeons led by Dr. William DeVries at the University of Utah replaced the badly diseased heart of Seattle dentist Barney Clark with an implanted Jarvik-7 artificial heart. Clark survived 112 days. In the 1980s about 70 people received Jarvik-7 implants, most of which were bridge implants for people awaiting DONOR HEARTS for transplant. The Jarvik-7 was far less than ideal as a permanent replacement for a human HEART, however, and Jarvik turned his attention in the 1990s to developing a more practical and effective design that would support, rather than replace, the heart to allow the heart to heal and recover. The Jarvik 2000 debuted as the first implantable LEFT VENTRICULAR ASSIST DEVICE (LVAD) and remains among the half-dozen LVADs currently involved in clinical research studies in the United States today.

See also BARNARD, CHRISTIAAN; COOLEY, DENTON; DEBAKEY, MICHAEL E.; DEVRIES, WILLIAM C.; HEART, ARTIFICIAL.

Jervell and Lange-Nielsen syndrome A rare genetic disorder in which there is congenital profound hearing loss along with abnormalities in the HEART's CONDUCTION PATHWAY. Most researchers consider Jervell and Lange-Nielsen syndrome a variation of LONG QT SYNDROME, which has very similar presentation and ELECTROCARDIOGRAM (ECG) findings. There is significant risk for SUDDEN CARDIAC ARREST (SCA).

Symptoms and Diagnostic Path

As with long QT syndrome, many people have no cardiac symptoms until CARDIAC ARREST or sudden cardiac arrest. When symptoms are present, they often include episodes of rapid HEART RATE (tachycardia) and SYNCOPE (fainting). EXERCISE and emotional stress often trigger symptoms. Diagnosis is primarily a combination of family history or gene analysis, ECG findings, and the presence of congenital sensorineural hearing loss.

Treatment Options and Outlook

Treatment might use ANTIARRHYTHMIA MEDICATIONS to restore and maintain a normal rhythm. When the ARRHYTHMIAS are pronounced, an IMPLANTABLE CARDIOVERTER DEFIBRILLATOR (ICD) is often the preferred treatment. The ICD automatically delivers an electrical shock to the heart when it goes into dangerous arrhythmias. It is also important to avoid triggers that encourage the arrhythmias. Key among these triggers are intense physical activity (such as competitive sports), jumping into cold water, and intense emotions. Family members and friends should know CPR (CARDIOPULMONARY RESUSCITATION). Although it is not possible to prevent the arrhythmias, with diligent management the person with Jervell and Lange-Nielsen syndrome can enjoy a fairly normal life.

Risk Factors and Preventive Measures

Because Jervell and Lange-Nielsen syndrome is genetic, genetic counseling is recommended for families in which the syndrome appears. The inheritance is autosomal recessive, meaning both parents must carry the mutated gene for the child to have the syndrome.

See also BRUGADA SYNDROME.

Kawasaki disease   See HEART DISEASE IN CHILDREN.

Kerlone   See BETAXOLOL.

Korotkoff sounds   Five kinds of arterial sounds heard through a STETHOSCOPE that provide the markers for a BLOOD PRESSURE reading. Russian physician Nicholai Korotkoff was the first to detect the sounds and correlate them to blood pressure. The sounds characterize the vibrational changes that occur in the walls of the arteries in response to the changing pressures of BLOOD flowing through them. In people who have stage 2 (severe) HYPER-TENSION (high blood pressure), the Korotkoff sounds may not accurately reflect systolic pressure, diastolic pressure, or both.

When taking a blood pressure measurement, the health-care provider places an inflatable cuff around the arm just above the elbow, and puts the stethoscope over the brachial artery on the inside of the arm in the bend of the elbow. The cuff is inflated until blood flow through the artery stops, and then the inflation is slowly released while the health-care provider listens through the stethoscope to the sounds of blood moving through the artery and watches the corresponding pressure readings on the SPHYGMOMANOMETER dial or gauge.

- The first sound, Korotkoff phase I, is a pronounced and loud tap; it marks systole (the ventricle's peak contraction).
- The second sound, Korotkoff phase II, is a loud whooshing sound; it marks the surge of blood pushed into the arteries with the systolic contraction.
- The third sound, Korotkoff phase III, is a soft tap.
- The fourth sound, Korotkoff phase IV, is a soft whooshing sound; it marks the end of the current contraction's surge of blood.
- The fifth sound, Korotkoff phase V, is silence; it marks diastole (the momentary pause when the ventricle is at rest before the next CARDIAC CYCLE begins) and the point at which the blood pressure cuff no longer restricts the flow of blood through the arm.

See also HEART RATE; PULSE; VITAL SIGNS.

labetalol A medication taken to lower BLOOD PRESSURE as a treatment for HYPERTENSION. Common brand names available in the United States include Normodyne and Trandate. Labetalol has a blended adrenergic receptor antagonist action, blocking alpha and beta adrenergic receptors to slow and strengthen the HEARTBEAT to lessen the HEART's workload as well as to dilate peripheral arteries and arterioles to lower blood pressure. Doctors frequently prescribe labetalol in combination with other medications to reduce blood pressure, such as DIURETIC MEDICATIONS, and recommend lifestyle modifications including low-salt diet and daily EXERCISE. Common side effects of labetalol, which often diminish after taking the medication for a few weeks, include gastrointestinal upset, SEXUAL DYSFUNCTION, fatigue, and orthostatic HYPOTENSION (a sudden drop in blood pressure upon rising). As with most ANTIHYPERTENSIVE MEDICATIONS it is important to taper off labetalol when stopping the medication to prevent rebound hypertensive crisis (rapid escalation of blood pressure).

See also ALPHA ANTAGONIST MEDICATIONS; BETA ANTAGONIST MEDICATIONS.

Laënnec, René (1781–1826) French physician who invented the STETHOSCOPE, a simple device that focuses and amplifies the sounds of the HEART and the lungs. The model Laënnec designed in 1816 was inspired by his impromptu rolling of a piece of paper into a funnel-like tube to listen to the chest of a corpulent female patient when attempts at AUSCULTATION (tapping the chest to listen for differences in sounds) produced little useful diagnostic information. Laënnec turned his paper prototype into various crafted wooden models featuring trumpet-shaped tubes with narrow flares at one end and wider flares at the other. The wide flare was placed against the patient's chest and the narrow flare to the physician's ear. Laënnec spent three years investigating the sounds his stethoscopes amplified and in 1819 published a discussion of his techniques and their diagnostic implications in *A Treatise on Diseases of the Chest and Mediate Auscultation*. Laënnec later turned his diagnostic explorations to studies of cirrhosis of the liver and of tuberculosis; he died of tuberculosis at age 45.

See also CORVISART, JEAN-NICHOLAS.

Lanoxin See DIGOXIN.

laser revascularization See TRANSMYOCARDIAL LASER REVASCULARIZATION (TMLR).

late potential study See SIGNAL-AVERAGED ELECTROCARDIOGRAM (SAECG).

lateral tunnel See FONTAN PROCEDURE.

left ventricular assist device (LVAD) An implantable mechanical pump that supplements the natural HEART's pumping action to increase its effectiveness when severe HEART DISEASE impairs the heart's function. The first LVADs were developed in the mid-1980s as alternatives to full artificial hearts, implanted as temporary bridge devices to support people waiting for HEART TRANSPLANTS. In 2002 the U.S. Food and Drug Administration (FDA) granted approval for use of LVADs as permanent treatment (destination therapy) for people in end-stage HEART FAILURE for whom other treatments have failed and heart transplant is not an option. Cardiovascular surgeons in the United States have implanted LVADs in several thousand people; there are a number of designs available including several that are completely internal with battery-operated control units placed beneath the skin of the abdomen. Other LVAD models are portable but connect to external drive units. Such models typically rely on AC electrical current (plug into an electrical outlet) and can be operated for a short time (six to eight hours) by a battery pack worn on the belt or in an over-the-shoulder pack. Some models are pneumatic (powered by pressurized air).

In general, an LVAD works by shunting BLOOD from the left ventricle to a pump unit. The cardiovascular surgeon inserts one cannula, or large tube, into the pulmonary vein to intercept oxygenated blood returning from the lungs to the left ventricle and inserts another cannula into the aorta to carry the blood from the LVAD pump unit into the body. The heart continues to beat and circulate blood to the lungs for oxygenation, but the LVAD does the main pumping work. This allows the damaged heart to rest and also delivers an adequate supply of oxygenated blood to the body's tissues; it often can sustain a person's cardiovascular functions for the time it takes to acquire a donor heart after being placed on the list for heart transplant.

Extensive research has shown that LVADs can provide a significantly higher QUALITY OF LIFE and can extend LIFE EXPECTANCY by one to three years or longer when implanted in people with end-stage heart failure. The risks associated with LVADs are those of any heart surgery, notably postoperative infection and thromboembolism (blood clots), as well as mechanical failure, which is rare but does occur. People who receive LVADs typically take ANTICOAGULANT MEDICATIONS to reduce the risk for blood clots. Unlike heart transplant, rejection is not a problem with an LVAD because its composition is entirely synthetic and does not activate the immune system. An LVAD sometimes is a viable treatment option when a donor heart is rejected. New LVAD designs are becoming smaller and quieter and have fewer moving parts.

See also DONOR HEART; CARDIOVASCULAR SYSTEM; HEART, ARTIFICIAL; LIVING WITH HEART DISEASE.

left ventricular ejection fraction (LVEF) A calculation of the percentage of BLOOD that leaves the left ventricle with each contraction. The normal value is 55 percent. Percentages lower than normal suggest damage to the myocardium (HEART muscle) such as can occur with CARDIOMYOPATHY, HEART FAILURE, HEART ATTACK, and VALVE DISEASE. A low LVEF indicates that the heart's pumping ability is compromised. Measurements obtained during ECHOCARDIOGRAM, DOPPLER ULTRASOUND of the heart, MAGNETIC RESONANCE IMAGING (MRI), and RADIONUCLIDE SCAN can provide the data the cardiologist uses to calculate LVEF. Doctors consider heart failure severe when LVEF drops below 35 percent. LVEF has emerged as the most useful predictor of cardiac arrest risk. When the LVEF drops below 35 percent, the risk of cardiac arrest climbs significantly. At this point the cardiologist may suggest a prophylactic IMPLANTABLE CARDIOVERTER DEFIBRILLATOR (ICD).

See also MEDICATIONS TO TREAT HEART DISEASE.

Lenegre-Lev disease An ARRHYTHMIA, sometimes called Lev disease, in which the HEART's CONDUCTION PATHWAY becomes scarred (fibrotic) and calcified over time, resulting in complete HEART BLOCK. Although in some people Lenegre-Lev disease is inherited, in most people it is idiopathic (develops for unknown reasons). Because Lenegre-Lev disease is progressive, it is most common in people over age 70.

Symptoms and Diagnostic Path

Some people experience PALPITATIONS or LIGHTHEADEDNESS and SYNCOPE with EXERCISE, though most people do not have symptoms and the arrhythmia is usually detected when an ELECTROCARDIOGRAM (ECG) is performed for another reason. The ECG is diagnostic.

Treatment Options and Outlook

A person who has no symptoms typically requires no treatment other than regular assessment. When symptoms exist, the preferred treatment is implantation of a PACEMAKER to restore a regular heart rhythm. A pacemaker typically ends symptoms and is a successful long-term therapy. After the heart rhythm is restored and stabilized, most people return to their regular daily activities without restriction.

Risk Factors and Preventive Measures

Because the causes of Lenegre-Lev disease are unknown, there are no known preventive measures.

See also BRUGADA SYNDROME; LONG QT SYNDROME.

Lescol See FLUVASTATIN.

lesion A defined and specified location of tissue damage. Lesions affecting the HEART are called cardiac lesions; they include myocardium (heart muscle tissue) damaged or destroyed by CORONARY ARTERY DISEASE (CAD), ISCHEMIC HEART DISEASE (IHD), CARDIOMYOPATHY, HEART FAILURE, and congenital malformations of the heart and great vessels. Sometimes doctors create therapeutic lesions, as in ABLATION (destruction of some of the nerve pathways in the heart to stabilize a serious ARRHYTHMIA). Lesions having cardiovascular significance can affect the arteries and veins, brain (as in damage due to TRANSIENT ISCHEMIC ATTACK [TIA] or STROKE), and kidneys (possibly affecting BLOOD PRESSURE, BLOOD volume, and ELECTROLYTE balance). Lesions can be temporary or permanent. The extent and nature of a cardiac or cardiovascular lesion is a determining factor when considering treatment options.

See also CARDIOVASCULAR DISEASE; HEART DISEASE IN CHILDREN.

life expectancy The average age to which people born in a particular year can expect to live. Life expectancy differs for men, women, and ethnicity. Death that occurs at an age earlier than life expectancy is considered premature; CARDIOVASCULAR DISEASE (CVD) is the leading cause of premature death in the United States. Health experts estimate that if the major preventable forms of CVD were eliminated, life expectancy among Americans would rise by nearly seven years. Improvements in living standards and medical care have extended life expectancy across all ages, sometimes dramatically; this is expressed as the average number of years of life remaining.

At present, having one major form of CVD shortens life expectancy by two to four years; having two or more major forms of CVD further shortens life expectancy though the extent of this depends on the forms of heart disease and other health factors such as smoking and diabetes. Reducing personal risk factors for heart disease increases life expectancy; WEIGHT MANAGEMENT, smoking cessation, and controlling BLOOD PRESSURE provide the most substantial gains.

See also DEATHS FROM HEART DISEASE; LIFESTYLE AND HEART HEALTH.

lifestyle and heart health Though heredity, congenital factors, and aging influence the development of heart disease, the most significant risk factors for heart disease correlate to lifestyle: smoking, OBESITY, high-fat diet, and physical inactivity. Many health experts believe that lifestyle management alone, started in early childhood with nutritious eating habits and daily EXERCISE, could prevent 90 percent or more of adult heart disease among people under age 70. Numerous studies support this contention, and American physician Dean Ornish has developed a lifestyle-based approach, proven through clinical research studies, that halts and even reverses CARDIOVASCULAR DISEASE (CVD).

Smoking

Cigarette smoking accounts for nearly 150,000 deaths from heart disease in the United States each year, making smoking the leading cause of heart disease. Another 35,000 Americans die from heart disease as a consequence of secondary, or environmental, smoke exposure (so-called passive smoking). The effects of cigarette smoking on the cardiovascular system are numerous and devastating.

- NICOTINE and other chemicals in cigarette smoke damage the cells that line the walls of the arteries, causing the arteries to stiffen and become less flexible.

SELECTED U.S. LIFE EXPECTANCY FIGURES

Year of Birth	Life Expectancy: Male		Life Expectancy: Female	
	At Birth	In 2000 (years remaining)	At Birth	In 2000 (years remaining)
2000	74.3 years	74.3 years	79.7 years	79.7 years
1980	70.0 years	55.3 years	77.4 years	60.3 years
1960	66.6 years	36.7 years	73.1 years	41.0 years
1940	60.8 years	19.9 years	65.2 years	23.1 years
1920	53.6 years	7.6 years	54.6 years	9.1 years
1900	46.3 years	2.4 years	48.3 years	2.7 years

Source: National Vital Statistics Report Vol. 51, No. 3, December 19, 2002

- Nicotine is a potent toxin that kills nerve cells in the blood vessels, reducing the ability of the arteries to respond to changes in BLOOD PRESSURE and blood volume. Nicotine also poisons other cells in the body including the cells of the heart.

- Nicotine is a stimulant that increases the HEART RATE.

- The tars and other residues in cigarette smoke damage cells and the structure of the lungs, blocking and collapsing the alveoli (clusters of lung tissue where oxygen–CARBON DIOXIDE exchange takes place).

- People who smoke have diminished lung capacity; smoking two packs of cigarettes a day (moderate smoker) can cut lung capacity in half.

In aggregate, these changes result in various cardiovascular consequences including ATHEROSCLEROSIS (arterial plaque accumulations along the inner walls of the arteries), HYPERTENSION (high blood pressure), CORONARY ARTERY DISEASE (CAD), peripheral vascular disease (PVD), HEART FAILURE, HEART ATTACK, and STROKE. Avoiding exposure to cigarette smoke, by not smoking and by staying out of environments where others smoke, eliminates cigarette smoking as a risk factor. Among adults who do smoke, stopping has immediate and profound beneficial effects. One year after quitting, a smoker's risk for heart disease is cut in half; 15 smoke-free years restore the body's systems and functions to nearly the same level of cardiovascular risk as an adult of comparable age and general health status who never smoked.

Obesity

Obesity, defined in medical terms as a BODY MASS INDEX (BMI) of 30 or higher (body weight greater than 20 percent above the determined healthy marker for height), runs a close second to cigarette smoking in terms of its correlations to heart disease. More than 61 million Americans are obese; another 70 million are overweight (BMI between 25 and 29.9; body weight 10 to 20 percent greater than the determined healthy marker for height).

Obesity directly raises the risk for heart disease by increasing the effort the heart must exert to pump blood throughout the body. Excess body fat compresses cardiovascular structures such as arteries and veins and can apply pressure to the heart as well. Obesity also correlates to increased levels of TRIGLYCERIDES (the primary component of body fat, or adipose tissue) and other lipids in the body. Among adults who have been obese for a number of years, the presence of some form of cardiovascular disease—hypertension, HYPERLIPIDEMIA, atherosclerosis, and coronary artery disease being the most common—is almost certain. Obesity also increases the risk for health conditions that contribute to heart disease, notably INSULIN RESISTANCE and type 2 DIABETES. More than 95 percent of people with type 2 diabetes are overweight or obese.

Even modest weight loss produces measurable improvements in cardiovascular health. A loss of 10 to 20 pounds can decrease blood pressure by

10 mm Hg. Some people who take medication for hypertension or type 2 diabetes are able to wean off the medication with weight loss of 10 to 20 percent. Metabolism increases with regular physical activity, which improves insulin sensitivity (makes cells more receptive to insulin). Modest weight loss also relieves pressure against cardiovascular structures and organs, improving their abilities to function.

Diet and Eating Habits

Health experts recommend that adults obtain 30 percent or fewer of their daily calories from dietary fats (and 10 percent or fewer from saturated fats), 15 percent from protein, and 55 percent from carbohydrates. Since 1980 average caloric intake from dietary fat has dropped among Americans from 40 percent to about 35 percent. Surveys show that people are more mindful of the need to watch dietary fat intake, even when they indulge in high-fat foods. Even fast-food offerings now include lower fat options (though many fast-food items remain less healthy choices). Overall the eating habits of Americans have improved considerably since the early 1960s when researchers issued the first warnings about the correlations between diet and heart disease. However, the average American eats too much (consumes too many calories) and eats the wrong balance of foods for optimal health. The high-fat staples of today's fast-food menus—pizza, burgers, and fries—that account for about 10 percent of the American diet comprised less than 2 percent of the daily diet of Americans in the 1960s.

Good nutrition is important for meeting the body's needs to repair tissues and stave off disease processes. Fruits and vegetables contain minerals, vitamins, antioxidants, and other nutrients vital to body function. Numerous studies show that a diet following the Mediterranean style of eating—high consumption of fruits and vegetables, moderate consumption of whole grain products and fish, low consumption of red meats—supports improved cardiovascular health by slowing the processes that contribute to atherosclerosis and coronary artery disease.

Exercise

The body requires a minimal level of physical activity to maintain its peak metabolic efficiency, yet about 40 percent of Americans get no physical activity in their daily lives. Regular exercise, even mild activity such as walking for 10 to 15 minutes, has innumerable benefits particularly for the cardiovascular system. Health experts recommend that adults engage in moderate physical exercise for 30 to 60 minutes a day, five days a week. Numerous studies show that such a level of exercise improves the functioning of the cardiovascular system and the pulmonary system. Aerobic exercise—activity that increases the heart rate and breathing rate for at least 10 minutes at a time—has the greatest cardiovascular benefit. Walking at a moderate pace for 20 to 30 minutes at a time is sufficient to generate measurable differences within just a few weeks. Regular exercise also improves insulin sensitivity and helps the body to burn fat for energy. Physical activity builds muscle bulk, which further increases the body's energy needs to contribute to weight loss. People who regularly exercise tend to look and feel healthier—in large part because they are.

See also AFRICAN AMERICANS AND CARDIOVASCULAR DISEASE; LYON DIET HEART STUDY; ORNISH PROGRAM; TOBACCO USE; WOMEN AND HEART DISEASE.

light-headedness   A sensation of DIZZINESS, wooziness, or feeling as though one is about to faint. There are many possible causes for light-headedness, including exhaustion, emotional distress, hunger, HYPOGLYCEMIA (low BLOOD sugar), and physical exertion. Transient light-headedness is a common symptom in people who have cardiac rhythm abnormalities. Many medications, especially ANTIHYPERTENSIVE MEDICATIONS, can cause light-headedness and orthostatic HYPOTENSION (a sudden drop in BLOOD PRESSURE upon rising) as side effects. By itself, light-headedness seldom signals any significant health concerns unless it continues for longer than two days without an identifiable cause. Some people who experience light-headedness also may feel nauseated or actually may faint (lose consciousness). The first time this happens, or if it happens frequently, a doctor should evaluate it. Sometimes it is helpful to change medication doses or times, or even change to different medications.

See also SYNCOPE.

lipid-lowering medications A category of medications doctors prescribe to decrease BLOOD levels of TRIGLYCERIDES and cholesterol, which are chemical structures collectively known as LIPIDS or fatty acids. Elevated blood lipid levels present a significant risk for various forms of CARDIOVASCULAR DISEASE (CVD), notably ATHEROSCLEROSIS and CORONARY ARTERY DISEASE (CAD). Lipid-lowering medications are most effective when integrated with lifestyle modifications including low-fat diet and daily physical EXERCISE. There are several classifications of lipid-lowering medications that act in different ways. The medication the doctor chooses to prescribe depends on a number of factors including the nature of the person's lipid elevations, extent of cardiovascular disease, and lifestyle habits. Some lipid-lowering medications are most effective in targeting very low-density lipoprotein (VLDL), low-density lipoprotein (LDL), or triglycerides, for example, and others have more modest effects to lower total cholesterol levels. Some also raise high-density lipoprotein (HDL), the "good" cholesterol.

Bile Acid Sequestrants

Bile acid sequestrants, also called bile acid resins, were the first lipid-lowering medications to become available. They work by binding with bile, which contains cholesterol, in the intestinal tract. The bile and cholesterol are then excreted from the body in the feces. The three bile acid sequestrants currently available in the United States are:

- CHOLESTYRAMINE, available in generic versions as well as the brand-name products Questran, Locholest, and Prevalite

- COLESTIPOL, available in generic versions as well as the brand-name product Colestid

- COLESEVELAM, available in generic versions as well as the brand-name product WellChol

Bile acid sequestrants alone typically reduce blood levels of LDL by about 20 percent, which often is enough in mild to moderate HYPERCHOLESTEROLEMIA to put LDL in the "normal" range and decrease total cholesterol by about 5 to 10 percent. Bile acid sequestrants have no effect on HDL. Some people experience a rise in blood levels of triglycerides when taking bile acid sequestrants, however, making it important to monitor blood lipid levels for the duration of the lipid-lowering therapy. Doctors sometimes prescribe a bile acid sequestrant in combination with another type of lipid-lowering medication, an HMG CoA REDUCTASE INHIBITOR MEDICATION (also called statin medications). This can decrease LDL levels by 40 percent or more and tends to offset any rise in triglycerides.

Bile acid sequestrants are available in powder form, which must be mixed with juice or soft foods such as applesauce, and tablets. It is important to drink an increased amount of water daily, as bile acid sequestrants can cause constipation and fecal impaction. They also can cause other forms of gastric distress including dyspepsia (upset or irritable stomach), nausea, and flatulence (gas). Bile acid sequestrants interact with numerous medications including many prescribed to treat heart disease. Among them are BETA ANTAGONIST MEDICATIONS and some DIURETIC MEDICATIONS taken to treat HYPERTENSION (high BLOOD PRESSURE) and HEART FAILURE, some ANTIARRHYTHMIA MEDICATIONS, and most ANTICOAGULANT MEDICATIONS taken to prevent blood clots.

Because they cause the body to excrete more of the lipids that normally serve as carriers for fat molecules (fatty acids cannot dissolve in the blood), bile acid sequestrants inhibit the absorption of fat soluble vitamins such as vitamin A, vitamin E, and vitamin K. A shortage of vitamin K can cause bleeding problems, which can become compounded in people who also are taking anticoagulant medications. Supplements of these nutrients, when the doctor recommends them, should be taken one hour before or six hours after the bile acid sequestrant dose.

HMG CoA Reductase Inhibitors (Statins)

HMG CoA reductase inhibitor medications block the action of an enzyme the liver requires to synthesize cholesterol, effectively curtailing cholesterol production. These drugs, also called statins, are the cornerstone of drug therapy for various forms of HYPERLIPIDEMIA. Doctors expect to see total cholesterol drop by about 25 percent and LDL by about 35 percent within two to three months of initiating statin therapy; aggressive lifestyle modifications (particularly an increase in daily exercise) can cause these cholesterol levels to decline even more. Statins also can raise HDL by 10 to 20 percent, further protecting the cardiovascular system.

Doctors consider prescribing statin lipid-lowering medications when high blood cholesterol levels, especially LDL and VLDL, do not come down as much as desired with lifestyle modifications such as low-fat diet and daily exercise. Doctors tend also to prescribe statins for people who have modestly elevated blood cholesterol levels but multiple other risk factors for heart disease such as smoking or family history. Health experts now recommend that nearly everyone who experiences a heart attack begin taking a statin medication afterward to prevent subsequent heart attacks (called secondary prevention); statins also have the ability to reduce inflammation in the walls of the arteries, which decreases arterial plaque accumulation.

Statins interact with numerous other medications and can cause gastrointestinal distress particularly at the onset of therapy. A very rare but potentially life-threatening side effect is RHABDO-MYOLYSIS, in which muscle tissue begins to rapidly break down and release large amounts of protein into the bloodstream. The excess of protein overwhelms the kidneys, which can experience damage and failure. Symptoms of rhabdomyolysis include extreme weakness and muscle pain and require emergency medical attention.

Fibric Acid Derivatives (Fibrates)

Fibric acid derivatives, or fibrates, block the liver from synthesizing the lipoproteins that serve as carriers for triglycerides, effectively limiting the level of triglycerides that can circulate in the bloodstream. This action also permits the liver to increase synthesis of HDL carriers, increasing the level of circulating HDL. The fibrates available in the United States include clofibrate (Atromid-S), FENOFIBRATE (Tricor), and GEMFIBROZIL (Lopid). These medications typically reduce triglycerides up to 60 percent and raise HDL about 25 percent. They have very little, and often no, effect on LDL and VLDL or may cause LDL/VLDL to increase. Doctors typically prescribe fibrates for people who have familial HYPERTRIGLYCERIDEMIA or elevated blood triglycerides levels without corresponding increases in total cholesterol or LDL/VLDL.

Sometimes doctors prescribe a fibrate in combination with a statin, particularly for people who have very high blood levels of both triglycerides and LDL/VLDL (as in familial hyperlipidemia). Such a combination appears to increase the risk for the rare side effect rhabdomyolysis; people taking the

LIPID-LOWERING MEDICATIONS			
Classification	**Medications**	**Example Brand Name Products**	**Therapeutic Benefit**
Bile acid sequestrant	Cholestyramine	Questran, Questran Light, Locholest, Prevalite	Reduce LDL 20 percent; reduce total cholesterol 5 to 10 percent
	Colestipol	Colestid	
	Colesevelam	WellChol	
HMG CoA reductase inhibitor (statin)	Atorvastatin	Lipitor	Reduce LDL/VLDL 35 percent, reduce total cholesterol by 25 percent, raise HDL by 10 to 20 percent
	Fluvastatin	Lescol	
	Lovastatin	Mevacor	
	Pravastatin	Pravachol	
	Simvastatin	Zocor	
Fibric acid derivative (fibrate)	Clofibrate	Atromid-S	Reduce triglycerides by 60 percent; raise HDL by 25 percent
	Fenofibrate	Tricor	
	Gemfibrozil	Lopid	

two kinds of medications should receive frequent and regular blood tests to measure the amount of protein in the blood as well as cholesterol and triglycerides levels. Clofibrate has the highest rate of side effects and generally is prescribed only when blood triglycerides levels are extremely high (over 5000) or other lipid-lowering medications have been ineffective. Common and relatively benign side effects of the fibric acid derivatives include gastrointestinal distress (which often goes away after a few weeks of taking the medication) and increased risk for developing gallstones.

See also ATHEROSCLEROSIS; CHOLESTEROL, BLOOD; LIFESTYLE AND HEART HEALTH; INFLAMMATION AND HEART DISEASE; MEDICATIONS TO TREAT HEAT DISEASE; NUTRITION AND DIET; PLAQUE, ARTERIAL.

lipids A classification of organic molecules (biochemicals), also called fatty acids. Lipids are essential for numerous functions within the body. They have primary roles in cell membrane development and maintenance, energy storage, and nutrient transport. There are three main kinds of lipids in the human body:

- TRIGLYCERIDES, the most abundant lipid found in body fat (adipose tissue) and a key source of cellular energy
- phospholipids, which are the essential structures of cell membranes
- sterols, which help to transport and dissolve fat-soluble substances and form the basis of other chemicals in the body such as hormones

Lipids are necessary for health and for life. They become health problems only when they are present in excess, as in conditions such as HYPERCHOLESTEROLEMIA and HYPERTRIGLYCERIDEMIA. During digestion dietary lipids are broken down into their core components, which the bloodstream then carries to the liver. The liver reassembles the components into the lipid structures the body needs, such as lipoprotein (lipids that combine with proteins) and cholesterol. Other lipids are formed through chemical interactions that take place in the blood and tissues. Many factors influence lipid synthesis (production) and metabolism (cellular consumption), including dietary lipids and physical activity.

See also ATHEROSCLEROSIS; CHOLESTEROL, BLOOD; EXERCISE; LIPID-LOWERING MEDICATIONS; NUTRITION AND DIET.

Lipitor See ATORVASTATIN.

lipoproteins See LIPIDS.

lisinopril A medication taken to treat HYPERTENSION (high BLOOD PRESSURE). Common brand names available in the United States include Prinivil and Zestril. Lisinopril is an ANGIOTENSIN-CONVERTING ENZYME (ACE) INHIBITOR MEDICATION that works by preventing the RENIN-ANGIOTENSIN-ALDOSTERONE (RAA) HORMONAL SYSTEM, one of the body's primary blood pressure regulation mechanisms, from raising blood pressure. Lisinopril, like other ACE inhibitors, dilates the peripheral arteries and arterioles to reduce the resistance blood encounters. Doctors often prescribe lisinopril in combination with a DIURETIC MEDICATION for optimal control of blood pressure, and frequently in combination with DIGOXIN to treat HEART FAILURE. There is growing evidence that ACE inhibitors such as lisinopril help to strengthen myocardial cell contractions following HEART ATTACK (MYOCARDIAL INFARCTION). CLINICAL RESEARCH STUDIES continue to explore this issue. Common side effects of lisinopril include headache, DIZZINESS, cough, orthostatic HYPOTENSION, and weakness. Rarely, ACE inhibitors can cause kidney distress or failure and angioedema (swelling into the tissues due to excess fluid).

See also ANGIOTENSIN-CONVERTING ENZYME; ANGIOTENSIN II RECEPTOR ANTAGONIST MEDICATIONS; ANTIHYPERTENSIVE MEDICATIONS; MEDICATIONS TO TREAT HEART DISEASE.

living will See ADVANCE DIRECTIVES.

living with heart disease More than 80 million adult Americans—about 36 percent of the population—live with some form of HEART DISEASE that

AMERICANS LIVING WITH HEART DISEASE

Form of Heart Disease*	Number of Americans
Overall	80 million
Angina pectoris	9.8 million
Coronary artery disease (CAD)/ ischemic heart disease (IHD)	16.8 million
Arrhythmias	4.3 million
Heart attack	7.6 million
Heart failure	5.7 million
Hypertension (high blood pressure)	73.6 million
Peripheral vascular disease (PVD)	8 million
Stroke	6.5 million

Source: American Heart Association: Heart Disease and Stroke Statistics Update 2009.
*Includes overlaps among those with multiple forms of heart disease.

ranges in severity from mild to incapacitating. Many of them have had to make adjustments in their lifestyles though continue to enjoy many of their favorite activities thanks in large part to incredible advances in medicine and technology over the last decades of the 20th century and first decade of the 21st century. At present about 80 percent of people of all ages who have some form of heart disease are able to work without restriction due to health considerations. For those between the ages of 50 and 60, however—considered the peak years for productivity and achievement—only about 40 percent who have diagnosed heart disease can continue employment without restriction. By age 70 and older, more than 80 percent of people with heart disease need help with the ACTIVITIES OF DAILY LIVING (ADLS)—the routine tasks of everyday life. About half a million Americans of working age who would like to be employed are unable to work because of their heart disease.

Lifestyle Management

Lifestyle management is essential for satisfactory quality of life. People who know they have heart disease may make lifestyle modifications to support improved cardiovascular health or may choose to forgo such changes. With adequate attention, lifestyle management of factors such as smoking, diet, and exercise can extend life as well as improve quality of life. Some people resist making changes

that they view as "taking the pleasure" out of life. This is a matter of perception; many more people are eager to implement changes that make it more likely they will live and enjoy favorite activities for longer.

People who have limiting heart disease, particularly end-stage HEART FAILURE and severely reduced CARDIAC CAPACITY following heart attack, may need additional assistance such as short-term care in a skilled nursing facility (SNF) or HOME HEALTH CARE nursing after hospital discharge and help with activities of daily living (ADLs). People who have had HEART ATTACKS should enter CARDIAC REHABILITATION programs after hospital discharge. Other health conditions such as diabetes and kidney disease can complicate the overall health picture.

When cardiovascular crisis strikes without warning, typically in people with undiagnosed heart disease, families often are unprepared for the additional care that becomes necessary. It can take several months to a year or longer for someone who has experienced a major cardiac event such as heart attack to reach a level of stability in everyday activities. A quarter of men and half of women who have heart attacks are unable to return to the lifestyles they had before their attacks. There may be cognitive as well as physical challenges. A support group can provide a venue for sharing information and experiences for people living with heart disease as well as for loved ones and caregivers.

It helps when other family members can make the same kinds of lifestyle changes as the person with heart disease. Perhaps the entire family can enjoy low-fat meals and take walks together after meals. All lifestyle modifications recommended for people recovering from heart attack or attempting to improve cardiovascular status are beneficial for people who do not have heart disease and can help prevent them from developing heart disease. The support and encouragement of loved ones can mean the difference between successful cardiac rehabilitation and repeated cardiovascular crises. If DIABETES is a contributing health factor, all people living in the household should attend diabetes education classes to learn about the disease of diabetes and successful strategies for health improvement and maintenance. Smoking cessation is crucial.

Medical Management

Most people with diagnosed heart disease of any kind take medications to treat their conditions. Some may take just a single medication, such as for mild hypertension or hyperlipidemia, with recommendations for lifestyle modifications. Many people who have heart disease have overlapping conditions and take multiple medications; cardiovascular drugs account for the second-largest segment of the pharmaceutical industry. Managing the medical care of the person with heart disease often requires coordinating medication schedules as well as other health-care needs such as doctors' appointments and follow-up or evaluatory tests.

Everyone who takes medications (for heart disease as well as for other medical conditions) should keep written records of what medications they take, the frequencies or times they take them, and the names of the doctors who prescribed them. Each time the doctor prescribes a new medication, it is important to ask the doctor or pharmacist whether the new medication will have any interactions with current medications. People with heart disease should receive regular medical checkups from their cardiologists, internists, or family practitioners that include blood pressure readings, blood cholesterol and triglycerides levels, and other relevant laboratory tests that can help to monitor cardiovascular status.

See also CARDIAC REHABILITATION; DEPRESSION; MEDICATION SIDE EFFECTS; ORNISH PROGRAM; STRESS AND HEART DISEASE; STRESS REDUCTION TECHNIQUES; STROKE; YOGA.

long QT syndrome (LQTS) A disorder of cardiac repolarization, often genetic, causing increased risk of CARDIAC ARREST. On an ELECTROCARDIOGRAM (ECG) the points that identify the electrical activity of this phase are labeled as Q, R, S, and T. The QT interval measures the length of time it takes the HEART to depolarize (discharge electrical current) and repolarize (recharge for the next cardiac cycle). Cardiologists typically measure the QT interval in milliseconds; a normal QT interval is 440 milliseconds (four-tenths of a second). Various factors can cause a somewhat prolonged QT interval, including other arrhythmias; in general, a QT interval longer than 480 milliseconds is considered diagnostic of long QT syndrome (LQTS). The extended polarization of myocardial (heart muscle) cells can result in erratic and extremely rapid contractions called TORSADES DE POINTES (TdP), a form of ventricular tachycardia.

Symptoms and Diagnostic Path

LQTS often presents no symptoms and is diagnosed incidentally when an ECG is conducted for other reasons or when the person experiences cardiac arrest and is resuscitated. Some people experience episodes of SYNCOPE (fainting), typically with physical exertion or emotional stress. In young people especially there often is not a cardiac evaluation because there are no other symptoms of heart disease and LQTS is relatively rare. However, LQTS is the leading cause of SUDDEN CARDIAC ARREST among young people. Health experts estimate that 50,000 Americans have LQTS, and that 3,000 die each year from sudden cardiac arrest.

Treatment Options and Outlook

In most people with LQTS BETA ANTAGONIST MEDICATIONS restore and maintain a normal heart rate. When this treatment is not effective, the cardiologist may place an IMPLANTABLE CARDIOVERTER DEFIBRILLATOR (ICD) to monitor the heart rhythm and deliver an electrical shock to return it to normal when necessary. Aside from avoiding medications known to sometimes cause LQTS, there is no way to prevent development of the acquired form. People who have LQTS should consider genetic evaluation to determine the probability of passing the disorder to their children.

Risk Factors and Preventive Measures

LQTS can be inherited or acquired; the diagnostic process and treatment options are the same for either. Researchers know of mutations that occur in six genes among people who have inherited forms of this disorder. There are two kinds of inherited LQTS: autosomal recessive (each parent has LQTS and carries the defective genes, and the child inherits both sets) and autosomal dominant (one parent has LQTS and passes the defective genes to his or her child). Those who have autosomal recessive LQTS also often are deaf; hearing is not affected in autosomal dominant LQTS. The mutations affect the functioning of ion channels (the pathways that electrically charged particles follow) in the myocardium.

Medication side effects are the most common cause of acquired LQTS. Among the medications that significantly increase the risk for LQTS are sotalol, dofetilide, erythromycin, promethazine, thorazine, droperidol, haloperidol, mellaril, and pentamadine. There are numerous other medications that people diagnosed with LQTS should avoid. The University of Arizona Health Services maintains a current listing of these medications at www.azcert.org.

See also BRUGADA SYNDROME; CONDUCTION SYSTEM; JERVELLE AND LANGE-NIELSEN SYNDROME; LIVING WITH HEART DISEASE; ROMANO-WARD SYNDROME.

Loniten   See MINOXIDIL.

loop diuretics   See DIURETIC MEDICATIONS.

Lopid   See GEMFIBROZIL.

Lopressor   See METOPROLOL.

losartan   A medication taken to treat HYPERTENSION (high BLOOD PRESSURE). Common brand names available in the United States include Cozaar. Losartan is an ANGIOTENSIN II RECEPTOR ANTAGONIST MEDICATION that works by blocking the action of the RENIN-ANGIOTENSIN-ALDOSTERONE (RAA) HORMONAL SYSTEM to raise blood pressure. It can take up to six weeks for losartan to achieve optimal effectiveness, though most people experience a drop in blood pressure within one or two weeks. Doctors often prescribe losartan in combination with a DIURETIC MEDICATION such as HYDROCHLOROTHIAZIDE for optimal blood pressure regulation. Losartan can cause gastrointestinal distress, headache, DIZZINESS, SLEEP DISTURBANCES, and dry mouth, though these side effects typically go away within a few weeks of taking the medication. Rare but serious side effects include kidney damage and failure, ventricular ARRHYTHMIAS, and HEART ATTACK or STROKE. Women who are pregnant should not take losartan, as angiotensin II receptor blockers are known to cause birth defects in the developing fetus.

See also ANGIOTENSIN-CONVERTING ENZYME (ACE) INHIBITOR MEDICATIONS; ANTIHYPERTENSIVE MEDICATIONS; ANGIOTENSIN II RECEPTOR; MEDICATIONS TO TREAT HEART DISEASE.

Lotensin   See BENAZEPRIL.

lovastatin   A medication taken to decrease elevated blood cholesterol and blood TRIGLYCERIDES levels. Common brand-name products available in the United States include Mevocor. Lovastatin belongs to the family of LIPID-LOWERING MEDICATIONS called HMG CoA REDUCTASE INHIBITOR MEDICATIONS or statins; it works by preventing the liver from synthesizing (producing) cholesterol. The statin medications also have an anti-inflammatory effect on the cells that line the walls of the arteries, helping to prevent the circumstances that encourage arterial plaque to accumulate and ATHEROSCLEROSIS to develop. Doctors often prescribe a statin medication such as lovastatin following HEART ATTACK (MYOCARDIAL INFARCTION) to reduce the risk for subsequent heart attacks. Lovastatin, like other lipid-lowering medications, achieves the greatest effect when combined with lifestyle modifications that include low-fat diet and daily EXERCISE.

Gastrointestinal side effects such as nausea, stomach irritation (dyspepsia), flatulence (gas), and CONSTIPATION are common when beginning treatment with lovastatin; these side effects typically go away after taking the medication for a few weeks. Lovastatin, like all HMG CoA reductase inhibitors, can interact with numerous medications, including the immunosuppressive drug CYCLOSPORINE (taken to prevent rejection after organ transplant), DIGOXIN, other classifications of lipid-lowering medications, and oral contraceptives (birth control pills). GRAPEFRUIT AND GRAPEFRUIT JUICE interfere with lovastatin. A very rare but life-threatening side effect is RHABDOMYOLYSIS, a condition in which muscle tissue breaks down. The resulting release of protein overwhelms the kidneys and can cause permanent kidney failure.

See also FENOFIBRATE; GEMFIBROZIL; INFLAMMA-TION AND HEART DISEASE; LIFESTYLE AND HEART HEALTH; MEDICATIONS TO TREAT HEART DISEASE; NUTRITION AND DIET; PLAQUE, ARTERIAL.

low blood pressure   See HYPOTENSION.

Lown-Ganong-Levine (LGL) syndrome   An ARRHYTHMIA classified as a paroxysmal supraventricular tachycardia (PSVT) involving an unknown ACCESSORY PATHWAY. LGL occurs in basically the same location in the HEART as WOLFF-PARKINSON-WHITE (WPW) SYNDROME, but the accessory pathway is not visible on ELECTROCARDIOGRAM (ECG).

Symptoms and Diagnostic Path

Symptoms are episodic and may include LIGHT-HEADEDNESS, DIZZINESS, PALPITATIONS, and occasionally SYNCOPE (fainting). Some people also experience DYSPNEA (difficulty breathing) and CHEST PAIN, particularly if they have underlying CORONARY ARTERY DISEASE (CAD). The diagnostic path includes ELECTROCARDIOGRAM (ECG) and BLOOD tests to evaluate electrolyte levels in the blood. The cardiologist may also request blood thyroid levels because hyperthyroidism (overactive thyroid) can cause many of the same symptoms, although it requires a different and noncardiac therapeutic course. Because the arrhythmia does not show up on conventional ECG, electrophysiology study (a CARDIAC CATHETERIZATION procedure in which the arrhythmia is provoked through electrical stimulation of the involved area of the heart) is necessary to make the diagnosis.

Treatment Options and Outlook

Treatment may be with medications such as beta blockers and calcium channel blockers or ABLATION. The cardiologist may also use intravenous ADENOSINE to restore a normal rhythm if TACHYCARDIA is present at the time of the examination.

Risk Factors and Preventive Measures

Because doctors do not know what causes Lown-Ganong-Levine syndrome, there are no identifiable risk factors or preventive measures.

See also BETA ANTAGONIST MEDICATIONS.

Lozol   See INDAPAMIDE.

lung capacity   The volume of air the lungs are capable of holding. The total lung capacity of a healthy adult is four to six liters (4,000 to 6,000 cubic centimeters). Body height influences lung size and hence lung capacity; men typically have greater lung capacity than women because men generally are taller than women. As well, people who live at higher altitudes have larger lung capacities because there is less oxygen in the air, so the lungs must take in more volume with each breath to achieve the needed oxygen content. Other variables that affect lung capacity are aerobic FITNESS, smoking, CARDIOVASCULAR DISEASE (CVD), pulmonary disease, and age. A device called a spirometer measures lung volumes (except residual volume, which must be calculated). Those commonly measured to determine lung capacity include:

- Tidal volume—the amount of air taken into the lungs with each normal breath; in a healthy adult, this is about 500 cubic centimeters.
- Vital capacity—the amount of air taken into the lungs on the first inspiration following a deep exhalation; it correlates to sex, age, and height.
- Residual volume—the amount of air remaining in the lungs after a deep exhalation; in a healthy adult, this is about 1,500 cubic centimeters (calculated).

Lung capacity diminishes with age as the lungs lose some of their elasticity, which limits their ability to expand and contract. Regular physical activity, particularly aerobic EXERCISE (exercise sustained over a period of time that increases the heart rate and breathing rate), even at modest levels helps to keep the lungs functioning at maximum capability and can increase lung capacity for nearly all people except those who have end-stage pulmonary or cardiovascular disease. When lung capacity decreases, the heart must work harder to move enough oxygen (via the blood) through the body. Severely compromised lung capacity, as occurs with advanced CHRONIC OBSTRUCTIVE PULMONARY DISEASE (COPD), can lead to right ventricular dysfunction and PULMONARY CONGESTION/PULMONARY

EDEMA; PULMONARY HYPERTENSION, and congestive HEART FAILURE.

See also AEROBIC CAPACITY; AGING, EFFECT ON CARDIOVASCULAR SYSTEM; CARDIOMYOPATHY; CARDIOVASCULAR SYSTEM; PULMONARY FUNCTION.

Lyme disease An infection caused by the bacterium *Borrelia burgdorferi,* which is transmitted by the bite of a deer tick. Mice and deer harbor the bacteria. Lyme disease gets its name from the location where the disease was first identified, the town of Old Lyme, Connecticut.

Symptoms and Diagnostic Path

The initial infection often is mild and produces vague symptoms including rash at the site of the tick bite, a low-grade fever, headache, and itching. Some people immediately experience joint inflammation and pain, muscle pain, and generalized stiffness as well as lethargy; others experience these symptoms months to years after the initial infection. Diagnosis is by blood tests that detect antibodies to *B. burgdorferi.* When Lyme disease goes undiagnosed and untreated, it becomes latent and resurfaces with secondary symptoms that can include involvement of the neurological system and the cardiovascular system.

Lyme disease that is not treated adequately in its secondary stage can again become latent and resurface years after the initial infection as tertiary disease. In this advanced stage of infection, symptoms are severe and damage to the cardiovascular and neurological systems can be permanent.

Treatment Options and Outlook

Treatment for the initial infection is antibiotics, which cures the disease and prevents complications.

Treatment for latent Lyme disease is with stronger antibiotics to eliminate the infection and appropriate therapy for secondary symptoms. Cardiovascular complications can include inflammation of the heart valves, ARRHYTHMIAS, CARDIOMYOPATHY, and HEART FAILURE. Often when the infection is cured the cardiovascular symptoms go away as well, though in some people the CARDIOVASCULAR DISEASE (CVD) becomes permanent.

Treatment for tertiary Lyme disease is high-dose injection of antibiotic, as well as appropriate interventions to manage other symptoms.

Risk Factors and Preventive Measures

People who live in areas where Lyme disease is prevalent—notably the Pacific coast, the Northeast, and the upper Midwest regions of the United States—should be aware of the early symptoms of Lyme disease, check themselves for tick bites during peak tick season (summer and early fall), and see their doctors for evaluation of any symptoms that could be Lyme disease. Early diagnosis and treatment is the most effective way to preclude more severe and possibly permanent complications. About 8 to 10 percent of people who develop secondary or tertiary Lyme disease have cardiovascular complications.

See also VALVE DISEASE.

Lyon Diet Heart Study A randomized, controlled clinical research study conducted in Lyon, France, that compared the effects of a typical Mediterranean diet to those of an unregulated diet with regard to cardiovascular consequences after a first HEART ATTACK. The final findings, reported in 1999, provided what researchers consider to be among the most conclusive evidence that diet can significantly reduce the risk for subsequent HEART DISEASE and heart attack after a first heart attack. All participants—study and control—had recently experienced one heart attack. Those who followed the Mediterranean diet—a diet with 30 percent or fewer calories from fat and 10 percent or fewer from saturated fat and high in vegetables, fruits, whole grains and products, and fish—had a 50 to 70 percent lower risk for repeated (recurrent) heart disease including heart attack at the final follow-up for the study, 46 months after its inception.

See also LIFESTYLE AND HEART HEALTH; LIVING WITH HEART DISEASE; NUTRITION AND DIET; OMEGA FATTY ACIDS.

magnesium A mineral that is essential for development and strength of the bones and teeth, muscle contractions, protein synthesis, nerve signal conduction, function of the immune system, numerous enzyme-based processes within the body including many related to CALCIUM, and proper function of the HEART. The average adult body contains a little more than an ounce of magnesium, about 95 percent of which is in the bones and teeth. Magnesium, like calcium and POTASSIUM, is an ELECTROLYTE (ionized substance) that can carry an electrical charge. The correct balance of magnesium in the body is crucial for HEART RATE and heart rhythm; abnormal magnesium levels can cause ARRHYTHMIAS, ineffective contractions, and other disturbances of heart function. The body can withdraw some magnesium from the bones but not usually enough to make up for significant depletion and not to the extent that it can withdraw calcium from the bones.

Most people receive adequate amounts of magnesium through dietary sources such as meats, nuts, dark green leafy vegetables, whole grains and whole grain products, and dairy products. Drinking water with a high mineral content also contains magnesium and can be a significant source for people who do not otherwise consume magnesium-rich foods. Many over-the-counter laxatives and antacids contain high levels of magnesium; chronic use of these products can cause magnesium excess. Magnesium depletion can occur with chronic alcohol abuse, kidney disease, and osteoporosis. DIURETIC MEDICATIONS and DIGOXIN, taken long-term, can cause magnesium depletion in many people, especially the elderly who may not eat many foods that are the natural sources for magnesium. As well the body becomes less efficient with age at extracting minerals from dietary sources, making it necessary to consume higher amounts of magnesium-rich foods.

Sometimes doctors recommend magnesium supplements for people who are taking digoxin and/or diuretic medications long-term, such as to treat HYPERTENSION (high BLOOD PRESSURE) or HEART FAILURE. It is important for people taking digoxin and other DIGITALIS medications to have periodic blood tests to measure magnesium levels. However, people who have HEART DISEASE should not take magnesium supplements unless their doctors recommend they do so. Low magnesium levels often cause muscle cramps and can cause arrhythmias. Depletion of calcium often accompanies magnesium depletion, as these minerals come from many of the same sources and interact in many body functions.

See also CALCIUM CYCLE; CARDIAC CYCLE; NUTRITION AND DIET.

magnetic resonance imaging (MRI) An imaging technology that allows doctors to examine inner organs and structures without invading the body. Magnetic resonance imaging (MRI) uses a combination of radiofrequency signals and magnetic signals to generate multidimensional images representing body structures and functions. During MRI the person lies flat on a table that moves inside a large tubelike structure. The outer ring of the tube contains powerful magnets that cause the hydrogen atoms in all of the body's cells to align in the same direction. The inner ring contains coils that emit radiofrequency signals that activate the hydrogen atoms. When the radiofrequency signals stop the atoms again realign themselves, sending radiofrequency signals back out to the MRI machine, which registers them and sends them to a computer that translates them into visual images. The various cells in the body realign at different and unique rates. MRI can produce extraordinarily high-resolution images that show minute variations in structure or function.

Cardiologists use MRI to help identify areas of tissue death following HEART ATTACK (MYOCARDIAL INFARCTION). MRI also can help to diagnose congenital malformations of the HEART; heart valve disease; tumors such as MYXOMAS or metastatic cancers; and inflammation or infection of the sac surrounding the heart (PERICARDITIS), the lining of the heart (ENDOCARDITIS) and the heart muscle itself (MYOCARDITIS). A new application of MRI is MRI angiography, sometimes referred to as MRA or three-dimensional (3-D) cardiac angiography, that combines MRI and the injection of contrast medium into the blood vessels to generate high-resolution images of blood flow.

MRI does not cause any discomfort or require any preparation (unless combined with angiography, in which case there can be discomfort from insertion of the IV needle for administering the contrast medium). It takes 15 minutes to an hour to complete an MRI of the heart, depending on the number of views the cardiologist wants. Some people find it difficult to lie still for this amount of time, or feel claustrophobic inside the MRI equipment. The radiologist may give a mild sedative when this is the case. Because the MRI magnets are very powerful, no metal objects, including eyeglasses and removable dental appliances, are permitted in the procedure room. People who have PACEMAKERS or IMPLANTABLE CARDIOVERTENDEFIBRILLATOR (ICDs) should not have MRI.

See also COMPUTED TOMOGRAPHY (CT) SCAN; ECHOCARDIOGRAM; ELECTRON BEAM COMPUTED TOMOGRAPHY (EBCT) SCAN; POSITRON EMISSION TOMOGRAPHY (PET) SCAN; SINGLE PHOTON EMISSION COMPUTED TOMOGRAPHY (SPECT) SCAN.

Marfan syndrome An inherited connective tissue disorder that affects nearly every body system including the HEART and CARDIOVASCULAR SYSTEM. In Marfan syndrome there is a mutation in the gene FBN1 on chromosome 15. This gene instructs the body's processes related to synthesis of fibrillin, a protein necessary for the formation of connective tissue throughout the body. As a result connective tissues are not as elastic or strong as they should be. The effects can be mild and barely perceptible, as occurs in about 25 percent of people who have Marfan syndrome, or significant. About one in 20,000 Americans have Marfan syndrome, which is autosomal dominant in its inheritance pattern (receiving the defective gene from either parent can cause the disorder). Researchers believe spontaneous mutation of the FBN1 gene also occurs (the gene becomes defective during the early phases of cell reproduction soon after conception).

Symptoms and Diagnostic Path

People with Marfan syndrome tend to be unusually tall and thin with features that are thin and elongated. They often have deformities of the spine (scoliosis) and rib cage (ribs that either sink in or bulge outward because the cartilage attaching them to the sternum is weakened). These physical traits along with other symptoms such as joints that easily dislocate and displaced lenses in the eyes typically are the first indications that cause doctors to investigate for Marfan syndrome. Some people with very mild expressions of the disorder may reach middle adulthood before being diagnosed.

About 90 percent of people with Marfan syndrome have cardiovascular consequences, which can begin in childhood or early adulthood and include:

- Aortic root dilation and dissection—Thinning, stretching, bulging, and rupturing of the aortic root, the broad base of the aorta where it arises from the heart's left ventricle.

- ANEURYSM—Weakening and rupturing of an arterial wall, typically the abdominal aorta though it can affect other major arteries in the body.

- CARDIOMYOPATHY and cardiomegaly—Stretching (dilation) and enlargement of the heart that can lead to HEART FAILURE.

- Malfunctioning and sometimes malformed heart valves; BICUSPID AORTIC VALVE (in which the aortic valve has two leaflets, or flaps, instead of the normal three) and MITRAL VALVE PROLAPSE (an improperly formed mitral valve) are common in people with Marfan syndrome.

- ARRHYTHMIAS that are related to the changes in conductivity of myocardial tissues.

There is no definitive test for Marfan syndrome; diagnosis is a process of eliminating other possible conditions and looking for symptoms and changes within the body known to be components of Marfan syndrome. The severity of symptoms varies among people.

Treatment Options and Outlook

Treatment targets specific problems that arise. For cardiovascular problems treatment may include surgery to repair malfunctioning valves and dilations or aneurysms; BETA ANTAGONIST MEDICATIONS to regulate HEART RATE; ANTICOAGULANT MEDICATIONS for people who have had VALVE REPAIR AND REPLACEMENT operations; and medications that strengthen the heartbeat to reduce the risk for heart failure. Untreated Marfan syndrome nearly always results in early death, typically before age 30; with appropriate treatment and diligent medical management, many people who have Marfan syndrome can enjoy relatively normal lives.

Risk Factors and Preventive Measures

Marfan syndrome is a genetic disorder. People who have Marfan syndrome have a 50 percent chance of passing the condition to a child. About 25 percent of Marfan syndrome occurs spontaneously (with no family history).

See also SURGERY TO TREAT CARDIOVASCULAR DISEASE.

margarine See NUTRITION AND DIET.

marijuana, effects on the heart A number of studies suggest that the risk for HEART ATTACK increases fourfold during the first hour of smoking marijuana among people who have HEART DISEASE, a direct result of marijuana's effect to raise HEART RATE and BLOOD PRESSURE. This risk is about the same increase in risk that a sedentary person faces if he or she were to suddenly engage in strenuous physical activity such as running. For people who do not have heart disease the increase is negligible,

as is the increased risk with running or other physical exertion for someone who has a high FITNESS LEVEL. Researchers are unsure what causes these elevations though they suspect a combination of the smoke's effect on the lungs (altering oxygen exchange) and the action of marijuana's primary chemical ingredient, tetrahydrocannabinol (THC). Some studies using an aerosol form of the drug produce results that are similar but not quite as intense.

See also COCAINE AND HEART ATTACK; DRUG ABUSE AND HEART DISEASE.

marrow See BLOOD.

Mavik See TRANDOLAPRIL.

maximum heart rate See HEART RATE.

mechanical circulatory support (MCS) The use of mechanical devices to supplement or take over the cardiovascular functions that supply the body with oxygenated BLOOD. Such use may be short-term (hours), as with the HEART-LUNG BYPASS MACHINE during OPEN-HEART SURGERY, or long-term, as with an artificial heart or ventricular assist device (days to months). These technologies have saved thousands of lives and make possible the highly sophisticated heart operations performed today. Mechanical circulatory support (MCS) devices include:

- Artificial heart, several models of which can be implanted in the chest to supplement in "piggyback" fashion or to replace a severely damaged natural heart, often as a "bridge" while waiting for a DONOR HEART for HEART TRANSPLANT. Other models are external, with cannulas connecting to the heart's great vessels.
- Heart-lung bypass machine, which reroutes blood from the heart's major arteries to the bypass machine and then back to the body to maintain circulation during open heart surgery so surgeons can stop the heart to operate on it.

- INTRA-AORTIC BALLOON PUMP (IABP) COUNTERPUL-SATION, in which a tiny device inserted into the aorta where it leaves the heart assists the heart in moving blood from the left ventricle into the body after severe damage to the heart such as can occur after HEART ATTACK (MYOCARDIAL INFARCTION) or in HEART FAILURE.

- LEFT VENTRICULAR ASSIST DEVICE (LVAD), which is implanted into the left ventricle to provide pumping support to move blood out into the body.

- RIGHT VENTRICULAR ASSIST DEVICE (RVAD), which is implanted into the right ventricle to provide pumping support to move blood to the lungs for OXYGENATION.

- Biventricular assist device (BVAD), which is implanted into both ventricles to provide full pumping support to the heart.

- Extracorporeal membrane oxygenation (ECMO), in which blood temporarily is shunted from a major peripheral artery and vein (such as the femoral vessels) to a machine that functions similarly to a heart-lung bypass machine; this significantly lessens the heart's workload to allow the heart and CARDIOVASCULAR SYSTEM to recover or to stabilize until surgery.

In 2003 the U.S. Food and Drug Administration (FDA) approved certain models of ventricular assist devices for permanent treatment of end-stage heart failure, allowing the devices to be used in people who are not candidates for heart transplant. Researchers are hopeful that continued improvements in micro-technology will make the use of MCS devices viable treatment options for other forms of HEART DISEASE, extending life expectancy and improving QUALITY OF LIFE for thousands more people who cannot, for various reasons, undergo extensive heart operations. Infection, blood clots, and mechanical failure are the primary risks of MCS.

See also HEART, ARTIFICIAL; HEART DISEASE IN CHILDREN; LIVING WITH HEART DISEASE, SURGERY TO TREAT CARDIOVASCULAR DISEASE.

mechanical heart   See HEART, ARTIFICIAL.

mechanical ventilation   The use of a machine to substitute for breathing, sometimes referred to as life support. For mechanical ventilation, the doctor passes a tube through the mouth and down the throat into the pharynx (entrance to the trachea); an inflated balloon holds the tube, called an endotracheal tube, in place. Air moving into and out of the lungs passes through the tube to the mechanical ventilation machine (occasionally referred to as a respirator). When mechanical ventilation is going to be long-term (longer than two weeks), the doctor may perform a tracheostomy (make a surgical incision from the outside of the neck into the trachea) and place a cuff to which the tube attaches.

Mechanical ventilation is used on a temporary basis during surgery to continue respiration when the anesthesiologist administers medications to relax or paralyze the muscles as well as following CARDIAC ARREST or STROKE when lung function does not resume. Long-term mechanical ventilation may be necessary when there is damage to the respiratory centers of the brain such as after stroke. After longer than about 72 hours on mechanical ventilation the body adjusts to the mechanical support, and it becomes necessary to wean the person from the ventilator (gradually reduce the ventilator's function). Infection, damage to the trachea or larynx (including the vocal cords), and ventilator dependence are the primary risks of mechanical ventilation.

See also CPR (CARDIOPULMONARY RESUSCITATION); MECHANICAL CIRCULATORY SUPPORT.

medication management   The oversight and coordination of multiple medications. CARDIO-VASCULAR DISEASE (CVD) often occurs in multiple forms, so doctors prescribe multiple medications for treatment. Many of these medications complement one another without creating adverse effects, though some cannot be taken together. Doctors and pharmacists recommend these basic guidelines for medication management:

- Take medications according to the doctor's instructions and the directions on the label. Call the doctor's office or pharmacist about missed doses, to determine whether to take a "make-up" dose or wait until the next scheduled dose.

- Know the medication's most common side effects, and report them, as well as any unusual health events that occur while taking the medication, to the doctor.

- Write a list of all medications being taken. Include the medication's name and strength, the dose and time the medication is taken, and the name of the prescribing doctor. All of this information is on the prescription label.

- Make two or three copies of the list: one copy for the person to carry in his or her wallet or purse; one copy to keep in an obvious location at home (such as taped on the inside of the medicine cabinet door or even the refrigerator door); and one copy for a significant other (spouse, adult child, close friend).

- Show the medication list to the doctor at each doctor's appointment. This is particularly important for people who receive care from several doctors.

- Use the list kept at home as a reminder to take medications as scheduled.

- Order medication refills a week before the medication will run out. If the medication is gone before it is refilled, talk to the pharmacist about getting a 24-hour supply until the refill can be prepared. It is important to take medications for heart disease on a continuous basis when they are prescribed that way.

- When traveling, take along enough doses of medications to cover the length of the trip plus an extra day or two. If the travel supply runs short, most pharmacies can provide a short supply of the medication by contacting the prescribing doctor or dispensing pharmacy, information that should be on the list of medications the person carries.

- Check with the doctor or pharmacist before taking any over-the-counter products, including herbal remedies and allergy/cold/flu products.

- Do not stop taking a medication unless the doctor instructs.

- Follow the doctor's instructions for tapering off the medication if appropriate.

- Women who are pregnant should make sure the prescribing doctor knows this, and check with their regular obstetricians before taking any new medications or making medication changes.

Medications are the mainstay of medical treatment for CVD and make possible a nearly normal quality of life for many people who have any or multiple CVD conditions.

See also LIFESTYLE AND HEART HEALTH; LIVING WITH HEART DISEASE; MEDICATION SIDE EFFECTS; MEDICATIONS TO TREAT HEART DISEASE.

medication side effects The unintended and usually undesired consequences of taking a medication. Any medication, prescribed or over-the-counter, can have side effects. Additional adverse reactions can occur when medications are taken in combination with one another. The majority of medication side effects, such as gastrointestinal upset or headache, are mild and perhaps annoying or frustrating though not harmful to health. Some side effects, such as RHABDOMYOLYSIS or ARRHYTHMIA, are serious or life-threatening. Nearly any medication can cause an allergic response, which can range from mild (rash) to significant (difficulty breathing) in someone who is hypersensitive to any of its ingredients; anaphylactic shock is a life-threatening allergic response.

Medications within the same classification have common side effects just as they have common benefits; any of the ANGIOTENSIN-CONVERTING ENZYME (ACE) INHIBITOR MEDICATIONS, for example, can cause cough, and any of the thiazide or loop DIURETIC MEDICATIONS can cause POTASSIUM depletion. Individual drugs also have unique side effects not shared by other medications in the same classification. It is important for the doctor to know what other medications, including over-the-counter products, a person is taking before prescribing new medications. Knowing what side effects are common with particular medications helps to identify them if they occur, to prevent more serious complications.

See also ALPHA ANTAGONIST MEDICATIONS; ANGIOTENSIN II RECEPTOR ANTAGONIST MEDICATIONS; BETA ANTAGONIST MEDICATIONS; CALCIUM CHANNEL ANTAGONIST MEDICATIONS; HMG CoA REDUCTASE INHIBITOR MEDICATIONS; LIPID-LOWERING MEDICATIONS; MEDICATION MANAGEMENT; MEDICATIONS TO TREAT HEART

DISEASE; NITRATE MEDICATIONS; SODIUM CHANNEL BLOCKING MEDICATIONS; THROMBOLYTIC MEDICATIONS.

medications to treat heart disease Medication therapy is the cornerstone of treatment for CARDIOVASCULAR DISEASE (CVD). Many medications have specific uses; a number of medications, or classifications of medications, have multiple applications. Because most people with forms of HEART DISEASE typically have more than one condition and because one form of heart disease may lead to others, doctors often prescribe cardiovascular medications in combinations. A diuretic ("water pill"), for example, causes the body to eliminate more fluid. This reduces BLOOD volume, lowering BLOOD PRESSURE. Lower blood pressure reduces the heart's workload, aiding conditions such as CARDIOMYOPATHY and HEART FAILURE. The increased elimination of fluid also relieves edema resulting from heart failure. The table above summarizes the common classifications of medications to treat heart disease.

Comprehensive information for the medication classifications and many of the individual medications appears in the respective entries throughout this book.

See also ANTIARRHYTHMIA MEDICATIONS; ANTIHYPERTENSIVE MEDICATIONS; DIURETIC MEDICATIONS; LIPID-LOWERING MEDICATIONS; MEDICATION MANAGEMENT; MEDICATION SIDE EFFECTS.

meditation A method of focusing the mind that relieves STRESS and contributes to a sense of calm and centeredness. When practiced regularly, meditation can help to maintain healthy BLOOD PRESSURE and HEART RATE. There are many forms of meditation; meditation can be part of religious or spiritual practices though is not itself either spiritual or religious. An easy and effective meditation is to sit quietly and comfortably, with legs and arms uncrossed, and focus on the breath—how each breath sounds and feels, to envision the life-giving oxygen flowing into every cell in the body. This single-minded focus quiets the mind and the thoughts. Daily meditation is a key component of the ORNISH PROGRAM for reversing HEART DISEASE.

See also MINDFULNESS; STRESS REDUCTION TECHNIQUES; YOGA.

Mediterranean diet See NUTRITION AND DIET.

mental status See COGNITIVE FUNCTION.

metabolic syndrome A constellation of symptoms related to INSULIN RESISTANCE that includes a number of cardiovascular disorders. Researchers consider metabolic syndrome, sometimes called syndrome X or insulin resistance syndrome, to be a disorder of insulin metabolism and estimate that it affects nearly 47 million Americans (about one in four).

Symptoms and Diagnostic Path

There is no definitive diagnostic finding for metabolic syndrome; doctors generally presume it exists when three or more of its component disorders are present. Key characteristics are

- BODY MASS INDEX (BMI) greater than 30
- Abdominal adiposity (an "apple" body shape) with a waist circumference of 35 inches or greater for women and 40 inches or greater for men
- Elevated fasting BLOOD GLUCOSE levels (100 mm/dL or greater)
- Elevated blood insulin levels
- Elevated blood cholesterol and TRIGLYCERIDES levels
- Elevated BLOOD PRESSURE (130/85 mm Hg or greater)

Typically total and low-density lipoprotein (LDL) cholesterol are high and high-density lipoprotein (HDL) cholesterol is low, creating a strong predisposition for the development of ATHEROSCLEROSIS and CORONARY ARTERY DISEASE (CAD). Often, people who have metabolic syndrome also have type 2 diabetes and HYPERTENSION (high blood pressure), for which they receive treatment, and OBESITY.

Treatment Options and Outlook

The most effective treatment approach for metabolic syndrome is lifestyle modification to achieve weight loss and ultimately healthy weight. There is encouraging evidence that lifestyle measures can be successful in reversing metabolic syndrome's components. When the various components reach levels of therapeutic significance, however, it becomes necessary to begin treatment with medications to lower blood glucose, blood lipids, and blood pressure because each of these conditions in itself has significant cardiovascular consequences.

COMMON MEDICATIONS FOR HEART DISEASE

Classification or Type	Example Medications	Prescribed to Treat
Alpha antagonist (blocker)	Doxazosin, prazosin, terazosin, clonidine, guanfacine, methyldopa	Hypertension
Angiotensin-converting enzyme (ACE) inhibitor	Benazepril, captopril, enalapril, fosinopril, lisinopril, moexipril, ramipril, trandolapril	Hypertension; heart failure; arrhythmias
Angiotensin II receptor antagonist (blocker)	Candesartan, eprosartan, irbesartan, losartan, telmisartan, valsartan	Hypertension
Anticoagulant	Aspirin, clopidogrel, cilostazol, dipyridamole, pentoxifylline, ticlopidine, warfarin	Deep vein thrombosis (DVT); mitral valve prolapse; prophylaxis following angioplasty, CABG, valve surgery, heart attack, or stroke
Beta antagonist (blocker)	Acebutolol, atenolol, betaxolol, bisoprolol, carteolol, carvedolol, labetalol, metoprolol, nadolol, penbutolol, pindolol, propranolol, sotalol, timolol	Hypertension; arrhythmias
Bile acid sequestrant	Cholestyramine, colestipol, colesevelam	Hypercholesterolemia
Calcium channel antagonist (blocker)	Amlodipine, diltiazem, nifedepine, verapamil	Hypertension; arrhythmias
Digitalis	Digoxin, digitoxin	Heart failure, atrial fibrillation
Fibric acid derivative (fibrate)	Clofibrate, fenofibrate, gemfibrozil	Hypertriglyceridemia
HMG CoA reductase inhibitor (statin)	Atorvastatin, fluvastatin, lovastatin, pravastatin, simvastatin	Hypercholesterolemia, hypertriglyceridemia, preventive for subsequent heart attack
Immunosuppressive	Azathioprine, cyclosporine, prednisone	Prevent organ rejection following transplant
Loop diuretic	Bumetanide, ethacrynic acid, furosemide, torsemide	Hypertension, congestive heart failure
Nitrate	Nitroglycerin, amyl nitrate, isosorbide	Angina
Phosphodiestrase inhibitor	Enoximone, milrinone	Congestive heart failure
Potassium channel antagonist (blocker)	Amiodarone, ibutilide, dofetilide	Atrial fibrillation, atrial tachycardia
Potassium-sparing diuretic	Amiloride, triamterene, spironolactone	Hypertension, congestive heart failure
Sodium channel antagonist (blocker)	Mexiletine, quinidine, procainamide, propafenone	Severe ventricular arrhythmia that does not respond to other treatments
Thiazide diuretic	Bendroflumethiazide, chlorothiazide, chlorthalidone, hydrochlorothiazide (HCTZ), hydroflumethiazide, methyclothiazide, metolazone, polythiazide, quinethazone, trichlormethiazide	Hypertension, congestive heart failure

In the presence of metabolic syndrome, conventional treatments for HEART DISEASE appear to be less effective. Blood lipid levels may remain elevated despite lifestyle modifications and LIPID-LOWERING MEDICATIONS, for example, and ANTIHYPERTENSIVE MEDICATIONS may fail to produce the anticipated drop in blood pressure. Treatment thus often must be more aggressive earlier than is typical in the progression of any of the conditions independently, especially with respect to controlling the glucose/insulin balance, and may require multiple medications in combination.

Because insulin has key roles in the metabolism of lipids and elevated blood lipid levels contribute significantly to HEART DISEASE, some doctors are choosing to begin oral antidiabetes medications earlier in people who have two or more components of metabolic syndrome. Research continues to investigate the correlations between insulin resistance and hypertension, and to explore other cardiovascular links with insulin.

Risk Factors and Preventive Measures

Increased body weight, in particular obesity (BMI of 30 or greater), is the most significant factor for metabolic syndrome and appears to set the stage for the cascade of symptoms that develop. Maintaining healthy weight through a balance of daily EXERCISE and nutritious eating appears to be highly effective in preventing metabolic syndrome and especially insulin resistance and type 2 diabetes. However, the continuing rise of overweight people and obesity has many health experts worried that metabolic syndrome might soon become a greater risk factor for heart disease than smoking.

See also BODY SHAPE AND HEART DISEASE; CHOLESTEROL, BLOOD; DIABETES AND HEART DISEASE; LIFESTYLE AND HEART HEALTH; NUTRITION AND DIET; TOBACCO USE.

metabolism The chemical actions and reactions that take place in the body to produce and release energy. There are two aspects to metabolism, anabolism and catabolism. Anabolic processes make or store energy, and catabolic processes expend energy; metabolism is the balance that exists between the two.

The body's two primary energy sources are oxygen and glucose (sugar). The HEART and CARDIOVASCULAR SYSTEM are responsible for delivering enough oxygen to the body's cells to meet their energy demands. With increased physical activity metabolism also increases, and the body's need for oxygen rises. Various physiological mechanisms cause BLOOD PRESSURE and HEART RATE to increase, which in turn increases the flow of BLOOD. Breathing rate increases as well, getting more oxygen into the bloodstream.

The rise in metabolic rate (the rate at which the body is using energy) also increases the amount of glucose that the cells use. With sustained exercise the body consumes the available blood glucose supply in 15 to 20 minutes and begins converting glycogen (the storage form of glucose) back to glucose. It also begins to use TRIGLYCERIDES, fatty acids circulating in the bloodstream (and also stored in body fat), for extended energy. Health and fitness experts measure the level of energy expenditure during exercise in terms of metabolic equivalents (METS) or kilocalories (commonly referred to simply as calories).

An aerobically fit, cardiovascularly healthy body can meet and maintain the oxygen needs of body tissues at moderate levels of exertion for an extended time. When the aerobic fitness level is low or there is CARDIOVASCULAR DISEASE (CVD) that

METABOLIC EQUIVALENTS (METS)

METs	Calorie Equivalent	Physical Intensity Level	Example Activities
1–3	3.5 kcal/minute	Low	Casual walking (strolling), gardening, vacuuming or sweeping
3–6	3.5–7 kcal/minute	Moderate	Brisk walking, raking leaves, pushing a power mower, walking up stairs, dancing, bicycling less than 10mph or on flat terrain
6+	7+ kcal/minute	Vigorous	Running, swimming laps, singles tennis, bicycling steep hills or greater than 10mph

impairs the heart's ability to function efficiently, the body can sustain moderate physical activity for a limited time. Shortness of breath becomes extreme, forcing the person to slow or stop the activity. Regular exercise at a moderate level of exertion helps the cardiovascular system and the body to develop a higher level of AEROBIC FITNESS even in the presence of cardiovascular disease; as is the cycle of such processes, a higher aerobic fitness level in turn helps the heart to function more efficiently.

Increasing the body's metabolic rate through physical activity is key to weight loss and WEIGHT MANAGEMENT. The higher the metabolic rate, the more energy (calories) the body uses. Energy use is highest during the period of physical activity or exercise, though it continues for an extended time as the metabolic rate remains higher than usual for up to six hours following an exercise session. A person who is physically fit has a higher metabolic rate at rest than does a person who is not physically fit, in part because regular physical activity builds muscle and muscle uses more energy than fat, and in part because the more efficiently the body's cells function the more consistent their energy use.

See also NUTRITION AND DIET; OBESITY; PHYSICAL FITNESS.

methyldopa A medication taken to treat HYPERTENSION (high BLOOD PRESSURE). A common brand name product is Aldomet. Methyldopa is an ALPHA ANTAGONIST MEDICATION that works by reducing the action of epinephrine on the heart and BLOOD vessels. Methyldopa causes peripheral arteries to dilate, decreasing resistance for blood flowing through them. It also causes the heart to slow the rate and force of its contractions. These effects in combination cause blood pressure to drop. Methyldopa targets alpha-2 receptors, which also are present in other smooth muscle tissue throughout the body. Among methyldopa's side effects are actions on these other tissues, causing problems such as ERECTILE DYSFUNCTION and urinary stress incontinence. Other side effects may include sleepiness when beginning methyldopa therapy (which usually subsides after taking the medication for a few weeks), headache, and gastrointestinal upset (dyspepsia, diarrhea, CONSTIPATION). Methyldopa can interact with numerous medications including monoamine oxidase inhibitor (MAOI) ANTIDEPRESSANT MEDICATIONS and anesthetic agents. People who have PHEOCHROMOCYTOMA should not take methyldopa. Methyldopa also can cause Parkinson-like symptoms such as slowed movement and gait disturbances, or aggravate symptoms in people who have Parkinson's disease. When stopping methyldopa, it is important to taper the dose downward over several weeks. Suddenly stopping this medication can cause hypertensive crisis (a rapid and dangerous spike in blood pressure) with significant risk for STROKE or HEART ATTACK.

See also ANTIHYPERTENSIVE MEDICATIONS; BETA ANTAGONIST MEDICATIONS; MEDICATION SIDE EFFECTS; MEDICATIONS TO TREAT HEART DISEASE.

metolazone A DIURETIC MEDICATION taken to treat mild to moderate HYPERTENSION (high BLOOD PRESSURE). Common brand name products available in the United States are Zaroxolyn and Mykrox; though both medications contain metolazone, they are not biochemically equivalent and cannot be substituted for one another. Doctors may prescribe metolazone as monotherapy to accompany lifestyle modifications in people who are newly diagnosed with hypertension or in combination with antihypertensive medications for optimal blood pressure regulation. Metolazone is a thiazide diuretic; it acts on the kidneys to increase the amount of fluid drawn from the bloodstream into the urine. This reduces BLOOD volume, which helps to lower blood pressure. Metolazone can cause POTASSIUM depletion when taken long-term; doctors often suggest eating foods high in potassium (such as bananas and raisins) or may prescribe potassium supplements for people who take metolazone longer than a few months. ASPIRIN can reduce the effectiveness of metolazone. Side effects, when they occur, generally are mild and include dizziness and headache.

See also MEDICATION SIDE EFFECTS; MEDICATIONS TO TREAT HEART DISEASE.

metoprolol A medication taken to treat ARRHYTHMIAS, HYPERTENSION (high BLOOD PRESSURE), and

ANGINA. Metoprolol is one of the BETA ANTAGO-NIST MEDICATIONS; common brand-name products include Lopressor and Toprol XL. Metoprolol blocks primarily beta-1 receptors in the HEART and in the BLOOD vessels, slowing and stabilizing the rate and force of the heart's contractions. Metoprolol also helps to reduce anxiety response and migraine headaches and sometimes is prescribed in low doses for these purposes. Common side effects include tiredness and SEXUAL DYSFUNCTION (diminished libido and ERECTILE DYSFUNCTION). These side effects may go away after taking metoprolol for several weeks; if they do not, the doctor may prescribe a different beta-blocker to achieve the desired therapeutic effect without the undesired side effects. Various medications interfere with metoprolol including cimetadine (Tagamet) and ORAL CONTRACEPTIVES (birth control pills).

See also ANTIHYPERTENSIVE MEDICATIONS; MEDICA-TIONS TO TREAT HEART DISEASE.

Mevacor   See LOVASTATIN.

mexiletine   A medication taken to treat life-threatening ventricular ARRHYTHMIAS (irregularities in the electrical impulses within the left ventricle) that do not respond to other medications. Mexiletine, available in the United States as the brand-name product Mexitil, is a SODIUM CHANNEL ANTAGONIST MEDICA-TION. It works by inhibiting or blocking the flow of sodium into myocardial (HEART muscle) cells, slowing their ability to contraction, and it also affects the Purkinje cells (part of the heart's electrical impulse network). Mexiletine can cause other ventricular or atrial arrhythmias, HEART BLOCK, life-threatening electrical irregularities in the heart, CARDIAC ARREST, and SUDDEN CARDIAC ARREST (SCA). Cardiologists sometimes prescribe mexiletine for short-term use after HEART ATTACK, until the heart stabilizes.

See also ANTIARRHYTHMIA MEDICATIONS; MEDICA-TION MANAGEMENT; MEDICATIONS TO TREAT HEART DISEASE; PREMATURE VENTRICULAR CONTRACTIONS (PVCs).

Mexitil   See MEXILETINE.

Micardis   See TELMISARTAN.

microinfarction   An interruption of BLOOD flow that is small enough to have little or no perceptible effect, often involving only a few cells, until the cumulative damage becomes significant. Microinfarctions can occur in any body tissue. Microinfarctions involving the myocardium (HEART muscle) may cause slight elevations of CTNI (CARDIAC TRO-PONIN I), an enzyme myocardial and other muscle cells release when they are damaged. MAGNETIC RESONANCE IMAGING (MRI) often can detect areas of microinfarction that other imaging procedures cannot. Treatment focuses on eliminating the circumstances causing the microinfarctions, typically CORONARY ARTERY DISEASE (CAD) in the heart and ATHEROSCLEROSIS (deposits of fatty acids and other substances that accumulate along the inner walls of the arteries) elsewhere in the body.

See also HEART ATTACK; ISCHEMIC HEART DISEASE (IHD); STROKE; TRANSIENT ISCHEMIC ATTACK (TIA).

mindfulness   Having awareness of the present moment. Mindfulness is a key concept of many STRESS REDUCTION TECHNIQUES including MEDITATION, BIOFEEDBACK, and YOGA. Stress affects health in numerous ways. Researchers believe that exposure to continued stress keeps the body in a constant state of "FIGHT OR FLIGHT," maintaining primal survival responses in continual readiness. The human body is not designed to exist in such a continued state and over time begins to adapt its functions to accommodate the "fight-or-flight" state as the new normal state. This places strain on nearly all body cells, tissues, and organ systems. Many researchers believe this strain contributes to increased numbers of free radicals in the body and a corresponding susceptibility to degenerative processes that lead to disease.

Mindfulness focuses the conscious thoughts on the state of the present. This has numerous meanings and contexts that might include awareness that one's PULSE is racing or HEART is pounding. Once such information becomes conscious knowledge, it is possible to take steps to change the situation. Often a short meditation can generate enough relaxation to slow heart rate. Mindfulness might also be an awareness that the body needs exercise, encouraging a decision to take a walk or bicycle ride, wash floors, or do yard work. Such activities benefit the body and the mind, improving physical fitness at the same time they provide relaxation and stress relief.

See also ANGER; PERSONALITY TYPES; STRESS AND HEART DISEASE.

minimally invasive cardiac surgery A method for conducting operations on the HEART that does not require OPEN-HEART SURGERY. Though not yet among the standard options for many surgical heart treatments, a number of cardiovascular surgeons are using minimally invasive cardiac surgery particularly for people who are not good candidates for ANGIOPLASTY or open-heart surgery because of health status but who would benefit from CORONARY ARTERY BYPASS GRAFT (CABG). During minimally invasive cardiac surgery the surgeon makes a number of small incisions in the chest, called ports, that go between the ribs and into the thoracic cavity. Fiberoptic scopes and miniature instruments pass through the ports and the surgeon views what he or she is doing on a video monitor similar to a television screen. The premise is much the same as that for the laparoscopic and arthroscopic procedures that have become commonplace for other kinds of operations. Recovery time is much faster as the sternum (breastbone) remains intact.

When the surgical repair is relatively uncomplicated, as in CABG for one or two coronary arteries on the front of the heart, the surgeon may choose to let the heart continue beating. For such procedures, called MIDCAB, the surgeon makes another incision directly over the coronary artery to be replaced and uses an artery from within the chest wall to construct the graft. Another method of minimally invasive cardiac surgery stops the heart, as in conventional CABG, and the surgeon completes the operation through the ports. For somewhat more extensive repairs the surgeon uses the ports to insert cannulas into the heart's arteries to connect to the HEART-LUNG BYPASS MACHINE, stops the heart, and performs the operation with instruments inserted through the ports. Surgeons are exploring techniques to adapt minimally invasive cardiac surgery for use in other operations such as valve repair and replacement.

See also SURGERY TO TREAT CARDIOVASCULAR DISEASE.

Minipres See PRAZOSIN.

ministroke See TRANSIENT ISCHEMIC ATTACK.

minoxidil A medication taken to treat moderate to severe HYPERTENSION (high BLOOD PRESSURE) that does not respond to aggressive therapy with other medications (the standard point of definition for "aggressive" being a diuretic in combination with two other ANTIHYPERTENSIVE MEDICATIONS). Minoxidil works by causing the peripheral arteries to dilate, reducing the resistance BLOOD encounters as it flows through them. Minoxidil has a high risk for PERICARDIAL EFFUSION, in which fluid fills the pericardium (space surrounding the HEART), which compresses the heart and causes a condition called cardiac TAMPONADE. Emergency treatment to draw off the fluid is essential; the heart can collapse under the pressure of the fluid and stop beating. Because of this risk, doctors typically administer minoxidil in conjunction with a loop DIURETIC MEDICATION for maximum fluid management and a BETA ANTAGONIST MEDICATION to regulate HEART RATE, often with the person hospitalized for close monitoring.

One side effect of minoxidil is that it promotes hair growth; some people who take oral minoxidil experience increased body hair about six weeks after starting treatment and that persists for as long as the medication is being taken. This side effect led to the development of topical minoxidil, available as the brand-name product Rogaine, which doctors prescribe to treat male-pattern baldness (alopecia) though it is effective for certain kinds of hair loss in women as well. Because small amounts of the drug can be absorbed through the skin, people who have hypertension or other forms of cardiovascular disease should not use topical minoxidil.

See also MEDICATIONS TO TREAT HEART DISEASE.

mitral regurgitation   See HEART MURMUR.

mitral stenosis   Narrowing of the opening between the left atrium and left ventricle. Mitral stenosis can cause MITRAL VALVE PROLAPSE (MVP) and mitral regurgitation. The severity of the problem depends on the extent of the narrowing and can have numerous consequences for HEART FUNCTION.

Symptoms and Diagnostic Path
When mitral stenosis causes significant malfunctioning of the mitral valve or impedes the flow of blood from the atrium to the ventricle, it can cause ARRHYTHMIAS, PULMONARY HYPERTENSION, and right HEART FAILURE. Symptoms usually occur when these consequences have become pronounced and typically include shortness of breath with exertion and when lying down, fatigue, cough when lying down, and perceptible CYANOSIS (bluish hue to the lips, nail beds, and skin).

Treatment Options and Outlook
Treatment involves managing the consequential conditions with appropriate medications such as ANTIARRHYTHMIA MEDICATIONS and DIURETIC MEDICATIONS, and surgically repairing the stenosis and replacing the mitral valve if necessary.

Risk Factors and Preventive Measures
Mitral stenosis can be congenital or develop as a consequence of scarring caused by inflammation such as from rheumatic fever or bacterial or viral infection.
    See also AORTIC REGURGITATION; AORTIC STENOSIS; CARDIOVASCULAR SYSTEM; HEART DISEASE; MARFAN SYNDROME; MITRAL REGURGITATION; RHEUMATIC HEART DISEASE; SURGERY TO TREAT CARDIOVASCULAR DISEASE; VALVE REPAIR AND REPLACEMENT.

mitral valve   See HEART.

mitral valve prolapse (MVP)   A condition in which the mitral valve, which separates the left atrium and left ventricle, is weaker than normal and bulges into the atrium with each ventricular contraction. It is one of the most common HEART disorders, affecting about 5 percent of Americans.

Symptoms and Diagnostic Path
Most people who have MVP do not have symptoms and may not even know they have it. When symptoms do occur, it is because the prolapsed mitral valve is allowing blood to backflow into the left atrium (called mitral valve regurgitation). Symptoms of MVP may include

- PALPITATIONS or the sensation of a racing HEARTBEAT
- shortness of breath (DYSPNEA), particularly with EXERCISE
- unusual tiredness or fatigue
- achy CHEST PAIN

AUSCULTATION (listening to the heart with a STETHOSCOPE) reveals MVP's characteristic clicking sounds, and sometimes a HEART MURMUR is detectable when there is regurgitation. ECHOCARDIOGRAM is the conclusive diagnostic procedure because it can show the prolapse in action. Electrocardiogram (ECG), EXERCISE STRESS test, and CARDIAC CATHETERIZATION may offer further diagnostic information to help determine the severity of the MVP. These procedures also help to conclusively rule out other possible causes of the symptoms.

Treatment Options and Outlook
When MVP produces no symptoms, there is usually no need for treatment. Even most diagnosed MVP requires only watchful waiting. Serious MVP with regurgitation generally responds to management with medications; among those commonly used to treat MVP are BETA ANTAGONIST MEDICATIONS, ANTIARRHYTHMIA MEDICATIONS, DIURETIC MEDICATIONS, and VASODILATOR MEDICATIONS. When MVP generates significant symptoms, surgery to repair or replace the mitral valve becomes a consideration. People diagnosed with MVP should check with their doctors about antibiotic prophylaxis before dental and surgical procedures because MVP increases the risk for bacterial ENDOCARDITIS.

Risk Factors and Preventive Measures
MVP can be the result of a congenital weakness or minor malformation of the mitral valve or develop following an infection, commonly rheumatic fever. Mitral valve prolapse is also commonly associated

with MARFAN SYNDROME and EBSTEIN'S ANOMALY. There are no known measures to prevent MVP.

See also LIVING WITH HEART DISEASE; RHEUMATIC HEART DISEASE; VALVE DISEASE; SURGERY TO TREAT CARDIOVASCULAR DISEASE; VALVE REPAIR AND REPLACEMENT.

moexipril A medication taken to treat HYPERTENSION (high BLOOD PRESSURE). Moexipril is an ANGIOTENSIN-CONVERTING ENZYME (ACE) INHIBITOR MEDICATION; common brand-name products include Univasc. Moexipril works by interfering with the RENIN-ANGIOTENSIN-ALDOSTERONE (RAA) HORMONAL SYSTEM, one of the body's primary mechanisms for BLOOD pressure regulation. Cardiologists sometimes prescribe ACE inhibitors for people who have had an initial HEART ATTACK (MYOCARDIAL INFARCTION) to reduce the risk for subsequent heart attacks. Moexipril and other ACE inhibitors also may have preventive effects against heart attack in people with severe ISCHEMIC HEART DISEASE (IHD) or HEART FAILURE.

Many people with mild to moderate hypertension can take moexipril as monotherapy in conjunction with lifestyle modifications such as daily physical EXERCISE and low-fat diet. Doctors often prescribe moexipril in combination with a DIURETIC MEDICATION for moderate to severe hypertension or to provide optimal blood pressure regulation. Like other ACE inhibitors, moexipril can cause various side effects, including headache, DIZZINESS, weakness, and persistent dry cough.

See also ANTIHYPERTENSIVE MEDICATIONS; ANGIOTENSIN II RECEPTOR ANTAGONIST MEDICATIONS; LIFESTYLE AND HEART HEALTH; MEDICATION MANAGEMENT; MEDICATION SIDE EFFECTS; MEDICATIONS TO TREAT HEART DISEASE.

Morgangni-Adams-Stokes disease See STOKES-ADAMS DISEASE.

mucocutaneous lymph node syndrome See KAWASAKI DISEASE.

multi-unit gated acquisition (MUGA) scan A nuclear medicine test that uses a radionuclide to assess the flow of BLOOD through the HEART. During the test, the radiologist starts an IV and injects a radionuclide, which emits gamma radiation that a gamma camera subsequently detects. As the radionuclide travels through the bloodstream and through the heart, the gamma camera picks up its trail. The MUGA scan can measure the ventricular filling volume and allow the cardiologist or radiologist to calculate the LEFT VENTRICULAR EJECTION FRACTION (LVEF) a key indicator of the heart's effectiveness. During the scan, an ELECTROCARDIOGRAM (ECG) also records the heart's electrical activity. Like other RADIONUCLIDE SCANS, a MUGA scan can be done as a stress test to show how the heart functions during exercise.

See also ADENOSINE STRESS TEST; DIPYRIDAMOLE STRESS TEST; DOBUTAMINE STRESS TEST.

murmur See HEART MURMUR.

Mustard procedure An operation to correct TRANSPOSITION OF THE GREAT ARTERIES (TGA), a serious congenital malformation of the HEART in which the arteries and veins originating from the heart are transposed, or reversed, such that the aorta arises from the right rather than the left ventricle and the pulmonary artery arises from the left rather than the right ventricle. The Canadian cardiovascular surgeon William Mustard (1914–87) developed the procedure, in which the surgeon applies synthetic patches to redirect the flow of BLOOD within the heart though allowing the great arteries to remain reversed and the ventricles to reverse roles. Thus left ventricle pumps blood to the lungs and the right ventricle pumps oxygenated blood to the body. Though the Mustard procedure is not commonly performed in the United States any longer, it was the primary corrective surgery for TGA in the 1960s and 1970s and remains the mainstay of surgical correction of TGA in many other countries today because it is easier to perform and does not require the extensive surgical recovery facilities that procedures to return the great vessels to their correct placements demand.

The thousands of people who received the Mustard procedure as infants 20 to 30 years ago now provide researchers with the opportunity to assess the long-term consequences of such significant interventions. More than three-fourths of them have survived at least 20 years; many have mild to moderate cardiovascular health concerns that require regular cardiology follow-up and some level of medical intervention, such as medication to regulate heart rate and to strengthen the heart's contractions. Though the right ventricle eventually thickens and enlarges to help it meet the demands of its role, it cannot entirely compensate because by design it is not as large or as muscular as the left ventricle. ARRHYTHMIAS and HEART FAILURE are the most common cardiovascular consequences that develop. Most people who have had the Mustard procedure can engage in normal activities, though cardiologists might recommend refraining from very strenuous physical activities to help preserve heart function as long as possible.

See also ARTERIAL SWITCH PROCEDURE; BIDIREC-TIONAL GLENN PROCEDURE; BLALOCK-TAUSSIG PROCE-DURE; CARDIOVASCULAR SYSTEM; FONTAN PROCEDURE; HEART DISEASE IN CHILDREN; NORWOOD PROCEDURE.

myocardial infarction (MI)   The death of myo-cardial (HEART muscle) cells. Acute MI results from the sudden blockage of the flow of BLOOD through the CORONARY ARTERIES to the heart, such as with a blood clot (EMBOLISM), and is the most common cause of CARDIAC ARREST. Dead heart cells cannot contract or conduct electrical impulses. As the infarcted area becomes large enough, it causes loss of heart function and ARRHYTHMIAS. Most often, MI is used to refer to the acute circumstance of heart attack.

Symptoms and Diagnostic Path
MI may occur without symptoms until SUDDEN CARDIAC ARREST. Most people do experience symp-toms, however, that may be intermittent (such as with exertion) and progressive or, with acute MI, fairly sudden. Symptoms of MI may include

- CHEST PAIN (ANGINA pectoris)
- shortness of breath (DYSPNEA), wheezing, or shal-low breathing
- nausea and queasiness

- unusual tiredness and fatigue
- anxiety
- fainting (SYNCOPE) or loss of consciousness
- sweating (DIAPHORESIS)

The chest pain of MI may range from vague discomfort to intense, crushing pain and may radiate to other parts of the upper body such as the left arm, either shoulder, jaw, and under the shoulder blades in the back. Often the discomfort feels like moderate to severe indigestion, which causes people to delay seeking medical attention. Such delay often results in severe heart damage or death that could have been prevented with early treatment. The key diagnostic tools are ELECTRO-CARDIOGRAM (ECG) and blood tests to evaluate CARDIAC ENZYME and C-REACTIVE PROTEIN levels. Further tests may include ECHOCARDIOGRAM and ANGIOGRAPHY to determine the cause and extent of damage to the heart.

Treatment Options and Outlook
Acute MI is a life-threatening medical emergency that requires urgent treatment. Time is of the essence in getting the person to a hospital; statistics show that most people who die of MI do so before getting to a hospital. Initial medical care concentrates on oxygen supplementation, thinning of blood to limit clot for-mation, calming of the heart with BETA ANTAGONIST MEDICATIONS, lowering of the BLOOD PRESSURE, and pain control. Once the person is stabilized, clots that have formed are treated with THROMBOLYTIC MEDICA-TIONS or cardiac catheterization procedures. Early administration of ASPIRIN (chewed, not swallowed) is appropriate when MI is suspected and can be given before medical aid arrives.

Risk Factors and Preventive Measures
MI is a consequence of progressive HEART DISEASE, whether or not symptoms of heart disease have been present or detected. People at highest risk for MI are those who have diagnosed heart conditions such as CAD. PERIPHERAL VASCULAR DISEASE (PAD), smoking, HYPERTENSION (high BLOOD PRESSURE), ele-vated blood lipid levels (cholesterol and TRIGLYCER-IDES), and DIABETES are also significant risk factors. Preventing the underlying heart conditions that

lead to MI is the most effective prevention. Lifestyle factors that are crucial include daily physical EXERCISE, nutritious eating, maintaining healthy weight, and not smoking. After heart disease is diagnosed, it is important to follow treatment recommendations and make lifestyle changes to support heart health. Having had one MI significantly increases the risk for a subsequent MI, which makes preventive measures both important and effective across the spectrum of heart health.

See also BLOOD TESTS TO DETECT HEART ATTACK; CARDIOGENIC SHOCK; CARDIOMYOPATHY; EMERGENCY CARDIOVASCULAR CARE (ECC); HEART FAILURE; INFLAMMATION AND HEART DISEASE; LIFESTYLE AND HEART HEALTH; LIVING WITH HEART DISEASE; MEDICATIONS TO TREAT HEART DISEASE; SURGERY TO TREAT CARDIOVASCULAR DISEASE.

myocardial perfusion imaging   See RADIONUCLIDE SCAN.

myocardial stunning and hibernation   The persistent dysfunction or lack of function of myocardial (HEART muscle) cells after a significant ischemic event such as HEART ATTACK (MYOCARDIAL INFARCTION). Myocardial stunning occasionally occurs after CARDIOVERSION or DEFIBRILLATION (therapeutic shocks to the HEART to restore normal heart rate). Technologies such as MAGNETIC RESONANCE IMAGING (MRI) and SINGLE PHOTON EMISSION COMPUTED TOMOGRAPHY (SPECT) now can distinguish "stunned" cells from necrotic (dead) cells, which often are intermixed in the location of the infarction. Cells that remain in a state of dysfunction for an extended time are said to be in hibernation. Researchers suspect a gene mutation that alters CTNI (CARDIAC TROPONIN I), a protein that has key functions in the CARDIAC CYCLE, though do not yet know what causes the cells to return to function; there is no predictability to the timing or even to knowing whether stunned cells will die or recover. Presently there are no medical interventions to stimulate stunned or hibernating myocardial cells to return to activity.

See also ANGIOGENESIS; HEART'S REGENERATIVE ABILITY; TRANSMYOCARDIAL LASER REVASCULARIZATION (TMLR).

myocarditis   An inflammation of the myocardium (HEART muscle) usually caused by bacterial or viral infection though sometimes a consequence of radiation therapy for cancer or an adverse drug reaction. Myocarditis is a serious condition that, without appropriate treatment, can have long-term consequences or lead to death.

Symptoms and Diagnostic Path
Most people diagnosed with myocarditis complain of CHEST PAIN and shortness of breath, symptoms for which doctors typically conduct ELECTROCARDIOGRAMS (ECGs). Some health experts believe it is likely that subclinical myocarditis (myocarditis without specific cardiac symptoms) often accompanies viral infections but is not detected. Myocarditis also is a cardinal feature of RHEUMATIC HEART DISEASE, which typically develops following infection with streptococcus bacteria elsewhere in the body (such as strep throat). Myocarditis is a leading cause of SUDDEN CARDIAC ARREST (SCA) in young people and especially in young athletes, with death occurring during or immediately after strenuous physical activity, and with the autopsy showing the myocardial inflammation. Because of this association with sudden cardiac arrest, doctors generally recommend bed rest during the acute phase of myocarditis and restricted physical activity until the heart's functions return to normal.

Diagnosis generally is by ECG, which shows the electrical disturbances to the heart's rhythm that the inflammation causes, and ECHOCARDIOGRAM, which can show the areas of inflammation. HEART BLOCK and BUNDLE BRANCH BLOCK, rhythm disorders affecting the transmittal of pulsing signals between the atria and the ventricles, occur in about 20 percent of people diagnosed with myocarditis and may continue for several months after the inflammation has resolved. Dilated CARDIOMYOPATHY (enlarged and weakened ventricle) also can develop when the inflammation and resulting ARRHYTHMIAS affect the left ventricle's ability to pump efficiently.

Treatment Options and Outlook
Treatment targets pain relief and cardiac symptoms. Antibiotics are therapeutic only when bacterial infection can be identified, which typically requires endocardial needle biopsy (removing a

small core of tissue from the heart); NONSTEROIDAL ANTI-INFLAMMATORY DRUGS (NSAIDS) and IMMUNO-SUPPRESSIVE MEDICATIONS do not seem to offer any therapeutic value and may exacerbate symptoms. It is difficult to predict whether recovery will be complete and uneventful; some people have continued HEART DISEASE after the inflammation resolves, especially when cardiomyopathy has developed. Rarely, damage to the heart is so substantial that HEART TRANSPLANT becomes the only viable treatment option.

Risk Factors and Preventive Measures

Though myocarditis is uncommonly diagnosed, health experts believe it is more prevalent than statistics suggest. About three-fourths of people who are diagnosed with myocarditis currently have, or recently had, viral infections of the upper respiratory system (sinusitis, laryngitis) or the lungs (bronchitis, pneumonia). This correlation strongly suggests the virus moves through the body to also infect the heart. When myocarditis is bacterial, the most common cause is streptococcus, which causes strep throat, rheumatic fever (a systemic strep infection), and rheumatic heart disease (strep infection involving the heart valves). Aside from general precautions to reduce the risk of viral infections (such as covering coughs and sneezes and frequent handwashing), it is not possible to prevent viral myocarditis. Prompt diagnosis and treatment of bacterial infections of the upper respiratory tract and lungs is the most effective means to curtail the spread of the infection to other locations in the body including the heart.

See also INFLAMMATION AND HEART DISEASE; MEDICATION SIDE EFFECTS; PERICARDITIS; VALVE DISEASE.

myocardium   See HEART.

myxoma   A benign (noncancerous) connective tissue tumor. Though tumors that originate in the HEART are rare, myocardial myxomas are the most common among them and most myxomas develop in the heart. About 80 percent of myo-cardial myxomas develop in the left atrium; most others develop in the right atrium. It is unusual, though not unheard of, for a myxoma to occur in a ventricle. Nearly always there is only a single myo-cardial myxoma; myxomas in other locations in the body can have multiple occurrences. About 10 percent of myxomas appear to be familial (inherited), though researchers have not yet identified the responsible genes.

A myxoma in the heart can protrude into the chamber where it is growing, causing distortions that affect valve function. These tumors also present a significant risk for BLOOD clots to form, as they cause the blood to swirl and pool within the atrium.

Symptoms and Diagnostic Path

Symptoms tend to be generally those of cardiac insufficiency—shortness of breath, mild CYANOSIS (bluish hue to the lips, fingernail beds, and skin), tiredness—with the notable exception that they worsen or improve with changes in position. This reflects the tumor's movement within the heart chamber; when the person is lying down the myxoma may "hang" into the pathway of the valve and retreat along the atrial wall when the person sits or stands. Right atrium myxomas can become quite sizable—five inches or larger—before they manifest any symptoms. There does not appear to be any way to prevent myxomas, which are rare to begin with, from developing. With a large myo-cardial myxoma, the cardiologist often can hear during AUSCULTATION (listening to the chest with a STETHOSCOPE) the tumor "flop" as blood flows through the atrium.

Diagnosis is by ECHOCARDIOGRAM and DOPPLER ULTRASOUND, two noninvasive procedures that use sound waves to generate images of the heart and the flow of blood through the heart and great vessels.

Treatment Options and Outlook

Treatment is surgery to remove the tumor and repair any damage to the heart valves. Most people make full and uneventful recoveries without residual consequences, though should take ANTI-BIOTIC PROPHYLAXIS for future invasive procedures including dental work and surgery, as repaired or replaced heart valves are vulnerable to infection.

Risk Factors and Preventive Measures

About 10 percent of myxomas are hereditary, and there is a family history of them. Women are more likely than men to develop a myxoma. Though surgery usually cures myxoma, it is possible for a myxoma to recur if tumor cells remain following surgery. A person who has a family history of myxoma should receive regular cardiology evaluations. There are no known preventive measures for myxoma.

See also CANCER OF THE HEART; CARDIOVASCULAR SYSTEM; EMBOLISM; SURGERY TO TREAT CARDIOVASCULAR DISEASE; VALVE DISEASE; VALVE REPAIR AND REPLACEMENT.

nadolol A medication taken to treat HYPERTEN-SION (high BLOOD PRESSURE). Nadolol belongs to the family of BETA ANTAGONIST MEDICATIONS; a common brand-name product in the United States is Corgard. Nadolol lowers BLOOD pressure by slowing the contractions of the HEART and dilating the peripheral arteries to reduce the resistance blood encounters as it flows through them. Nadolol blocks both beta-1 and beta-2 receptors, so it also affects other smooth muscle tissues in the body. Nadolol has a long half-life, which means it stays active in the body for an extended time and can be taken once a day. Side effects generally are mild and may include tiredness or weakness when beginning nadolol therapy and ERECTILE DYSFUNC-TION in men as a result of the beta-blocking effect on the smooth muscle tissue of the genitourinary system.

See also ALPHA ANTAGONIST MEDICATIONS; ANTIHY-PERTENSIVE MEDICATIONS; MEDICATION SIDE EFFECTS; MEDICATIONS TO TREAT HEART DISEASE.

narrow therapeutic index (NTI) An identifier for a medication whose effective level and toxic level in the body are very close together, making precise dosing and close monitoring essential. Many medications taken to treat HEART DISEASE are narrow therapeutic index (NTI) drugs, notably DIGITALIS preparations (DIGOXIN and DIGITOXIN), some of the NITRATE MEDICATIONS, and WARFARIN (Coumadin). Other NTI medications include antiseizure medications, thyroid HORMONE replacement medications, and some other hormone replacement medications such as those taken to treat Addison's disease.

NTI medications represent one of the few circumstances in which the subtle differences that may exist in formulations of medications from different manufacturers can affect the level of the drug in the person's body. Although generic and brand-name medications contain the same amounts of the same active ingredients, their inactive ingredients typically differ. This affects the ways in which the medications become absorbed into the bloodstream and consequently their concentrations and desired therapeutic levels.

Pharmacists and doctors generally recommend that prescriptions for NTI medications consistently be the same brand-name product, such as Coumadin (for prescribed warfarin) or Lanoxin (for prescribed digoxin), or consistently be from the same manufacturer when generic products are dispensed. Whether generic or brand name does not matter; what is important is staying with the same product for the duration of therapy with the medication. The pharmacist can check dispensing records to verify this consistency.

See also MEDICATION SIDE EFFECTS; MEDICATIONS TO TREAT HEART DISEASE.

neurotransmitter A chemical in the body that conducts electrical impulses between nerve cells (neurons). There are dozens of neurotransmitters in the body; some are primarily active in the nervous system and brain and others in the peripheral body. Neurons produce the neurotransmitters that they need to convey the signals they carry. A neurotransmitter binds with receptor sites that act to create "bridges" between neurons. Some neurotransmitters, such as EPINEPHRINE and NOR-EPINEPHRINE, function as HORMONES in that they have actions on tissues in the body other than neurons. Some neurotransmitters are excitatory (they stimulate neuron activity) such as epinephrine, which binds to adrenergic receptors in the myocardium (HEART muscle) and sets in motion the cycle of events that generates a cardiac contraction. Other neurotransmitters are inhibitory (they block neuron activity) such as acetylcholine, which slows muscle cell contractions. ARRHYTHMIAS and HYPERTENSION (high BLOOD PRESSURE) can result when there are imbalances in the neurotransmitters affecting the heart and CARDIOVASCULAR SYSTEM.

See also CALCIUM CYCLE; CARDIAC CYCLE; HEART RATE.

New York Heart Association (NYHA) classification system See HEART FAILURE.

niacin A vitamin-B complex, also called nicotinic acid or niacinamide, taken to lower blood cholesterol levels as a treatment for mild HYPERCHOLESTEROLEMIA and HYPERLIPIDEMIA, typically recommended when blood cholesterol levels are higher than normal but not high enough to warrant therapy with LIPID-LOWERING MEDICATIONS, and lifestyle modifications are not lowering lipid levels as rapidly as the doctor would like to see, as well as sometimes in conjunction with lipid-lowering medications for increased effect. Niacin, also called nicotinic acid, is the vitamin B3 form; niacinamide is the active form. All have comparable actions and effects. Common brand-name products available in the United States include Nicobid, Niaspan (a long-acting form), and Nicotinex. Some niacin preparations are available as over-the-counter products. In the high doses necessary to affect blood cholesterol levels niacin preparations can cause the peripheral arteries to dilate, which can result in skin flushing and accompanying sensation of feeling hot and sometimes nauseated. People who have HYPERTENSION (high BLOOD PRESSURE) generally should not take niacin preparations unless their doctors specifically advise them to do so.

See also CHOLESTEROL, BLOOD; GARLIC AND GARLIC OIL; LIFESTYLE AND HEART HEALTH; NUTRITION AND DIET.

nicardipine A medication taken to treat HYPERTENSION (high BLOOD PRESSURE) and ANGINA. Nicardipine (Cardene) is a CALCIUM CHANNEL ANTAGONIST MEDICA-

TION; it works by slowing the flow of calcium into myocardial (HEART muscle) cells to delay initiation of the CALCIUM CYCLE, which in turn reduces the rate and force of the heart's contractions. Doctors often prescribe nicardipine in combination with a DIURETIC MEDICATION for optimal BLOOD pressure control, or in combination with a BETA ANTAGONIST MEDICATION when both hypertension and angina are present. GRAPEFRUIT AND GRAPEFRUIT JUICE interfere with nicardipine's absorption and should not be consumed while taking this medication, though other citrus fruits do not. Common side effects include headache, DIZZINESS, peripheral EDEMA (especially involving the legs and feet), dry mouth, and CONSTIPATION. Less common but more serious side effects include ARRHYTHMIAS and HEART BLOCK.

See also ANTIHYPERTENSIVE MEDICATIONS; MEDICATION SIDE EFFECTS; MEDICATIONS TO TREAT HEART DISEASE.

nicotine An addictive chemical that is the active ingredient in tobacco products and in some smoking cessation products such as nicotine gum and nicotine patches. Nicotine's primary action is in the brain, where it causes the release of the NEUROTRANSMITTER, DOPAMINE. Dopamine facilitates nerve signals related to sensations of pleasure. Nicotine causes the release of peripheral dopamine as well, which is a precursor for the other hormones, NOREPINEPHRINE and EPINEPHRINE. All three HORMONES stimulate cardiovascular functions and cause HEART RATE and BLOOD PRESSURE to rise. Nicotine appears to damage the cells that line the inner walls of the arteries, helping to establish the conditions that allow ATHEROSCLEROSIS (accumulations of arterial plaque) to develop at an accelerated rate. People who have HYPERTENSION or CORONARY ARTERY DISEASE (CAD) who want to use nicotine-based smoking cessation products should first check with their doctors.

See also SMOKING AND HEART DISEASE; TOBACCO USE.

nifedipine A medication taken to treat HYPERTENSION (high BLOOD PRESSURE) and ANGINA, including variant (Prinzmetal) angina. Doctors also sometimes prescribe nifedipine to treat CORONARY ARTERY SPASM. Nifedipine is a CALCIUM CHANNEL ANTAGONIST MEDICATION; common brand-names include Procardia and Adalat. Nifedipine works by slowing the CALCIUM CYCLE that initiates contraction of the myocardial (HEART muscle) cells to reduce the rate and force of the heart's pumping action. Through this action, nifedipine reduces the heart's oxygen needs and consumption. Some people experience a short-term increase in the number and intensity of anginal episodes when first beginning to take nifedipine; this typically goes away within two weeks as the medication reaches peak BLOOD levels. Side effects, which also often resolve within a few weeks of taking the medication, include nausea, CONSTIPATION, headache, flushing of the skin, and sleep disturbances. Rarely nifedipine causes ARRHYTHMIAS and HEART FAILURE.

See also ANTIHYPERTENSIVE MEDICATIONS; MEDICATION SIDE EFFECTS; MEDICATIONS TO TREAT HEART DISEASE; NITRATE MEDICATIONS.

nimodipine A medication taken to reduce damage to the brain resulting from cerebrovascular bleeding due to hemorrhagic STROKE (often resulting from congenital ANEURYSM). Common brand-name products include Nimotop. Nimodipine is a CALCIUM CHANNEL ANTAGONIST MEDICATION that works by relaxing the smooth muscle cells of peripheral artery walls and slowing their contraction response, helping to keep the arteries from going into spasm. Unlike other calcium channel blockers, nimodipine has little effect on myocardial (HEART muscle) cells. This medication seems to have a stronger effect on the arteries of the brain than on the arteries elsewhere in the body. Doctors typically prescribe nimodipine for 21 days following the initial cerebral hemorrhage, during which time the damaged arteries in the brain are healing. After 21 days, there is little therapeutic value to continuing the medication. Common side effects include headache, HYPOTENSION (low BLOOD PRESSURE), and ARRHYTHMIAS (typically bradycardia, or a slowed HEART rate).

See also ANTIHYPERTENSIVE MEDICATIONS; CARDIOVASCULAR SYSTEM; MEDICATIONS TO TREAT HEART DISEASE; TRANSIENT ISCHEMIC ATTACK (TTA).

nisoldipine A medication taken to treat HYPERTENSION (high BLOOD PRESSURE). Common brand-name products available in the United States include Sular. Nisoldipine belongs to the family of drugs called CALCIUM CHANNEL ANTAGONIST MEDICATIONS; it acts by slowing the CALCIUM CYCLE responsible for smooth muscle cell contraction. It has a negligible effect on myocardial (muscle) cells though has a significant effect on smooth muscle cells in the walls of the arterioles, the body's tiniest arteries, reducing the resistance BLOOD encounters as it flows through them and causing the body's blood pressure regulatory mechanisms to lower blood pressure. Doctors often prescribe nisoldipine in combination with other ANTIHYPERTENSIVE MEDICATIONS to treat moderate to severe hypertension. Taking nisoldipine with high-fat foods increases its absorption into the bloodstream; taking it with GRAPEFRUIT AND GRAPEFRUIT JUICE decreases its absorption and metabolism. Common side effects include headache and peripheral EDEMA (swelling in the arms and legs as a result of fluid retention). Nisoldipine has a mild diuretic effect and so may increase urine production. There is some concern that nisoldipine may increase the risk of HEART ATTACK in people who have moderate to serious CORONARY ARTERY DISEASE (CAD); research continues to examine this apparent correlation.

See also DIURETIC MEDICATIONS; MEDICATION SIDE EFFECTS; MEDICATIONS TO TREAT HEART DISEASE.

nitrate medications Organic nitrate compounds that have a vasodilator effect, taken to treat or prevent attacks of ANGINA (CHEST PAIN originating from the HEART). The three nitrate medications used in the United States are NITROGLYCERIN (in various forms), ISOSORBIDE (dinitrate and mononitrate), and amyl nitrite. Nitrate medications act directly on the peripheral BLOOD vessels, causing them to dilate and relax. Nitrates have a more intense effect on the veins, slowing the rate at which blood returns to the heart and correspondingly decreasing the heart's workload without directly affecting the myocardium (heart muscle) itself. The reduction in workload, or pumping effort, quickly lowers the myocardium's oxygen consumption, relaxing the demand on the coronary arteries to supply the heart with blood.

Sublingual (under the tongue) forms of nitrate medications are effective within minutes, producing relief that lasts 30 to 60 minutes. Longer acting nitrates, such as isosorbide and nitroglycerin patches or extended release capsules, aim to prevent angina attacks from occurring by keeping the peripheral blood vessels, and to lesser extent the CORONARY ARTERIES, dilated. The therapeutic value of this approach is inconsistent, however, as the body rather rapidly develops nitrate tolerance and then ceases to respond to nitrate medications. Generally, the body must be "nitrate-free" for 10 to 12 hours after a nitrate medication dose for the next dose to be effective. For this reason, dosing for long-acting nitrate products is typically daily for six to eight hours of nitrate coverage to provide the necessary nitrate break.

Nitrate toxicity (taking too much nitrate in too short a period of time), though uncommon, can result in serious and even life-threatening HYPOTENSION (low blood pressure). Severe hypotension causes reflex sinus tachycardia (very rapid heart contractions) in an effort to compensate by pumping more blood through the body. Though the response generally is short-lived as nitrates dissipate from active form very quickly, for someone with moderate to severe HEART FAILURE or CORONARY ARTERY DISEASE (CAD) the reflex tachycardia can be sufficient stress to the heart to cause CARDIAC ARREST. Mild to moderate overdose amounts of nitrate medications typically result in headache that subsides as the drug dissipates from the body. The most common scenario for overdose occurs with the unintended combination of nitrate medications. Of particular concern are the PDE5 INHIBITOR MEDICATIONS used to treat ERECTILE DYSFUNCTION that are also nitrate-based formulations. Men who take nitrate medications for angina should not take PDE5 inhibitors. Another rare circumstance under which nitrate toxicity can occur is among people who handle dynamite and other explosives that contain nitroglycerin. It is important to follow appropriate handling procedures including the use of protective clothing (gloves) to prevent nitroglycerin from becoming absorbed through the skin.

See also ATHEROSCLEROSIS; MEDICATION SIDE EFFECTS; MEDICATIONS TO TREAT HEART DISEASE.

nitroglycerin A medication taken to treat ANGINA. There are numerous brand-name products available in the United States. Nitroglycerin causes rapid and pronounced, but short-lived, dilation of the veins. This effect significantly slows the return of BLOOD to the HEART, reducing the heart's preload (amount of pumping effort necessary after each contraction) and relieving the myocardium's oxygen needs. Nitroglycerin also has a moderate effect to dilate the CORONARY ARTERIES and coronary arterioles, increasing the blood supply to the myocardium (heart muscle). Several forms of nitroglycerin are available, including:

- Sublingual tablets are placed under the tongue at the onset of an anginal attack; they dissolve slowly and enter the bloodstream immediately through the mucosal tissues of the mouth.

- Transdermal patches, such as Nitra-Du, are applied to the skin where they deliver a steady release of nitroglycerin absorbed through the skin into the body tissues and ultimately into the bloodstream.

- Translingual sprays deliver a metered dose of nitroglycerin under the tongue, where the drug is absorbed into the bloodstream in a manner similar to the absorption of sublingual nitroglycerin.

- Topical ointments are applied in measured amounts to the skin surface. They take longer to enter the bloodstream than sublingual or translingual forms though they produce an effect that lasts up to four hours. Topical nitroglycerin often helps to prevent attacks of angina when it is applied in advance of physical exertion that could trigger them.

- Extended release capsules take about 45 minutes to produce an effect, which lasts for six to eight hours. The intent of the extended release formulas is to prevent anginal attacks; however, as the body develops a tolerance to nitroglycerin there is some question as to whether this is an effective therapeutic approach.

The most common side effect of nitroglycerin products in any formulation is headache. The PDE5 inhibitors medications to treat erectile dysfunction cannot be taken in conjunction with nitroglycerin as sildenafil also is nitrate-based; combining sildenafil with other NITRATE MEDICATIONS can cause a potentially life-threatening drop in blood pressure.

See also CARDIOVASCULAR SYSTEM; HYPOTENSION.

nitroprusside   A medication administered intravenously to treat hypertensive crisis (a critically dangerous spike in BLOOD PRESSURE) in an emergency setting. Nitroprusside's effect is immediate and short-lived. Doctors sometimes give nitroprusside in cardiovascular crisis due to severe left HEART FAILURE and during HEART ATTACK (MYOCARDIAL INFARCTION) to help stabilize the body's hemodynamics. A metabolic by-product of nitroprusside is cyanide, a chemical that binds with iron in HEMOGLOBIN in the red BLOOD cells and prevents the hemoglobin from binding with oxygen. Doctors must carefully monitor for this effect, which is temporary but can have serious consequences if the cyanide binding becomes extensive. People who are moderate to heavy smokers are at greater risk for complications from cyanide binding, as cigarette smoke contains cyanide. A residual level of cyanide remains bound to iron in the hemoglobin of red blood cells in smokers, lowering the threshold for cyanide toxicity.

See also TOBACCO USE.

Nitrostat   See NITROGLYCERIN.

nonsteroidal anti-inflammatory drugs (NSAIDs)   A classification of medications that reduce swelling and relieve pain. NSAIDs act on hormone-like chemical messengers called PROSTAGLANDINS, which convey impulses between body tissues and the brain that are related to numerous functions, including inflammation in response to injury, the perception of pain, and the aggregation (clumping together) of platelets at the onset of COAGULATION (the clotting process). Injury and swelling cause tissues to release prostaglandins, sending pain signals to the brain. NSAIDs work by blocking the actions of enzymes (forms of cyclooxygenase commonly referred to as COX-1 and COX-2) that are key to prostaglandin's production.

There remains debate among researchers and doctors as to whether NSAIDs are helpful, harmful, or neutral with regard to their effects on CARDIOVASCULAR DISEASE (CVD). Some studies suggest that NSAIDs, like ASPIRIN (also considered an NSAID by classification), are beneficial because of their mild anticoagulant effect. Other studies seem to link NSAIDs with a higher rate of HEART ATTACK and STROKE among people who have heart disease. However, NSAIDs are commonly prescribed to treat PERICARDITIS.

Most NSAIDs nonselectively block COX-1 and COX-2. Aspirin, pharmacologically classified as an NSAID, primarily blocks COX-1, the form of cyclooxygenase that allows platelet aggregation to occur. Doctors routinely advise people with high risk for HEART DISEASE or heart attack, or who have heart disease or have had a heart attack, to take low-dose aspirin daily as a mild anticoagulant. Research in the late 1990s and early 2000s suggests that when a person takes both aspirin and another NSAID routinely, such as for chronic arthritis or other pain, the NSAID replaces the aspirin in blocking COX-1 activity. It appears, however, that unlike aspirin, an NSAID can relinquish its inhibitory effects. So after bumping aspirin, the NSAID releases the COX-1 again. This raises concern that regular NSAID use in people taking aspirin therapy may negate the benefits of the aspirin.

The most frequent side effect of NSAIDs is gastrointestinal distress, particularly dyspepsia (stomach irritation and upset). Taking high doses of NSAIDs for extended periods of time can cause irreversible liver and kidney damage and failure. Doctors typically evaluate routine blood tests to monitor for these rare but serious occurrences in people who take prescription NSAIDs for chronic conditions such as osteoarthritis and rheumatoid arthritis. People who routinely take over-the-counter NSAIDs, particularly when also taking aspirin therapy, when diagnosed with any form of heart disease, or when at high risk for heart disease, should talk with their doctors about alternatives that present a lower cardiovascular risk.

See also ANTICOAGULANT MEDICATIONS; ATHEROSCLEROSIS; CORONARY ARTERY DISEASE (CAD); LIVING WITH HEART DISEASE.

COMMON NONSTEROIDAL ANTI-INFLAMMATORY DRUGS (NSAIDS) AVAILABLE IN THE UNITED STATES

NSAID	Common Brand-Name Products	Typically Taken to Treat
Prescription:		
Diclofenac	Cataflam, Voltaren	Osteoarthritis, rheumatoid arthritis, ankylosing spondylitis, menstrual cramps
Diflunisal	Dolobid, generic diflunisal	Gout, osteoarthritis, rheumatoid arthritis, moderate pain
Etodolac	Lodine	Gout, osteoarthritis, rheumatoid arthritis
Fenoprofen	Nalfon, generic fenoprofen	Osteoarthritis, general pain
Ibuprofen	Advil, Motrin, Trendar, generic ibuprofen	Osteoarthritis, menstrual cramps, headache, mild to moderate pain, fever, musculoskeletal injuries
Indomethacin	Indocin	Gout, rheumatoid arthritis
Ketoprofen	Orudis, Oruvail, generic ketoprofen	Osteoarthritis, menstrual cramps, headache, mild to moderate pain, fever, musculoskeletal injuries
Meclofenamate	Meclomen, generic meclofenamate	Heavy menstrual bleeding and cramps, osteoarthritis, mild to moderate pain
Nabumetone	Relafen	Osteoarthritis, rheumatoid arthritis, ankylosing spondylitis
Naproxen	Naprosyn, Naprelan, generic naproxen	Osteoarthritis, menstrual cramps, headache, mild to moderate pain, fever, musculoskeletal injuries
Oxaprozin	Daypro, generic oxaprozin	Osteoarthritis, rheumatoid arthritis, bursitis, tendonitis, general pain
Phenylbutazone	Cotylbutazone, generic phenylbutazone	Gout
Piroxicam	Feldene, generic piroxicam	Osteoarthritis, menstrual cramps
Sulindac	Clinoril, generic sulindac	Gout, osteoarthritis, rheumatoid arthritis, bursitis, tendonitis
Tolmetin	Tolectin, generic tolmetin	Osteoarthritis, rheumatoid arthritis
Over-the-Counter:		
Aspirin	Numerous proprietary, store, and generic brands	General pain and inflammation, fever, anticoagulant therapy
Ketoprofen	Orudis KB, Oruvail, generic ketoprofen	General pain and inflammation, menstrual cramps, osteoarthritis, musculoskeletal injuries, headache, dental pain
Ibuprofen (200 mg strength)	Advil, Exedrin IB, Motrin IB, generic ibuprofen	General pain and inflammation, menstrual cramps, osteoarthritis, musculoskeletal injuries, headache, dental pain
Naproxen (220 mg strength)	Anaprox, Aleve, generic naproxen	General pain and inflammation, menstrual cramps, osteoarthritis, musculoskeletal injuries, headache, dental pain

norepinephrine A chemical the body produces that acts as a HORMONE and as a NEUROTRANSMITTER. Norepinephrine's primary role in the body is to regulate BLOOD PRESSURE, which it does by stimulating receptors in peripheral arteries and arterioles causing them to contract. This increases the resistance blood encounters when it flows through them, triggering the sequence of events that causes the heart to increase the rate and force of its contractions. This mechanism of blood pressure regulation is continuous, keeping blood pressure at a level that meets the body's needs for blood at all activity levels, and takes place without conscious awareness or involvement of the conscious brain.

The medulla of the adrenal gland and certain nerve endings in the sympathetic nervous system produce norepinephrine. Doctors sometimes administer norepinephrine as a drug during CARDIAC ARREST or SHOCK along with other resuscitative measures in an attempt to rapidly raise blood pressure. The body's stress response also activates the release of norepinephrine, which stimulates parts of the brain as well as increases cardiovascular activity. Norepinephrine is chemically related to other neurotransmitters, notably DOPAMINE and EPINEPHRINE, and also has actions in the brain and nervous system.

See also CATECHOLAMINES; RENIN-ANGIOTENSIN-ALDOSTERONE (RAA) HORMONAL SYSTEM; STRESS AND HEART DISEASE.

Normodyne See LABETALOL.

Norpace See DISOPYRAMIDE.

Norwood procedure The first of three stages of surgical correction for significant congenital malformations of the HEART such as HYPOPLASTIC LEFT HEART SYNDROME (HLHS), in which the left ventricle is missing or so severely underdeveloped that it is nonfunctional. With these malformations the heart is unable to pump oxygenated BLOOD to the body. The Norwood procedure, named after physician William Norwood who developed it in 1981 to treat HLSH, creates a two-chamber heart. Though this does not restore normal cardiovascular function, it does allow the heart to pump oxygenated blood to the body at a level adequate to support a nearly normal life. Pediatric cardiovascular surgeons typically perform the Norwood procedure within the first week or two of life, as the congenital malformations are life-threatening.

Procedure

For the Norwood procedure, the surgeons first cut the pulmonary artery away from the right ventricle and place a patch to close the opening. They then split and widen the aorta, which usually also arises from the right ventricle as the left ventricle is too undeveloped to support it, using a donor graft aortic segment (ALLOGRAFT). This strengthens the aorta so it can support blood flow going out to the body. The surgeons next connect the pulmonary artery to the base of the aorta so that some of the blood the ventricle pumps goes to the lungs.

Risks and Complications

The Norwood procedure is very high risk because the heart defects are so severe and the operation must be done within the first two weeks of life. One in four infants does not survive the surgery. Bleeding, infection, ARRHYTHMIAS, and failure of the right ventricle to function in its modified configuration are among the most significant complications. The infant continues to have inadequate OXYGENATION and greatly compromised cardiovascular function. However, the three in four infants who do survive have good prospects for successful follow-up surgeries that will provide much improved, though not normal, cardiac function.

Outlook and Lifestyle Modifications

The Norwood procedure is palliative, intended to improve oxygenation while the baby grows strong enough to withstand the necessary subsequent operations (usually the BIDIRECTIONAL GLENN PROCEDURE and the FONTAN PROCEDURE). The baby still has significantly impaired cardiac function and circulation and takes numerous medications to support and strengthen the heart. Care of the infant until the remaining operations can be completed is complex and requires dedicated effort.

In subsequent procedures surgeons will place shunts to create a direct flow of blood from the superior vena cava and the inferior vena cava, the major veins that bring blood back to the heart, to the pulmonary artery (bidirectional Glenn procedure and Fontan procedure). This allows natural gravitational flow to drain the unoxygenated blood into the lungs. The oxygenated blood returns to the heart's single ventricle via the pulmonary veins, flows to the ventricle, and is pumped out through the aorta.

See also BLALOCK-TAUSSIG PROCEDURE; DAMUS-KAYE-STANSEL PROCEDURE; HEART DISEASE IN CHILDREN;

HEART TRANSPLANT; SURGERY TO TREAT CARDIOVASCULAR DISEASE.

Nurses' Health Study A large-scale examination, funded by the U.S. National Institutes of Health (NIH), implemented in 1976 to study the long-term effects of ORAL CONTRACEPTIVES, diet, and lifestyle on the overall health of women. There now are two study groups, the original 122,000 nurses who enrolled in the 1976 study and the addition of 115,000 younger nurses in 1989. Study participants complete comprehensive health questionnaires every two years and provide BLOOD and tissue samples as requested. The Nurses' Health Study remains ongoing and issues reports of its findings as they are relevant. Though the Nurses' Health Study does not exclusively focus on cardiovascular health, a number of its findings address health matters related to risk factors for, as well as prevention and development of, CARDIOVASCULAR DISEASE (CVD). Such information is particularly insightful as many clinical research studies that focus on CVD have predominantly male populations; findings from studies such as the Nurses' Health Study provide information unique to women.

See also HORMONE REPLACEMENT THERAPY (HRT); LIFESTYLE AND HEART HEALTH; NUTRITION AND DIET.

nutritional supplements Products such as VITAMIN AND MINERAL SUPPLEMENTS and herbal remedies taken to increase or augment the nutrients the body receives. Nutritional supplements are exempt from U.S. regulations governing testing and demonstrated evidence of effective actions. The U.S. Food and Drug Administration (FDA) does have the authority to regulate nutritional supplement labeling and prohibits manufacturers from making claims about a product's effectiveness in the absence of verifiable clinical results. People who are taking medication for any form of heart disease should check with their doctors before taking any herbal remedies or nutritional supplements, including vitamin and mineral products. Some MEDICATIONS TO TREAT HEART DISEASE interact with nutrients such as iron and vitamin C, for example.

Most health experts agree that only people who are unable to obtain needed nutrients through dietary sources need to take nutritional supplements, unless there is a health condition or side effect of a medication that causes a depletion of specific nutrients. Health experts generally believe that though vitamin and mineral supplements may benefit people who have such deficiencies, supplements cannot precisely replicate vitamins and minerals and the interactions among them to present the body with what might otherwise come from nature. In other words, what comes from a bottle does not have the same actions in the body as what comes from the land. Whether this is of significance when considering the benefits of nutritional supplements remains a topic of debate.

See also COMPLEMENTARY THERAPIES; LIFESTYLE AND HEART HEALTH; MEDICATION MANAGEMENT; MEDICATION SIDE EFFECTS.

nutrition and diet The body's metabolic needs and the foods consumed to meet them. Nutrition and diet are essential to health and, when inadequate or inappropriate, contribute to disease. Many health experts believe that as much as 80 percent of disease in contemporary Western society relates to disparities between nutrition and diet.

Nutrition

Nutrition is what the body *needs*. The substances that are of value to the body from the foods consumed are called nutrients; they fall into five general categories.

- **Carbohydrates** are sugars that come primarily from plant sources and processed foods. They are the body's primary source of energy. They break down easily in the intestines and enter the bloodstream quickly. Natural food sources of carbohydrates include fruits, vegetables, and grains. Processed foods such as baked goods are the most common dietary source of carbohydrates.
- **Fats** come from animal and plant sources. Plant-based monounsaturated and polyunsaturated fats such as canola oil and olive oil help to raise high-density lipoprotein (HDL), the "good" cholesterol that helps keep lipids in the bloodstream from accumulating along the inner walls of the arteries. Animal-based saturated fats, trans fats

(found to limited extent in animal fats and primarily in processed fats such as margarines), and hydrogenated fats (processed fats with added hydrogen molecules to stabilize them in solid form at room temperature) provide the body with the components to synthesize LDL. The body needs a certain level of dietary fat, as lipids (fatty acids in the blood) are essential for many cell functions as well as to transport fat-soluble nutrients such as certain vitamins.

- **Proteins** come from animal sources and plant sources. Proteins are the fundamental building blocks of cells and tissues that are themselves comprised of amino acids arranged in various formations. Digestion breaks down dietary proteins into their constituent amino acids, which then enter the bloodstream. The body reassembles the amino acids into the proteins it needs. In addition to forming numerous body structures, proteins serve as transports for nutrients and genetic encoding, as antibodies, and in the body's fluid balance mechanism that is crucial for maintaining appropriate blood pressure.

- **Fiber** comes from plant sources. It provides the bulk that holds plants together, and it provides the bulk necessary to move digestive waste through the large intestine. Different kinds of fiber have the ability to absorb water and bind with bile acids, helping to keep dietary fats from entering the bloodstream.

- **Vitamins and minerals** are abundant in foods that come from natural sources, and as supplements added to processed foods such as dairy products, breads, and cereals. The more highly processed a food is, however, the less nutritional value (including vitamins and minerals) it has. Vitamins and minerals often need each other to become active in the body, such as calcium and vitamin D. Many minerals are ions, or chemicals capable of storing an electrical charge. These play crucial roles in communication among nerve cells and in the contractions of the heart.

Diet

Diet is what the body *gets*. Diet may or may not meet the body's nutritional needs. Through the processes of digestion and metabolism the body disassembles, reorganizes, and reassembles the carbohydrates, fats, and proteins from the foods that enter the body into forms that it can use. These are not always in the proportions that the body needs, however. Protein builds muscle because dietary sources of protein provide the body with the source material, or building blocks, that it needs to synthesize (produce) protein to manufacture new muscle cells. If dietary consumption provides the body with more protein than it needs, it converts the extra protein to storage forms of energy (primarily fat) because this is all it can do with substances that become excess calories. In the current typical Western diet, sources of dietary protein tend to be animal-based, making them high in fat as well. All calories that enter the body become expended or stored energy, regardless of their source. The optimal diet is one that meets the body's nutritional and caloric needs in balance, so the body needs and uses what enters through diet.

Eating Habits

How people eat is as significant as *what* they eat. Many people eat far more than their bodies require, and far more than they realize they consume. The portion size that forms the basis for a food's nutritional analysis may be a third to a half of the amount a typical person consumes. A 20-ounce bottle of soda, for example, actually contains 2.5 servings according to the label but most people drink the entire bottle. Most restaurant portions are two to four times the appropriate serving size, and when eating at home many people pay little attention to how much food they put on their plates. In general, one serving is the amount of food that fits in the palm of the hand; one serving of meat is the size of a deck of cards. All of these excesses add up to excess calories, excess body fat, excess body weight, and health problems such as DIABETES, HYPERTENSION (high BLOOD PRESSURE), and high blood cholesterol and blood TRIGLYCERIDES levels (setting the stage for ATHEROSCLEROSIS and CORONARY ARTERY DISEASE [CAD]). OBESITY, the leading health problem arising from excess caloric intake, has become a close second (and many health experts believe has surpassed) smoking as a risk factor for heart disease.

Eating habits are learned behaviors, which means it is possible to change them. Most people are unaware of what and how much they eat simply because they act from habit when eating. Often, the process of becoming aware is enough to catalyze a change in those habits. People attempting to make dietary changes tend to view healthful eating habits as depriving them of the foods they enjoy. However, nearly any food can be part of a nutritious eating pattern as long as it accounts for an appropriate amount and percentage of calories. Few foods are inherently "bad." Instead, it is important to look overall at food options and portion sizes to make choices that support cardiovascular (and overall) health and that deliver the nutrients the body needs.

American Heart Association's "Dietary Guidelines for Healthy Americans"

For many years the American Heart Association's step 1 and step 2 diets were the benchmarks for nutritional standards to prevent heart disease (step 1) and to modify lifestyle to help treat heart disease (step 2). In 2000 the American Heart Association issued a revised approach, "Dietary Guidelines for Healthy Americans," that simplifies nutritional recommendations to outline a single standard of heart-healthy eating habits for all adults and replaces its former step 1 diet. In general, the AHA's guidelines call for eating:

- At least five servings of fruits and five servings of vegetables every day; the more, and the more varied, the better. Fruits and vegetables are high in vitamins, minerals, antioxidants, and innumerable nutrients that the body needs.

- Fish, and particularly fatty fish such as salmon and tuna, at least two meals every week. Fish is high in OMEGA FATTY ACIDS, which help to lower LDL and VLDL, and low in fat and cholesterol.

- Skinless poultry, legumes, lean meats, and non-fat or low-fat dairy products, and fats and oils with less than two grams of saturated fat per tablespoon such that calories from saturated fat and trans fat combined comprise 10 percent or less, on average, of daily calorie consumption.

- Minimal sugar and other nutritionally empty calories (snack foods, soda, candy).

- Less than 2,400 milligrams of SODIUM daily.

- Enough calories to balance the calories expended. The AHA suggests a simple formula of multiplying one's desired weight by 15 for people who are active and by 12 for people who are sedentary to determine the average number of dietary calories per day that are appropriate.

The AHA guidelines also recommend 30 minutes of sustained EXERCISE daily to help maintain the body's energy balance and metabolic efficiency (particularly relative to lipid production and metabolism). Walking is generally adequate for most people to achieve this goal. Regular exercise reduces the risk for diabetes, a significant cause of heart disease, and for hypertension.

Therapeutic Lifestyle Change (TLC) Diet

The National Heart, Lung, and Blood Institute (NHLBI), through its National Cholesterol Education Program (NCEP), has developed the Therapeutic Lifestyle Change (TLC) diet for people who have high blood cholesterol (HYPERCHOLESTEROLEMIA, HYPERTRIGLYCERIDEMIA, or HYPERLIPIDEMIA), ATHEROSCLEROSIS, CORONARY ARTERY DISEASE (CAD), and who also may have INSULIN RESISTANCE or DIABETES (which are key risk factors for HEART DISEASE). The TLC diet arose from the NCEP's revised recommendations for dietary and blood cholesterol levels issued in its May 2001 *Third Report of the Expert Panel on Detection, Evaluation, and Treatment of High Blood Cholesterol in Adults*, known as the Adult Treatment Panel III (ATP III).

The American Heart Association has adopted the TLC diet as its recommended nutrition plan for people who have or are at high risk for heart disease. The TLC diet emphasizes:

- Increasing consumption of fruits, vegetables, and whole grains and whole grain products to consume 10 to 25 grams of soluble fiber and two grams plant stanols and sterols daily. Soluble fiber (such as oat bran and oatmeal provide) directly absorbs cholesterol in the small intestine, lowering the amount of dietary cholesterol that makes it into the bloodstream. Plant stanols and sterols have chemical structures similar to cholesterol that bind with the protein carriers that transport lipids into the bloodstream, but the liver cannot use these structures to manufacture cholesterol, which forces it to draw lipids, primarily from LDL and VLDL, from the bloodstream instead. This contributes to lowering blood cholesterol levels.

- Limiting to 7 percent or less of daily calories the consumption of foods that contribute to increased levels of LDL and VLDL. Such foods include saturated fats and trans fats, found in the highest concentrations in animal-based foods (such as meats) and in processed foods such as baked goods.

- Limiting dietary cholesterol to no more than 200 mg daily.

- Maintaining a balance among calories consumed, on average, that is 50 to 60 percent carbohydrate, 25 to 35 percent fat (including saturated fat, and no more than one-third of which comes from monounsaturated and two-thirds from polyunsaturated), and 15 percent protein.

- Consuming a daily calorie amount that maintains a healthy weight.

- Daily physical exercise that expends a minimum of 200 calories of energy; more for those who need to lose weight to achieve a healthy BODY MASS INDEX (BMI).

The TLC diet is similar to the Mediterranean diet, which is based on the eating habits of people from the Mediterranean region and emphasizes high consumption of vegetables, fruits, whole grains and whole grain products, and fish. A dietary focus on such foods is inherently low in fats and processed foods, the primary culprits when it comes to dietary challenges for people who have heart disease. As well, the Mediterranean diet embraces the Mediterranean lifestyle, which is one of simplicity by modern standards and one of regular, moderate physical activity. There is much clinical evidence that the Mediterranean way of eating supports cardiovascular health and can reduce some risks for heart disease when followed consistently and accompanied by daily physical exercise (as the TLC diet recommends).

Food Substitutes and "Diet" Foods

Food manufacturers are continually searching for ways to bolster sales of their products, and replacing "unhealthy" ingredients with "healthy" ones has become one approach touted as allowing people to continue eating former favorites. Most health and nutrition experts recommend that people apply a framework of moderation to their eating habits that allows them to incorporate small amounts of former favorites rather than looking for ways to replace them, in keeping with the emphasis on increasing the amounts of vegetables, fruits, and whole grains and whole grain products in the daily diet.

- Salt substitutes typically contain POTASSIUM instead of sodium, which offers a similar taste of saltiness. People who take potassium-sparing diuretic medications can develop HYPERKALEMIA (elevated blood potassium), a potentially dangerous imbalance of ELECTROLYTES essential to the CARDIAC CYCLE, when using such substitutes.

- Fat substitutes replace fat in processed foods such as baked goods and snack items with substances made of proteins, carbohydrates, or fat molecules that are too large for the human digestive system to absorb (such as olestra). Though they replace the fat, often they increase the total calories, making them a questionable choice for people concerned with weight loss.

- Sugar substitutes, or artificial sweeteners, use products such as aspartame and saccharin to impart a taste of sweetness. Those that the FDA has approved for use have no apparent harmful effects, though people who have a metabolic disorder called phenylketonuria (PKU) cannot consume products containing aspartame.

"Diet" foods may contain combinations of fat substitutes and sugar substitutes and attempt to preserve the perception of favorite foods without the same numbers of calories. For the most part, such products really are nothing like the originals they purport to replace and contain enough calories that portion size remains a significant factor. In most situations a small portion of the "real" food is a better alternative for people who must have those favorite foods, accounting for its nutrient balance by making adjustments in other foods consumed.

The United States Department of Agriculture (USDA) permits food manufacturers to label their products as "heart-healthy" when those products meet certain criteria for saturated fat, trans fat, total fat, cholesterol, and sodium levels. Foods claiming to be low-fat, reduced fat, or fat-free similarly must meet certain criteria. Even so, it is important to carefully read product labels as such criteria compare the low-fat or reduced fat product to the regular version of the product, not to a uni-form standard of fat content. Even products that meet the criteria to claim they are fat-free can contain enough fat that, when consumed in amounts greater than the labeled portion size, they contribute a measurable quantity of dietary fat.

See also CHOLESTEROL, BLOOD; LIFESTYLE AND HEART HEALTH; LIVING WITH HEART DISEASE; ORNISH PROGRAM.

oat bran   See NUTRITION AND DIET.

obesity   Body weight greater than 20 percent over the healthy weight for a person's height or a BODY MASS INDEX (BMI) of 30 or greater. Obesity is a risk factor for many health conditions, notably type 2 DIABETES and numerous forms of CARDIOVASCULAR DISEASE (CVD) including ATHEROSCLEROSIS, HYPERTENSION (high BLOOD PRESSURE), CORONARY ARTERY DISEASE (CAD), CARDIOMYOPATHY (enlargement and weakening of the HEART), and HEART FAILURE. Many health experts believe obesity now rivals cigarette smoking as the most significant modifiable risk factor for HEART DISEASE.

The steady increase in the numbers of obese Americans over the past decade alarms health-care providers. Nearly two-thirds of the U.S. adult population is overweight and over a third is obese. Many factors contribute to obesity, though the bottom line is deceptively simple: more calories consumed than expended. Only one in five Americans participates in regular, moderate EXERCISE. Two in five Americans participate in no physical exercise other than what is necessary to carry out their regular daily activities. The American Heart Association reports that physical inactivity is nearly comparable to smoking or high blood cholesterol as a risk factor for CAD and correlates to more than a twofold increase in the likelihood of developing CAD.

Obesity stresses the cardiovascular system in a number of ways. Excess body fat puts pressure on internal organs and against BLOOD vessels, raising the resistance blood must flow against to circulate through the body. This causes the heart to work harder—HEART RATE and the heart's force of contractions both increase. Correspondingly, BLOOD PRESSURE rises. As well, excess body fat signals excess lipids in the bloodstream. Over time these responses have a high likelihood of developing into cardiovascular health problems such as atherosclerosis, hypertension, cardiomyopathy, and CAD. The likelihood of INSULIN RESISTANCE and type 2 DIABETES increases dramatically with obesity as well, both of which are additional risk factors for cardiovascular disease.

Weight loss and WEIGHT MANAGEMENT can mitigate many of these cardiovascular risks and effects. Numerous clinical studies have demonstrated that modest weight loss can lower blood pressure and improve blood cholesterol and blood triglycerides levels, particularly when the weight loss is the result of lifestyle changes such as lowering the amount of fat in the diet and increasing the amount of physical exercise.

See also BODY SHAPE AND HEART DISEASE; INFLAMMATION AND HEART DISEASE; LIFESTYLE AND HEART HEALTH; WAIST CIRCUMFERENCE.

occlusion   An obstruction that creates a partial or complete blockage in a structure such as an artery. Nearly all arterial occlusions occur from accumulations of arterial plaque that build up along the inside walls of the arteries, gradually narrowing the opening for BLOOD flow. This narrowing is called STENOSIS. As plaque accumulates, it irritates the wall of the artery, causing it to become inflamed, and also forms an irregular surface. These circumstances can cause blood clots to develop. The clot may become large enough to block the artery at the point of stenosis, or may break away from the plaque and lodge elsewhere in another artery.

An occlusion in one of the CORONARY ARTERIES can cause ANGINA (CHEST PAIN), ischemia (lack of oxygen to an area of tissue), CORONARY ARTERY

SPASM, and HEART ATTACK (MYOCARDIAL INFARCTION). An occlusion in one of the carotid arteries in the neck can cause TRANSIENT ISCHEMIC ATTACKS (TIAs), particularly when the occlusion occurs in conjunction with CAROTID STENOSIS, or STROKE if the occlusion grows large enough. An occlusion also may block any of the smaller arteries in the brain, causing stroke, or a peripheral artery, generally causing pain and swelling. DEEP VEIN THROMBOSIS (DVT) occurs when an occlusion results from a clot that forms in a vein, typically one of the inner veins of the legs. DVT develops when blood flow through the vein becomes occluded by pressure, such as when sitting with pressure against the back of the legs for extended periods of time.

Doctors typically use imaging technologies such as ULTRASOUND or DOPPLER ULTRASOUND to diagnose venous occlusions and may use ANGIO-GRAM, CARDIAC CATHETERIZATION, MAGNETIC RESONANCE IMAGING (MRI), or COMPUTED TOMOGRAPHY (CT) SCAN to diagnose arterial occlusions. Treatment depends on the occlusion's location, cause, and extent of damage. For arterial occlusions causing heart attack or stroke, doctors can sometimes administer THROMBOLYTIC MEDICATIONS—"clot busters"—that break up the clot causing the occlusion. Further treatment generally includes anticoagulant medications to help prevent future clots from forming, as well as whatever measures are appropriate to remedy or manage the underlying condition. This might include CAROTID ENDARTERECTOMY for carotid artery occlusions resulting from carotid stenosis, or ANGIOPLASTY or CORONARY ARTERY BYPASS GRAFT (CABG) for coronary artery occlusions resulting from CORONARY ARTERY DISEASE (CAD). Surgeons sometimes perform ATHERECTOMY to open the artery and remove the occlusion or angioplasty to replace a damaged segment of artery as treatment for peripheral artery occlusions.

See also ATHEROSCLEROSIS; EMBOLISM; PLAQUE, ARTERIAL; THROMBOLYSIS.

Olean See NUTRITION AND DIET.

olestra See NUTRITION AND DIET.

omega fatty acids Forms of dietary lipids that are the base structures for PROSTAGLANDINS and as such play key roles in the actions of platelets (the red BLOOD cells that initiate the clotting sequence) in the bloodstream. Chemists designate these fatty acid chains as "omega" as a convention of naming chemical structures using Greek letters combined with numbers to identify the locations of specific chemical bonds.

Some forms of omega fatty acids, notably omega-3 and omega-6, have come into prominence for their roles in cardiovascular health and disease. These two appear to work in tandem, with omega-3 fatty acids inhibiting platelet aggregation (the tendency of platelets to become sticky and clump together) and omega-6 fatty acids encouraging platelet aggregation and hence clot formation. When dietary consumption of these fatty acids is balanced, their actions in the body are balanced.

Both omega-3 and omega-6 fatty acids are essential fatty acids, which means the body requires them to function but must acquire them from dietary sources outside the body. Omega-3 fatty acids include eicosapentaenoic acid (EPA), docosahexaenoic acid (DHA), and alpha-linolenic acid (ALA). Fatty fish such as salmon, mackerel, tuna, and sardines contain high levels of EPA and DHA. Soybeans, canola, walnuts, flaxseeds and their oils are high in alpha-linolenic acid. The most common dietary omega-6 fatty acids are linoleic acid, found in vegetable oils, and arachidonic acid, found in meats.

Current dietary recommendations advise adults to include fish containing omega-3 fatty acids in at least two meals each week. The American Heart Association (AHA) further suggests that people with high blood TRIGLYCERIDES levels, which present a significant risk for ATHEROSCLEROSIS and CORONARY ARTERY DISEASE (CAD), talk with their doctors about taking omega-3 supplements as well. However, more than three grams a day of omega-3 fatty acids, from all sources combined, could cause prolonged bleeding because of omega-3's role in inhibiting platelet aggregation.

Most people who follow the AHA's "Dietary Guidelines for Healthy Americans" and who replace meats with other protein sources such as fish will inherently increase their dietary omega-3 fatty acid consumption and reduce their omega-6 fatty acid consumption. This will bring blood triglycerides levels down in all but those who have familial lipid disorders, possibly eliminating the need to take LIPID-LOWERING MEDICATIONS.

There has been some concern that fish high in omega-3 fatty acids also contain contaminants such as mercury and other heavy metals that could cause health problems in people who consume large quantities of contaminated fish. The AHA's recommendation of fish for two meals each week is well within the consumption guidelines established by the Environmental Protection Agency (EPA) for such contaminants; most health experts do not consider there to be any appreciable health risk from following the AHA recommendation. Some doctors recommend omega-3 supplements for people who have significant cardiovascular disease or who have had heart attacks. Because it is possible to take too much of such supplements or to create interactions with some medications taken to treat heart disease, it is important to first check with a doctor.

See also CHOLESTEROL, BLOOD; HYPERLIPIDEMIA; NUTRITION AND DIET.

open-heart surgery The common term for surgical procedures in which surgeons open the chest to expose the HEART. The most frequently performed open-heart operation is CORONARY ARTERY BYPASS GRAFT (CABG), in which surgeons replace diseased or damaged CORONARY ARTERIES with new arteries crafted from BLOOD vessels harvested elsewhere in the body or from synthetic materials. Surgeons also perform open-heart procedures to correct congenital malformations of the heart, repair or replace heart valves, and attempt to improve severe CARDIOMYOPATHY and HEART FAILURE. Open-heart operations require that the surgeon bypass the heart, connecting its great arteries to cannulas (large tubes) that reroute blood to a HEART-LUNG BYPASS MACHINE.

Open-heart surgery is considered among the most significant medical achievements of the 20th century. Before the heart-lung bypass machine, surgeons could open the chest to get to the heart though they could not stop the heart to operate on it. This limited the kinds of operations surgeons could perform. Experimentation with machines that could take over the oxygenation and pumping of blood began in the 1930s, though it was the late 1950s before researchers developed heart-lung bypass machines and procedures for routing blood through them that allowed consistent perfusion. Once surgeons could safely stop the heart, they could open it to repair congenital heart malformations, diseased heart valves, and occluded coronary arteries. Refinements in technology and in surgical techniques in the last half of the 20th century have made open-heart operations among the most commonly performed surgical procedures in the United States.

Procedure

For open-heart surgery, the surgeon must first cut through the sternum (breastbone), then spread apart the ribs to expose the heart. After connecting large tubes called cannulas to the heart's main arteries to reroute blood flow to the heart-lung bypass machine, the surgeon bathes the heart in a cooled solution that slows and then stops its contractions. After the operation is finished, the heart often starts beating again on its own when the flow of blood is restored; if it does not, the surgeon administers a measured electrical charge to initiate contractions.

Risks and Complications

The two most significant risks of open-heart surgery are that the heart will not restart and that the person is unable to wean from the cardiopulmonary bypass. Other risks and complications include excessive bleeding during or after surgery, infection, and failure of the procedure.

Outlook and Lifestyle Modifications

The outlook of open-heart surgery depends on the underlying cardiovascular situation, the complexity of the operation, and the person's general health and strength. Everyone who undergoes open-heart surgery benefits from lifestyle modifications that include nutritious (and often low-fat) eating habits, daily EXERCISE, and WEIGHT MANAGEMENT.

Most people report that the discomfort they feel during the recovery period comes from the sternum healing, which can take up to several months to be complete. Depending on the kind of operation, most people can return to their normal activities within two months of their surgeries. Nearly 700,000 open-heart operations are performed in the United States each year; 90 percent of them are for CABG.

See also BATISTA HEART FAILURE PROCEDURE; HEART TRANSPLANT; SURGERY TO TREAT CARDIOVASCULAR DISEASE; VALVE REPAIR AND REPLACEMENT.

oral contraceptives HORMONE-based medication a woman takes to prevent pregnancy, also called birth control pills. Most oral contraceptives contain a mix of ESTROGEN and progesterone that regulates a woman's menstrual cycle to suppress ovulation. Studies conducted over the 40 years since the birth control pill made its debut show an appreciable increase in risk for thromboembolic STROKE (stroke caused by blood clots blocking blood vessels) among women who take oral contraceptives and have one or more of these factors:

- age 35 or older
- smoke cigarettes
- uncontrolled or undiagnosed HYPERTENSION (high BLOOD PRESSURE)
- frequent migraine headaches

For women who are healthy and have none of these factors, which comprises the majority of women taking oral contraceptives, there is no increased risk for cardiovascular complications. For women who have one or more of these factors, the risk for cardiovascular and cerebrovascular problems, especially venous blood clots (which can result in stroke), increases.

Cardiovascular risk further appears related to the amount of estrogen in the oral contraceptive. The first generation of oral contraceptives that came into use in the early 1960s contained what by contemporary standards were high amounts of estrogen, typically 50 to 60 micrograms. Most birth control pills prescribed today contain 20 to 35 micrograms of estrogen, although higher estrogen pills remain available as some women require

higher doses of estrogen to suppress ovulation. The greater the amount of estrogen in the oral contraceptive, the higher the risk for cardiovascular complications—a risk that increases exponentially as other factors enter into the picture as well, such that many doctors will not prescribe oral contraceptives containing estrogen for women who are age 35 or older, smoke, have hypertension, and have frequent migraines.

Age, smoking, and hypertension are themselves significant risk factors for heart disease; researchers do not clearly understand how oral contraceptives further influence cardiovascular risk. There is growing evidence that taking oral contraceptives when OBESITY and DIABETES, also independent risk factors for heart disease, are present also increases the risk of heart disease. Most health experts believe, and research findings seem to support, that oral contraceptives have no influence on cardiovascular risk among women who have no risk factors for cardiovascular disease.

See also HORMONE REPLACEMENT THERAPY; LIFESTYLE AND HEART DISEASE; WOMEN AND HEART DISEASE.

organ donation See DONOR HEART.

Ornish program A lifestyle modification approach to treating and reversing HEART DISEASE. American physician Dean Ornish developed the approach, which emphasizes an integration of four key components: diet, EXERCISE, MEDITATION and YOGA, and a support network of family and friends.

- **Diet** The Ornish program advocates a low-fat, plant-based diet featuring whole foods such as fruits, vegetables, grains, and legumes, including soybeans.
- **Exercise** The Ornish program incorporates moderately intense exercise (boosting HEART RATE to 50 to 80 percent of maximum heart rate) for 30 minutes at a time every day or for one hour three times a week.
- **Stress relief and relaxation** The Ornish program incorporates meditation and yoga (or variations such as prayer) as methods to clear

the mind and relax the body, helping to relieve physical and mental or emotional stress.

- **Support network** The Ornish program encourages developing close personal relationships to generate a sense of being connected and loved.

Its integrated approach makes the Ornish program unique among lifestyle modification methods for HEART disease. It truly represents a complete shift in lifestyle for nearly everyone who adopts it. A number of clinical studies have affirmed the ability of the Ornish program to make measurable differences in cardiovascular disease. It is one of the only lifestyle modification programs covered by Medicare. There are now Ornish programs in locations throughout the United States.

See also LIFESTYLE AND HEART HEALTH; NUTRITION AND DIET.

orthopnea Shortness of breath or difficulty breathing that occurs while lying down and is relieved when sitting up or standing. Orthopnea is a key symptom of moderate to severe congestive HEART FAILURE. When lying down there is less resistance for BLOOD to return to the HEART from the lower body, increasing the volume of blood that flows through the heart and the lungs. In heart failure the heart's capacity to pump blood is diminished, and fluid begins to collect in the lungs, further increasing the pressure against which the heart must work. The lungs cannot fully inflate because of the fluid, and the heart cannot pump enough blood through the body to meet the oxygen needs of tissues. When sitting up or standing blood drains, with help from gravity, into the lower extremities and the heart is able to pump more efficiently to relieve the fluid buildup in the lungs. Uncontrolled HYPERTENSION (high BLOOD PRESSURE), CORONARY ARTERY DISEASE (CAD), VALVE DISEASE, and congenital heart malformations are the most common reasons heart failure develops. Treatment targets relieving the accumulation of fluid and improving the underlying condition, if possible, that is responsible for establishing the conditions of heart failure. This might include treatment with DIURETIC MEDICATIONS and ANTIHYPERTENSIVE MEDICATIONS.

See also MEDICATIONS TO TREAT HEART DISEASE; PULMONARY CONGESTION/PULMONARY EDEMA; PULMONARY HYPERTENSION.

Oslo Study Diet and Antismoking Trial One of the early studies that provided conclusive evidence of the role lifestyle, particularly eating habits and TOBACCO USE, has in the development, treatment, and prevention of HEART DISEASE. The study, conducted in the early 1970s, enrolled 1,200 men who had HYPERCHOLESTEROLEMIA (elevated blood cholesterol levels) but otherwise were healthy. Half of the group (the study group) received instruction and follow-up regarding lifestyle modifications, namely following a low-fat diet and smoking cessation. The other group (the control group) received no such instruction or follow-up. After five years total blood cholesterol levels had dropped 13 percent in the study group and only 3 percent in the control group. After eight and a half years, the men in the control group had experienced twice as many CARDIAC EVENTS as the men in the study group. These findings were among the first to provide a scientific foundation for lifestyle intervention as a form of treatment for early heart disease, as well as a form of prevention for those who had not yet developed physiological evidence of heart disease.

See also CHOLESTEROL, BLOOD; CORONARY PRIMARY PREVENTION TRIAL; FRAMINGHAM HEART STUDY; HELSINKI HEART STUDY; WOMEN'S HEALTH INITIATIVE.

overweight See OBESITY.

oxidation The biochemical process through which oxygen combines with other substances within a cell, at the molecular level, to generate energy. Oxidation is a normal function of metabolism. Among the waste by-products of oxidation are molecular structures called FREE RADICALS. The body in balance has a number of processes for eliminating free radicals. The body in imbalance accumulates free radicals, which many health experts believe contribute to diseases that develop over time such as CARDIOVASCULAR DISEASE (CVD).

Most molecules have structures that allow them to bind with specific other molecules to form functional units. Free radicals, as waste by-products, are irregularly and inconsistently formed. They are incomplete, leaving them free to bind with whatever other molecules they bump into first. When a free radical binds with a normal molecule, the resulting structure has no functional purpose. It floats around, like a molecular dust particle. It can settle where it has no effect and eventually become either assimilated into a cell or eliminated from the body with other waste, or it can disrupt cellular functions on any number of levels. Dietary nutrients called ANTIOXIDANTS, enzymes that are components of vitamins, play key roles in neutralizing free radicals. Antioxidants are easy binding partners for free radicals. Once the binding occurs, the free radical becomes "garbage in waiting" for elimination from the cell and from the body.

Individually, free radicals are fairly harmless, but in aggregrate as they accumulate over time, they can wreak havoc with cellular, and consequently tissue and organ, functions. Many health experts believe this leads to the kind of damage to cells and tissues that results in diseases associated with aging, such as ATHEROSCLEROSIS and CORONARY ARTERY DISEASE (CAD). Research to explore the role of antioxidants has so far failed to yield conclusive findings, though prevailing medical opinion is that a nutritious diet that supplies the body with needed nutrients, including antioxidants, helps the body to neutralize and eliminate free radicals to reduce the potentially damaging consequences of oxidation.

See also COENZYME Q-10.

oxygenation The process of getting oxygen into the BLOOD. Oxygen is a vital energy source for cells and without it they cannot function. Some cells can sustain for 10 minutes or longer when deprived of oxygen; others, such as brain cells and myocardial (HEART muscle) cells, succumb within minutes without oxygen. Oxygenation takes place as a gas exchange across membranes. In the lungs, the membranes line the alveoli and through them oxygen enters the bloodstream, attaching to the HEMOGLOBIN in red blood cells, and carbon dioxide leaves. Pressure facilitates this exchange, with each gas moving in the direction of lower pressure. A similar exchange takes place within the capillary

beds, where the oxygen leaves the hemoglobin in the blood and enters the cells that need to use it for energy.

Many factors can affect or impair oxygenation, particularly CARDIOVASCULAR DISEASE (CVD) such as CORONARY ARTERY DISEASE (CAD) and HEART FAILURE, which puts increased stress on the heart and CARDIOVASCULAR SYSTEM to boost circulation in compensation. HEART RATE and BLOOD PRESSURE both increase, as does the force of the heart's contractions. These responses can be physiologically appropriate, such as when the body's oxygen needs increase during physical activity, and return to normal when oxygen demand does. Or they can reflect cardiovascular or pulmonary disease, in which the heart cannot pump an adequate supply of oxygenated blood through the body. When oxygenation becomes inadequate the most obvious indication is shortness of breath; other symptoms may include tightness in the chest and ANGINA. Prolonged inadequate oxygenation is called HYPOXIA.

See also DYSPNEA; SCHEMIC HEART DISEASE (IHD); OXYGEN THERAPY; PULMONARY SYSTEM.

oxygen therapy The administration of oxygen by face mask or nasal cannula (small tubes that rest in the entrance to the nostrils) to raise the percentage of oxygen in the BLOOD as a treatment for HYPOXIA (insufficient oxygen). Short-term oxygen therapy is common during and after surgery, during treatment for HEART ATTACK and sometimes stroke, and in any health situation in which blood oxygen levels are lower than normal. People who have health conditions such as severe HEART FAILURE or CHRONIC OBSTRUCTIVE PULMONARY DISEASE (COPD) may receive long-term oxygen therapy using portable oxygen tanks or a room-based device called an oxygen separator, which extracts and concentrates oxygen from atmospheric (room) air and redispenses it. Some portable oxygen therapy units are small enough to be worn in a bag that hangs from the shoulder, or that fit onto a small wheeled dolly. This greatly improves mobility and QUALITY OF LIFE for people with end-stage heart and lung diseases.

Pure oxygen is quickly harmful to the body in most situations and can result in oxygen toxicity, causing PULMONARY EDEMA (fluid accumulations in the lungs) and damage to lung tissues. Because of this, oxygen therapy mixes oxygen with atmospheric air. Atmospheric air is 21 percent oxygen; oxygen therapy typically delivers between 28 and 40 percent oxygen. An oxygen tank contains compressed oxygen that is released from the tank using a regulator that adjusts flow rate, which helps determine the concentration of oxygen the person receives. People who are critically ill with cardio-pulmonary collapse sometimes require higher concentrations of oxygen, which must be administered under careful control and observation (typically in a hospital intensive care unit) to minimize toxicity. Oxygen also is explosive and flammable, so people using oxygen therapy must take care to stay away from burning objects such as cigarettes.

See also CARDIOVASCULAR SYSTEM; HEMOGLOBIN; OXYGENATION; PULMONARY SYSTEM.

pacemaker An electronic device that overrides the HEART's natural pacing mechanisms, which have become dysfunctional, to maintain an adequate rate and rhythm of HEARTBEAT. Pacemakers run from long-life batteries and most are implanted, though cardiologists sometimes use external pacemakers when the need is temporary or until an internal pacemaker can be implanted. The pacemaker consists of two components, the pacing unit and the pacing wires. In a surgical procedure, the cardiologist inserts one or two pacing wires into a vein in the chest and threads them through to the heart. Electrodes on the ends of the wires make contact with the wall of the right ventricle (single chamber pacemaker) or with the wall of the right atrium and the wall of the right ventricle (dual chamber pacemaker). The wires attach to the pacing unit, or control unit, which is about the size of a pager and is sewn into a pocket of muscle tissue usually in the chest area. The pacing unit contains the electronics and batteries that discharge a mild electrical current through the electrodes to stimulate the heart's CARDIAC CYCLE. Many pacemakers also have sensing electrodes that detect whether the heart's natural pacemaker, the SINOATRIAL (SA) NODE, releases a pacing signal and suppresses the pacemaker's discharge when the SA signal is adequate. A pacemakers only increase the rate of the heart. It cannot prevent heartbeats or lower the heart rate.

The first pacemakers were developed in the 1950s, an outgrowth of radio technology that evolved during World War II. Medical historians credit Wilson Greatbatch, an electrical engineer, with inventing the modern implantable pacemaker. Greatbatch's designs were the first to be implanted in humans in the 1960s; one of the first patients to receive a Greatbatch pacemaker lived more than 30 years with the device regulating his heart as a treat-ment for HEART BLOCK. Today cardiologists implant more than 150,000 pacemakers a year to treat a range of ARRHYTHMIAS.

People who have pacemakers should carry pacemaker ID cards, which contain pertinent information about the pacemaker model, settings, and date of implantation. Typically the cardiologist's office provides or arranges for this ID card.

See also CARDIAC RESYNCHRONIZATION THERAPY (CRT); CONDUCTION PATHWAY; ENTERTAINMENT MAPPING; IMPLANTABLE CARDIOVERTER DEFIBRILLATOR (ICD); SICK SINUS SYNDROME; SURGERY TO TREAT CARDIOVASCULAR DISEASE; TWIDDLER'S SYNDROME.

pacemaker syndrome A dysfunction of the HEART's rhythm in a person who has an implanted PACEMAKER, in which the atria (heart's upper chambers) and the ventricles (heart's lower chambers) no longer function in synchronization because the pacemaker regulates ventricular contraction. This is called atrioventricular (AV) dyssynchrony, and there are many reasons it can occur, ranging from deterioration of heart function to improper pacemaker settings.

Symptoms and Diagnostic Path
Symptoms of pacemaker syndrome are numerous and correspond to multiple aspects of heart function. They include

- LIGHT-HEADEDNESS, DIZZINESS, and SYNCOPE (fainting)
- difficulty breathing (DYSPNEA), especially when lying down
- fatigue and weakness
- PALPITATIONS
- restlessness and anxiety

The diagnostic path begins with a physical examination during which the doctor may recognize exaggerated pulsations in the veins of the neck. An ELECTROCARDIOGRAM (ECG) typically shows abnormal timing between the atrial and ventricular contractions. After ruling out other possible pacemaker issues such as malfunction, improper settings, and low battery, the pattern of symptoms makes diagnosis straightforward.

Treatment Options and Outlook

Treatment may be as simple as reprogramming the device; although sometimes it is necessary to implant another pacing lead.

Risk Factors and Preventive Measures

The most common scenario for pacemaker syndrome is ventricular pacing. Continuing deterioration of heart function can contribute to shifts in the heart's natural electrical activity. Close monitoring is important to detect and correct problems such as AV dyssynchrony before significant symptoms develop.

See also AUSCULTATION; CONDUCTION PATHWAY; VENTRICULAR TACHYCARDIA.

pace mapping   A method to identify the precise points of dysfunction in the HEART that permit aberrant electrical activity, causing significant ventricular ARRHYTHMIAS, primarily VENTRICULAR TACHYCARDIAS and premature ventricular contractions (PVCs). After identifying these points, the cardiologist can use ABLATION to destroy the reentry circuit and restore the heart's normal conduction.

Procedure

Pace mapping is done when the arrhythmia is severe, does not respond to other treatment, or other treatment causes intolerable side effects, such as when an IMPLANTABLE CARDIOVERTER DEFIBRILLATOR (ICD), which delivers an electrical shock directly to the heart when it detects tachycardia, activates frequently. This causes considerable discomfort. The cardiologist may suggest pace mapping and ablation as a more permanent solution.

Pace mapping with ablation takes about four hours and is performed with the person under IV sedation. Most people have the procedure done on an inpatient basis. Preparation requires fasting (nothing to eat or drink) for eight hours before the scheduled procedure time.

Pace mapping is done as a CARDIAC CATHETERIZATION procedure in which the cardiologist threads a very thin, flexible catheter through a vein (such as the femoral vein in the groin) and into the heart. The catheter's tip detects electrical activity in the heart, which it transmits to a monitor. When the catheter detects an area of abnormal electrical activity, the cardiologist can release a brief burst of radiofrequency energy that destroys a small number of myocardial cells. After these cells are destroyed, they can no longer conduct electricity. The cardiologist may use several catheters at different locations of the heart depending on the reentry circuits.

Risks and Complications

Risks include bleeding, clot formation, injury to the heart from the catheters, and further arrhythmias. Among the complications that can arise from these risks are STROKE, MYOCARDIAL INFARCTION (MI), HEART FAILURE, and CARDIOGENIC SHOCK. The underlying arrhythmias are usually life-threatening, however, which itself establishes risk for many of these same complications.

Outlook and Lifestyle Modifications

Most people remain in the hospital until the cardiologist determines they are stable. The cardiologist will provide instructions for follow-up care and monitoring.

The person must lie flat for a period of time after the procedure to make sure there is no bleeding at the insertion site and that there are no arrhythmias.

See also ACCESSORY PATHWAY.

palliation, staged   The sequence of three surgical procedures to repair HYPOPLASTIC LEFT HEART SYNDROME (HLHS) and other serious congenital heart malformations in which the HEART is nonfunctional in its current structure:

- the NORWOOD PROCEDURE, performed within 10 days of birth
- the BIDIRECTIONAL GLENN PROCEDURE, performed when the infant is around six months old
- the FONTAN PROCEDURE, done when the child is two to three years old

Staged palliation is a permanent remedy for these serious heart malformations, though it does not restore the heart to a normal structure or functional configuration. For HLHS, for example, in which there is no functional left ventricle, the surgeon often constructs a two-chamber heart. Though these surgical reconstructions are now the standard of treatment for serious congenital heart malformations, surgeons have only been performing them since the late 1970s so do not yet know the lifetime consequences of such repairs. For the most part, people who had staged palliation as infants and who are now in their 20s and 30s are able to enjoy relatively normal activities in their lives.

See also CARDIOVASCULAR SYSTEM; HEART DISEASE; HEART DISEASE IN CHILDREN; HEART TRANSPLANT; SURGERY TO TREAT CARDIOVASCULAR DISEASE.

palpitations Awareness of the HEARTBEAT, often as a sense of feeling the HEART "pounding" or of skipped beats. Most episodes of palpitations are benign and do not indicate any underlying heart problem. Stress (physical and emotional), EXERCISE, physical exertion, anxiety, and stimulants such as CAFFEINE and NICOTINE are the most common causes of palpitations. Some people have palpitations when they take decongestant medications such as pseudoephedrine, particularly in combination with caffeine or nicotine. Reducing stimulant intake generally ends palpitations related to their use within a few days to a week. HYPERTHYROIDISM (overactive thyroid), which can occur as a condition or as a result of taking too much thyroid supplement to treat hypothyroidism (underactive thyroid), also can cause palpitations. Palpitations sometimes occur with ANEMIA, MITRAL VALVE PROLAPSE (MVP), and occasionally signal ARRHYTHMIAS (irregularities in the heartbeat) such as PREMATURE VENTRICULAR CONTRACTIONS (PVCs) that require further medical assessment and may need treatment.

Diagnosis focuses on finding and eliminating or treating the underlying causes of the palpitations. The doctor often has the person wear a HOLTER MONITOR to collect a 24-hour ELECTROCARDIOGRAM (ECG) and keep a diary of palpitations that occur. The doctor compares the diary with the data of the ECG to see if there are any correlations between symptoms and the heart's activity. Treatment then targets any identified cardiac problems. When diagnostic investigation fails to turn up physical explanations for palpitations, stress and anxiety are most likely the precipitating factors. STRESS REDUCTION TECHNIQUES such as BIOFEEDBACK, MEDITATION, YOGA, and GUIDED IMAGERY can help to reduce the negative effects of stress. Sometimes the doctor may choose to prescribe an ANTI-ANXIETY MEDICATION, depending on the circumstances, for short-term or situational stress.

See also STRESS AND HEART DISEASE.

para-Hisiam pacing See ELECTROPHYSIOLOGY STUDY.

paroxysmal hypertension See HYPERTENSION.

patent ductus arteriosus (PDA) Failure of the ductus arteriosus, a normal opening between the pulmonary artery and the aorta in the circulatory system of the unborn child, to close after birth. The mother's BLOOD supply provides OXYGENATION to the fetus. Because the lungs do not function until after birth, fetal circulation bypasses the lungs to go directly from the right ventricle to the left atrium. Exposure to oxygen when the lungs begin to function at birth causes the ductus arteriosus to close, normally within 24 hours of birth. When the ductus arteriosus remains open, or patent, some of the blood flow from the HEART recirculates to the lungs without going to the rest of the body. The PDA causes the heart to pump a mix of oxygenated and unoxygenated blood out to the body, which may not be enough oxygen to meet the body's needs.

PDA is one of the most common birth defects affecting the heart, accounting for about 10 percent of congenital heart malformations. It is more common in premature infants and often appears in constellations of congenital malformations such as TETRALOGY OF FALLOT. In some infants the ductus arteriosus spontaneously closes after a period of months. Among those in which it remains open, medication or surgery becomes necessary. Untreated PDA results in PULMONARY HYPERTENSION and HEART FAILURE, often in childhood though occasionally not until adulthood. Medical treatment is injection of the NONSTEROIDAL ANTI-INFLAMMATORY DRUG (NSAID) indomethacin (Indocin), which is effective in closing the PDA in about 80 percent of infants with PDA. The indomethacin blocks the actions of prostaglandins, hormonelike chemicals in the body that maintain the patency of the ductus arteriosus. Surgery to close the PDA is necessary when medication is ineffective or not an appropriate treatment choice.

When significant congenital malformations of the heart, such as tetralogy of Fallot or TRANSPOSITION OF THE GREAT ARTERIES (TPA), also are present, cardiologists usually administer prostaglandin E1 (PGE1) to keep the ductus arteriosus open until surgeons can safely repair the heart's structural defects. Maintaining the PDA open allows the heart to receive at least minimal oxygenation from the blood mixing between the pulmonary artery and the aorta.

See also ARTERIAL SWITCH PROCEDURE; BIDIRECTIONAL GLENN PROCEDURE; BLALOCK-TAUSSIG PROCEDURE; FONTAN PROCEDURE; MUSTARD PROCEDURE; NORWOOD PROCEDURE.

PDE5 inhibitor medications   A class of medications prescribed to treat ERECTILE DYSFUNCTION. Those currently available in the United States are sildenafil (Viagra), vardenafil (Levitra), and tadalafil (Cialis). These medications work by blocking the action of the enzyme phosphodiesterase type 5 (PDE5). Such inhibition extends the action of another enzyme, guanosine monophosphate (cGMP), that allows the penis to become erect. Nitric oxide naturally present in the body activates the release of cGMP and also causes the BLOOD vessels in the penis to expand.

The elevated levels of nitric oxide that PDE5 inhibitors permit can cause blood vessels throughout the body to dilate and relax, causing blood pressure to drop. Men who are taking NITRATE MEDICATIONS for ANGINA and other cardiovascular conditions should not take these medications, as the combined actions of these drugs to increase nitric oxide levels in the body can cause precipitous and even fatal drops in BLOOD PRESSURE. Though many men who have HEART DISEASE can safely take PDE5 inhibitors, it is crucial to let the prescribing physician know what other medications are being taken.

An occasional side effect with PDE5 inhibitors is a change in visual perception in which a bluish hue discolors vision, sometimes accompanied by blurred vision. This is brought about by the effect on the blood vessels in the retina and can last up to several days and can be problematic for men whose jobs require accurate color vision (such as pilots). Other side effects may include headache and orthostatic or postural HYPOTENSION (sudden drop in blood pressure upon changing positions). There also is an increased risk of HEART ATTACK and STROKE when taking PDE5 inhibitors, regardless of underlying HEART DISEASE.

See also MEDICATION SIDE EFFECTS; MEDICATIONS TO TREAT HEART DISEASE.

pear body shape   See BODY SHAPE AND HEART DISEASE.

pentoxifylline   A ANTICOAGULANT MEDICATION taken to slow the clotting action of the BLOOD. Pentoxifylline, available in the United States as the brand-name product Trental, works by decreasing platelet aggregation (the clumping together of platelets that is the first phase of COAGULATION) and by decreasing fibrinogen levels in the blood, reducing the blood's ability to construct clots. Doctors commonly prescribe pentoxifylline to treat INTERMITTENT CLAUDICATION and as a prophylactic (preventive) measure to help prevent subsequent STROKE or HEART ATTACK. Pentoxifylline is chemically similar to CAFFEINE and can have similar adverse effects on the body, including agitation, feeling jittery, and ARRHYTHMIAS. Pentoxifylline can lower the effectiveness of some ANTIHYPERTENSIVE MEDICATIONS.

See also BLOOD; HYPERTENSION.

percutaneous transluminal coronary angioplasty (PCTA)   See ANGIOPLASTY.

pericardial effusion   An abnormal collection of fluid between the pericardium (the protective sac surrounding the HEART) and the myocardium (heart muscle). A thin film of fluid lubricates the space between the heart and the pericardium, protecting the heart from friction as it beats. Pericardial effusion develops when there is an irritation of the pericardium such as PERICARDITIS, injury to the chest and structures in proximity to the heart, or bleeding following surgery or from a dissecting aneurysm of the aorta. The volume of fluid increases in an effort to reduce the irritation. The pericardium does not stretch or flex, however, so the excess fluid compresses inward against the heart. This compression quickly interferes with the heart's normal function, causing arrhythmias and limiting the heart's mechanical ability to contract.

Symptoms and Diagnostic Path

The symptoms of pericardial effusion may come on gradually or suddenly, depending on the amount of fluid and the rate at which it is accumulating, and include:

- difficulty breathing, painful breathing, or shortness of breath, especially when lying down (DYSPNEA)
- CHEST PAIN
- cough without symptoms of upper respiratory infection
- unusual tiredness or fatigue
- LIGHT-HEADEDNESS, fainting (SYNCOPE)
- PALPITATIONS or rapid HEARTBEAT

ECHOCARDIOGRAM typically confirms the diagnosis. Other diagnostic procedures might include ELECTROCARDIOGRAM (ECG), blood tests, and COMPUTED TOMOGRAPHY (CT) scan.

Treatment Options and Outlook

Mild pericardial effusion with no evidence of TAMPONADE (pressure-induced ARRHYTHMIAS and interference with the heart's function) often responds well to treatment with NONSTEROIDAL ANTI-INFLAMMATORY DRUGS (NSAIDs) to relieve the underlying inflammation causing the increased fluid (which is the heart's attempt to relieve the irritation). For more severe pericardial effusion, treatment is to drain the fluid (pericardiocentesis). Pericardial effusion can become chronic, depending on the cause.

Risk Factors and Preventive Measures

Viral infections (including HIV), bacterial infections elsewhere in the body, autoimmune disorders, and heart surgery increase the risk for pericardial efusion. Pericardial effusion also can develop without apparent cause. There are no known methods to prevent pericardial effusion.

See also AORTIC ANEURYSM; CARDIOVASCULAR SYSTEM.

pericarditis   An inflammation of the thin, tough, membranous sac that encases and protects the myocardium (HEART muscle). There are numerous possible causes for pericarditis, including viral or bacterial infection, metastatic cancer, kidney failure, PERICARDIAL EFFUSION, and radiation therapy. Inflammatory disorders such as systemic lupus erythematosus and rheumatoid arthritis sometimes cause an inflammatory response in other locations including the pericardium. Medications for which pericarditis is a known side effect include HYDRALAZINE (Apresoline), taken to treat HYPERTENSION (high BLOOD PRESSURE) and HEART FAILURE; penicillin, taken to treat bacterial infections; PROCAINAMIDE (Pronestyl), taken to treat ARRHYTHMIAS; and phenytoin (Dilantin), taken to prevent seizures.

Symptoms and Diagnostic Path

The main symptom of pericarditis is a sharp, achy pain in the chest that persists over time. There may be difficulty breathing (DYSPNEA), and many people have a cough. Diagnostic procedures may include blood tests, chest X-ray, ELECTROCARDIOGRAM (ECG), ECHOCARDIOGRAM, and COMPUTED TOMOGRAPHY (CT) SCAN of the chest. The doctor will also ask about recent viral and bacterial infections, HEART ATTACK or heart surgery, radiation therapy to the chest, and other health issues. Echocardiogram and CT scan are the most likely to confirm the diagnosis.

Treatment Options and Outlook

Treatment targets the underlying cause as well as attempts to relieve discomfort. NONSTEROIDAL ANTI-INFLAMMATORY DRUGS (NSAIDs) are commonly prescribed for this purpose. Most people feel markedly better within two weeks and are fully recovered within three months. In some people, however, pericarditis may be chronic.

Risk Factors and Preventive Measures

Men have greater risk for pericarditis. Although many of the causes of pericarditis are known, there are no measures to prevent most pericarditis. However, pericarditis is often idiopathic (the cause remains unknown). Early diagnosis and treatment help to minimize complications such as pericardial effusion and cardiac TAMPONADE.

See also CANCER OF THE HEART; ENDOCARDITIS; CARDIOVASCULAR SYSTEM.

peripheral vascular disease (PVD) A form of CARDIOVASCULAR DISEASE (CVD) that affects structures and functions of the CARDIOVASCULAR SYSTEM other than the HEART and its structures. Most commonly affected are the arteries and veins in the legs and feet. The most serious and common form of PVD is peripheral vascular disease (PAD), in which deposits of fatty acids and other material collect along the walls of the arteries in the extremities (primarily the legs). PAD may also affect the arteries that supply organs such as the kidneys, intestines, and stomach. Most people who have PVD also have other forms of CVD, notably CORONARY ARTERY DISEASE (CAD) and increased risk for MYOCARDIAL INFARCTION (MI), STROKE, and pulmonary EMBOLISM (BLOOD clot in the lungs) due to the potential for fragments of accumulated arterial plaque to break away and enter the bloodstream.

Symptoms and Diagnostic Path

About half of people who have PVD have no symptoms and do not know they have the condition. When symptoms are present, they may include:

- pain, cramping, numbness, burning, aching, or tingling in the feet, legs, and sometimes buttocks
- difficulty walking
- EDEMA (fluid accumulation and swelling)
- toes and feet that are pale or bluish and cool to the touch
- intolerance of cold temperatures (air or water)
- ERECTILE DYSFUNCTION in men

Cramping and pain that develops with walking and goes away with rest is called INTERMITTENT CLAUDICATION and is a hallmark of PVD. The diagnostic path begins with a detailed health history and physical examination. The doctor will check the PULSE at various points along the arms, legs, and feet. The doctor may also take BLOOD PRESSURE readings on both arms as well as both legs. Diagnostic procedures may include DOPPLER ULTRASOUND, ANGIOGRAPHY (an imaging procedure using dye injected into the arteries), and MAGNETIC RESONANCE IMAGING (MRI).

Treatment Options and Outlook

When narrowing of the arteries is severe, the preferred course of treatment is ANGIOPLASTY (surgery to open blocked arteries), often with placement of STENTS to help keep the arteries open. Extensive blockage of peripheral arteries may require surgery to create a graft to bypass the damaged area, a procedure similar to CORONARY ARTERY BYPASS GRAFT (CABG). Other treatments include PENTOXIFYLLINE and CILOSTAZOL when intermittent claudication is present, and ANTICOAGULANT MEDICATIONS such as ASPIRIN or WARFARIN (Coumadin) to reduce the risk for clot formation. Lifestyle measures to improve PVD include daily physical EXERCISE, nutritious eating, no smoking, and WEIGHT MANAGEMENT (weight loss if necessary).

PVD is a leading cause of disability among people age 50 and older, primarily because it reaches an advanced state before treatment begins, and limits activity for about half of people who develop it. However, early diagnosis, appropriate treatment, and lifestyle modifications can significantly improve QUALITY OF LIFE and permit a fairly normal lifestyle. Untreated PVD can result in permanent damage, including gangrene necessitating amputation.

Risk Factors and Preventive Measures

Having DIABETES (type 1 or type 2) significantly raises the risk for PVD because diabetes damages peripheral nerves and blood vessels, which interferes with circulation. Other risk factors include age, smoking, OBESITY, HYPERTENSION (high blood pressure), and physical inactivity. Infections can also damage the blood vessels, causing inflammation, narrowing (STENOSIS), and stiffness. Daily exercise (especially walking), nutritious eating, weight management, and not smoking are the most significant measures for preventing PVD and heart disease in general.

See also ATHEROSCLEROSIS; DEEP VEIN THROMBOSIS (DVT); CLAUDICATION; INFLAMMATION AND HEART DISEASE; LIFESTYLE AND HEART HEALTH; LIVING WITH HEART DISEASE; MEDICATIONS TO TREAT HEART DISEASE; PLAQUE, ARTERIAL; RAYNAUD'S SYNDROME; SURGERY TO TREAT CARDIOVASCULAR DISEASE; TOBACCO USE.

Persantine See DIPYRIDAMOLE.

personality types Patterns of behavior. Researchers have long explored the correlations between personality characteristics and health. Numerous surveys have noted for decades that people who live the longest appear to have cheery, positive dispositions. Though such observations are difficult to quantify, some researchers have drawn converse correlations as well between hostile, negative outlooks and health problems and disease. True objective data are scant in supporting either premise, though many health experts believe them to be valid at least to some extent.

The classic "coronary personality" arising from early investigations of personality correlations to HEART DISEASE was dubbed type A. Researchers classified type A personality as aggressive, action-oriented, short-tempered, and achievement-driven—the iconoclastic power executive. In contrast is the type B personality featuring a calm, measured, and composed disposition. Many health-care providers felt that the majority of people with heart disease, particularly CORONARY ARTERY DISEASE (CAD), fell into the type A category, and in 1981 an advisory panel appointed by the U.S. National Institutes of Health (NIH) added type A personality as an independent risk factor for CAD. Subsequent, more stringently designed studies have failed to substantiate this correlation. Health experts have backed away from personality type, in itself, as a risk factor for illness and disease. However, the general relationship between emotional state and health or disease is well accepted among health experts and supported by clinical research studies.

The precise mechanisms by which emotional traits and responses influence wellness and illness, and in particular heart disease, are not well understood. The physiological responses that cause BLOOD PRESSURE and HEART RATE to rise are also activated during emotional stress (broadly defined to include aggression). Levels of EPINEPHRINE, NOREPINEPHRINE, and other HORMONES increase with emotional stress, having direct consequence on the cardiovascular system. The type A personality comprises classically "high stress" traits and reactions; the type B personality comprises classically "laid-back" characteristics and responses. Recent research suggests the influence of personality on heart disease is more narrowly focused on DEPRESSION and emotional distress, resulting in classification of a personality type D. The foundation of this personality type D is negative emotion, and some studies show a correlation between it and the likelihood of repeat HEART ATTACK. Further research remains necessary to determine the extent of this and other personality-based factors in the development and progression of heart disease. Nonetheless, doctors encourage people to engage in STRESS REDUCTION TECHNIQUES to mitigate the effects of stress on health. Most health experts feel there are potentially great benefits and few health risks associated with attempts to achieve a positive outlook on life and to approach the complexities of everyday life with a greater sense of calm.

See also EMOTIONS AND HEART DISEASE; MEDITATION; STRESS AND HEART DISEASE; YOGA.

physical fitness The performance capability of the HEART, lungs, and musculoskeletal structures, encompassing five areas.

- Aerobic endurance—the ability of the cardio-pulmonary system to efficiently and effectively circulate oxygenated BLOOD throughout the body for an extended time.
- Muscle strength—the ability of the muscles to perform against resistance for short periods of time.
- Muscle endurance—the ability of the muscles to perform against resistance for an extended time.
- Flexibility—the range of motion the joints permit.
- Muscle-to-fat ratio (lean body mass)—the percentage of muscle tissue compared to the percentage of fat tissue.

Physical fitness is the consequence of efforts to maintain the body's functional capacity and strength through EXERCISE and regular physical activity and is a factor in measuring overall cardiovascular health. Health experts recommend at least 30 minutes a day of light to moderate physical activity such as walking and 60 to 90 minutes three days a week of vigorous exercise as the minimum standard for adults to maintain appropriate physical fitness.

See also AEROBIC CAPACITY.

plaque, arterial Accumulations of fatty acid deposits and BLOOD cells that collect along the inner walls of the arteries. These accumulations form occlusive structures called ATHEROMAS that narrow and constrict the channels of the arteries to restrict blood flow. This restriction results in the cardiovascular disease ATHEROSCLEROSIS. Atherosclerosis often is secondarily named for its location. CORONARY ARTERY DISEASE (CAD) identifies arterial plaque accumulations in the CORONARY ARTERIES that supply the heart muscle (myocardium). PERIPHERAL VASCULAR DISEASE (PVD) identifies arterial plaque accumulations in the distant, or peripheral, arteries. CAROTID STENOSIS identifies atherosclerosis that has narrowed the passageway through the carotid arteries that supply the brain and head with blood.

Arterial plaque accumulations typically begin when fatty acids in the blood lodge against the inside wall of an artery. Researchers speculate that tiny tears in the inner surface of the arterial wall release substances that attract platelets, fibrin, and other components of the body's clotting mechanism. The resulting clot that forms protrudes into the flow of blood, creating a swirl that allows heavier substances such as fatty acids to settle out of the blood. As well, various particles in the blood (red blood cells, white blood cells, platelets) attach to the protrusion. Even after the tear heals the site attracts further substances from the blood and the accumulation continues. Cigarette smoking and a diet high in saturated fats accelerate the accumulation.

Very low-density lipoprotein (VLDL) cholesterol and low-density lipoprotein (LDL) cholesterol are especially sticky and adhere to the accumulation more easily than does high-density lipoprotein. The flow of blood through the artery compresses the accumulated particles into a hard-packed layer known as plaque. Arterial plaque that accumulates in the coronary arteries has an unusually high concentration of CALCIUM, making the atheromas detectable with a form of sophisticated imaging technology called ELECTRON BEAM COMPUTED TOMOGRAPHY (EBCT) SCAN. This calcium concentration makes the plaque brittle and susceptible to breaking away from the walls of the arteries, posing significant risk for STROKE and HEART ATTACK.

As arterial plaque accumulations contribute to various cardiovascular diseases, diagnostic efforts focus on identifying those diseases. Nutritious eating habits and regular physical exercise help to minimize the formation of arterial plaque. Some people have gene mutations that cause elevated fatty acids in the blood; when this is the case, nutrition and activity are especially important. The most effective approach to treating the cardiovascular diseases that result from arterial plaque is to prevent the plaque from forming and accumulating in the first place. Once it settles into the arteries; intervention to remove it is difficult.

Lipid-lowering medications and therapies to lower blood cholesterol and TRIGLYCERIDES levels prevent further accumulation of plaque though usually cannot completely regress plaque that is already present. CHELATION THERAPY, a treatment in which chemicals injected into the bloodstream attract and bind with certain minerals so those minerals can be removed from the body, long has been a tantalizing theory though is so far an unproven nonsurgical treatment for reducing arterial plaque accumulations.

See also ANGIOPLASTY; CHOLESTEROL, BLOOD; CAROTID ENDARTERECTOMY; CORONARY ARTERY BYPASS GRAFT (CABG); GARLIC AND GARLIC OIL; HERBAL REMEDIES; INFLAMMATION AND HEART DISEASE; STENT.

Plavix   See CLOPIDOGREL.

Pletal   See CILOSTAZOL.

polycythemia   An overproduction of BLOOD cells, especially red blood cells, that can develop as a consequence of numerous health conditions in which the body does not receive adequate OXYGENATION.

The primary risk of this overproduction is a thickening of the blood, significantly raising the risk for blood clots that can cause DEEP VEIN THROMBOSIS (DVT), HEART ATTACK, and STROKE.

Polycythemia vera, also called primary polycythemia, is an inherited form of polycythemia in which the bone marrow produces too many of all three kinds of blood cells—red blood cells, white blood cells, and platelets—as a result of gene mutations. As well, platelets (blood cells responsible for clotting) often are abnormally formed. Secondary polycythemia also develops in people who travel from low altitudes to unusually high altitudes (more than 5,000 feet above sea level), to help the body compensate for the reduced oxygen content of the air.

Symptoms and Diagnostic Path

The symptoms of polycythemia vera tend to become apparent in midlife, even though the condition has always been present, and may include headache, itchy skin, and DYSPNEA (shortness of breath or difficulty breathing). Blood tests, notably hematocrit (percentage of red blood cells in the blood), make the diagnosis. Because secondary polycythemia is adaptive, it typically does not cause symptoms; the proportion of red blood cells in the blood readjusts when returning to a lower altitude.

Treatment Options and Outlook

Treatment for polycythemia vera is phlebotomy, the removal of blood. This is usually done one unit at a time (the same amount of blood collected when donating blood) until the hematocrit returns to normal. Once treatment becomes necessary it is an ongoing process, the timing of which depends on how quickly the red cell count goes back up. Untreated polycythemia vera can cause fatal heart attack or stroke. Controlled polycythemia vera typically has no effect on QUALITY OF LIFE.

Risk Factors and Preventive Measures

Polycythemia vera is a genetic disorder that affects proportionately more men than women. There are no known preventive measures.

See also ANEMIA.

positron emission tomography (PET) scan   A noninvasive imaging technology that combines radio-nuclides with computed tomography to generate three-dimensional images of internal organs and structures such as the HEART and the CORONARY ARTERIES. For this diagnostic procedure, the radiologist injects a radioactive solution, most often glucose that contains a radionuclide "tag," into the vein of the person undergoing evaluation. As the solution travels through the body the radionuclides are absorbed into cells and naturally break apart, or decay, at a known rate. This process generates a form of emitted radiation called gamma rays; a special camera called a gamma camera detects the accumulations of gamma rays in varying concentrations in the tissues being studied.

Damaged tissue, such as occurs during attacks of ISCHEMIA or after HEART ATTACK, absorbs the radionuclides in different concentrations than healthy tissue. The patterns of gamma radiation accumulations present dimensional pictures of the damage. A PET scan of the heart can take 45 minutes to two hours to complete, depending on the kinds of images the cardiologist wants to generate. PET scan often is done in combination with an EXERCISE STRESS TEST, helping to shape decisions about treatment and particularly whether CORONARY ARTERY BYPASS GRAFT (CABG) or ANGIOPLASTY are appropriate options. The radiation exposure of PET scanning is minimal, as the radionuclide decays very rapidly and is gone from the body within a few hours. PET scan results are highly reliable except in people who have INSULIN RESISTANCE or DIABETES. These health conditions interfere with cell metabolism and in particular glucose uptake, presenting an inaccurate picture of radionuclide absorption.

See also COMPUTED TOMOGRAPHY (CT) SCAN; MAGNETIC RESONANCE IMAGING (MRI); SINGLE PHOTON EMISSION COMPUTED TOMOGRAPHY (SPECT) SCAN.

postmenopausal estrogen therapy   See HORMONE REPLACEMENT THERAPY (HRT).

post-myocardial infarction cardiac remodeling   A molecular process by which myocardial (HEART muscle) cells reconfigure their structures and functions to compensate for damage that occurs to the heart following HEART ATTACK (myocardial infarction) and with progressive HEART FAILURE. Such changes often include increasing the cell's electrical sensitivity and metabolic rate and are apparent as enlargement of the myocardium in the area of the damage (typically the left ventricle, the right ventricle, or both ventricles). Angiotensin II plays a key role in cardiac remodeling; blocking its actions with the use of ANGIOTENSIN II RECEPTOR ANTAGONIST MEDICATIONS and ANGIOTENSIN-CONVERTING ENZYME (ACE) INHIBITOR MEDICATIONS appears to limit CARDIOMYOPATHY resulting from cardiac remodeling. This decreases the likelihood of subsequent cardiac events and progressive damage to the heart.

See also CARDIOVASCULAR DISEASE (CVD); CARDIOVASCULAR SYSTEM.

postural orthostatic tachycardia syndrome (POTS)
A condition in which moving to a standing position after lying down results in a sudden increase in HEART RATE (tachycardia). The effect is a temporary inability of the HEART to effectively pump BLOOD, causing blood to pool in the lower extremities and not get to the brain. This results is LIGHT-HEADEDNESS and fainting (SYNCOPE). The person subsequently sits or lies down, which helps blood return to the heart. Doctors do not know what causes POTS but believe it is a dysfunction of the AUTONOMIC NERVOUS SYSTEM.

Symptoms and Diagnostic Path
The characteristic symptoms of POTS are lightheadedness and fainting when standing up after lying down and often also with physical exertion (such as lifting) and exercise. Other symptoms may include

- nausea
- difficulty breathing
- headache
- anxiety
- feeling shaky and weak
- chills or flushing
- blurred vision or other visual disturbances

Most people also experience ongoing fatigue and difficulty sleeping. Because these symptoms can indicate various forms of CARDIOVASCULAR DISEASE (CVD), the diagnostic path typically includes ELECTROCARDIOGRAM (ECG) and blood tests to evaluate CARDIAC ENZYMES and ELECTROLYTES. The conclusive diagnostic procedure is the TILT TABLE TEST, in which the person lies on a table that moves. The diagnosis is confirmed when moving the table from the supine (lying flat) to an upright position causes a change in heart rate of 30 beats per minute or more or heart rate rises to 120 beats per minute or more within 10 minutes of being upright, without a drop in blood pressure.

Treatment Options and Outlook
There is no standardized treatment approach for POTS. Treatment depends on the particular constellation and severity of symptoms and typically combines lifestyle measures and medications. Medications may include BETA ANTAGONIST MEDICATIONS (beta blockers), although in some people these medications make symptoms worse. The steroid fludrocortisone (Florinef), which causes the body to retain fluid and SODIUM, provides relief for some people. Other medications that may help include certain ANTIARRHYTHMIA MEDICATIONS, selective serotonin reuptake inhibitor (SSRI) medications

(a class of ANTIDEPRESSANT MEDICATIONS), and VASO-CONSTRICTOR MEDICATIONS (notably midodrine).

Lifestyle measures such as increased fluid consumption, adequate sleep, and regular EXERCISE to maintain good muscle tone help to reduce the frequency and severity of POTS episodes for many people. Because positional changes typically cause or exacerabate symptoms and make many exercise activities difficult, riding a stationary bicycle is a good choice for many people. This form of activity minimizes positional changes while providing aerobic benefit and strengthening the legs in particular. Cardiovascular fitness improves the heart's effectiveness and efficiency, and good muscle tone and strength in the legs improves circulation (especially the ability of the veins to return blood to the heart).

Effective control of symptoms is often a process of trial to find the combination that works best for the individual. Keeping a journal of symptoms can help to identify precipitating activities or times during which symptoms are more likely or more severe. In many people POTS improves over time and ultimately goes away, although for some people it remains a chronic and disabling condition.

Risk Factors and Preventive Measures

About 80 percent of people who have POTS are women of menstruating age, most commonly those in their teens and early 20s. However, researchers do not know what this implies. Many people develop POTS after health conditions such as viral infections, trauma, and major surgery, and also after childbirth. Again, the correlations are unclear. There are no known methods for preventing the development of POTS.

See also FITNESS LEVEL; LIFESTYLE AND HEART HEALTH; LIVING WITH HEART DISEASE; MEDICATIONS TO TREAT HEART DISEASE.

potassium A chemical capable of carrying an electrical charge that is essential for normal HEART function and rhythm. Potassium is an ELECTROLYTE, or ion, that facilitates electrical activity in the heart as well as in the contraction of muscle cells, smooth and skeletal, throughout the body. Researchers have identified a correlation between blood potassium levels and BLOOD PRESSURE; when blood potassium levels are below normal, blood pressure rises, and when blood potassium levels are slightly elevated, blood pressure drops. However, blood potassium levels that are too high cause dangerous ARRHYTHMIAS (irregularities in the heartbeat) that can stop the heart from beating. Some DIURETIC MEDICATIONS taken to treat HYPERTENSION (high blood pressure) cause potassium depletion; other medications taken to treat heart disease may cause potassium levels in the body to increase. It is important to know whether medications influence the body's potassium levels, particularly for those who have hypertension or other forms of CARDIOVASCULAR DISEASE (CVD).

Foods that are high in potassium include dried beans and lentils, bananas, cantaloupe and other melons, tomatoes, spinach, meats, seafood and fish, milk and dairy products, berries, prunes and prune juice, and baked potatoes. Many salt substitute products that are low in sodium are high in potassium. Many people with potassium depletion, such as from diuretics, can adequately increase potassium through diet. Occasionally doctors choose to prescribe potassium replacement tablets, generally for people who cannot, for various reasons, make up lost potassium through diet. People taking medications that increase potassium retention in the body need to limit consumption of foods high in potassium.

See also CALCIUM CYCLE; HYPERKALEMIA; HYPOKALEMIA; MAGNESIUM; NUTRITION AND DIET; SODIUM.

power of attorney See ADVANCE DIRECTIVES.

pravastatin A LIPID-LOWERING MEDICATION taken to reduce blood cholesterol and blood triglycerides levels as treatment for HYPERCHOLESTEROLEMIA, HYPERTRIGLYCERIDEMIA, and HYPERLIPIDEMIA. Pravastatin (Pravachol) belongs to the family of HMG CoA REDUCTASE INHIBITOR MEDICATIONS, also referred to as statins. These drugs work by blocking the action of 3-hydroxy-3-methyl-glutaryl coenzyme-A reductase (HMG CoA), an enzyme the liver needs to produce cholesterol. The reduction of newly produced (synthesized) cholesterol forces the body to withdraw cholesterol from the bloodstream, generating a two-prong approach to lowering blood levels of fatty acids. Recent research indicates that pravastatin and other HMG CoA reductase inhibitors prolong the success of heart transplant after surgery. These medications also appear to improve survivability after HEART ATTACK and CORONARY ARTERY BYPASS GRAFT (CABG).

Pravastatin, like other HMG CoA reductase inhibitors, interacts with numerous other medications and especially should not be taken in combination with lipid-lowering medications in the fibric acid family (clofibrate, FENOFIBRATE, GEMFIBROZIL). Gastrointestinal side effects (dyspepsia, nausea, flatulence, and diarrhea or CONSTIPATION) are common when first beginning the medication though typically wane after taking pravastatin for several weeks. Less commonly pravastatin's side effects can include hemolytic ANEMIA, liver damage, and serious skin disorders. A very rare, life-threatening side effect is RHABDOMYOLYSIS, a breakdown of muscle tissue that sends excessive amounts of protein into the bloodstream. This protein can overwhelm the kidneys, causing kidney damage and failure.

See also ATORVASTATIN; CHOLESTEROL, BLOOD; FLUVASTATIN; LOVASTATIN; SIMVASTATIN; TRIGLYCERIDES, BLOOD.

prazosin An ANTIHYPERTENSIVE MEDICATION taken to treat HYPERTENSION (high BLOOD PRESSURE). Brand-name products commonly prescribed in the United States include Minipress. Prazosin belongs to the drug family of ALPHA ANTAGONIST MEDICATIONS; it works by preventing EPINEPHRINE and NOREPINEPHRINE from stimulating receptors in the veins and peripheral arterioles. The peripheral vessels contain sensors for one of the body's blood pressure regulation mechanisms; this blockade causes these BLOOD vessels to dilate and relax, lowering the resistance blood encounters when flowing through them.

Doctors prescribe prazosin alone to treat mild to moderate hypertension or in combination with other antihypertensives or DIURETIC MEDICATIONS to treat moderate to significant hypertension. Many people experience HYPOTENSION (low blood pressure) when beginning treatment with prazosin or

when increasing the prazosin dose; blood pressure stabilizes after a week or two of taking the medication. Other side effects may include headache, drowsiness, fatigue, and palpitations; these, too, generally abate after taking the medication for several weeks.

See also DOXAZOSIN; MEDICATIONS TO TREAT HEART DISEASE; TERAZOSIN.

pregnancy and heart disease Numerous changes take place in a woman's body during pregnancy that affect her CARDIOVASCULAR SYSTEM. A woman's BLOOD volume increases by 50 percent or more by the middle of the pregnancy's second term. The percentage of red blood cells within the blood, which carry oxygen, increases to accommodate the need to oxygenate the fetus's body. Hormonal changes cause the pregnant woman's blood vessels, especially veins, to relax, increasing the effort the HEART must put forth to push blood through the body and return it to the heart for OXYGENATION. The heart's workload correspondingly intensifies by as much as 50 percent, raising BLOOD PRESSURE and HEART RATE and in some women resulting in a temporary enlargement of the heart.

Some women have various forms of HEART DISEASE when they become pregnant, such as HYPERTENSION (high blood pressure) and congenital heart disorders. Some women develop temporary heart conditions during pregnancy that go away after the baby's birth. Other women develop, or find that the physical strain of pregnancy reveals existing but previously undiagnosed, heart and cardiovascular disorders that will remain after pregnancy. Managing cardiovascular care during pregnancy requires careful coordination between the woman's cardiologist and obstetrician, as some medications ordinarily used to treat heart conditions are not safe to take during pregnancy because they may harm the developing fetus.

Congenital Heart Conditions
Women who are of childbearing age in the early 2000s are the first generation of women for whom surgical repair of congenital heart malformations was a treatment standard. Many will have uneventful pregnancies and return to the

cardiovascular status they had before pregnancy. A woman who has a significant congenital malformation, such as HYPOPLASTIC LEFT HEART SYNDROME (HLHS) or TETRALOGY OF FALLOT, should consult with an obstetrician who specializes in high-risk pregnancies and with a cardiologist when planning a pregnancy, to accommodate to the best extent possible the implications and ramifications for her health as well as for the health of her baby. These consultations should include discussions of:

- Current medications and their known effects during pregnancy, especially on the fetus. For many medications taken to treat heart disease, doctors do not know the effects on the unborn child's development either during pregnancy or later in life.
- Expectations about cardiovascular status during and after pregnancy. Given the strain pregnancy places on the body, what additional factors should the woman with congenital heart disease consider?
- Possible complications for the woman, for the pregnancy, and for the fetus, and options for addressing them.

Doctors know that a woman who gives birth to a child with a serious congenital heart malformation (such as tetralogy of Fallot) has at least a 10 percent chance of a second child having a similar malformation, pointing to a genetic connection. As this is the first generation of women with surgically repaired congenital malformations to reach childbearing age, there are less data about the risk a woman faces who herself has a serious congenital heart malformation for giving birth to children who also have congenital heart malformations. The most common congenital heart malformations—PATENT DUCTUS ARTERIOSUS (PDA) and septal defects—do not appear to have a genetic basis. However, new knowledge and understanding of the genetic influences for health conditions and disorders emerges nearly weekly, and continuing research is likely to reveal many answers over the coming years. A geneticist can help a woman who has a congenital heart disorder evaluate the potential role of genetics in her health and assess the risk

that her congenital malformation is hereditary and could be passed on to her children.

Hypertension, Arrhythmias, and Murmurs

Typically a woman's blood pressure increases 8 to 10 percent by the middle of pregnancy, remaining at that level through the remainder of her pregnancy and returning to normal within six weeks of delivery. There are no health consequences from this; it is the normal course of pregnancy and helps to efficiently circulate the increased blood volume in the woman's body during pregnancy. About 5 percent of pregnant women develop a more serious complication, preeclampsia, in which blood pressure becomes elevated above 140/90 mm Hg and there is protein present in the urine (proteinuria). Proteinuria indicates that the kidneys are not functioning properly, often as a consequence of microscopic damage from the hypertension. When detected and treated, preeclampsia usually can be kept in check until it is safe to deliver the baby. Occasionally preeclampsia progresses to eclampsia, which is a medical emergency requiring prompt delivery of the baby to safeguard the lives of both mother and child. Though maternal deaths in childbirth are uncommon in the United States, eclampsia accounts for about 16 percent of them.

Occasional ARRHYTHMIAS and HEART MURMURS also are common in pregnancy. The vast majority are benign, require no treatment, and disappear following delivery. These changes reflect the increased demand on the heart and cardiovascular system during pregnancy. A woman who enters pregnancy with diagnosed disorders of rhythm or heart valve disease and who is receiving treatment for them will need continued treatment during pregnancy, though it may be necessary to change to medications that are safe for the developing fetus.

Cardiomyopathy and Heart Failure

Hypertrophic CARDIOMYOPATHY is a hereditary form of heart disease in which the heart becomes thickened and enlarged, which reduces its efficiency. About 90 percent of women who have hypertrophic cardiomyopathy when they become pregnant have uneventful pregnancies and deliveries, with minimal health complications for them or their babies. Though symptoms of cardiomyopathy, such as shortness of breath resulting from reduced CARDIAC OUTPUT and FATIGUE may temporarily worsen, the woman's cardiovascular status most often returns to its pre-pregnancy state within a few weeks of delivery. Occasionally HEART FAILURE, a common consequence of cardiomyopathy, develops, requiring aggressive treatment after delivery to prevent further deterioration of the heart. Some medications normally used to treat the usual type of dilated cardiomyopathic heart failure, notably ANGIOTENSIN-CONVERTING ENZYME (ACE) INHIBITOR MEDICATIONS, cannot be taken during pregnancy because they can damage the developing fetus. The physiological stress of pregnancy also can cause a dilated nonhypertrophic cardiomyopathy to develop. This is more likely to occur in women who enter pregnancy with existing hypertension or DIABETES.

Diabetes

Diabetes presents an increased risk for various forms of CARDIOVASCULAR DISEASE (CVD) and can be a factor in pregnancy in two ways: it can be present and diagnosed at the time a woman conceives, and it can develop during pregnancy (gestational diabetes). Careful monitoring and management of blood glucose (sugar) levels are essential in either case, as are lifestyle measures to maintain nutritious eating habits and weight management that is healthy for both mother and child. As hypertension and cardiomyopathy can develop either as a consequence of the physiological demands of pregnancy or the progression of diabetes, having diabetes when pregnant exacerbates the risk. Doctors will carefully monitor heart function during pregnancy.

See also HEREDITY AND HEART DISEASE; NUTRITION AND DIET; WOMEN AND HEART DISEASE.

premature ventricular contraction (PVC) An irregular contraction of the HEART that typically occurs early in the CARDIAC CYCLE, causing the ventricle to contract out of rhythm. PVCs are very common and the vast majority of the time are harmless though they can be alarming when they are noticeable. Though electrical stimulation of the myocardium (heart muscle) typically begins

with the SINOATRIAL (SA) NODE, all myocardial cells are capable of initiating electrical signals (which is what happens in some ARRHYTHMIAS such as FIBRILLATION). Ordinarily the SA node's impulse is strong enough to override any errant signals other myocardial cells generate, causing the cells to contract in the patterns that produce the heart's pumping action. Occasionally these errant signals gain enough momentum to initiate a contraction, which manifests as an early beat or sometimes an extra or ECTOPIC HEARTBEAT.

PVCs can sometimes be symptoms of underlying HEART DISEASE such as CARDIOMYOPATHY and CORONARY ARTERY DISEASE (CAD), or of drug interactions or other health conditions such as thyroid disorders, and should be evaluated to rule out such causes. CAFFEINE, NICOTINE, and decongestant medications taken for colds and flu also can cause PVCs. Basic diagnostic tests generally include an ELECTROCARDIOGRAM (ECG), HOLTER MONITOR to record a 24-hour ECG, and sometimes an EXERCISE STRESS TEST. The results of any of these may indicate the need for further, focused diagnostic procedures. Treatment targets any identified underlying heart disease as well as reducing consumption of any substances that could be stimulating the heart (such as caffeine and nicotine), and may include ANTIARRHYTHMIA MEDICATIONS for persistent PVCs. ABLATION may be a treatment option for frequent, highly symptomatic PVCs.

See also ANXIETY; ATRIOVENTRICULAR (AV) NODE; COLD/FLU MEDICATION AND HYPERTENSION; CARDIOVASCULAR SYSTEM; HEART BLOCK; PALPITATIONS.

primary pulmonary hypertension (PPH) See PULMONARY HYPERTENSION.

Prinivil See LISINOPRIL.

procainamide An ANTIARRYTHMIA MEDICATION taken to treat irregularities in the heartbeat. Common brand-name products in the United States include Pronestyl, Procanabid, and Procan SR. Procainamide is a SODIUM CHANNEL BLOCKING MEDICATION, categorized as a class I antiarrhythmic. It slows the rate at which electrical impulses move through myocardial (heart muscle) cells by blocking the flow of SODIUM, an ion (ELECTROLYTE) necessary for myocardial cells to contract. This in turn slows and stabilizes the rate of contractions of the heart. Doctors typically prescribe procainamide to treat sustained ventricular tachycardia (a pattern of rapid and ineffective contractions) that is causing symptoms and has failed to respond to treatment with other antiarrhythmia medications.

Procainamide can cause serious side effects, including additional and potentially fatal arrhythmias and a complex of symptoms that resemble systemic lupus erythematosus (SLE), an autoimmune disorder affecting connective tissue throughout the body. Because of procainamide's risk for causing life-threatening ARRHYTHMIAS, people often are hospitalized when beginning treatment with the medication so doctors can monitor HEART RATE and rhythm and initiate emergency cardiac measures if necessary to restore normal rhythm. People who have third degree HEART BLOCK, PREMATURE VENTRICULAR CONTRACTIONS (PVCs), chronic respiratory disorders such as asthma or CHRONIC OBSTRUCTIVE PULMONARY DISEASE (COPD), SLE, myasthenia gravis, or liver or kidney disease should discuss the risks of procainamide in depth with their cardiologists before taking this medication.

See also MEDICATIONS TO TREAT HEART DISEASE; MEXILETINE; PROPAFENONE; QUINIDINE.

Procan SR See PROCAINAMIDE.

Procardia See NIFEDIPINE.

propafenone An ANTIARRHYTHMIA MEDICATION taken to treat irregularities of the heartbeat. Brand-name products available in the United States include Rhythmol. Propafenone is a SODIUM CHANNEL BLOCKING MEDICATION, categorized as a class I anti-arrhythmic. Propafenone works by blocking the flow of SODIUM, an ion necessary for myocardial (HEART muscle) cells to contract. This slows the rate at which electrical impulses move through the heart and particularly through the His-Purkinje system, slowing and stabilizing the HEART RATE and rhythm. Like other class I antiarrhythmic medications, propafenone carries a high risk for causing other, and potentially fatal, arrhythmias. Doctors typically prescribe it only to treat sustained ventricular tachycardia (a pattern of rapid, ineffective contractions) that does not respond to other antiarrhythmia medications and is potentially life-threatening. Propafenone also has a mild beta antagonist (blocker) effect, acting in a limited though direct way on the cells of the heart and the arterial walls to slow their ability to contract as well. Other possible side effects of propafenone include DIZZINESS, headache, FATIGUE, and ANGINA.

See also BETA ANTAGONIST MEDICATIONS; MEDICATIONS TO TREAT HEART DISEASE; MEXILETINE; PROCAINAMIDE; QUINIDINE.

propanolol A medication taken to treat HYPERTENSION (high BLOOD PRESSURE), ANGINA, certain ARRHYTHMIAS, and HEART FAILURE. Doctors also sometimes prescribe propanolol to treat migraine headaches, essential tremor, and anxiety and panic disorders. Common brand-name products available in the United States include Inderal. Propanolol is a nonselective BETA ANTAGONIST MEDICATION; it blocks beta-1 and beta-2 receptors in the smooth muscle cells of the HEART and the BLOOD vessels. This effect causes the heart to contract more slowly and efficiently, and the arteries to dilate and allow more blood to flow through them. In combination, these actions result in lower blood pressure. Establishing an appropriate therapeutic dose is a challenge with propanolol and other beta-blockers in that individuals respond uniquely to the medication and there is no consistent correlation between a dosage amount and its effect in the body. Dosing is a matter of titration (gradually increasing the dose) until the desired effects are achieved. Common side effects with propanolol include SLEEP DISTURBANCES and vivid dreams, headache, tiredness, moodiness, and gastrointestinal distress (primarily nausea). Most side effects subside after a few weeks of taking propanolol. Doctors often prescribe propanolol in combination with other ANTIHYPERTENSIVE MEDICATIONS and DIURETIC MEDICATIONS to provide optimal blood pressure reduction.

See also ALPHA ANTAGONIST MEDICATIONS; MEDICATIONS TO TREAT HEART DISEASE.

prostaglandins Hormonelike chemicals in the body that play key roles in various processes within the body including facilitation of pain signals, inflammation response, and COAGULATION (clot formation). There are numerous prostaglandins, only a few of which affect cardiovascular function. Prostaglandin I2 (PGI2), for example, initiates platelet aggregation (the clumping together of platelets) to set in motion the process of coagulation. Prostaglandins D, E2, and F act on the smooth muscle tissue of the walls of the blood vessels to cause them to constrict, which raises BLOOD PRESSURE. Prostaglandin D is implicated as a contributing factor to the changes that take place in myocardial (HEART muscle) cells in HEART FAILURE. An increase in prostaglandin E1 (PGE1) maintains a PATENT DUCTUS ARTERIOSUS (PDA) in a newborn (an open channel between the pulmonary artery and the aorta) who has serious congenital heart malformations and is being explored as a beneficial treatment for serious heart failure.

Researchers are unsure what causes prostaglandin production in the body to increase; many variables likely are at play. NONSTEROIDAL ANTIINFLAMMATORY DRUGS (NSAIDs) suppress prostaglandin production. Aspirin is particularly effective in suppressing prostaglandins D, E, and F—the forms associated with CARDIOVASCULAR DISEASE (CVD); many people take ASPIRIN therapeutically and preventively for CORONARY ARTERY DISEASE (CAD), PERIPHERAL VASCULAR DISEASE (PVD), and other forms of HEART DISEASE. Other NSAIDs do not seem as effective as aspirin for this purpose, though they do exert some suppressive effect, especially on platelet aggregation; additional therapeutic effects are under investigation.

See also HEART DISEASE IN CHILDREN; INFLAMMATION AND HEART DISEASE.

protein See NUTRITION AND DIET.

pseudoephedrine A decongestant medication, typically available over-the-counter without a doctor's prescription, that is a common ingredient in cold and flu medications. There are numerous brand-name and store-brand products in addition to generic formulations; among the most common are Sudafed, Genaphed, PseudoGest, Novafed, Afrin Extended Release, and Drixoral NonDrowsy Formula. Pseudoephedrine is an adrenergic agonist medication; it stimulates EPINEPHRINE receptors primarily in the nasal and bronchial passages (nose and airways) though also throughout the body when taken systemically. In some people, or when taken for a prolonged period of time, pseudoephedrine elevates BLOOD PRESSURE, increases HEART RATE, and can cause PALPITATIONS or other irregular heart rhythms. People who have heart disease, particularly HYPERTENSION (high blood pressure) or CORONARY ARTERY DISEASE (CAD), should not take oral pseudoephedrine; nasal spray products generally do not produce systemic response. Oral pseudoephedrine can interact with various prescription medications; a pharmacist can provide advice about specific combinations.

See also COLD/FLU MEDICATION AND HYPERTENSION; EPHEDRA.

pulmonary artery See CARDIOVASCULAR SYSTEM.

pulmonary artery banding An operation to reduce the flow of BLOOD from the HEART to the lungs as a means of preventing PULMONARY CONGESTION and pulmonary vascular disease due to PULMONARY HYPERTENSION (elevated pressure within the blood vessels of the lungs) resulting from congenital heart defects.

Procedure

In this operation the surgeon places a wide band around the pulmonary artery and tightens it until achieving the appropriate reduction in blood flow. Pulmonary artery banding may be the first of multiple operations to correct a complex of congenital heart malformations or a palliative procedure when the malformations cannot be completely corrected with surgery. The operation typically is performed before the child is two years old and often in the first six months of life.

Risks and Complications

Pulmonary artery banding can cause complications later in life; it requires regular monitoring and follow-up care. Sometimes additional operations become necessary as the child grows, as the band can become too tight or too loose.

Outlook and Lifestyle Modifications

While pulmonary artery binding is highly effective as a temporary or interim measure, children who undergo pulmonary artery banding have significant congenital heart malformations that affect cardiovascular function lifelong. These malformations often restrict activity to some degree, even after comprehensive repair or reconstruction.

See also ARTERIAL SWITCH PROCEDURE; BIDIRECTIONAL GLENN PROCEDURE; BLALOCK-TAUSSIG PROCEDURE; HEART DISEASE IN CHILDREN; FONTAN PROCEDURE; NORWOOD PROCEDURE.

pulmonary atresia   A congenital HEART malformation in which the valve between the right ventricle and the pulmonary artery, the pulmonary valve, fails to form and there is no outlet for BLOOD to pass from the right ventricle into the pulmonary artery and to the lungs. Pulmonary atresia often does not become apparent until after birth, as before birth the lungs of the fetus do not function (the mother's blood supplies the fetus with oxygen). A natural opening, the ductus arteriosus, connects the pulmonary artery directly with the aorta to circulate blood through the unborn baby's body. The pressure changes that occur within the cardiopulmonary system when the newborn begins breathing after birth cause the ductus arteriosus to begin to close, typically within 24 to 72 hours of birth.

Symptoms and Diagnostic Path

Most oxygenation problems are obvious very quickly after birth, with the infant acquiring a dusky blue hue to the skin and showing other signs of limited oxygenation. Diagnosis of pulmonary atresia may include ECHOCARDIOGRAM and CARDIAC CATHETERIZATION, procedures that help doctors to determine the extent of malformation present and to take measures to improve the flow of oxygenated blood.

Treatment Options and Outlook

Some oxygen continues to get into the baby's system through the mingling of blood that the ductus arteriosus allows; when doctors suspect pulmonary atresia or other anomalies of structure they administer injections of PROSTAGLANDIN E2 (PGE2), a hormonelike chemical that prevents the ductus arteriosus from closing. When this structure remains open, it is called a PATENT DUCTUS ARTERIOSUS (PDA). Surgery is necessary to create a pulmonary valve to restore the normal flow of blood between the heart and lungs.

Risk Factors and Preventive Measures

Pulmonary atresia often occurs in combination with other heart malformations; the repair process may require multiple operations over the child's first two years of life. In the majority of those born with pulmonary atresia, surgery is a successful remedy that, though it may not restore normal function to the heart, allows a relatively normal life. Children born with congenital heart malformations such as pulmonary atresia will require lifelong monitoring and care from cardiologists who specialize in such conditions.

See also ATRIOVENTRICULAR (AV) CANAL DEFECT; BICUSPID AORTIC VALVE; COARCTATION OF THE AORTA; DOWN SYNDROME, HEART MALFORMATIONS ASSOCIATED WITH; EBSTEIN'S ANOMALY; EISENMENGER'S SYNDROME; HEART DISEASE; HEART DISEASE IN CHILDREN; HYPOPLASTIC LEFT HEART SYNDROME (HLHS); PROSTAGLANDINS; SINGLE VENTRICLE; TETRALOGY OF FALLOT; TRANSPOSITION OF THE GREAT ARTERIES (TGA); TRISCUSPID ATRESIA.

pulmonary congestion/pulmonary edema   A condition in which lung tissue becomes saturated with fluid, interfering with OXYGENATION of the BLOOD. There are numerous causes for pulmonary edema; among the most common are congestive HEART FAILURE secondary to HYPERTENSION, coronary HEART DISEASE (CHD), cardiomyopathies, ARRHYTHMIAS, and valvular HEART diseases. PULMONARY HYPERTENSION and progressive lung diseases such as CHRONIC OBSTRUCTIVE PULMONARY DISEASE (COPD) and emphysema that damage the structures within the lungs (primarily the alveoli) where oxygen exchange takes place are among the most common causes of right heart failure, which causes congestion of the liver. Pulmonary edema also can cause heart failure, as the pressure against which the right heart must pump blood to get it to the lungs becomes too high for the right ventricle to accommodate.

Resistance, or the pressure that blood encounters when it flows through the blood vessels, ordinarily is so low in the blood vessels of the lungs that the force of the left ventricle's contractions to pump blood out to the body creates sufficient momentum to send blood to the right heart or to the lungs if the right heart is nonfunctional. Surgical remedies for serious congenital heart malformations such as HYPOPLASTIC LEFT HEART SYNDROME (HLHS) and TETRALOGY OF FALLOT take advantage of this natural tendency by creating shunts between the great arteries of the heart that bypass a nonfunctional right ventricle. When resistance increases in the blood vessels of the lungs, the structures and mechanisms of the cardiopulmonary system are ill-equipped to adapt. The right ventricle, which pumps blood to the lungs, is not as thick or muscular as the left ventricle, which pumps blood to the body. When the pressure within the blood vessels in the lungs becomes higher than the right ventricle's ability to counter, the heart cannot generate enough pumping force to adequately move blood through the lungs.

Pressure is a key mechanism for regulating the amount of fluid in the blood. When pressure inside the blood vessels becomes significantly higher than the pressure outside the blood vessels, fluid leaves the blood and accumulates in the tissues; fluid follows the path of least resistance. When this occurs in the tissues of the lungs, the tiny sacs where oxygen exchange takes place, the alveoli, cannot function properly and not enough oxygen gets into the blood. A secondary risk is infection, causing pneumonia.

Symptoms and Diagnostic Path

Symptoms of pulmonary edema include shortness of breath, difficulty breathing, coughing, tiredness, and occasionally a sensation of tightness in the chest or chest pain. Chest X-ray typically shows fluid accumulation in the tissues of the lungs.

Treatment Options and Outlook

Treatment combines drawing additional fluid out of the body in the urine with DIURETIC MEDICATIONS and treating the underlying health condition. Pulmonary edema can be acute (a response to a specific circumstance) or chronic (occurring over an extended period of time). Chronic cardiovascular conditions or chronic pulmonary conditions nearly always accompany chronic pulmonary edema. Medications and lifestyle modifications (such as decreased SODIUM consumption) to control the volume of fluid in the body help to minimize pulmonary edema.

Risk Factors and Preventive Measures

Pulmonary congestion and pulmonary edema develop as consequences of underlying heart disease and lung disease. Taking appropriate measures to reduce the risks for these underlying conditions and diligent compliance with treatment once underlying conditions are diagnosed are the most effective measures for prevention.

See also BIDIRECTIONAL GLENN PROCEDURE; EDEMA; FONTAN PROCEDURE; CARDIOVASCULAR SYSTEM; NORWOOD PROCEDURE; PULMONARY SYSTEM; SMOKING AND HEART DISEASE.

pulmonary function See LUNG CAPACITY.

pulmonary hypertension Chronic elevation of the pressure in the pulmonary artery that leads from the heart's right ventricle to the lungs that arises when changes to the BLOOD vessels within the lungs causes increased resistance to the flow of blood. Pulmonary hypertension that has no identifiable cause is called primary pulmonary hypertension (PPH). Pulmonary hypertension can develop secondary to other health conditions such as congenital heart disease, pulmonary embolism (blood clot in the lung), sickle-cell ANEMIA, and CHRONIC OBSTRUCTIVE PULMONARY DISEASE (COPD). Doctors manage secondary pulmonary hypertension by treating the causative conditions though they sometimes need to prescribe medications specifically to treat the pulmonary hypertension. Untreated pulmonary hypertension causes right

HEART FAILURE, which also can cause pulmonary artery pressure to increase.

Symptoms and Diagnostic Path

Pulmonary hypertension can exist for many years without symptoms or detection. When symptoms do occur they tend to be vague and generalized and may include tiredness, shortness of breath especially with exertion (DYSPNEA), and PALPITATIONS. Measuring pulmonary artery BLOOD PRESSURE is invasive, requiring insertion of a catheter through a blood vessel and into the heart. Diagnosis most frequently is by exclusion, ruling out other possible causes. CARDIAC CATHETERIZATION helps with this process of elimination as well as provides an opportunity to measure pulmonary artery pressure and often is done when more obvious potential causes of symptoms are not responsible.

There is an association between pulmonary hypertension and appetite suppressant medications that are chemically related to amphetamines. Cocaine use, HIV/AIDS, and RAYNAUD'S SYNDROME (a disorder affecting the circulation of blood in the fingers and toes) are also associated with pulmonary hypertension, though the extent to which any of these associations actually cause pulmonary hypertension remains unknown.

Treatment Options and Outlook

Treatment typically involves taking DIURETIC MEDICATIONS to help the body drain off excess fluid and making lifestyle choices to support cardiovascular health, notably smoking cessation if that is a factor and exposure to environmental irritants that affect lung function. It may also be necessary to take medications to strengthen the efficiency of the heart's contractions. Once primary pulmonary hypertension develops it can be managed though not cured; secondary pulmonary hypertension may resolve when the underlying condition does though the longer pulmonary hypertension is present the more likely there is permanent damage to the small blood vessels within the heart. HEART-LUNG TRANSPLANT is sometimes an option, albeit one of significant risk, when pulmonary hypertension develops as a result of congenital heart malformations or is so severe as to restrict daily life activities.

Risk Factors and Preventive Measures

Because the causes of pulmonary hypertension are poorly understood, there are few preventive measures aside from smoking cessation and other lifestyle measures to prevent HEART DISEASE. Researchers believe that 10 percent or more of primary pulmonary hypertension has hereditary (genetic) components.

See also COCAINE AND HEART ATTACK; HEART DISEASE; LIFESTYLE AND HEART HEALTH; LIVING WITH HEART DISEASE; MEDICATIONS TO TREAT HEART DISEASE; SMOKING AND HEART DISEASE.

pulmonary stenosis A congenital HEART malformation in which the pulmonary artery, which carries BLOOD from the heart's right ventricle to the lungs for oxygenation, is narrowed. Often pulmonary stenosis occurs in combination with other structural malformations involving the heart's chambers, great vessels, and valves. Untreated pulmonary stenosis results in right HEART FAILURE, though this usually does not become apparent until adulthood when the heart is no longer able to compensate. Pulmonary stenosis can result from narrowing or malformation of the pulmonary valve (valvular pulmonary stenosis, the most common presentation), above the pulmonary valve along the pulmonary artery (supravalvular pulmonary stenosis), or, least commonly, below the pulmonary valve affecting the structure of the right ventricle. Rarely, pulmonary stenosis develops later in life as a consequence of RHEUMATIC HEART DISEASE.

Symptoms and Diagnostic Path

Pulmonary stenosis produces a characteristic HEART MURMUR that doctors generally can detect by listening to the heart with a STETHOSCOPE; ECHOCARDIOGRAM and imaging technologies such as COMPUTED TOMOGRAPHY (CT) SCAN or MAGNETIC RESONANCE IMAGING (MRI) can confirm its presence and help determine its seriousness.

Treatment Options and Outlook

Nearly always treatment is to widen the stenosis surgically, which sometimes can be done with balloon VALVULOPLASTY (CARDIAC CATHETERIZATION in which a tiny balloon is guided into the heart and inflated to stretch apart the leaflets of the pulmonary valve) or an open-heart operation to reconstruct the valve or the area of the stenosis (and to repair any other malformations that are present).

Risk Factors and Preventive Measures

Pulmonary stenosis is a congenital heart defect that may have genetic or hereditary correlations. There are no known preventive measures for pulmonary stenosis.

See also ANTIBIOTIC PROPHYLAXIS; AUSCULTATION; CARDIOVASCULAR SYSTEM; SURGERY TO TREAT CARDIOVASCULAR DISEASE; VALVE REPAIR AND REPLACEMENT.

pulmonary system   The organs, structures, and functions within the body that oxygenate the BLOOD. These include the trachea (windpipe), bronchi, bronchioles, lungs, alveoli, and extensive capillary beds that infiltrate lung tissue. The primary function of the pulmonary system is to bring air into the lungs so the lungs can extract oxygen from it. There is an intimate integration between the pulmonary system the heart, and the CARDIOVASCULAR SYSTEM. Air enters the trachea through the nose or mouth and travels through the branchlike network of airways (the bronchi and bronchioles) into the alveoli deep within the lungs.

Ancient physicians believed air breathed into the body traveled directly to the HEART and was carried throughout the body by the blood vessels, not an entirely inaccurate perception in a most basic sense. Seventeenth-century physician William Harvey's accurate description of the structures and functions of the heart and circulatory system, published in 1628, and Italian physiologist Lazzaro Spallanzani's similarly precise description in the 1790s of gas exchange within the lungs opened the door for other scientists to explore the separate yet interrelated structures and functions of the cardiovascular and pulmonary systems, including the role of the blood.

From each RESPIRATORY CYCLE (a completed round of inhalation and exhalation) healthy lungs are able to extract enough oxygen to support four CARDIAC CYCLES. The heart's right ventricle pumps unoxygenated blood through the pulmonary artery to the lungs. The blood circulates through the network of capillaries, releasing CARBON DIOXIDE and other metabolic wastes and picking up oxygen. The oxygenated blood returns to the heart via the left atrium, and the left ventricle pumps it out to the body. The respiratory rate generally increases or decreases in synchronization with the heart rate to meet the body's need for oxygen.

The Airways

The trachea, or windpipe, is a thick, sturdy tube made of rings of cartilage that slightly expand and contract with breathing. The cartilage rings of the trachea help to keep it rigid and open during breathing and movement. Though a direct blow to the throat can injure the trachea, causing partial or complete collapse, the trachea is a substantial structure that can withstand considerable pressure. Connecting the cartilage rings are bands of fibrous tissue.

The trachea extends from the back of the throat to just below the top of the sternum, becoming slightly wider as it descends. From behind the aortic arch at the top of the heart, the trachea branches into two tubes, the bronchi, one of which goes to each lung. Each bronchus branches into smaller and smaller tubes extending deeper into the lungs; the smallest branches are no bigger in diameter than a hair and are called bronchioles. The bronchioles open into the alveoli, clusterlike air sacs where gas exchange (oxygen and carbon dioxide) takes place.

The Lungs

The lungs snuggle the heart, one to either side. A protective double-layer membrane, the pleura, encases each lung. A thin layer of fluid allows the lungs to move without friction as they expand and contract during breathing. The right lung has three lobes: upper, middle, and lower. The left lung has two lobes, upper and lower, creating space to accommodate the heart. Each lobe performs essentially the same functions. Inner lung tissue consists of fibrous strands linking together thousands of alveolar clusters. The rib cage contains and protects the lungs and provides the rigidity necessary to support the dynamic pressures of breathing.

The Mechanics of Breathing

The pulmonary system is closed and pressurized; respirations occur as the smooth muscle tissue of the rib cage and the diaphragm (a flat muscle that forms the bottom of the chest cavity) contract and relax. Contraction pulls the ribs apart, expanding the lungs. Relaxation allows the rib cage to return to its normal position. Expansion creates pressure that pulls air into the lungs; relaxation allows air to leave the lungs. Each breath starts when the rib muscles (intercostal) contract, which pulls air through the nose. Air enters the nasal passages and is warmed and moistened as it passes through the sinuses. At the top of the trachea is a small flap called the epiglottis that keeps food and fluid from entering the trachea. As the air gets to the back of the throat the epiglottis lifts and the air drops down the trachea.

The air travels through the bronchi and bronchioles until it reaches the alveoli. A very thin membrane lines each alveolus; the capillary beds entwine on the other side of the membrane. Oxygen from inhaled air passes across the membrane and binds with HEMOGLOBIN molecules on the red blood cells. At the same time carbon dioxide crosses the membrane from the blood and enters the air. This exchange, too, is pressure-driven. With inhalation the air pressure of the atmosphere is greater than the air pressure within the alveoli so oxygen encounters less resistance moving to the blood. Conversely with exhalation air pressure within the alveoli is higher than in the atmosphere so carbon dioxide encounters less resistance moving from the blood. The carbon dioxide level in the blood is one of the key triggers that signals the autonomic nervous system to stimulate contractions of the intercostal (rib) muscles, initiating a respiratory cycle.

See also ANEMIA; BLOOD GASES; CHRONIC OBSTRUCTIVE PULMONARY DISEASE (COPD); CIRCULATION; HARVEY, WILLIAM; OXYGENATION; OXYGEN THERAPY; PULSE OXIMETRY.

pulse An observable passage of BLOOD through the arteries that represents the heart's contractions. Most often the pulse is felt with the fingertips and can be detected in any artery that is near enough to the skin. Common pulse points that cardiologists usually palpate (feel) or ausculate (listen to with a STETHOSCOPE) are:

- radial arteries at the wrists
- brachial arteries at insides of the elbows
- carotid arteries in the neck
- temporal arteries at the sides of the forehead
- femoral arteries in the groin
- popliteal arteries at the backs of the knees
- dorsal pedis arteries on the tops of the feet

The characteristics of the pulse provide important diagnostic information about a range of cardiovascular diseases. Doctors note a pulse's rate, rhythm, force, delays, and other features. The pulse of a person who has a healthy cardiovascular system is consistent in its rate, rhythm, and force at various pulse points.

When taking the pulse, it is important to use one or two fingers pressed firmly against the pulse

PULSE CHARACTERISTICS AS SYMPTOMS OF HEART DISEASE

Pulse Characteristic	May Be a Symptom of
Rate regular though slower than 60 beats per minute	Bradycardia; heart block; hypothyroidism
Rate regular though faster than 100 beats per minute	Tachycardia; atrial or ventricular arrhythmias; hyperthyroidism
Irregular and rapid, with beats closer and further apart without apparent pattern	Cardiomyopathy; sinus arrhythmias; heart failure; coronary artery disease (CAD); atrial flutter and fibrillation
Irregular and slow, with beats closer and further apart without apparent pattern	Heart block
Rate and rhythm irregular	Sinus node disorders; tachycardia-bradycardia syndrome
Visible pounding ("water hammer" pulse, Corrigan's sign) at the pulse point	Aortic insufficiency (damage to the aortic valve)
Irregular force (some beats are weak, some beats are strong)	Long QT syndrome; left heart failure
Strong during exhalation, weak during inhalation	Pericarditis; pericardial effusion; cardiac tamponade
Regular though weak	Aortic stenosis; pericardial effusion

point so the full pad of the fingertip is in equal and firm contact with the skin. The thumb has a palpable pulse, so should not be used to take the pulse. To take a pulse, count the number of beats that occur in one minute, timed with a clock or watch. Some people count the beats for 15 or 30 seconds, then multiply the result by four or two to get the number of beats in 60 seconds. This is less accurate, and may not reveal irregularities in rhythm and force of the heartbeat. Medications, physical activity, and TOBACCO USE can temporarily alter pulse characteristics.

See also AUSCULTATION; HEARTBEAT; HEART RATE.

pulse oximetry   A method for monitoring the percentage of oxygen in the BLOOD. A pulse oximeter is a device that fits over the end of a finger. Two wavelengths of light emanate from the oximeter and penetrate the HEMOGLOBIN being circulated in the blood, as detected when the blood pulses through the small arteries at the ends of the fingers. The hemoglobin, the protein in the red blood cells that carries oxygen, absorbs one wavelength but not the other. A computer processor calculates the difference between the two wavelengths and then determines the saturation point of the hemoglobin. A desirable pulse oximetry reading is 95 percent or higher. A reading lower than 95 percent indicates that the body's tissues are not receiving adequate oxygen.

See also BLOOD GASES, ARTERIAL; OXYGENATION; OXYGEN THERAPY.

P-wave   See ELECTROCARDIOGRAM (ECG).

quality of life The ability to participate in and enjoy the activities and events of daily life that provide pleasure, satisfaction, and joy. HEART DISEASE can have a minimal to a significant effect on a person's quality of life, depending on the extent to which it limits favorite activities. Treatment for HEART disease can have equally significant effects.

Assessing quality of life incorporates both objective and subjective measures. General assessment tools include questionnaires such as the Sickness Impact Profile (SIP) and the Short Form Health Survey (SF-36). These questionnaires elicit responses about the effects of health and illness on physical, social, emotional, relationship, and work dimensions of daily living. Some employers and insurers use the SIP and SF-36 in their processes for determining disability status. Numerous disease-specific questionnaires attempt to evaluate similar aspects with regard to the nature of illness, such as HYPERTENSION (high BLOOD PRESSURE), HEART FAILURE, and post-HEART ATTACK status.

Heart disease is a leading cause of disability in the United States; inherent in this distinction is limitation of activities. Nearly a quarter of men and half of women who have heart failure are New York Heart Association (NYHA) classification category III or IV—partially or fully disabled as a consequence of their heart failure. Stroke leaves 30 percent of its survivors with permanent disabilities and unable to return to jobs and activities in which they participated before their strokes. Most people who have heart disease are able to return to functional lives; whether that establishes an acceptable quality of life is a matter of subjective perception.

See also DEATHS FROM HEART DISEASE; LIFESTYLE AND HEART HEALTH; LIVING WITH HEART DISEASE.

Questran See CHOLESTYRAMINE.

quinapril An ANGIOTENSIN-CONVERTING ENZYME (ACE) INHIBITOR MEDICATION taken to treat HYPERTENSION (high BLOOD PRESSURE). Common brand-name products available in the United States include Accupril. Quinapril works by preventing the synthesis of angiotensin II, a powerful vasoconstrictor, to block its actions to raise blood pressure. Doctors may prescribe quinapril alone for mild hypertension and in combination with a DIURETIC MEDICATION for moderate hypertension. Doctors also prescribe quinapril to treat congestive HEART FAILURE, usually in combination with DIGOXIN. Possible side effects include tiredness, orthostatic HYPOTENSION, ARRHYTHMIAS, gastrointestinal distress (nausea, vomiting, diarrhea, or CONSTIPATION), and angioedema (fluid retention resulting in swelling), particularly of the lips and mouth. Angioedema is a medical emergency when it interferes with breathing or swallowing.

See also ANGIOTENSIN II RECEPTOR ANTAGONIST MEDICATIONS; ANGIOTENSIN-CONVERTING ENZYME; ANTIHYPERTENSIVE MEDICATIONS; BENAZE-PRIL; CAPTOPRIL; ENALAPRIL; FOSINOPRIL; LISINOPRIL; MOEXIPRIL; RAMIPRIL; TRANDOLAPRIL.

Quinidex See QUINIDINE.

quinidine A medication taken to treat ARRHYTHMIAS (irregularities of the HEARTBEAT). Common brand-name products available in the United States include Cardioquin, Quinidex, and Quinaglute Dura Tabs. Quinidine is a SODIUM CHANNEL BLOCKING MEDICATION, categorized as a class I antiarrhythmic, that regulates the heart's rhythm by inhibiting the flow of sodium through myocardial (HEART muscle) cells. Such inhibition slows and stabilizes the rate and force of the heart's contractions. Doctors prescribe quinidine to treat a spectrum of arrhythmias including atrial flutter and fibrillation, symptomatic PREMATURE VENTRICULAR CONTRACTIONS (PVCs), and ventricular tachycardia that is not the result of HEART BLOCK. People who have LONG QT SYNDROME or heart block should not take quinidine as the medication exacerbates the arrhythmia. Possible side effects include headache, lethargy, new arrhythmias, and disturbances of blood composition.

See also ANTIARRHYTHMIA MEDICATIONS; ATRIAL FIBRILLATION; MEDICATIONS TO TREAT HEART DISEASE; MEXILETINE; PROCAINAMIDE; PROPAFENONE.

Q-wave   See ELECTROCARDIOGRAM (ECG).

QRS internal   See ELECTROCARDIOGRAM (ECG).

QT internal   See ELECTROCARDIOGRAM (ECG).

QTc internal   See ELECTROCARDIOGRAM (ECG).

radial artery   See CARDIOVASCULAR SYSTEM.

radiofrequency catheter ablation   A method for permanently eliminating certain ARRHYTHMIAS. Done as a CARDIAC CATHETERIZATION procedure, radiofrequency catheter ablation uses a brief burst of radiofrequency heat to necrotize, or kill, myocardial (HEART muscle) cells that are conducting or originating errant electrical impulses. The ablation targets a small and precisely defined area of cells. The death of the cells interrupts the pathway for the electrical impulses, helping to restore the heart's normal electrical pathways.

Procedure

Radiofrequency catheter ablation usually requires an overnight stay in the hospital. For the procedure, the cardiologist inserts a catheter into a BLOOD vessel near the surface of the skin and threads it through to the desired location within the heart using FLUOROSCOPY (moving X-rays) for guidance. The person is sedated for comfort during the procedure, and the cardiologist uses a local anesthetic to numb the area where the catheter is inserted. The discharge of radiofrequency heat, which is similar to the microwave energy, is painless. Radiofrequency catheter ablation is the treatment of choice for supraventricular tachycardia, an arrhythmia of rapid and uncoordinated contractions of the atria, and a treatment option for ATRIAL flutter and FIBRILLATION.

Risks and Complications

Radiofrequency catheter ablation is the treatment of choice for supraventricular tachycardia and for atrial flutter, arrhythmias characterized by rapid and regular impulses in the top chambers of the heart. For these conditions, the procedure's risks are minimal, and it is more than 90 percent successful in permanently resolving the arrhythmias. Radiofrequency catheter ablation is also a treatment option for atrial fibrillation and many ventricular arrhythmias, although both the risks and the success rates are typically less favorable. An overnight stay in the hospital following the procedure is necessary to monitor for arrhythmias, which are an uncommon but potentially serious complication of radiofrequency catheter ablation. It is also possible for there to be injury to the blood vessels through which the catheter passes; this complication is also uncommon.

Outlook and Lifestyle Modifications

Radiofrequency catheter ablation frequently is a permanent solution for common atrial and some ventricular arrhythmias, after which no lifestyle modifications are necessary. Some arrhythmias may return, requiring further treatment including repeat radiofrequency catheter ablation.

See also CARDIOVERSION; PACEMAKER.

radionuclide scan   An imaging procedure in which a solution tagged with radioactive isotopes is administered, usually by intravenous injection, to provide visualization of cardiovascular functions. The isotopes follow the solution, often glucose, on its course into the tissues and cells. As the isotopes deteriorate (a normal process) they discharge harmless radiation that specialized cameras can detect. A computer assembles the patterns of radioactivity into multidimensional images that the doctor then interprets to assess the extent of damage or disease present in the HEART and BLOOD vessels. Radionuclide scanning often is done in combination with an

EXERCISE STRESS TEST to examine the cardiovascular system both at rest and under the stress of moderately intense physical activity (real or pharmaceutically induced).

Some people experience discomfort during the injection of the radioactive solution. Some people also feel chest discomfort such as ANGINA and shortness of breath (DYSPNEA) when the cardiologist also is using an injected drug such as DIPYRIDAMOLE to assess cardiovascular response during simulated exercise. Such discomfort is temporary.

Procedure

A radionuclide scan of the heart takes about an hour to conduct, though the radioactive solution may be administered via IV up to an hour before the start of the scan. Commonly, two sets of scans are done four to six hours apart.

Risks and Complications

There is no risk from the radioactivity of the isotopes; they completely deteriorate within a few hours.

Outlook and Lifestyle Modifications

Radionuclide scans are diagnostic. It is common to feel tired after the procedure even into the next day. However, most people quickly return to their usual activities.

See also ADENOSINE STRESS TEST; COMPUTED TOMOGRAPHY (CT) SCAN; DIPYRIDAMOLE STRESS TEST; DOBUTAMINE STRESS TEST; MAGNETIC RESONANCE IMAGING (MRI); POSITRON EMISSION TOMOGRAPHY (PET) SCAN; SINGLE PHOTON EMISSION COMPUTED TOMOGRAPHY (SPECT) SCAN.

ramipril A medication taken to treat HYPERTENSION (high BLOOD PRESSURE). Brand-name products available in the United States include Altace. Ramipril is an ANGIOTENSIN-CONVERTING ENZYME (ACE) INHIBITOR MEDICATION; it works by preventing the body's production of the vasoconstrictor chemical angiotensin II. Doctors prescribe ramipril alone to treat mild hypertension and in combination with a DIURETIC MEDICATION (commonly a thiazide diuretic) to treat moderate hypertension. Doctors also prescribe ramipril after a HEART ATTACK (MYOCARDIAL INFARCTION) to reduce the risk for subsequent heart attacks and to mitigate post-heart attack HEART FAILURE.

Side effects that can occur when taking ramipril include headache, FATIGUE, and nausea. Some people experience a persistent, dry cough that lingers even after switching to a different medication. Rare but serious side effects include ARRHYTHMIAS, ANGIOEDEMA, and heart attack or STROKE. Women should not take ramipril or other ACE inhibitors during pregnancy, as these medications can cause serious injury and death to the fetus (particularly in the second and third trimesters of pregnancy).

See also ANGIOTENSIN II RECEPTOR ANTAGONIST MEDICATIONS; ANTIHYPERTENSIVE MEDICATIONS; MEDICATIONS TO TREAT HEART DISEASE.

rauwolfia A chemical family of alkaloids that act on the sympathetic nervous system to slow the nerve impulses that direct BLOOD PRESSURE. Rauwolfia derivatives include reserpine, serpentine (also called rauwolfia serpentina), and deserpidine. They are taken to treat HYPERTENSION (high blood pressure). Because rauwolfia alkaloids have far-reaching systemic effects as a result of their actions on nerve pathways and a low level for toxicity, doctors do not commonly prescribe them.

Rauwolfia compounds interact with numerous other medications and some foods; they cannot be taken within two weeks of taking monoamine oxidase inhibitor (MAOI) ANTIDEPRESSANT MEDICATIONS or selective MAOIs (such as selegiline) taken to treat Parkinson's disease. Rauwolfia alkaloids can also cause Parkinson-like neuromuscular symptoms including tremors and movement difficulties. These medications are associated with potentially life-threatening bradycardia (slowed heart rate) and pheochromocytoma (a rare adrenal tumor that

RAUWOLFIA ALKALOIDS	
Rauwolfia Derivative	**Common Brand-Name Products**
Deserpidine	Harmony
Reserpine	Serpasil, Serpalan
Serpentine (rauwolfia serpentina)	Raudixin, Rauval, Rauverid, Wolfina

causes excessive production of EPINEPHRINE and NOREPINEPHRINE, resulting in episodes of extremely high blood pressure).

See also ANTIHYPERTENSIVE MEDICATIONS; ARRHYTHMIA; MEDICATIONS TO TREAT HEART DISEASE; PAROXYSMAL HYPERTENSION.

Raynaud's syndrome A disorder of the peripheral BLOOD vessels of the hands and feet in which the body's response to cold is exaggerated, resulting in partial to complete shutdown of the blood supply to the fingers and toes. The primary symptoms include discoloration of the skin and discomfort or pain of the fingers and toes, reflecting the diminished blood supply. In some people Raynaud's syndrome also may involve the nose and outer portions of the ears (especially the earlobes). About 10 to 20 percent of adults in the United States have Raynaud's syndrome; the disorder is most common in women between the ages of 20 and 45. The condition also is called Raynaud's phenomenon and Raynaud's disease.

Symptoms and Diagnostic Path

Raynaud's syndrome presents symptoms episodically or in the form of attacks, typically brought on by exposure to cold temperatures. Such exposure activates the normal body mechanisms that constrict peripheral blood vessels to return more blood to the body's core, preserving warmth. In Raynaud's syndrome this mechanism causes over-constriction of the arterioles, resulting in spasms that completely shut down the flow of blood. Attacks may occur with every exposure to cold or without apparent pattern. Emotional stress also can initiate attacks in some people.

Diagnosis includes blood tests to look for evidence of inflammatory response within the body, which shows up as elevations of certain kinds of blood cells.

Treatment Options and Outlook

Treatment is primarily preventive and nonmedical, with emphasis on keeping the extremities as well as the body core warm when exposed to cold temperatures so as to mitigate the body's protective mechanisms. When an attack takes place, prompt efforts to warm the fingers and toes (such as going indoors, taking a warm bath or shower, or getting near a heat source) can lessen the symptoms and duration of the attack. Careful management of DIABETES, when present, and smoking cessation are also key preventive measures. When attacks are frequent and symptoms severe, doctors may prescribe VASODILATOR MEDICATIONS such as ALPHA ANTAGONIST MEDICATIONS or topical NITROGLYCERIN to help relax the blood vessels; medications are not always effective.

Risk Factors and Preventive Measures

Researchers are uncertain what causes this disorder. There appear to be associations with connective tissue disorders such as lupus erythematosus (systemic and discoid) and rheumatoid arthritis, though this is not consistent. About 10 percent of people who have Raynaud's syndrome have other health conditions affecting the flow of blood to the extremities, such as PERIPHERAL VASCULAR DISEASE (PVD) and vascular deterioration of DIABETES. Medications that cause vasoconstriction (constrict the blood vessels and reduce blood flow) also can cause symptoms of Raynaud's syndrome. Such medications include BETA ANTAGONIST MEDICATIONS taken to treat HYPERTENSION (high BLOOD PRESSURE), ergotamine derivatives taken to treat migraine headaches and Parkinson's disease, and cold/flu medications that contain decongestants (commonly pseudoephedrine). There is a high correlation between long-term cigarette smoking and Raynaud's syndrome.

See also NICOTINE; SMOKING AND HEART DISEASE.

red blood cell See BLOOD.

reentry A dysfunction of conductivity within the HEART in which electrical impulses shortcut the normal CONDUCTION SYSTEM and thereby form a rapid looping of electrical activation. Reentry is the most common cause of tachyarrhythmias that require treatment, including ATRIAL FIBRILLATION, VENTRICULAR TACHYCARDIA, and some forms of ventricular fibrillation. Common reentry locations include:

- AV node reentry, in which errant electrical impulses from a loop involving two "limbs" of the AV node and the atria themselves
- AV reentry, in which errant impulses form a loop involving an ACCESSORY PATHWAY and the normal conduction pathway
- scar reentry, in which errant impulses loop around dead tissue in the heart, such as a previous surgical scar (incisional reentry) or scar from a previous HEART ATTACK (as in ischemic ventricular tachycardia)
- bundle branch reentry, in which errant impulses form a loop going down one of the bundle branches and back up another, typically seen only in very small diseased and dilated hearts

Reentry can also be classified by the size of the electrical "loop" that is involved. Macroreentry involves large areas of myocardium (heart tissue), as in the types of reentry in the preceding list. Microreentry circuits involve only a minuscule area, as in atrial tachycardia and atrial fibrillation.

Arrhythmias caused by reentry are often treated with ABLATION to destroy the conductivity of the dysfunctional cells, returning the heart to its normal conduction pathway.

See also ANTIARRHYTHMIA MEDICATIONS; RADIO-FREQUENCY CATHETER ABLATION; SURGERY TO TREAT CARDIOVASCULAR DISEASE.

rehabilitation, cardiac   See CARDIAC REHABILITATION.

renin-angiotensin-aldosterone (RAA) hormonal system   One of the body's primary mechanisms for regulating BLOOD PRESSURE. Specialized cells within the kidneys continuously monitor the volume and pressure of BLOOD as it flows through its filtering structures (the glomeruli). When blood pressure drops, these cells release the enzyme renin into the bloodstream. There, renin encounters a protein called angiotensinogen that the liver produces and that always circulates in the bloodstream. Angiotensinogen is an inactive precursor for the angiotensin proteins. When renin interacts

with angiotensinogen, the renin cleaves, or splits, angiotensinogen molecules into smaller molecules, one of which is angiotensin I. Angiotensin I also is inert. When the blood's circulation takes angiotensin I to the lungs, however, it encounters ANGIOTENSIN-CONVERTING ENZYME (ACE). ACE cleaves angiotensin I, producing the active protein angiotensin II. Angiotensin II acts in multiple ways to increase blood pressure:

- It stimulates the adrenal cortex to release aldosterone, a HORMONE that causes the kidneys to increase the amount of SODIUM and fluid retained in the blood. This increases blood volume.
- It binds with receptors in the arterioles, the body's smallest arteries, and causes them to constrict (tighten and narrow). This increases the resistance blood encounters when it flows through the arterioles, causing the HEART to intensify the force of its contractions.
- It stimulates the pituitary gland to release antidiuretic hormone (ADH), which causes the kidneys to retain additional fluid in the blood. This further increases blood volume.
- It causes myocardial cells to thicken, increasing myocardial mass (causing the heart to enlarge). This gives the heart greater pumping capacity and efficiency.

In health, the RAA hormonal system maintains the blood pressure in intricate balance, making continual adjustments. When CARDIOVASCULAR DISEASE (CVD) interferes with the heart's ability to move blood efficiently through the body to meet the body's OXYGENATION needs, the changes that the RAA hormonal system initiate can become permanent and hypertension results. Two classifications of ANTIHYPERTENSIVE MEDICATIONS, ANGIOTENSIN-CONVERTING ENZYME (ACE) INHIBITOR MEDICATIONS and ANGIOTENSIN II RECEPTOR ANTAGONIST MEDICATIONS, lower blood pressure by interrupting the RAA cycle. ACE inhibitor medications appear to also have therapeutic value for treating heart failure and for decreasing the risk of subsequent heart attacks after a first HEART ATTACK.

See also HEART DISEASE; MEDICATIONS TO TREAT HEART DISEASE.

reserpine See RAUWOLFIA.

respiratory cycle A sequence of inhalation and exhalation. The level of CARBON DIOXIDE in the BLOOD signals the medulla, a structure in the brain that regulates vital functions such as breathing, to initiate a respiratory cycle. The medulla sends nerve signals to the smooth muscles in the chest (intercostal, or rib, and the diaphragm), causing them to contract. This expands the chest cavity, lowering air pressure within the lungs. When the pressure within the lungs becomes less than the atmospheric pressure outside the lungs, air flows down the trachea and into the lungs. Oxygen molecules cross from the air into the bloodstream. As the chest wall muscles relax, the chest cavity contracts to reverse the pressure. Carbon dioxide molecules leave the blood and enter the air, which is then exhaled. An adult at rest typically completes 12 to 20 respiratory cycles per minute, a pace that is roughly a one-to-four ratio with the CARDIAC CYCLE (one respiratory cycle for every four cardiac cycles).

See also CARDIOVASCULAR SYSTEM; HEART; PULMONARY SYSTEM.

restenosis Repeated narrowing of an artery after ANGIOPLASTY or CORONARY ARTERY BYPASS GRAFT (CABG) to open an OCCLUSION. About a third of people who undergo balloon angioplasty, in which a tiny balloon is inserted into the blocked artery and inflated to compress against the artery's wall, the ATHEROMA (hardened accumulation of arterial plaque) causing occlusion experience restenosis within six months of the procedure. People with DIABETES have a higher risk for restenosis, though restenosis can occur in anyone. At present there are few other ways to determine who will have restenosis.

See also ATHEROMA; ATHEROSCLEROSIS; CAROTID ENDARTERECTOMY; CAROTID STENOSIS; CORONARY ARTERY DISEASE; STENT.

resting heart rate See HEART RATE.

rhabdomyolysis A very rare though potentially life-threatening disorder in which the body metabolizes (breaks down) muscle tissue at a rate that puts excess protein (myoglobin) and cellular toxins into the bloodstream, which strains and can shut down the kidneys. Rhabdomyolysis can occur with traumatic crush injuries and burns, in chronic alcoholism, and with prolonged inactivity resulting in muscle atrophy (wasting). It also is an uncommon side effect of certain medications, notably HMG CoA REDUCTASE INHIBITOR MEDICATIONS (statins) taken to lower BLOOD lipid (CHOLESTEROL and TRIGLYCERIDES) levels. There is increased and significant risk of rhabdomyolysis when taking an HMG CoA reductase inhibitor in combination with another family of LIPID-LOWERING MEDICATIONS, fibric acid derivatives (fibrates).

Symptoms of rhabdomyolysis may not appear until the condition begins to cause kidney damage. Early symptoms include muscle weakness and pain, darkened (tea-colored) urine, and indications of ELECTROLYTE imbalance such as confusion and disorientation. The damage to the kidneys interferes with their ability to maintain the body's electrolyte balance; hypokalemia (insufficient POTASSIUM) and hypocalcemia (insufficient CALCIUM) often develop early in the course of disease. Diagnosis is by blood tests that measure the presence of myoglobin; treatment includes intravenous fluids to help relieve the strain on the kidneys and other supportive measures as necessary including kidney dialysis for renal failure.

See also MEDICATION SIDE EFFECTS; MEDICATIONS TO TREAT HEART DISEASE.

Rhesus (Rh) factor See BLOOD.

rheumatic heart disease Damage to the HEART, particularly the valves, that occurs as a complication of rheumatic fever. Rheumatic fever is a systemic infection caused by streptococcus A bacteria that typically develops following untreated strep throat infection. Though more common in those under age 15, rheumatic fever can infect anyone at any age. In rheumatic fever the infection commonly attacks connective tissue throughout the body and can leave residual damage in any organ or structure. In rheumatic HEART DISEASE the infection attacks the heart valves, leaving them scarred and distorted. This damage is permanent, though it may not be noticeable for months to years after the infection. Damaged heart valves do not open and close properly, affecting the ability of the heart to pump blood.

Symptoms and Diagnostic Path

Symptoms of rheumatic heart disease are those of inadequate OXYGENATION and may include shortness of breath (DYSPNEA), PALPITATIONS, fainting episodes (SYNCOPE), and persistent tiredness or FATIGUE.

Treatment Options and Outlook

Often surgery is necessary to replace the damaged valves. Left untreated, the valve damage can cause more extensive damage to the heart, resulting in CARDIOMYOPATHY and HEART FAILURE.

Risk Factors and Preventive Measures

Rheumatic heart disease was once a leading cause of disabling heart disease and of death due to heart disease; current antibiotic treatment for strep throat has greatly reduced its occurrence. Fifteen thousand Americans died from rheumatic heart disease in 1950 compared to 3,500 in 2000. Rheumatic heart disease continues to account for the majority of operations to repair or replace heart valves.

See also ANTIBIOTIC PROPHYLAXIS; VALVE DISEASE; VALVE REPAIR AND REPLACEMENT.

right ventricular assist device (RVAD)   An implantable pump that mechanically supplements the heart's right ventricle in severe right HEART FAILURE. An RVAD may be a bridge device to improve cardiovascular function while awaiting HEART TRANSPLANT, a short-term support to allow the right ventricle to recover and heal itself sufficiently to resume function, or a permanent treatment for end-stage heart failure when heart transplant is not a viable option. Doctors may use a temporary RVAD to help wean a person from cardiopulmonary support following OPEN-HEART SURGERY. There are various models of RVADs, all of which are self-contained and run on long-life batteries. There is an increased risk for blood clots and infection following implantation of an RVAD; doctors commonly prescribe ANTIBI-

OTIC PROPHYLAXIS and ANTICOAGULANT MEDICATIONS. Though the severity of HEART DISEASE typically is disabling, most people who receive an RVAD are able to enjoy a reasonable QUALITY OF LIFE and take fewer medications than before the implant.

See also HEART, ARTIFICIAL; LEFT VENTRICULAR ASSIST DEVICE (LVAD); MECHANICAL CIRCULATORY SUPPORT.

Romano-Ward syndrome   An inherited ARRHYTHMIA that is a form of LONG QT SYNDROME (LQTS), also called LQTS-1 and autosomal dominant LQTS. It differs from LQTS primarily in its inheritance pattern, which is autosomal dominant (only one parent having the mutated gene can pass the disorder to a child).

Symptoms and Diagnostic Path

A person with Romano-Ward syndrome may have no symptoms, although the arrhythmia still exists. Some people experience episodes of SYNCOPE (fainting), while for others the first indication of a problem is CARDIAC ARREST or SUDDEN CARDIAC ARREST. Diagnosis is by ELECTROCARDIOGRAM (ECG), which shows a prolonged QTc interval; genetic testing may also be done to identify the specific mutations. Most people are diagnosed before young adulthood, often because a parent has the disorder.

Treatment Options and Outlook

As with other forms of LQTS, treatment is with ANTIARRYTHMIA MEDICATIONS or IMPLANTABLE CARDIOVERTER DEFIBRILLATOR (ICD). BETA ANTAGONIST MEDICATIONS (beta blockers) are often successful in preventing symptoms in younger people. The risk for cardiac arrest and sudden cardiac arrest remains high even with such treatments, however. People who have any form of LQTS including Romano-Ward syndrome should avoid strenuous EXERCISE (including competitive sports), sudden intense EMOTION, and medications and other substances known to prolong the QTc interval. The Web site www.azcert.org (also accessible through www.qtdrugs.org) maintains a current list of drugs that prolong the QTc interval.

Risk Factors and Preventive Measures

Romano-Ward syndrome is inherited; doctors recommend genetic consultation for people who know it is in their families. A child has a 50 percent likelihood of inheriting the mutated genes from a parent who has the disorder.

See also LIVING WITH HEART DISEASE; MEDICATIONS TO TREAT HEART DISEASE; SHORT QT SYNDROME.

Ross procedure An operation to correct AORTIC STENOSIS (narrowing of the aortic valve between the left ventricle and the aorta) that occurs as a congenital malformation of the aortic valve or develops later in life as a consequence of disease such as RHEUMATIC HEART DISEASE or infection.

Procedure

Named after the English surgeon who developed the procedure, Donald Ross, the Ross procedure is an OPEN-HEART SURGERY. It replaces the damaged aortic valve with the person's own pulmonary valve and replaces the harvested pulmonary valve with an ALLOGRAFT valve (donor valve). Ross discovered that a transplanted pulmonary valve has fewer risks for rejection and complications and also will grow when the procedure is performed on a child. As well, the pulmonary valve is similar in construction to the aortic valve. The Ross procedure is about 90 percent effective in establishing a permanent resolution of the aortic stenosis.

Risks and Complications

Key risks associated with the Ross procedure are excessive bleeding during surgery, difficulty weaning from CARDIOPULMONARY BYPASS, postoperative infection, thromboembolism (blood clot), and failure of the grafts. The Ross procedure has fewer complications than synthetic grafts. As with other forms of valve disease, there is increased risk for infection (notably ENDOCARDITIS) and thromboembolism. Because the new valves are the person's own tissue, there is no risk of rejection and no need for anticoagulation therapy.

Outlook and Lifestyle Modifications

The Ross procedure has good long-term success, with about half of people who undergo it living 15 years or longer without graft failure. When the operation takes place in childhood, the valves tend to grow as the child grows. Graft failure requires another surgery to replace the failing valves. Antibiotic prophylaxis before any invasive procedure (including dental) is necessary to prevent endocarditis.

See also ANTIBIOTIC PROPHYLAXIS; CARDIOVASCULAR SYSTEM; HEART; VALVE DISEASE; VALVE REPAIR AND REPLACEMENT.

R-wave See ELECTROCARDIOGRAM (ECG).

S

S-A node See SINOATRIAL (SA) NODE.

salt See SODIUM.

saunas and high blood pressure See HYPERTENSION.

second-degree heart block See HEART BLOCK.

Sectral See ACEBUTOLOL.

septal defect A congenital malformation of the HEART in which there is an abnormal opening in the septum, or wall, between the heart's chambers. A septal defect allows oxygenated and unoxygenated BLOOD to mix in the heart, reducing the level of oxygen in the blood pumped out to the body. There are three general kinds of septal defects:

- Atrial septal defect (ASD) is an abnormal opening between the two upper chambers, the atria.
- Ventricular septal defect (VSD) is an abnormal opening between the two lower chambers, the ventricles.
- Atrioventricular canal defect (AVCD), also called atrioventricular septal defect (AVSD), occurs when the opening is between an atrium and a ventricle or when there are multiple openings in the septum.

Symptoms and Diagnostic Path

Many septal defects are detected at birth or within the first two weeks of life because they can be heard during AUSCULTATION (listening to the heart with a STETHOSCOPE). Minor septal defects may escape detection until a later routine examination and the doctor hears the abnormal movement of blood, sometimes in adolescence or even adulthood. VSDs and AVCDs are almost always detected in childhood. Diagnostic procedures to confirm the diagnosis may include chest X-ray, ELECTROCARDIO-GRAM (ECG), and ECHOCARDIOGRAM.

Treatment Options and Outlook

Surgery to close the opening is the preferred treatment for most septal defects. Doctors might leave very small defects unrepaired, as these are likely to close on their own over time. Large septal defects left untreated can have serious cardiovascular consequences, leading to CARDIOMYOPATHY, HEART FAIL-URE, and PULMONARY HYPERTENSION. Some people may need to take DIURETIC MEDICATIONS or other medications to support the heart's pumping efficiency, though most make full and complete recoveries from surgery and need no further treatment. Sometimes an ASD is not detected until adulthood, in which case there already may be some damage to the heart or pulmonary hypertension. Cardiologists often opt to repair the ASD to prevent further deterioration of cardiovascular status, and then use medications to treat any heart disease that has developed.

Risk Factors and Preventive Measures

Some septal defects occur in association with other heart malformations, such as TETRALOGY OF FAL-LOT and EISENMENGER SYNDROME, that are far more significant and require immediate treatment. There are no known measures to prevent septal defects.

See also CARDIOVASCULAR SYSTEM; HEART DISEASE; HEART DISEASE IN CHILDREN; MEDICATIONS TO TREAT

HEART DISEASE; SURGERY TO TREAT CARDIOVASCULAR DISEASE.

septum See HEART.

sexual activity and heart disease Many people who have HEART DISEASE worry that sexual activity will worsen their conditions or cause another HEART ATTACK or STROKE. Most, however, are able to continue sexual activity with no increased risk to health, though they may need to make some adjustments to accommodate changes to physical capabilities. In general, the physical exertion and cardiovascular response of sexual intercourse are comparable to walking up two flights of stairs at a moderately brisk pace. Most people with heart disease who can do this without becoming short of breath or experiencing ANGINA (CHEST PAIN) can engage in sexual activity without worry or harm to their HEART health. Even those who cannot often are able to find ways to express sexual intimacy that are safe for cardiovascular well-being. Though some people are uncomfortable discussing sexual activity with their cardiologists, these are common concerns and cardiologists are accustomed to addressing them. As each individual's health situation is unique, it is best to talk through any concerns with the doctor.

Just as heart disease requires adjustment and adaptation in other aspects of life, sometimes it is necessary to make accommodations for sexual activity such as:

- choosing positions that are less physically demanding, and using pillows or cushions for added support
- planning sex for times when both partners are rested and relaxed
- waiting for three hours after eating before having sex (digestion diverts BLOOD to the gastrointestinal system)

The partner of the person who has heart disease also often feels anxiety and fear about resuming sexual activity, especially after heart attack or stroke. When couples can discuss these worries, they can work together to find solutions that both partners find acceptable. Sometimes just being able to talk about one's concerns in this regard greatly eases them, and anxiety about sex subsides.

Some MEDICATIONS TO TREAT HEART DISEASE, notably BETA ANTAGONIST MEDICATIONS, can cause ERECTILE DYSFUNCTION (difficulty obtaining or maintaining an erection sufficient for sexual intercourse) in men and diminished libido (sex drive) in men and women alike. Sometimes it is possible to switch to a different medication that causes fewer such side effects. When this is not the case, other approaches to managing erectile dysfunction might be appropriate. As yet there are few medical approaches to improve physical sexual response for women; a gynecologist often can offer suggestions as well as determine whether there are factors other than heart disease that could be the problem.

Doctors typically recommend waiting for about four weeks after heart attack or heart surgery to resume sexual activity, primarily to give the body a chance to heal. This is a common recommendation following most significant medical interventions and operations regardless of the body system involved that often has little to do with cardiovascular health. Recent research shows that the risk of having a heart attack doubles during sex for everyone, regardless of cardiovascular status—to about one in a million, a miniscule risk. Health experts agree that the benefits of a loving, intimate sexual relationship are much greater than the potential risks of sexual activity.

See also LIVING WITH HEART DISEASE; SEXUAL DYSFUNCTION.

sexual dysfunction A collective term for difficulties engaging in or enjoying sexual activity. Sexual dysfunction can affect both men and women. Diminished libido (sex drive) can result in lowered interest in sex. HEART DISEASE that impairs the circulation of BLOOD, such as PERIPHERAL VASCULAR DISEASE (PVD), can cause damage to nerves and blood vessels, reducing the body's physical ability to respond sexually. HYPERTENSION (high BLOOD PRESSURE) also can damage peripheral nerves and arteries. Diabetes, a common cause of hypertension, damages nerves and blood vessels as well. It is common to feel fearful and worried about the effects the physical excitation of sex might have on the heart and CARDIOVASCULAR SYSTEM. Such anxiety makes it difficult to relax and remain centered in the pleasure of sexual activity.

MEDICATIONS TO TREAT HEART DISEASE sometimes are to blame for changes that affect the body's sexual response. Those that relax smooth muscle tissue, such as ALPHA ANTAGONIST MEDICATIONS and BETA ANTAGONIST MEDICATIONS, to treat HYPERTENSION and ANGINA also can relax smooth muscle tissue in the genitals, causing ERECTILE DYSFUNCTION in men and reduced sexual response in women.

Though HEART DISEASE and some medications taken to treat heart disease can result in sexual dysfunction, it is important to have a doctor's examination to rule out other causes for which there are remedies. Talking about worries and concerns often helps to alleviate anxiety and also helps partners to express their desire for intimacy. As well, there are a number of treatment approaches to help with erectile dysfunction. It is important to talk with the cardiologist before taking any medications, such as sildenafil or alprostadil, as there may be interactions with medications being taken for heart disease.

See also DIABETES AND HEART DISEASE; LIVING WITH HEART DISEASE; PDE5 INHIBITOR MEDICATIONS; SEXUAL ACTIVITY AND HEART DISEASE.

shock, cardiovascular   See CARDIOGENIC SHOCK.

shortness of breath   See DYSPNEA.

sibutramine   An appetite suppressant medication taken to facilitate weight loss in OBESITY. The brand-name product available in the United States is Meridia. Sibutramine works by extending the availability of NEUROTRANSMITTERS in the brain that facilitate nerve signals for satisfaction and pleasure, which has the effect of diminishing one's interest in eating. This medication is most effective when used as part of a weight loss approach that includes controlled diet and daily physical EXERCISE. Side effects

that can occur with sibutramine include headache, CONSTIPATION, DEPRESSION, and mood swings. Sibutramine also can increase BLOOD PRESSURE and HEART RATE, particularly in combination with other medications that can have similar effects such as over-the-counter decongestants, and cause PALPITATIONS. In people who already have HYPERTENSION (high BLOOD PRESSURE) or other forms of HEART DISEASE, these cardiovascular side effects can cause cardiovascular symptoms to worsen. It is important to thoroughly understand the potential benefits and risks of taking sibutramine with regard to individual cardiovascular status.

See also COLD/FLU MEDICATION AND HYPERTENSION; LIFESTYLE AND HEART HEALTH; NUTRITION AND DIET; WEIGHT MANAGEMENT.

sickle-cell anemia   See ANEMIA.

sick sinus syndrome   See TACHYCARDIA-BRADYCARDIA SYNDROME.

signal-averaged electrocardiogram (SAECG)   A specialized ELECTROCARDIOGRAM (ECG) that uses computer technology to enhance and analyze electrical signals the HEART produces that an ordinary ECG does not capture, and to clean up distortion that comes from extraneous electrical signals (such as from muscle contractions during breathing and movement). Doctors most often use SAECG to assess the potential for dangerous ARRHYTHMIAS following damage to the heart (such as after HEART ATTACK) by searching for areas of delayed conduction (called late potentials) that scar tissue can cause. SAECG also is helpful in diagnosing arrhythmic right ventricular dysplasia. There is no special preparation for an SAECG; an ordinary 12-lead ECG collects the electrical signals.

See also CARDIOVASCULAR SYSTEM; SUDDEN CARDIAC ARREST (SCA).

silent ischemia   See ISCHEMIA.

simvastatin   A LIPID-LOWERING MEDICATION taken to treat HYPERCHOLESTEROLEMIA, HYPERLIPIDEMIA, and HYPERTRIGLYCERIDEMIA. Simvastatin belongs to the family of HMG CoA REDUCTASE INHIBITOR MEDICATIONS commonly referred to as statins. Available in the United States as the brand-name product Zocor, simvastatin works by blocking the action of 3-hydroxy-3-methyl-glutaryl coenzyme-A reductase (HMG CoA), an ENZYME the liver needs to synthesize cholesterol. This has the twofold effect of decreasing the amount of cholesterol the liver produces and forcing the body to draw from lipids already in the bloodstream to meet its needs for cholesterol and other fatty acids. HMG CoA reductase inhibitors also have an inflammation-suppressing effect on the walls of the arteries, helping to reduce the irritation that attracts platelets and other cells to collect at the site.

As with other statins, gastrointestinal distress (dyspepsia, nausea, diarrhea, CONSTIPATION) is common when beginning treatment with simvastatin though usually resolves within a few weeks of taking the medication. Simvastatin interacts with numerous other medications including some that are commonly prescribed to treat heart disease and should not be taken in combination with lipid-lowering medications called fibrates (GEMFIBROZIL, clofibrate, FENOFIBRATE). The latter can result in a rare but potentially fatal complication called RHABDOMYOLYSIS in which the body metabolizes muscle tissue, which sends toxic levels of protein and other cellular substances into the bloodstream; this can cause kidney damage and failure. Simvastatin also reduces the effectiveness of ORAL CONTRACEPTIVES (birth control pills) and some antibiotics.

See also ATHEROSCLEROSIS; CHOLESTEROL, BLOOD; INFLAMMATION AND HEART DISEASE; MEDICATIONS TO TREAT HEART DISEASE.

single photon emission computed tomography (SPECT) scan

A sophisticated imaging procedure that uses radionuclides to create computer-generated, three-dimensional images of organs and body structures. SPECT can help cardiologists to "see" the functioning of the myocardium (HEART muscle) and coronary arteries in a noninvasive way. The procedure is similar to a COMPUTED TOMOGRAPHY (CT) SCAN, with the injection of radioactive isotopes to provide enhanced images. There is minimal danger from the radioactive isotopes; they disintegrate rapidly after being injected into the body. Sensors within the scanner detect this disintegration and use it to generate images. Metabolic functions draw the isotopes into cells; uptake is dense in healthy tissue and meager in damaged tissue such as might occur following HEART ATTACK. SPECT is most useful when combined with results from ELECTROCARDIOGRAM (ECG), ECHOCARDIOGRAM, and other imaging studies. SPECT is usually combined with an exercise stress test or pharmacological stress testing (such as DOBUTAMINE or DIPYRIDAMOLE). Some people feel claustrophobic while in the tunnel-like CT scanner.

See also ADENOSINE STRESS TEST; DIPYRIDAMOLE STRESS TEST; DOBUTAMINE STRESS TEST; ELECTRON BEAM COMPUTED TOMOGRAPHY (EBCT) SCAN; MAGNETIC RESONANCE IMAGING (MRI); RADIONUCLIDE SCAN.

single ventricle

See HYPOPLASTIC LEFT HEART SYNDROME (HLHS).

sinoatrial (SA) node

A cluster of nerve and myocardial muscle cells located at the junction between the superior vena cava and the right atrium that functions as the heart's natural PACEMAKER. In a healthy HEART the myocardial muscle cells of the SA node spontaneously contract 60 to 100 times a minute. Their contractions stimulate the SA node's nerve cells to generate an electrical impulse that dissipates through the right atrium, initiating a wave of contraction that surges through the right atrium to start a CARDIAC CYCLE. Doctors call this pattern, in which the SA node initiates the heart's pacing signals, normal sinus rhythm. In SICK SINUS SYNDROME and certain ARRHYTHMIAS, the SA node is dysfunctional and the heart's electrical signals originate elsewhere such as the atrioventricular (AV) node or the purkinje network, or, rarely, within a cluster of cells in the myocardium that becomes electrically hyperactive. The SA node can malfunction for numerous reasons, key among them being congenital defects in the node's structure and damage to the atrial wall as a consequence of HEART ATTACK. Some people have SA node dysfunctions without symptoms; doctors usually do not treat these dysfunctions. SA node problems that cause symptoms generally require implantation of an electronic pacemaker to take over the role of the SA node in originating the heart's pacing signals.

See also ACCESSORY PATHWAY; CARDIOVASCULAR SYSTEM; CONDUCTION SYSTEM.

sinus arrest See TACHYCARDIA-BRADYCARDIA SYNDROME.

sinus arrhythmia See TACHYCARDIA-BRADYCARDIA SYNDROME.

sinus bradycardia See TACHYCARDIA-BRADYCARDIA SYNDROME.

sinus rhythm See SINOATRIAL (SA) NODE.

sinus tachycardia See TACHYCARDIA-BRADYCARDIA SYNDROME.

sirolimus An IMMUNOSUPRESSIVE MEDICATION taken after organ transplant to prevent rejection. It works by inhibiting the body's production and activation of T-lymphocytes, the immune system's "attack" cells and by blocking the development of antibodies (substances that identify tissues as invaders the immune system must attack). The commmon brand-name product available in the United States is Rapamune. Sirolimus has numerous potential side effects, one of the most important being susceptibility to infection as a consequence of suppressed immune system activity. Other common side effects include gastrointestinal distress (nausea, vomiting, flatulence, diarrhea), mood swings, tachycardia (rapid HEARTBEAT), and disorders of the bone marrow and BLOOD such as ANEMIA and THROMBOCYTOPENIA. Sirolimus also interacts with numerous other medications and causes a wide range of abnormal laboratory test results.

See also HEART TRANSPLANT; HEART-LUNG TRANSPLANT.

sleep disturbances Difficulty sleeping as a consequence of HEART DISEASE or of MEDICATIONS TO TREAT HEART DISEASE is common. Some studies suggest that as well, sleep disturbances such as sleep apnea may be early clues that heart disease is developing. Many medications disturb the body's natural rhythms, causing sleepiness during the day and insomnia during the night. When the source of sleep disturbance is a medication, changing to a different drug usually resolves the problem. Sometimes a particular medication provides the optimal therapeutic effect, however, or it takes a certain combination of medications to fully achieve control of symptoms. Even medications that cause drowsiness can interfere with sleep and the body's circadian rhythm (cycle of sleep and wakefulness).

Lying down can present significant stress for a heart that already is struggling to meet the body's oxygenation needs; sleep problems are common in congestive HEART FAILURE and some forms of CARDIOMYOPATHY as the heart cannot accommodate the additional pressure of the change in position. As well, lying down can affect valve function when the heart's valves are damaged or when there is a FIBROELASTOMA (a loosely attached tumor on or near a heart valve that shifts position to block a valve's movement.

Insomnia

The inability to fall or stay asleep at night is one of the most common sleep disturbances among adults. The likelihood of insomnia increases with age; some studies suggest that more people than not suffer from insomnia after age 65. Though everyone has sleepless nights, insomnia is a chronic problem that can have serious consequences for health as well as quality of life. Sleep apnea and medication side effects are common causes of insomnia, though often there is no clearly identifiable explanation. Sometimes a sleep analysis conducted through a sleep center can pinpoint contributing circumstances.

Health experts disagree about the value of sleep medications to treat insomnia, as such medications have numerous side effects and interactions with other medications. As well, because such drugs alter brain chemistry they can inadvertently worsen rather than improve insomnia. Though some people find a glass of wine relaxing, alcohol generally is not a good choice as a sleep aid as its initial effect is stimulatory. Because alcohol also is a central nervous system depressant it can exacerbate other sleep problems such as sleep apnea.

Daytime Sleepiness

Daytime sleepiness is almost always the consequence of inadequate nighttime sleep or the side effect of medications. It can range from drowsiness and the desire to take naps to lack of energy and a hazardous inability to remain awake. When medications are to blame, shifting their dosage schedules or if possible changing to other medications often eliminates the problem. Efforts to improve sleep quality during the night also are helpful.

Restless Leg Syndrome

Restless leg syndrome is characterized by the sensation of "crawling" skin and muscle twitches, sometimes violent, in the legs. Often the person who has restless leg syndrome is unaware of the extent to which he or she thrashes about at night though wakes in the morning feeling tired and unrested. PERIPHERAL VASCULAR DISEASE (PVD), in which circulation particularly in the legs and feet is impaired, and DIABETES are associated with restless leg syndrome. Doctors believe the resulting damage to the fine nerves and BLOOD vessels interrupts or otherwise distorts electrical signals from the brain to the muscle cells. Medications to improve blood flow to the legs and to inhibit muscle contractions are among the common treatment approaches.

Sleep Apnea

Sleep apnea is a condition in which a person experiences repeated lapses in breathing. This deprives the body of oxygen, causing restlessness and sometimes wakefulness. The person who has sleep apnea breathes fitfully, sounding as though he or she stops breathing and then gasps for air. The gasping awakens the person at least partway, though often without conscious recollection of it in the morning. People who have sleep apnea often snore loudly, with silence marking the periods of apnea. In addition to interrupting the flow of oxygen to organs and structures throughout the body sleep apnea disrupts the sleep cycle, preventing the person from entering the dream stages of rapid eye movement (REM) sleep. REM sleep is the most restful phase of the sleep cycle.

Most sleep apnea is primarily mechanical, occurring when there is an impediment to the flow of air into the trachea. These forms of sleep apnea often are associated with OBESITY, in which extra layers of tissue compress the throat when lying down. Some sleep apnea is neurological in nature, reflecting a problem with the nerve signals from the brain that initiate a RESPIRATORY CYCLE.

There are various treatments for sleep apnea, though unfortunately there is no single treatment certain to work, and some work only for a while. Many people have loose tissue in the backs of their throats that falls across the top of the trachea when lying down. Such people often receive at least temporary relief from laser surgery that burns away a small amount of excess tissue at the back of the throat. Other people benefit from using a continuous positive airway pressure (CPAP) machine at night, which pressurizes the airways to keep them open. CPAP often is useful for those whose sleep apnea is neurological, as it can be programmed to regularly deliver inhalations. Weight loss and exercises to strengthen the muscles of the throat area are also helpful for most people who have sleep apnea regardless of its cause.

There is a correlation between sleep apnea and cardiovascular problems such as CORONARY ARTERY DISEASE (CAD), HEART FAILURE, STROKE, and HEART ATTACK. Researchers are uncertain whether the sleep apnea is a symptom of heart disease or contributes to its development; a combination of both is likely.

Improving Sleep Quality

Methods to improve sleep quality depend to an extent on the nature of sleep disturbance. Nearly always, relaxation methods and changes in lifestyle offer some improvement. These include:

- regular physical EXERCISE, ideally in the middle to late afternoon
- eating a light rather than a heavy evening meal
- avoiding stimulants such as CAFFEINE, NICOTINE, and alcohol within six hours of bedtime

- taking a warm, relaxing bath or shower 30 minutes before going to bed
- getting up and out of bed if not asleep in 30 minutes
- reserving the bedroom environment for sleep and sex only
- darkening the bedroom and listening to relaxing music or "white noise" devices when falling asleep

See also LIFESTYLE AND HEART HEALTH; PULMONARY SYSTEM.

smokeless tobacco   See TOBACCO USE.

smoking and heart disease   Cigarette smoking is the leading cause of HEART DISEASE in the United States and accounts for one-third of the deaths due to heart disease. Its effects on the cardiovascular system are numerous and toxic; cigarette smoke contains more than 4,000 identified chemicals that are detrimental to health. Among them are:

- CARBON MONOXIDE, which bumps oxygen to bind with HEMOGLOBIN in the blood. This reduces by as much as half the amount of oxygen the BLOOD can carry to organs and tissues, including the HEART, throughout the body. The decreased supply of oxygen to the heart can cause ISCHEMIC HEART DISEASE (IHD) and corresponding ANGINA.
- Tar, a resinous residue that coats the insides of the alveoli (tiny sacs in the lungs where oxygen exchange takes place). This blocks the exchange of oxygen for carbon dioxide across their membranes and eventually causes their collapse.
- More than 40 identified carcinogens (chemicals known to cause cancer) including those that cause small cell lung carcinoma, a deadly form of cancer that develops almost exclusively in people who smoke, used to smoke, or are extensively exposed to secondhand smoke (such as by living in a household where others smoke). The carcinogens in cigarette smoke also cause liver, pancreatic, stomach, and colorectal cancers and are contributing factors in breast cancer.

- NICOTINE, an addictive and toxic stimulant that constricts blood vessels and damages the cells of the arterial walls. Nicotine's VASOCONSTRICTION effect causes blood pressure to rise; its effect as a central nervous system stimulant increases the rate and force of the heart's contractions. Nicotine irritates the walls of the arteries causing inflammation that activates the body's inflammatory response, the first stage in the development of arterial plaque. These actions begin with the first puff of cigarette smoke that enters the lungs and linger for 20 to 40 minutes after the last.

Cigarette smoking doubles a person's risk for HEART ATTACK or STROKE, compounding the effects of other risk factors. The longer a person smokes and the heavier the habit (packs per day), the more extensive the risk for developing HYPERTENSION (high BLOOD PRESSURE), ATHEROSCLEROSIS (occlusive accumulations of arterial plaque along the inner walls of the arteries), and CORONARY ARTERY DISEASE (CAD). Though cigarette smoking's contribution as a risk factor for heart disease diminishes with SMOKING CESSATION, damage already caused is permanent and requires appropriate medical treatment.

Secondhand Smoking

Secondhand smoking, also called passive smoking or environmental smoking, is the circumstance of those who do not smoke breathing the cigarette smoke from those who do smoke. It was identified as a major health concern in the 1980s and still today accounts for a significant percentage of chronic respiratory infections, asthma, and ear infections in children who live with adults who smoke. In adults secondhand smoke can cause the same diseases as it causes in those who smoke, including heart disease and cancer. Public health experts estimate that secondhand smoking accounts for 46,000 heart disease deaths in nonsmokers each year in the United States. Smoking is prohibited in nearly all public buildings and workplaces in the United States as an effort to protect nonsmokers from the health hazards of secondhand smoke.

Smoking Cessation

No matter how long a person has smoked, studies continue to reinforce that there are health benefits from quitting. The immediate cardiovascular effects are improved oxygen supply to the heart and reduced irritation to the arteries. Long-term, the risk for developing heart disease returns to about the same level as that for a nonsmoker in 10 years. The addictive nature of nicotine makes it difficult to simply quit smoking. Many smokers are more successful in their efforts to quit when they follow structured programs to gradually reduce their bodies' needs for nicotine. Nicotine supplements (nicotine patches and gums) can help to ease the physical dependence and minimize withdrawal symptoms. Hypnosis and behavior modification therapy can help address the behavior patterns associated with smoking.

See also CARDIOVASCULAR SYSTEM; LIFESTYLE AND HEART HEALTH; PULMONARY SYSTEM.

snuff See TOBACCO USE.

sodium An ELECTROLYTE essential for many functions within the body including the contractions of the HEART. Sodium is an ion, a chemical capable of carrying an electrical charge, and is essential for the initiation of myocardial (heart muscle) cell contraction in the CARDIAC CYCLE. At the start of the cardiac cycle sodium fills the myocardial cells, facilitating their receipt of nerve signals instructing them to contract. When the sodium level reaches a certain point, the cells exchange sodium for CALCIUM ions; when the calcium level reaches a certain point the cell contracts. At the end of the contraction sodium again returns to the cells and the cycle begins anew.

Sodium also is integral to the body's fluid balance, which is an important element of BLOOD PRESSURE regulation. Sensors in the glomeruli of the kidneys detect the level of sodium and water in the BLOOD and adjust the amount of sodium the kidneys retain in the bloodstream. The retained sodium draws additional water into the bloodstream as well, increasing blood volume and hence blood pressure. When the kidneys excrete more sodium, this draws water from the bloodstream into the urine, reducing blood volume and hence blood pressure.

Sodium is the primary ingredient in table salt (known chemically as sodium chloride). Doctors often recommend that people who have hypertension (high blood pressure) reduce their salt intake to lower the amount of sodium that enters the body. This helps to prevent additional water from being drawn into the bloodstream. DIURETIC MEDICATIONS often taken to treat hypertension work by causing the kidneys to withhold less sodium.

See also POTASSIUM; RENIN-ANGIOTENSIN-ALDOSTERONE (RAA) HORMONAL SYSTEM.

sodium channel blocking medications Medications taken to treat ARRHYTHMIAS (irregularities of the HEARTBEAT), notably ATRIAL FIBRILLATION. Some class I ANTIARRHYTHMIA MEDICATIONS are used to treat severe ventricular arrhythmias (such as ventricular tachycardia) but themselves can have potential dangerous side effects. Sodium channel blockers commonly prescribed in the United States include:

- MEXILETINE (Mexitil)
- lidocaine
- PROCAINAMIDE (Pronestyl)
- PROPAFENONE (Rythmol)
- QUINIDINE (Cardioquin, Quinidex)

These medications have narrow therapeutic indexes, which means that the margin between the therapeutic, or helpful, amount of the drug and the lethal amount of the drug is very small. The most significant as well as the most frequent side effects of sodium channel blockers are the worsening of the existing arrhythmia or the development of new and serious arrhythmias. People taking sodium channel blockers require regular monitoring to detect such side effects before they cause CARDIAC ARREST or SUDDEN CARDIAC ARREST.

See also MEDICATIONS TO TREAT HEART DISEASE; MEDICATION SIDE EFFECTS; NARROW THERAPEUTIC INDEX (NTI).

sonogram See ULTRASOUND.

sphygmomanometer   The technical name for the device used to measure BLOOD PRESSURE. It consists of a gauge that reports the pressure of BLOOD in millimeters of mercury (mm Hg) and an inflatable cuff that goes around an extremity, usually the upper arm. The cuff also can be placed at other locations on the arms or legs to obtain blood pressure readings at different sites if desired, which doctors sometimes do when evaluating peripheral circulation. The cuff is inflated until it cuts off the flow of BLOOD through the artery, then slowly released while listening to the PULSE through a STETHOSCOPE. The first sound heard identifies SYSTOLE, the peak of the CARDIAC CYCLE when the left ventricle contracts to send blood into the body. The last sound heard is DIASTOLE, the trough of the cardiac cycle when the HEART is momentarily at rest. The English scientist Stephen Hales developed the first crude sphygmomanometer, consisting of a catheter inserted into the aorta and a glass-enclosed column of mercury, in 1733. Most sphygmomanometers today are electronic.

See also HALES, STEPHEN; CARDIOVASCULAR SYSTEM.

spironolactone   A POTASSIUM-sparing DIURETIC MEDICATION ("water pill") taken to treat congestive HEART FAILURE and HYPERTENSION (high BLOOD PRESSURE). Common brand-name products in the United States include Aldactone. Spironolactone has a mild diuretic effect, acting on the kidneys to block sodium reabsorption though permit potassium reabsorption. The reduction in retained SODIUM serves to draw additional fluid from the BLOOD, reducing blood volume to lower blood pressure and decrease the heart's workload. Doctors may prescribe spironolactone in combination with other diuretic medications or with ANTIHYPERTENSIVE MEDICATIONS that lower blood pressure through mechanisms other than fluid reduction. Possible side effects include gastrointestinal distress and drowsiness. Spironolactone also can result in hyperkalemia (too much potassium in the blood) and hyponatremia (not enough SODIUM in the blood), creating ELECTROLYTE imbalance that affects the heart's ability to maintain a normal rhythm.

See also ARRHYTHMIAS; MEDICATIONS TO TREAT HEART DISEASE.

staged palliation   See PALLIATION, STAGED.

statin medications   See HMG CoA REDUCTASE INHIBITOR MEDICATIONS.

stenosis   A narrowing or constricture of a BLOOD vessel that occurs as a result of a congenital malformation or an occlusion that develops. A stenosis slows the flow of blood through the artery and also can create a pattern of turbulence within the blood flow that contributes to the formation of blood clots (COAGULATION). Stenosis is the key problem arising from ATHEROSCLEROSIS and CORONARY ARTERY DISEASE (CAD). In cardiovascular disease, the surgeon can clear or replace stenosed segments of arteries through ANGIOPLASTY, ATHERECTOMY, and bypass graft surgery. For reasons cardiologists and researchers do not fully understand, an artery in which a stenosis is repaired tends to restenose in a relatively quick fashion. About half of coronary artery blockages repaired using angioplasty, for example, restenose within six months. A small springlike device, called a STENT, inserted into the area of the stenosis can help to prolong the effects of surgical correction.

Congenital stenosis most often affects the great arteries of the heart, notably the aorta. Surgical correction of such malformations is essential to regain and maintain normal heart function. These corrections typically are permanent and successful.

See also AORTIC STENOSIS; CAROTID STENOSIS; CORONARY ARTERY BYPASS GRAFT (CABG); HEART DISEASE.

stent   A tiny, springlike mesh "tunnel" inserted into an area of STENOSIS (narrowing) in an artery to maintain the blood vessel's patency (keep the channel open for blood flow). The stent is compressed when the cardiovascular surgeon inserts it and then springs open when deployed to apply pressure against the walls of the artery. Most coronary ANGIOPLASTY procedures now employ stents to delay restenosis. The stent, in its compressed form, is threaded through a blood vessel at the end of a catheter, then placed into position with guidance from FLUOROSCOPY. Once deployed, the stent holds open the area of the stenosis. Many stents now in use are drug-eluting stents; they release medications directly into the site of the stenosis to help prevent additional accumulations of arterial plaque, the most common reason for restenosis.

See also CARDIAC CATHETERIZATION; CORONARY ARTERY BYPASS GRAFT (CABG); SURGERY TO TREAT CARDIOVASCULAR DISEASE.

step diet   See NUTRITION AND DIET.

sternal pain   Pain in the breastbone, or sternum, after OPEN-HEART SURGERY. It is necessary to cut through the sternum to expose the HEART. After surgery, the sternum is stapled back together. It takes longer for this sternal wound to completely heal, up to six months, than for the rest of the healing that takes place after open-heart surgery; it takes six to eight weeks for the sternum to be strong enough to support activities such as driving. There are many nerve endings in the periosteum (the thin layer of protective tissue that covers bone), which causes the pain. The sternum is an important support structure for the cage in which the organs of the pulmonary system reside and function; each breath pressures the sternum.

Sternal pain tends to have a sharp quality most evident with inhalation (taking a breath in). The natural tendency is to guard against this pain by taking shallow breaths; this does not support healing or recovery. After surgery hospital staff will provide instructions for deep breathing and incentive spirometry, methods for increasing expansion of the lungs. The sharpness of sternal pain fades within two weeks of surgery, though discomfort can remain a factor (particularly when breathing) for quite some time following. NONSTEROIDAL ANTI-INFLAMMATORY DRUGS (NSAIDs) often are effective in reducing sternal pain.

See also CORONARY ARTERY BYPASS GRAFT (CABG); SURGERY TO TREAT CARDIOVASCULAR DISEASE.

stethoscope   A device for listening to the sounds of the HEART, BLOOD vessels, and lungs that is the mainstay of preliminary diagnosis in contemporary Western medicine. The French physician René Laënnec invented the first stethoscope, a simple tube, in 1816. There have been many variations on the device's design through the decades since its invention, among the most popular being models that folded. The modern design of dual earpieces and a single flexible tube with a diaphragm at the end came into popular use in the early 20th century. When placed in firm contact with the skin, the stethoscope's diaphragm collects and amplifies sound signals that the listener can hear through the earpieces. Certain functions have characteristic sounds—for example, the "lupp-dubb" of the normally beating heart. Deviations from known sounds help doctors to more narrowly focus their diagnostic efforts. The stethoscope also is used to listen to the sounds of blood flowing through the arteries when taking BLOOD PRESSURE readings.

See also CORVISART, JEAN-NICHOLAS; LAËNNEC, RENÉ.

Stokes-Adams disease   A HEART disorder in which the heart's electrical impulses become interrupted, slowing the heart's contractions and reducing the flow of oxygenated blood to the body. This disorder is named for the two Irish physicians who first identified the complex of symptoms that characterize the disorder, William Stokes (1804–78) and Robert Adams (1791–1875). The condition is less commonly called transient ARRHYTHMIA and cardiogenic SYNCOPE.

Symptoms and Diagnostic Path
The most common symptom of Stokes-Adams disease is SYNCOPE (fainting), which results from temporary inadequate BLOOD flow to the brain. Some people experience seizures during syncopal episodes or profuse sweating right before fainting. There is no predictability to the syncopal episodes. Diagnosis can be difficult because the irregularities in the HEARTBEAT are present only immediately before and during a syncopal episode. By the time the person receives medical attention the episode is over and conventional ELECTROCARDIOGRAM (ECG)

is normal. Echocardiogram may detect congenital defects in the heart's structure that are capable of altering the heart's electrical activity. Ambulatory ECG (HOLTER MONITOR) over 24 hours is the most conclusive diagnostic procedure because it can detect abnormalities in the heart's electrical system whether or not such irregularities produce symptoms.

Treatment Options and Outlook

ANTIARRHYTHMIA MEDICATIONS may control Stokes-Adams episodes in some people, notably when the episodes are mild and fairly infrequent. However, when episodes are frequent or extended or medications are not effective, a PACEMAKER is necessary to regulate the heart's electrical impulses. With such regulation, the episodes subside. Untreated Stokes-Adams can be fatal.

Risk Factors and Preventive Measures

Stokes-Adams disease is more common in people over age 60, although it can affect younger people in whom heart problems might not be an initial concern. The disorder sometimes develops following a HEART ATTACK that results from blocked blood flow through the coronary arteries that cuts off blood supply and oxygen to a portion of the heart (MYOCARDIAL INFARCTION). Stokes-Adams disease is also associated with inflammation and infection involving the heart such as MYOCARDITIS and ENDOCARDITIS and with RHEUMATIC HEART DISEASE (RHD). Often, however, the cause remains unknown. There are no known measures to prevent Stokes-Adams disease.

streptokinase   A THROMBOLYTIC MEDICATION given to dissolve BLOOD clots that have already formed in an artery or vein. Streptokinase is an enzyme that increases the body's production of plasmin, a substance that breaks down fibrinogen, the core substance of blood clots. It acts very rapidly upon injection, producing thrombolytic effects within minutes. It is most effective when administered within four to six hours of the onset of a HEART ATTACK or STROKE. As well, the body produces antibodies that are effective for about six months following the administration of streptokinase, during which time the immune system will inactivate the drug. Streptokinase must be given at least six months from any previous dose. Streptokinase cannot be administered when hemorrhagic stroke is suspected and must be used with great caution in people taking ANTICOAGULANT MEDICATIONS.

See also COAGULATION; MEDICATIONS TO TREAT HEART DISEASE.

stress and heart disease   The correlation between HEART DISEASE and stress remains a topic of debate among health experts. A U.S. National Institutes of Health (NIH) advisory panel designated stress, as expressed through type A personality (aggressive, driving personality), as an independent risk factor for CORONARY ARTERY DISEASE (CAD) in 1981 after reviewing numerous observational studies that identified a higher rate of heart disease in people with high stress lifestyles. Since then, however, researchers have been unable to establish a conclusive, objective link between stress and heart disease or to identify and understand the mechanisms through which stress contributes to the development of heart disease. Current research suggests that stress may have a greater influence on recovery from, rather than development of, HEART ATTACK or STROKE. The NIH and other health organizations have subsequently reclassified stress as a contributing, rather than independent, risk factor for heart disease.

Most health experts believe stress plays some role in the development of disease in general. The physiological responses stress elicits cause changes in cell activity and body functions, upsetting the body's HOMEOSTASIS (ability to maintain itself in balance). Stress activates the release of cortisol and EPINEPHRINE, for example, two of the hormones that cause BLOOD PRESSURE to rise and HEART RATE to increase. The body is not intended to function over the long term at such an elevated level, though researchers do not clearly understand what happens when it does so. Elevated cortisol and epinephrine levels are associated with HYPERTENSION (high blood pressure), though whether as cause or effect is uncertain. Stress also appears to have an effect on the body's handling of FREE RADICALS, the molecular particles remaining as metabolic waste by-products that scientists suspect are responsible for health conditions that develop over time such as cancer, DIABETES, and heart disease.

Stress, emotional or physical, is a difficult factor to quantify because it is highly variable among individuals. People respond differently to similar situations and employ a spectrum of STRESS REDUCTION TECHNIQUES to help them cope with emotionally stressful circumstances. Objective measures can assess the effectiveness of such techniques with regard to lowering blood pressure, heart rate, and breathing rate, which presumably restores the body to a nonstress level of function. Multiple factors, from genetics to lifestyle, influence physical stress—wear and tear on the body over time—in ways that support health or foster disease. Doctors know that changing lifestyle factors alters their effects on the body. Smoking, for example, stresses the body in numerous ways to cause health problems; smoking cessation ends those stresses and their corresponding health problems, except when damage has already occurred (which sometimes is difficult to ascertain). Much study remains to be done to determine the full scope of stress on health and disease.

See also PERSONALITY TYPES; LIFESTYLE AND HEART HEALTH.

stress reduction techniques Methods to mitigate the health consequences of everyday stress and to aid in relaxation. There are numerous stress reduction techniques as well as many activities that result in stress reduction though that is perhaps not their intent, such as EXERCISE. As much as is possible, it helps to organize and simplify daily responsibilities and functions into predictable and manageable patterns. This is a major challenge for many adults who are balancing work and family and may require enlisting the assistance of coworkers and family members. Though sometimes it is not possible or practical to change certain stress factors, often changing the way one responds to those factors can reduce the amount of stress they generate. It is important to set aside "self" time and to consider this time as much inviolable as the time dedicated to other responsibilities. Though objective research substantiating the effects of stress on

health and disease is not conclusive, most health experts believe excessive stress is a significant contributing factor to many health conditions, including HYPERTENSION (high BLOOD PRESSURE) and other forms of HEART DISEASE.

Some methods for relaxation and stress reduction include:

- GUIDED IMAGERY, in which one might follow the directions of a tape recording to clear the mind and focus on a particular image or scene
- MEDITATION, in which one consciously considers and then releases the thoughts in the mind
- prayer, in which there is communication with the divinity of one's choosing
- TAI CHI, a structured form of Eastern martial arts that combines slow, graceful movement with meditation
- visualization, a process of seeing in one's mind a perception of healing and health
- YOGA, which combines structured physical movements that emphasize flexibility and balance with meditation.

As well, nutritious eating habits and daily physical exercise help the body to function optimally for health and are general lifestyle measures that help prevent heart disease.

See also ANTIOXIDANT; BIOFEEDBACK; FREE RADICALS; LIFESTYLE AND HEART HEALTH; NUTRITION AND DIET; OXIDATION.

stroke A "brain attack" in which a BLOOD clot blocks the flow of blood through an artery in or supplying the brain, or in which a blood vessel leaks blood into the brain. A stroke can cause temporary or permanent damage to any part of the brain, resulting in disrupted physical and cognitive functions. Strokes that affect the BRAIN STEM can be fatal, as the brain stem is largely responsible for regulating the body's basic survival functions such as HEART RATE, BLOOD PRESSURE, and breathing. Stroke remains the leading cause of disability in the United States. Independent of other forms of heart disease, stroke is the third leading cause of death accounting for about 280,000 deaths each year.

Ischemic stroke Ischemic stroke, also called cerebral infarction, results when there is an obstruction within an artery that cuts the flow of blood, and hence the oxygen supply, to a portion of the brain. When deprived of oxygen for much longer than four to six minutes, brain cells die and the brain cannot replace them. The majority of ischemic strokes result from atherosclerosis in which fragments of arterial plaque (deposits of fatty acids and other substances that accumulate along the inside walls of the arteries) break away and travel through the bloodstream until they can no longer pass through an artery and they become lodged. They block the flow of blood beyond the point of occlusion. The extent of damage depends on the location of the occlusion and the amount of brain tissue the blocked vessel ordinarily serves. When the blood supplies a large portion of the brain, the damage can be substantial or even fatal.

Hemorrhagic stroke Hemorrhagic stroke, sometimes called intracerebral hemorrhage, occurs when an arterial wall dissects (splits apart) within the brain and allows blood to leak into an area of brain tissue. Hemorrhagic stroke has the effect of flooding brain cells, literally drowning them. About 12 percent of strokes are hemorrhagic; 40 percent of hemorrhagic strokes are fatal. In addition to the other warning signs of stroke, sudden and severe headache, often accompanied by nausea and vomiting, is a common symptom of hemorrhagic stroke and indicates increasing intracranial pressure (pressure within the skull). However, generally it is not possible to tell from a person's symptoms whether a stroke is ischemic or hemorrhagic.

Hypertension and stroke HYPERTENSION (high blood pressure) is the most common cause of stroke, particularly when it coexists with atherosclerotic disease and DIABETES. As blood flows through the arteries the atherosclerotic accumulations generate turbulence that causes the blood to swirl and pool. Pooling encourages clots to develop. As well, the turbulence chips away at the atheroma, causing it to erode. The fragments float through the bloodstream until they no longer can pass through a blood vessel. Phagocytes, specialized "cleaner" blood cells, attack and consume the fragments. The larger the fragment the longer this

process takes, and the more likely there will be damage to the cells deprived of blood because of the vessel's occlusion. In the arterioles, the body's tiniest arteries, this damage generally is minimal and the surrounding cells can compensate for cells that are lost. When these arterioles are in the brain, the small occlusions can cause TRANSIENT ISCHEMIC ATTACKS (TIAs), sometimes called mini or micro strokes, that produce short-term symptoms. Small occlusions can occur without causing symptoms as well, and are called silent cerebral infarctions or silent strokes; though without symptoms, the damage to the brain can become significant over time. In larger arteries occlusions can have disastrous consequences.

Hypertension also sets the stage for hemorrhagic stroke, with the increased pressure against the walls of the arteries causing tissue deterioration and loss of elasticity. This lessens the artery's ability to withstand the continual pulsating bursts of pressure against its walls, and the layers of the artery's walls can begin to separate or can outright rupture. The larger the artery in which this occurs, the more rapid and serious the damage, though even small arteries can release significant amounts of blood before the body's clotting mechanisms activate to slow and stop the blood flow. Maintaining control of blood pressure through medications and lifestyle helps to minimize the risk of stroke, though having hypertension is a major risk factor for stroke.

Symptoms and Diagnostic Path

Warning signs announce that most strokes are taking place, though often people do not recognize or acknowledge them until the stroke is well under way. It is important to know and respond to the symptoms of stroke, which include any sudden:

- weakness or numbness, especially on just one side of the body
- loss of balance or "stagger" when walking
- difficulty speaking or understanding what others are saying
- blurred or double vision
- severe headache, especially when accompanied by nausea and vomiting

It is crucial to seek emergency medical attention at the first indication that a stroke might be occurring. Not all strokes display all the warning signs.

Treatment Options and Outlook

Early intervention and treatment are essential to minimize the damage and consequences of stroke. Detection and treatment with thrombolytic medications within several hours of the onset of an ischemic stroke can restore circulation to the brain before permanent damage occurs.

The most effective treatment for most ischemic strokes is early intervention with THROMBOLYTIC MEDICATIONS ("clot busters") that, when injected into the bloodstream, act immediately to dissolve the clot. This relieves the occlusion and restores blood flow, typically within seconds to minutes. Such medications include STREPTOKINASE and TISSUE PLASMINOGEN ACTIVATOR (TPA), which must be administered within three hours of the onset of the stroke to be effective. Beyond this window of time, the clot is firmly established and thrombolytic medications are ineffective in dissolving it.

Thrombolytic medications are not helpful in hemorrhagic stroke and in fact can worsen bleeding as they interfere with the clotting process. It is essential for doctors to determine whether a stroke is hemorrhagic or ischemic before administering thrombolytic medications. The imaging procedure COMPUTED TOMOGRAPHY (CT) SCAN is highly effective for this purpose. Treatment for hemorrhagic stroke depends on the extent of the bleeding and whether there is a dangerous increase in intracranial pressure. When the latter occurs, doctors may choose surgical intervention to attempt to drain the collecting blood to relieve pressure. Medications to reduce the brain's fluid levels also may be used for this purpose. Often, treatment is supportive while the body attempts to contain and absorb the hemorrhage.

Rehabilitation can be prolonged even when damage from the stroke seems moderate. Some areas of the brain can learn to take over functions from damaged parts of the brain, while other losses such as speech are more difficult to replace or accommodate. With diligent effort and a guided rehabilitation program, about 60 percent of people who experience strokes can return to productive lives. However, recovery can take time; 20 to 30 percent of people still require institutional care (skilled nursing facility or long-term care facility) three months after their strokes. About 30 percent have permanent disabilities as a result of their strokes.

Risk Factors and Preventive Measures

Stroke can strike anyone at any age. However, certain circumstances increase the risk for stroke. They include:

- hypertension
- cigarette smoking
- other heart disease, particularly ATHEROSCLEROSIS, CORONARY ARTERY DISEASE (CAD), PERIPHERAL VASCULAR DISEASE (PVD), and CAROTID STENOSIS (carotid artery disease)
- physical inactivity
- age
- DIABETES
- kidney disease
- family history of stroke
- previous stroke, TIAs, or HEART ATTACK
- African-American heritage
- ATRIAL FIBRILLATION

Some risk factors, such as age and race, cannot be changed. This makes it all the more important to mitigate lifestyle risk factors by maintaining a healthy weight, getting daily physical exercise, eating a nutritious diet, and keeping other health conditions (especially diabetes and hypertension) under tight control.

See also AFRICAN AMERICANS AND CARDIOVASCULAR DISEASE; AMERICANS WITH DISABILITIES ACT (ADA); DIABETES AND HEART DISEASE; LIFESTYLE AND HEART HEALTH; QUALITY OF LIFE; SMOKING AND HEART DISEASE; TRANSIENT ISCHEMIC ATTACK (TIA).

stroke volume The amount of BLOOD the HEART pumps to the body with each contraction. Stroke volume correlates to AEROBIC CAPACITY; the higher one's level of aerobic capacity the greater the stroke volume. Diminished stroke volume accompanies forms of HEART DISEASE in which the heart's pumping capacity becomes reduced, such as CARDIOMYOPATHY, VALVE DISEASE, and HEART FAILURE. Stroke volume also drops when HEART ATTACK (MYOCARDIAL INFARCTION) damages or scars myocardial tissue of the left ventricle.

Cardiologists commonly measure stroke volume in one of three ways:

- CARDIAC CATHETERIZATION is the only direct, and the most precise, means of measuring stroke volume. It is an invasive procedure that requires a catheter to be inserted through a blood vessel and placed in the right ventricle. Sensors in the catheter's tip record the temperature of the volume of blood when the ventricle is full and the temperature of the residual blood after a contraction ejects that volume. Cardiologists then use mathematical formulas to calculate stroke volume from the data required. Because there are risks inherent in cardiac catheterization, doctors use this method only when doing the procedure for other diagnostic or therapeutic purposes.

- DOPPLER ULTRASOUND, which uses high-frequency sound waves to track the flow of blood, is noninvasive though indirect. Cardiologists use mathematical formulas to calculate stroke volume from data the Doppler ultrasound provides. This method is precise enough for clinical purposes though generally not used in research applications.

- Impedance cardiography measures the varying rates at which electromagnetic impulses travel through different kinds of tissues. Electrodes placed on the outside of the chest and neck collect data about the resistance the impulses encounter. Fluids convey different resistance than solid structures, allowing cardiologists to use mathematical formulas to calculate stroke volume. This method is precise enough for clinical purposes though generally not used in research applications.

Doctors use stroke volume as one measurement that helps to assess improvements in cardiac function following CORONARY ARTERY BYPASS GRAFT (CABG) and other operations on the heart. It also is one of the variables used to calculate total CARDIAC OUTPUT.

See also CARDIAC CYCLE; ECHOCARDIOGRAM; CARDIOVASCULAR SYSTEM; LEFT VENTRICULAR EJECTION FRACTION (LVEF).

ST-segment   See ELECTROCARDIOGRAM (ECG).

subaortic stenosis   See AORTIC STENOSIS.

subendocardial ischemia   See ISCHEMIC HEART DISEASE (IHD).

subepicardial ischemia/transmural ischemia   See ISCHEMIC HEART DISEASE (IHD).

sudden cardiac arrest (SCA)   Unexpected and complete cessation of HEART function (CARDIAC ARREST) that results in death within minutes. Most people who experience SCA are found after death has already occurred, though some people receive CPR (cardiopulmonary resuscitation) or EMERGENCY CARDIOVASCULAR CARE (ECC) without success. Often the loss of heart function occurs so quickly that there is no opportunity to respond to symptoms before death is imminent.

Many people who succumb to SCA have diagnosed HEART DISEASE though are not expected to die at the time SCA strikes. Others are found to have HEART DISEASE at autopsy (examination of the body after death), and in some, there is no clear identification of damage to the heart. SCA accounts for 250,000 deaths in the United States each year, most of which are due to CORONARY ARTERY DISEASE (CAD). The remainder of SCAs are due to ARRHYTHMIAS. There really is no way to predict or prevent SCD, though people with certain disorders of rhythm such as LONG QT SYNDROME (LQTS) are at increased risk. SCA also is related to cocaine use.

Health experts believe that widespread availability of AUTOMATED EXTERNAL DEFIBRILLATORS (AEDs) may help to increase the survival rate among those who experience SCA by administering lifesaving electrical shock to reorganize the heart's electrical activity into a functional pattern. Because death so rapidly follows the onset of symptoms (which often are not perceptible until the person collapses and loses consciousness), the greatest success in revival occurs in witnessed attacks. Resuscitative efforts initiated 10 minutes or longer after the attack begins seldom succeed.

SCA is nearly always due to a malignant ventricular arrhythmia such as ventricular tachycardia or ventricular fibrillation. By some accounts, SCA is the number one cause of death in the United States. Treatment for people who do survive SCA typically includes an IMPLANTABLE CARDIOVERTER DEFRIBRILLATOR (ICD), which can detect future episodes of such arrhythmias and immediately deliver an electrical shock to restore the heart's rhythm. Some people who have HEART FAILURE have increased risk for SCA and may benefit from prophylactic ICD implantation.

See also BRUGADA SYNDROME; CHAIN OF SURVIVAL; COCAINE AND HEART ATTACK; COMMOTIO CORDIS; DEATHS FROM HEART DISEASE.

Sular   See NISOLDIPINE.

superior vena cava   See CARDIOVASCULAR SYSTEM.

supraventricular tachycardia   See ARRHYTHMIA.

surgery to treat cardiovascular disease   The medical discipline of operating on the HEART and BLOOD vessels. In casual use, the term *surgery* applies to the operations as well as the discipline. Surgeons in the United States perform 6 million cardiovascular operations each year. Operations on the heart may repair or replace diseased heart valves, replace occluded CORONARY ARTERIES, reconstruct congenital malformations of the heart, and replace the heart itself through HEART TRANSPLANT or HEART-LUNG TRANSPLANT. The rib cage and sternum encase the heart in a sturdy, protective shell that limits access to the heart. Typical surgical methods use different approaches to enter this shell; these include:

- CARDIAC CATHETERIZATION, in which the cardiologist inserts a catheter into a peripheral blood vessel near the surface of the skin and threads the catheter to the heart using moving X-ray (FLUOROSCOPY) for guidance. The CARDIOLOGIST can then pass tiny instruments through the catheter. Cardiologists may use cardiac catheterization to operate on the coronary arteries, to place an occlusive device to correct a PATENT DUCTUS ARTERIOSUS (PDA), and for minor operations on the heart valves.

- Minimally invasive surgery, in which the surgeon makes several small (one-inch or less) incisions between the ribs and inserts an endoscope and endoscopic instruments. Surgeons may use minimally invasive SURGERY for less complex operations such as a single CORONARY ARTERY BYPASS GRAFT (CABG).

- Closed-heart surgery, in which the surgeon opens the chest to expose the heart though does not stop the heart to perform the operation. Surgeons often can use closed heart operations for correcting minor congenital malformations of the heart such as COARCTATION OF THE AORTA and certain shunts.

- OPEN-HEART SURGERY, in which the surgeon opens the chest, connects the great vessels of the heart to cannulas that carry blood to a HEART-LUNG BYPASS MACHINE, and stops the heart from beating for the duration of the operation. Surgeons must use open-heart surgery for operations to replace heart valves, correct or reconstruct major congenital malformations, CABG involving two or more coronary arteries, and other complex operations that are possible only when the heart is not moving.

The surgical method the surgeon chooses to use depends on multiple variables, key among them being the nature of the operation and the health status of the person. The surgeon should discuss the benefits and risks of surgery in general as well as of the specific procedure and approach. Hospitals require this as an element of INFORMED CONSENT.

Risks of Cardiovascular Surgery

Risk is inherent in any kind of surgery. General risks include bleeding during or after the operation, infection, and failure of the operation to correct the identified problem. There also are risks involved with receiving anesthesia, which can include allergic or adverse response to the anesthetic agents. Additional risks specific to cardiovascular surgery include HEART ATTACK or STROKE from blood clots dislodged into the bloodstream, and inability to restart the heart following open-heart surgery. As well, each individual has unique risks relative to his or her personal health situation. A person who is critically ill following heart attack has a much greater risk for dying during or immediately after surgery than a person who is reasonably healthy except for the cardiovascular problem for which surgery is necessary. It is essential to fully understand the risks of cardiovascular surgery on an individual basis.

No operation can correct an adverse situation to perfection; it also is important to understand the limitations of cardiovascular surgery. CABG may need to be repeated in five to 15 years, for example, or even sooner if there is rapid RESTENOSIS. People who receive graft or prosthetic heart valves will need ANTIBIOTIC PROPHYLAXIS before dental and surgical procedures. Those who undergo heart transplant or heart-lung transplant must take IMMUNOSUPPRESSIVE MEDICATIONS for the remainder of their lives, which increases their susceptibility to infection.

Benefits of Cardiovascular Surgery

Cardiovascular surgery extends life and improves QUALITY OF LIFE for millions of Americans each year. Thousands of children grow to adulthood that several decades ago would have died in early infancy as a consequence of congenital HEART DISEASE. Open-heart surgery is one of the major medical advances of the 20th century and makes it possible for hundreds of thousands of people to enjoy active lives that otherwise would be cut short by heart diseases such as RHEUMATIC HEART DISEASE, which was the leading cause of death due to heart disease among adults in the 1950s. The benefits of a particular cardiovascular operation are unique to the individual, however, and always should outweigh the risks in the perception of the surgeon as well as the person having the operation.

Recovery from Cardiovascular Surgery

Most cardiovascular procedures require an overnight stay in the hospital to permit monitoring for postoperative bleeding or other complications as well as for ARRHYTHMIAS or other cardiac consequences that may develop; some operations may require a hospital stay of a week or longer. Recovery may take a few weeks to several months, depending on the operation and one's general health condition, though many people return to a reasonable level of function within several weeks. Some people experience residual limitations, such as shortness of breath with strenuous EXERCISE, while others find the limitations that defined their lives before surgery disappear when recovery is complete. A positive outlook and diligent attention to lifestyle habits that promote cardiovascular health are crucial for the best possible outcomes.

See also ABDOMINAL AORTIC ANEURYSM; ANGIOPLASTY; ARTERIAL SWITCH PROCEDURE; ATHERECTOMY; BIDIRECTIONAL GLENN PROCEDURE; CARDIOMYOPLASTY; CAROTID ENDARTERECTOMY; ENDARTERECTOMY; FONTAN PROCEDURE; NORWOOD PROCEDURE; VALVE REPAIR AND REPLACEMENT.

syncope　The clinical term for fainting. Syncope is a temporary loss of consciousness resulting from inadequate oxygen reaching the brain. When cardiovascular in nature, syncope typically occurs as a result of HYPOTENSION (low BLOOD PRESSURE), ARRHYTHMIAS (irregularities affecting the HEARTBEAT), or CAROTID STENOSIS (narrowing of the carotid arteries that carry BLOOD through the neck to the head and brain). Syncope also is a key symptom of STOKES-ADAMS DISEASE, a disorder characterized by transient arrhythmias. There also are numerous non-cardiovascular causes of syncope including MEDICATION SIDE EFFECTS.

Neurocardiogenic Syncope

Neurocardiogenic syncope, also called neurally medicated syncope and vasovagal syncope, occurs when there is a dysfunction in the brain centers responsible for regulating blood pressure. The dysfunction may involve the BRAIN STEM, medulla, or nerve paths. Neurocardiogenic syncope is a disorder of the AUTONOMIC NERVOUS SYSTEM that affects cardiovascular functions such as blood pressure and HEART RATE. Doctors do not know what initiates syncopal episodes, which may vary in frequency and often are brought on by circumstances such as standing from a prone or sitting position. Neurocardiogenic syncope often begins in late adolescence or early adulthood.

It appears that in many people who have this disorder, the brain's mechanisms for regulating blood pressure fail to sense the change in gravitational pull when the person stands up, allowing BLOOD to drop to the lower extremities without initiating a rise in blood pressure and heart rate to maintain appropriate circulation. The resulting inadequate blood supply to the brain causes temporary loss of consciousness, during which the person typically slumps into a prone position. This restores normal circulation, and the person regains consciousness. Doctors often use a TILT TABLE TEST to diagnose neurocardiogenic syncope, instigating in a controlled setting the kinds of positional changes that typically cause syncopal episodes. Other diagnostic procedures include ELECTROCARDIOGRAM (ECG) and EXERCISE STRESS TEST to determine whether arrhythmias are present. Syncope associated with arrhythmias typically occurs with either very rapid or very slow heart rates, due to disorders in the heart's electrical system. Though an ECG can diagnose these abnormalities, it can be difficult to capture the pertinent findings on ECG as they are often very transient. Cardiologists often need to perform extended ECG monitoring or even implant an ECG recording device to secure this diagnosis. Treatment depends on the diagnostic findings and may include medications to regulate blood pressure.

Arrhythmic Syncope

Syncope associated with arrhythmias typically occurs with ventricular bradycardia, an extraordinarily slow HEART rate, or atrial or ventricular FIBRILLATION, an extraordinarily rapid heart rate and rhythm that an ECG usually can determine. Syncope is usually an indication of a number of disorders involving the heart's electrical pacing system. Treatment targets the specific disorder and may range from medications to regulate heart rate and rhythm (ANTIARRHYTHMIA MEDICATIONS) to an implanted PACEMAKER or IMPLANTABLE CARDIOVERTER DEFIBRILLATOR (ICD).

Orthostatic Hypotension

Orthostatic hypotension—a sudden drop in blood pressure upon rising—is a frequent cause of syncope and can occur whether or not HEART DISEASE is present though is more common when there is underlying cardiovascular disease. It is often a side effect of medications taken to treat HYPERTENSION (high blood pressure). Often it is possible to control syncope due to orthostatic hypotension by rising slowly, which allows the body more time to adjust to the change in position. Orthostatic hypotension becomes more common with increasing age and is a side effect of many medications, including MEDICATIONS TO TREAT HEART DISEASE.

See also HEART AND CARDIOVASCULAR SYSTEM; LIGHT-HEADEDNESS.

syndrome X See METABOLIC SYNDROME.

systolic dysfunction Abnormal or impaired contraction that can affect any of the HEART's chambers though most commonly affects the left ventricle. Systole is the point in the CARDIAC CYCLE of the heart's most forceful contraction in which the right ventricle pumps BLOOD to the lungs and the left ventricle pumps blood into the aorta for distribution throughout the body. Systole is the first or top number in a BLOOD PRESSURE reading, representing the apex of the heart's function. The force of systole is an important factor in determining the volume of blood the heart sends out with each contraction. Left ventricular dysfunction is significant because it means the heart's ability to pump blood out to the body is impaired. This either can cause or be the result of HEART FAILURE, often accompanied by left ventricle hypertrophy (thickening of the left ventricle wall) as the heart attempts to compensate for the impaired function. Systolic dysfunction can arise from electrical disturbances of the heart that cause ARRHYTHMIAS or from scarring and other tissue damage due to HEART ATTACK (MYOCARDIAL INFARCTION).

Symptoms and Diagnostic Path

The key symptom of systolic dysfunction is difficulty breathing or shortness of breath (DYSPNEA) with EXERCISE or when lying down. The dyspnea during exercise is significant enough to limit activity. People who have systolic dysfunction may get tired very quickly, feel fatigued, and have a persistent cough. The diagnostic path typically includes ELECTROCARDIOGRAM (ECG) and blood tests to measure blood cell counts and electrolyte levels. LEFT VENTRICULAR EJECTION FRACTION (LVEF) is the primary means by which cardiologists determine whether systolic dysfunction exists; an LVEF of 40 percent or less indicates systolic dysfunction, mild to severe HEART FAILURE. Other diagnostic procedures the doctor might consider, based on the person's unique health history and presentation of symptoms, include ECHOCARDIOGRAM and stress test, either exercise or pharmaceutical.

Treatment Options and Outlook

Treatment includes medications such as DIGOXIN and ANGIOTENSIN-CONVERTING ENZYME (ACE) INHIBI-TOR MEDICATIONS, sometimes taken in combination, to strengthen the force of each contraction and decrease the load the heart faces with each beat to improve the heart's pumping efficiency. Other medications may be prescribed as well, depending on the extent of overall HEART DISEASE that exists. Systolic dysfunction typically is one of several cardiovascular conditions present. Systolic dysfunction tends to be progressive even with treatment, however, leading to heart failure.

Risk Factors and Preventive Measures

CORONARY ARTERY DISEASE (CAD) and ISCHEMIC HEART DISEASE (IHD) are the leading causes of systolic dysfunction. The presence of other CARDIOVASCULAR DISEASE (CVD) such as hypertrophic CARDIOMYOPATHY, AORTIC STENOSIS, and untreated or poorly controlled chronic HYPERTENSION are additional risk factors. Preventing or diagnosing and appropriately treating these underlying conditions can improve cardiac function.

See also CARDIOVASCULAR SYSTEM; DIASTOLE; DIASTOLIC DYSFUNCTION; MEDICATIONS TO TREAT HEART DISEASE.

systolic pressure   See BLOOD PRESSURE.

tachycardia   See ARRHYTHMIA.

tachycardia-bradycardia syndrome   An ARRHYTH-MIA disorder in which there are alternating periods of tachycardia (rapid HEART RATE) and bradycardia (slow heart rate) typically as a dysfunction of the sinus node and often in conjunction with ATRIAL FIBRILLATION. These specialized clusters of cells—the SINOATRIAL (SA) NODE, which originates the heart's electrical impulses, and the ATRIOVENTRICULAR (AV) NODE, which regulates electrical activity between the atria and the ventricles—control the HEART's rhythm. Other names for this syndrome include bradycardia-tachycardia syndrome and sick sinus syndrome.

Symptoms and Diagnostic Path

Symptoms of tachycardia-bradycardia syndrome may include PALPITATIONS, difficulty breathing (DYSPNEA), mental confusion, LIGHT-HEADEDNESS or SYNCOPE (fainting), and FATIGUE. Because the arrhythmias are episodic, the diagnostic path uses both ELECTROCARDIOGRAM (ECG) and HOLTER MONITOR (an ECG worn for 48 to 72 hours) to determine what is happening with electrical activity in the heart. Because symptoms could indicate other forms of HEART DISEASE, the diagnostic path also often includes a comprehensive cardiovascular examination incorporating BLOOD tests, stress testing, and other procedures.

Treatment Options and Outlook

For most people who have tachycardia-bradycardia syndrome, the preferred treatment is a PACEMAKER to take over regulation of the heart's electrical activity. ANTIARRHYTHMIA MEDICATIONS or ABLATION may be necessary to treat the tachycardia.

With treatment most people return to their usual activities.

Risk Factors and Preventive Measures

Tachycardia-bradycardia syndrome most often occurs in people over the age of 70 and is most likely the result of age-related degeneration that takes place within the heart. It may also accompany other forms of heart disease such as CORONARY ARTERY DISEASE (CAD), ISCHEMIC HEART DISEASE (IHD), and CARDIOMYOPATHY. Treatment of any underlying cardiovascular conditions may prevent the development of further symptoms. Lifestyle factors to mitigate the risk for heart disease in general are also helpful for maintaining heart health.

See also AGING, CARDIOVASCULAR EFFECTS OF; EXERCISE STRESS TEST; MEDICATIONS TO TREAT HEART DISEASE; SURGERY TO TREAT CARDIOVASCULAR DISEASE.

tai chi   An ancient form of martial arts that uses slow, deliberate movements to develop breathing, coordination, and balance. Tai chi is typically a group activity; many community centers and senior centers sponsor classes and sessions. Several studies suggest that tai chi helps to lower BLOOD PRESSURE and strengthen HEART RATE without increasing stress on the HEART. As well, tai chi is an excellent STRESS REDUCTION TECHNIQUE whose movements can be performed anywhere, whether with a group or alone, as a form of MEDITATION. The best way to learn and perform tai chi is through organized classes that can teach the proper movements and flow of the postures. Though its movements are slow and graceful, tai chi stimulates the heart and CARDIOVASCULAR SYSTEM. Some rehabilitation programs incorporate tai chi for people recovering from HEART ATTACK and especially STROKE because movements can be adapted to accommodate physical limitations.

See also EXERCISE; LIFESTYLE AND HEART HEALTH; LIVING WITH HEART DISEASE; QUALITY OF LIFE; YOGA.

tamponade, cardiac Constriction of the HEART to the extent that it can no longer have an effective beat. Cardiac tamponade typically develops as a consequence of PERICARDIAL EFFUSION. In either condition fluid accumulates between the pericardium and the myocardium (heart muscle), gradually compressing the heart until it has ineffective contractions and cannot expand. Common causes include bleeding into the pericardium, such as following cardiovascular surgery, renal failure, malignancy, and trauma.

Symptoms include extreme shortness of breath and sharp pain originating in the chest (symptoms that often emulate those of HEART ATTACK). Chest X-ray and ECHOCARDIOGRAM generally can show the fluid accumulation to confirm the diagnosis. Cardiac tamponade is a life-threatening crisis that requires emergency treatment to relieve the fluid and the pressure, usually by draining it from the pericardial sac with a needle and syringe. Treatment also is necessary to manage the underlying cause. The effects of coexisting or causative conditions notwithstanding, most people recover from cardiac tamponade that is immediately and appropriately treated. Untreated cardiac tamponade quickly leads to ventricular FIBRILLATION (erratic, rapid, and dysfunctional contractions of the ventricles) and death.

See also CARDIOVASCULAR SYSTEM; SURGERY TO TREAT CARDIOVASCULAR DISEASE.

target heart rate See HEART RATE.

Taussig, Helen (1898–1986) The first pediatric cardiologist (specialist in HEART conditions in children). Taussig is most noted for her work to develop an operation to correct "blue baby syndrome," in which cyanosis (bluish hue to the skin) indicates the body is not receiving adequate OXYGENATION. After struggling to overcome the learning disorder

dyslexia, Taussig earned an undergraduate degree from the University of California-Berkeley in 1921 and her medical degree from Johns Hopkins University School of Medicine in 1927 and then turned her focus to research. Using the then-revolutionary technology of FLUOROSCOPY (moving X-rays), one of the earliest imaging procedures, Taussig was able to determine that "blue babies" had heart malformations that prevented blood from traveling to the lungs for oxygenation.

In collaboration with surgeon Alfred Blalock and surgical technician Vivien Thomas, Taussig developed the operation known today as the BLALOCK-TAUSSIG PROCEDURE to repair the malformations and restore pulmonary circulation. Thomas invented many of the specialized instruments the new operation required and tested the operation on numerous animals, and Blalock performed the perfected operation on two children in 1944. The procedure revolutionized treatment for congenital heart malformations and remains the mainstay of surgical correction for a number of heart defects. In 1954 Taussig received international recognition for her work in pediatric cardiology when she received the Albert Lasker Award for Clinical Medical Research. Her alma mater, Johns Hopkins University School of Medicine, made Taussig the first woman to be appointed a full professor. Taussig also received the U.S. Medal of Freedom from President Lyndon B. Johnson in 1964 and became the first woman president of the American Heart Association in 1965.

See also BLALOCK, ALFRED; THOMAS, VIVIEN.

telmisartan A medication taken to treat HYPERTENSION (high BLOOD PRESSURE). Brand-name products available in the United States include Micardis. Telmisartan is an ANGIOTENSIN II RECEPTOR ANTAGONIST MEDICATION that works on the RENIN-ANGIOTENSIN-ALDOSTERONE (RAA) HORMONAL SYSTEM to prevent ANGIOTENSIN II, an enzyme the body produces that functions as a powerful vasoconstrictor, from binding with receptors in the walls of the arterioles, the smallest of the body's arteries. This blockade keeps the arterioles relaxed, reducing the resistance blood encounters when flowing through them and maintaining a lower blood pressure. Doctors sometimes prescribe telmisartan in combination with other antihypertensive medications and diuretic medications ("water pills"). Side effects with telmisartan, as with other angiotensin II receptor antagonists, are uncommon. Women who are in the second or third trimester of pregnancy should not take telmisartan as it crosses the placental barrier and is known to cause problems such as HYPOTENSION (low blood pressure) and kidney failure in the unborn child that can result in fetal death or in death of the infant shortly after birth. Telmisartan can interact with DIGOXIN, taken to treat ARRHYTHMIAS and HEART FAILURE, and the anticoagulant ("blood thinner") WARFARIN, taken to prevent blood clots.

See also ANGIOTENSIN-CONVERTING ENZYME (ACE) INHIBITOR MEDICATIONS; ANTICOAGULANT MEDICATIONS; DIURETIC MEDICATIONS; MEDICATION SIDE EFFECTS; MEDICATIONS TO TREAT HEART DISEASE.

tetralogy of Fallot A constellation of four congenital HEART malformations that constitutes a complex and significant deformation of the heart. Its major malformations appear in varying degrees of severity and require surgical reconstruction. Though rare, tetralogy of Fallot accounts for about 10 percent of congenital heart malformations and occurs more commonly in children with Down syndrome. It is possible for the malformations to be mild enough to escape detection at birth though nearly always the defect causes symptoms by early childhood. The malformations include:

- VENTRICULAR SEPTAL DEFECT (VSD), an abnormal opening in the wall (septum) that divides the right and left ventricles. This allows unoxygenated and oxygenated BLOOD to mix, reducing the oxygen level of the blood the left ventricle pumps out to the body.

- PULMONARY STENOSIS, in which the passage from the right ventricle into the pulmonary artery is narrow and constricted. The pulmonary valve also may be deformed. Sometimes called right ventricular stenosis, this malformation limits the volume of blood the heart can pump to the lungs for OXYGENATION.

- Aortic valve positioned above the VSD rather than in the left ventricle, allowing blood from both ventricles to enter the aorta. This allows unoxygenated blood from the right ventricle to mix with oxygenated blood from the left ventricle, creating diminished oxygen levels in the blood that the aorta carries out to the body.

- Right ventricular hypertrophy, in which the right ventricle is overdeveloped, making its walls thick and stiff. This restricts its pumping capability and further limits the volume of blood the heart sends to the lungs. In combination with the pulmonary stenosis, right ventricular hypertrophy leads to HEART FAILURE as the right ventricle cannot maintain an adequate supply of blood to the lungs.

Symptoms and Diagnostic Path
The primary symptom of tetralogy of Fallot is CYANOSIS, a bluish hue to the skin and especially the lips and nail beds, that signals inadequate oxygen supply to the body's tissues. There might also be shortness of breath. These symptoms commonly appear during crying or feeding in an infant and during physical activity if the child is older at the time of diagnosis. Doctors sometimes call these symptoms "tet spells." Diagnostic imaging procedures such as ECHOCARDIOGRAM and COMPUTED TOMOGRAPHY (CT) SCAN reveal the specific malformations, which vary widely in their severity.

Treatment Options and Outlook
Treatment for tetralogy of Fallot is surgical reconstruction of the malformations, usually performed in stages during the child's first two or three years of life when the syndrome is diagnosed in infancy. Most children who undergo reconstructive surgery are able to resume normal activities and grow to adulthood with few cardiovascular problems. Close monitoring throughout life is necessary, as is ANTIBIOTIC PROPHYLAXIS for dental and surgical procedures.

As the first generation of those to receive operations for tetralogy of Fallot and other extensive congenital heart malformations is now in adulthood, doctors are not certain of the long-term implications of such extensive surgical repairs. It is likely there are increased risks for heart failure, valve malfunctions, and other disturbances of heart function though the overall outlook remains excellent.

Risk Factors and Preventive Measures

Down syndrome and family history of tetralogy of Fallot increase the risk for a child to be born with this congenital disorder. There are no known preventive measures.

See also BIDIRECTIONAL GLENN PROCEDURE; CARDIO-VASCULAR SYSTEM; CYANOTIC CONGENITAL HEART DISEASE; DOWN SYNDROME AND HEART DISEASE; FONTAN PROCEDURE; HEART DISEASE IN CHILDREN; NORWOOD PROCEDURE; TRANSPOSITION OF THE GREAT ARTERIES (TGA).

thallium   See RADIONUCLIDE SCAN.

thallium stress test   See RADIONUCLIDE SCAN.

third-degree heart block   See HEART BLOCK.

Thomas, Vivien (1910–1985)   The surgical technician who worked with pioneering pediatric cardiologist Helen Taussig and surgeon Alfred Blalock to develop the technique and invent many of the specialized instruments that made possible surgical repair of septal defects and other congenital HEART malformations to treat "blue baby syndrome." Thomas conducted extensive research to perfect the techniques and instruments, and in 1944 he was part of the surgical team that performed the first septal defect repair on a young child at Johns Hopkins University hospital. Thomas later became supervisor of the surgical research laboratories at Johns Hopkins and worked closely with Blalock to invent numerous surgical instruments and techniques, many of which remain in use in cardiovascular surgery today.

See also BLALOCK, ALFRED; BLALOCK-TAUSSIG PROCEDURE; CYANOTIC, CONGENITAL HEART DISEASE; HEART DISEASE IN CHILDREN; TAUSSIG, HELEN.

thrombocythemia   A disorder of the BLOOD in which the bone marrow produces too many platelets, the blood cells responsible for initiating COAGULATION (clotting). This results in abnormal clotting that produces both excessive bleeding and the formation of blood clots in blood vessels throughout the body, with significantly increased risk for HEART ATTACK (MYOCARDIAL INFARCTION) and STROKE as well as DEEP VEIN THROMBOSIS (DVT). Thrombocythemia belongs to a classification of blood conditions called myeloproliferative disorders.

The doctor uses blood tests that measure the numbers of the different blood cells and bone marrow biopsy to make the diagnosis. Treatment depends on the severity of symptoms and may include taking medications that suppress platelet production or aggregation (the tendency for platelets to stick together, which is the first step in clot formation). Some people have few symptoms and can manage the disorder with ASPIRIN therapy. Plateletpheresis, in which platelets are withdrawn from the blood, may be necessary when symptoms are severe. Thrombocythemia is a lifelong condition after it develops; doctors do not know how and why it occurs though it is more common in people over age 50 and in women.

See also ANEMIA; ANTICOAGULANT MEDICATIONS; THROMBOCYTOPENIA; THROMBOPHILIA.

thrombocytopenia   A disorder of the BLOOD in which there are too few platelets, the blood cells that initiate COAGULATION (the formation of blood clots). Thrombocytopenia can occur as a primary condition, secondary to other health conditions, or as a side effect of certain medications (including heparin administered as therapy to prevent the formation of blood clots following HEART ATTACK, STROKE, or surgery). The bone marrow manufactures platelets, which it releases into the bloodstream. The spleen, an organ of the circulatory system located in the left upper abdomen under the lower ribs, extracts a third of the platelets from circulation and stores them until the body needs them to replenish circulating levels of platelets or to respond to bleeding.

Thrombocytopenia can result when the bone marrow produces too few platelets, as might occur with some cancers of the blood such as leukemia and lymphoma, or when the spleen fails to release enough platelets into circulation. Aplastic ANEMIA also affects platelet production. Some autoimmune disorders, such as systemic lupus erythematosus (SLE) and AIDS, destroy platelets. Blood tests diagnose thrombocytopenia; bone marrow biopsy (an examination of cells extracted from the bone marrow) helps to determine the cause. Treatment targets the underlying condition, if one exists, and also includes efforts to raise the platelet count. Such efforts may incorporate medications to stimulate platelet production and suppress the immune system as well as surgery to remove the spleen. People who have thrombocytopenia should not take ASPIRIN or NONSTEROIDAL ANTI-INFLAMMATORY DRUGS (NSAIDs), as these medications impair platelet aggregation and delay clotting. Thrombocytopenia raises the risk for hemorrhagic stroke, the less common though more deadly form of stroke caused by bleeding into brain tissue. Most thrombocytopenia resolves with treatment, though sometimes the condition is chronic.

See also IMMUNOSUPPRESSIVE MEDICATIONS; THROMBOCYTHEMIA; THROMBOPHILIA.

thromboembolism   See EMBOLISM.

thrombolytic medications   Enzyme-based biopharmaceuticals administered intravenously to dissolve blood clots that have formed in the arteries or veins. When given within three hours of a HEART ATTACK or an ischemic STROKE thrombolytic medications can effectively mitigate the effects of the event, sometimes averting both damage and symptoms. These drugs work by converting plasminogen, an inert protein in the bloodstream, to plasmin, an active enzyme that dissolves fibrin.

Fibrin is a sticky, threadlike substance that becomes activated from fibrinogen during the COAGULATION process. It forms a web that catches platelets and other blood cells, accumulating them into a semisolid structure that dams the flow of blood. Other chemicals activated as part of the coagulation process draw the fluid from this structure, causing it to harden. During the time the fibrin is semisolid, plasmin can dissolve it. After the fibrin hardens, other body mechanisms become activated to slowly dismantle the clot as the healing process progresses. Plasmin is not effective on

hardened fibrin, which is why treatment must begin within a few hours of the onset of the attack (heart attack or stroke).

Thrombolytic medications derive from natural sources; many are genetically engineered (recombinant) proteins designed to activate plasmin from plasminogen. Though they act in similar ways when administered, each has unique characteristics and properties. Those commonly used in the United States include lanoteplase, reteplase, staphylokinase, STREPTOKINASE, tenecteplase, TISSUE PLASMINOGEN ACTIVATOR (tPA), and UROKINASE.

See also ANTICOAGULANT MEDICATIONS; ATHERECTOMY; CORONARY ARTERY BYPASS GRAFT (CABG).

thrombophilia   A disorder in which the BLOOD coagulates (clots) abnormally fast. Some forms of thrombophilia are inherited and are gene mutations that affect the body's production and use of clotting factors (proteins that are integral to the coagulation process). Other forms of thrombophilia develop secondary to health conditions such as cancer or systemic lupus erythematosus (SLE). HEART FAILURE and HEART ATTACK (MYOCARDIAL INFARCTION) also create an increased risk for thrombophilia, which itself creates an increased risk for heart attack and STROKE.

Blood tests can diagnose disorders involving clotting factors; ECHOCARDIOGRAM or DOPPLER ULTRASOUND can pinpoint the location of thromboemboli (blood clots that occlude blood vessels). Treatment is primarily preventive and typically incorporates ANTICOAGULANT MEDICATIONS in combination with regular physical activity, especially walking, to strengthen the muscles supporting peripheral blood vessels and keep blood from pooling. When there is a large thromboembolus that is detected early, the doctor may choose to use an injected thrombolytic medication to dissolve the clot.

See also COAGULATION; EMBOLISM; THROMBOCYTHEMIA; THROMBOCYTOPENIA.

thrombosis   See EMBOLISM.

ticlopidine   A medication taken to treat CLAUDICATION (pain in the legs with walking). Common brand-name products available in the United States include Ticlid. Ticlopidine is a platelet aggregate inhibitor medication; it works by preventing platelets from sticking together in the first stage of COAGULATION (clot formation). Ticlopidine cannot dissolve a clot that already has formed, though it can help to prevent subsequent clots from forming in the blood vessels. Gastrointestinal distress, especially nausea and diarrhea, is a common side effect particularly at the onset of treatment. In many people this distress subsides as the medication is taken over time though about 10 percent of people have significant enough gastrointestinal distress that they cannot take the medication. Ticlopidine also can cause abnormalities in the blood including THROMBOCYTOPENIA (shortage of platelets) and, as its purpose is to delay coagulation, excessive bleeding.

See also DIABETES AND HEART DISEASE; MEDICATIONS TO TREAT HEART DISEASE; PERIPHERAL VASCULAR DISEASE (PVD).

tidal volume See LUNG CAPACITY.

tilt table test A noninvasive procedure that helps to diagnose certain kinds of ARRHYTHMIAS, HYPOTENSION (low BLOOD PRESSURE), and other cardiovascular conditions to evaluate the cardiovascular implications of SYNCOPE (fainting episodes).

Procedure

The tilt table test places a person in a prone position for baseline readings of blood pressure, heart rate, and ELECTROCARDIOGRAM (ECG). Then the table tips the person, held securely in place with safety straps, into a position of 30 degrees for a period of time (comparable to lying on a steep hill) and then to 60 or 70 degrees for a period of time (nearly upright). The person's head is always upright during a tilt table test; the premise is to expose the body's blood pressure and HEART RATE regulatory mechanisms to the physiological stresses of changing from lying down to being upright. Sometimes the test is repeated after administering an intravenous injection of isuprel or a similar drug to simulate the physiological changes of moderate EXERCISE.

Risks and Complications

Some people feel chest tightness or even CHEST PAIN as a result of the medications administered during the tilt table test or as a consequence of arrhythmias and other cardiovascular function changes that occurred. These complications are short-lived.

Outlook and Lifestyle Modifications

Because the tilt table test evokes symptoms, DIZZINESS and nausea may persist for 15 to 30 minutes after the procedure. Most people return to normal after that time and are able to again engage in their usual activities.

See also EXERCISE STRESS TEST.

timolol A medication taken to treat HYPERTENSION (high BLOOD PRESSURE). Timolol belongs to the BETA ANTAGONIST MEDICATIONS family of drugs; common brand-name products available in the United States include Blocadren. Timolol is a nonselective beta-blocker, which means it affects smooth muscle tissue throughout the body as well as within the HEART and CARDIOVASCULAR SYSTEM. Doctors often prescribe timolol in combination with other ANTIHYPERTENSIVE MEDICATIONS, particularly thiazide DIURETIC MEDICATIONS, and lifestyle modifications to establish optimal control of blood pressure. Common side effects include weakness, tiredness, SEXUAL DYSFUNCTION (ERECTILE DYSFUNCTION in men and diminished libido in men and women), stress incontinence in women, and SLEEP DISTURBANCES (notably, vivid dreams). As these side effects tend not to resolve over time, when they are intolerable it often is preferable to change to a different beta-blocker or a different kind of antihypertensive.

See also ALPHA ANTAGONIST MEDICATIONS; ANGIOTENSIN-CONVERTING ENZYME (ACE) INHIBITOR MEDICATIONS; ANGIOTENSIN II RECEPTOR ANTAGONIST MEDICATIONS; CALCIUM CHANNEL ANTAGONIST MEDICATIONS; EXERCISE; LIFESTYLE AND HEART HEALTH.

tissue plasminogen activator (tPA) An enzyme-based biopharmaceutical agent administered intravenously or intra-arterially to dissolve BLOOD clots that form in blood vessels. In the United States doctors use tPA primarily to treat HEART ATTACK and ischemic STROKE. Like other THROMBOLYTIC MEDICA-TIONS, tPA must be administered within the first few hours after the stroke begins. It acts to convert plasminogen to plasmin, an enzyme that dissolves fibrin in newly formed blood clots (thrombi). When administered early in the course of a heart attack or stroke, tPA can minimize and often prevent permanent damage by rapidly restoring blood flow to reduce the number of cells affected by HYPOXIA (lack of oxygen) as a result of the occluding clot (thromboembolus). Doctors typically administer tPA in combination with ANTICOAGULANT MEDICA-TIONS to stop clots from re-forming and to prevent new clots from developing.

The action of tPA is nondiscriminatory; that is, it dissolves newly formed fibrin in any clot anywhere in the body. This creates the risk of bleeding or hemorrhage (extensive blood loss), particularly in a person who recently has had surgery or a major wound. In stroke especially, there is the potential that minor hemorrhagic activity also has taken place in the brain; tPA will dissolve clots that have formed to seal off leaking blood vessels as well as those that may be blocking blood vessels. Doctors typically use computed tomography (CT) scan to determine whether a stroke is ischemic, as are 80 percent of strokes, or hemorrhagic. People over age 70 have a greater risk of bleeding with tPA therapy.

See also COAGULATION; STREPTOKINASE; THROMBO-SIS; UROKINASE.

tobacco use The leading cause of HEART DISEASE in the United States. About 43.4 million American adults smoke cigarettes—about 22 percent of men and 17 percent of women. Another 5 million use smokeless tobacco products such as chewing tobacco and snuff. Though heart disease is most widely associated with cigarette smoking, all forms of tobacco use introduce NICOTINE into the body, an addictive chemical that has numerous effects on the structures and functions of the HEART and CAR-DIOVASCULAR SYSTEM. Cigarette smoke compounds the problem by affecting the ability of the lungs to deliver oxygen to the blood. There is no habit that has greater deleterious effects on cardiovascular health and health overall. Tobacco use offers no

health benefits and accounts for nearly 450,000 deaths in the United States each year.

The advent of mass production of cigarettes in the 1940s launched cigarette smoking as an accessible habit; mass marketing presented that habit as trendy and sophisticated. Millions of Americans took it up. By the early 1960s health experts knew cigarette smoking accounted for numerous health problems, and in 1964 the U.S. Surgeon General Terry Luther, M.D., issued the first, and milestone, surgeon general's advisory on the health risks of cigarette smoking. In 1965 the U.S. Congress passed the Federal Cigarette Labeling and Advertising Act and in 1969 the Public Health Cigarette Smoking Act. Smoking among American men declined from 52 percent in 1965 to 28 percent 30 years later, in 1995, a decline that continues.

Though 80 percent of those who smoke start before age 18, smoking among youth and Americans overall is steadily dropping. About half of all those who ever have smoked have stopped. About 80 percent of workplaces in the United States now are smoke-free, though heart disease attributable to secondhand, or environmental, smoke claims the lives of 46,000 Americans, deaths due to heart disease, each year. Public health officials continue to emphasize education efforts to discourage people from starting tobacco use and smoking cessation efforts to help people quit smoking. Those who stop tobacco use experience an immediate decrease in their risks for developing heart disease; after 15 years of not smoking, former smokers have relatively the same risk for heart disease as those who never smoked.

See also LIFESTYLE AND HEART HEALTH; PERIPH-ERAL VASCULAR DISEASE (PVD); SMOKING AND HEART DISEASE.

torsades de pointes A form of VENTRICULAR TACHYCARDIA characterized by variability of the QRS interval, an electrical pattern of the HEART on an ELECTROCARDIOGRAM (ECG). It is associated as a severe adverse effect with certain medications as well as a number of gene mutations and is a significant risk with LONG QT SYNDROME (LQTS). Treatment with conventional ANTIARRHYTHMIA MEDICATIONS commonly prescribed for ventricular tachycardia can cause fatal ARRHYTHMIAS when taken by a person who has torsades de pointes; an ECG can distinguish torsades de pointes from other forms of ventricular tachycardia. Torsades de pointes can progress to ventricular fibrillation without symptoms or notice; ventricular fibrillation is a life-threatening emergency.

Women are three times more likely than men to develop torsades de pointes though researchers are uncertain of the reason for this. Those who have family histories of SUDDEN CARDIAC ARREST or LQTS also are at increased risk for torsades de pointes. ELECTROLYTE imbalances also may exist with torsades de pointes. Treatment may include electrolyte replacement, adrenergic agonist medications, or BETA ANTAGONIST MEDICATIONS. When medications fail to regulate rhythm, an IMPLANTABLE CARDIO-VERTER DEFIBRILLATOR (ICD) may be necessary.

See also DEFIBRILLATION; EMERGENCY CARDIOVAS-CULAR CARE; MEDICATION SIDE EFFECTS; MEDICATIONS TO TREAT HEART DISEASE; PACEMAKER.

torsemide   A POTASSIUM-sparing DIURETIC MEDICA-TION taken to treat HYPERTENSION (high BLOOD PRES-SURE) and congestive HEART FAILURE and related EDEMA (fluid retention). Common brand-name products available in the United States include Demadex. The potassium-sparing diuretics have a mild to moderate action on the glomeruli of the kidneys, causing the kidneys to pass SODIUM and water in the urine but retain potassium to maintain better electrolyte balance. The most common side effect when initiating torsemide therapy, as with diuretic therapy in general, is excessive urination. This is a consequence of the medication's action on the kidneys; urine volume and frequency sta-bilize over the course of six to eight weeks, which resolves this effect. Other common side effects include headache, DIZZINESS, and nausea; these also resolve in most people after taking torsemide for several weeks. Doctors may prescribe torse-mide in combination with other MEDICATIONS TO TREAT HEART DISEASE. Torsemide's potassium-spar-ing effect can lead to HYPERKALEMIA (elevated blood potassium levels), which can cause ARRHYTHMIAS.

See also ANTIHYPERTENSIVE MEDICATIONS; MEDICA-TION SIDE EFFECTS.

total cavopulmonary connection   See FONTAN PROCEDURE.

trandolapril   An ANGIOTENSIN-CONVERTING ENZYME (ACE) INHIBITOR MEDICATION taken to treat HYPER-TENSION (high BLOOD PRESSURE). In the United States trandolapril is available as the brand-name product Mavik and in combination with the CAL-CIUM CHANNEL ANTAGONIST MEDICATION verapamil in the brand-name product Tarka. Trandolapril low-ers blood pressure by blocking a step in the body's primary blood pressure regulatory mechanism, the RENIN-ANGIOTENSIN-ALDOSTERONE (RAA) HORMONAL SYSTEM. Side effects, when they occur, include DIZ-ZINESS, diarrhea, and persistent cough. Trandolapril, like other ACE inhibitors, can cause serious injury, birth defects, and death in an unborn child; women who are pregnant should not take trandolapril. Doctors often prescribe trandolapril in combination with other MEDICATIONS TO TREAT HEART DISEASE, such as DIURETIC MEDICATIONS and medications to treat HEART FAILURE and ARRHYTHMIAS.

See also ANGIOTENSIN II RECEPTOR ANTAGONIST MEDICATIONS; ANTIHYPERTENSIVE MEDICATIONS; MEDI-CATION SIDE EFFECTS.

tranquilizers   See ANTIANXIETY MEDICATIONS.

transesophageal echocardiography (TEE)   See ECHOCARDIOGRAM.

trans-fatty acids   See NUTRITION AND DIET.

transient ischemic attack (TIA)   A mini, or micro, STROKE. TIAs may occur without symptoms or may cause minor symptoms such as momentary loss of cognitive function or movement. TIAs occur when tiny BLOOD clots occlude the arterioles and small arteries within the brain, interrupting the flow of blood. Because the areas affected are small (and may be only a few cells), the damage, though permanent, is not obvious. It is, however, cumulative. TIAs are a significant risk factor for STROKE, in which a larger thromboembolism blocks the flow of blood to a larger area of the brain and produces symptoms. A third of people who have TIAs have a major stroke within five years of the onset of the TIAs. COMPUTED TOMOGRAPHY (CT) SCAN can confirm that TIAs are taking place. As most TIAs are ischemic (caused by clots or occlusions), doctors typically prescribe ASPIRIN therapy or ANTICOAGULANT MEDICATIONS to help prevent blood clots from forming as well as attempt to treat other HEART DISEASE such as ATHEROSCLEROSIS and CORONARY ARTERY DISEASE (CAD), both of which increase the risk for TIAs and stroke because of the accumulations of arterial plaque.

See also HEART ATTACK; PLAQUE, ARTERIAL; THROMBOLYSIS.

transmyocardial laser revascularization (TMLR)

A surgical treatment for severe ISCHEMIC HEART DISEASE (IHD) in which the cardiologist uses a specialized laser to infuse the myocardium (HEART muscle) with multiple tiny channels that, when they heal, function as pseudo-arteries to increase the flow of blood to myocardial cells. TMLR often is performed in conjunction with CORONARY ARTERY BYPASS GRAFT (CABG) to improve the outcome, or can be performed as a separate procedure when CABG is not a viable option. TMLR is an option for people who do not receive relief from ANGINA through medications. Its risks are the same as for any other surgery, and it can provide long-term though not always complete relief from angina. There is some evidence that TMLR may encourage ANGIOGENESIS (the growth of new blood vessels) that further improves myocardial perfusion.

See also ANGIOPLASTY; MEDICATIONS TO TREAT HEART DISEASE; SURGERY TO TREAT CARDIOVASCULAR DISEASE.

transposition of the great arteries (TGA)

A serious congenital malformation of the HEART in which the originations of the HEART's major arteries are reversed. The aorta arises from the right instead of the left ventricle, causing the heart to pump unoxygenated blood returning from the body back out to the body without going to the lungs. The pulmonary artery arises from the left instead of the right ventricle, which pumps oxygenated blood coming from the lungs back to the lungs without going to the body. Nearly always there are atrioventricular septal defects (openings in the septa, or walls, separating the heart's chambers) that allow oxygenated blood and unoxygenated blood to mix in the ventricles, so the blood going out to the body carries a minimal amount of oxygen. Often other malformations are present as well. Though TGA is a rare defect, it accounts for about 10 percent of congenital heart malformations and is the most common form of CYANOTIC CONGENITAL HEART DISEASE.

Symptoms and Diagnostic Path

Doctors nearly always detect TGA within a few hours of birth as the infant clearly is not receiving adequate OXYGENATION. ECHOCARDIOGRAM confirms the presence of the malformations and the diagnosis.

Treatment Options and Outlook

Treatment is surgery, which may consist of a series of operations depending on the extent of the malformations. After surgical correction of the malformations the heart functions normally and the child enjoys a normal lifestyle. In adulthood those who have had surgical corrections for TGA are at increased risk for other forms of HEART DISEASE though monitoring and follow-up care help to identify and treat other heart conditions before they become significant.

Risk Factors and Preventive Measures

TGA is significantly more common in males. No risk factors or preventive measures are known.

See also ARTERIAL SWITCH PROCEDURE; BIDIRECTIONAL GLENN PROCEDURE; BLALOCK-TAUSSIG PROCEDURE; CARDIOVASCULAR SYSTEM; FONTAN PROCEDURE; HEART DISEASE IN CHILDREN; LIVING WITH HEART DISEASE; NORWOOD PROCEDURE; PALLIATION, STAGED; TETRALOGY OF FALLOT.

traveling with heart disease Many people with HEART DISEASE want to enjoy local and distant travel though are concerned about the effects of sitting for prolonged periods of time or traveling in areas where health-care services are limited.

Though heart disease may shape to some extent one's travel destinations and means of transportation, taking basic precautions can make travel both possible and enjoyable.

- Take enough medication to cover half again the length of time of the intended travel. Most pharmacies will provide additional quantities of medications to accommodate travel plans.
- Plan for changes in time zones to keep medications on schedule. When such changes are extreme, such as if traveling from the U.S. West Coast to Europe, discuss with the cardiologist or pharmacist how to best accommodate medication dosages.
- Ask the prescribing doctor for extra written prescriptions to carry in case it becomes necessary to obtain additional medications. The prescriptions should include full contact information for the doctor in case a pharmacy needs to clarify or verify the prescription, or, in the case of travel to another country, make substitutions.
- Carry medications in their original, pharmacy-labeled containers.
- Plan itineraries that allow adequate time for movement and rest. Inactivity raises the risk for blood clots and other circulatory problems.

Other challenges when traveling include maintaining nutritious, low-fat eating habits and continuing daily physical EXERCISE. These important efforts may require creative ingenuity though are especially important when travel involves sitting for extended periods of time (such as when flying or riding in a car, train, or bus). As often as possible it is good to stand up and walk around. When this is not possible, periodically lifting one foot from the floor and moving the foot and leg, then repeating with the other, helps to maintain good blood flow and reduce the risk for DEEP VEIN THROMBOSIS (DVT) and EDEMA.

See also LIFESTYLE AND HEART HEALTH; QUALITY OF LIFE.

triamterene A POTASSIUM-sparing DIURETIC MEDICATION taken to treat HYPERTENSION (high BLOOD PRESSURE), HEART FAILURE, and EDEMA. In the United States triamterene alone is available as the brand-name product Dyrenium and in a combination with HYDROCHLOROTHIAZIDE (a thiazide diuretic) as the brand-name products Dyazide and Maxzide. Triamterene alone is a mild to moderate diuretic that acts on the glomeruli of the kidneys to decrease SODIUM and water reabsorption, allowing more sodium and water to pass in the urine. Combination products that include hydrochlorothiazide produce a stronger diuretic action and allow some potassium to be released along with sodium and water. Dizziness and fatigue are among the common side effects. Triamterene, like other potassium-sparing diuretics, can allow blood potassium levels to become too high, in which case potentially dangerous ARRHYTHMIAS may result.

See also ANTIHYPERTENSIVE MEDICATIONS; MEDICATIONS TO TREAT HEART DISEASE.

tricuspid atresia A congenital malformation of the HEART in which the triscupid valve between the right atrium and the right ventricle fails to develop, resulting in there being no opening between the two chambers and no way for BLOOD returning from the body to enter the right ventricle. It is among the more common congenital heart malformations and a cause of "blue baby" syndrome. About 20 percent of infants born with triscupid atresia have other heart malformations such as SINGLE VENTRICLE, in which there is just one ventricle instead of the normal two ventricles, or TRANSPOSITION OF THE GREAT ARTERIES (TGA), in which the heart's arteries and veins arise from the incorrect chambers. Often there is at minimum an ATRIAL SEPTAL DEFECT (ASD) in which an abnormal opening exists in the wall (septum) that separates the two atria. This opening creates a channel that allows unoxygenated blood to pass directly from the right atrium to the left atrium where it mixes with oxygenated blood returning to the left atrium from the lungs. The oxygen content of the blood the left ventricle pumps to the body hence is diminished though often is adequate to meet the body's basic needs.

Symptoms and Diagnostic Path

It is possible for triscupid atresia to escape detection at birth and then become apparent several months later, typically when the infant is being evaluated for failure to grow. Rarely, undiagnosed triscupid atresia can persist until adulthood, although substantial damage occurs to the heart and lungs as a result. Often there are electrical disturbances in the ELECTROCARDIOGRAM (ECG) as the conduction pattern through the heart is altered. Imaging technologies such as ECHOCARDIOGRAM, COMPUTED TOMOGRAPHY (CT) SCAN, and MAGNETIC RESONANCE IMAGING (MRI) can aid in diagnosis. CARDIAC CATHETERIZATION with FLUOROSCOPY (moving X-ray), though invasive, allows a conclusive diagnosis.

Treatment Options and Outlook

Treatment is surgery to repair the malformations that are present, in an attempt to restore as normal function as possible to the heart. When serious malformations are present surgery is extensive and takes place through a series of operations over the child's first three years of life. The extended outcome of corrective surgery depends on the extensiveness of the malformations; many children are able to participate in most activities except strenuous physical exercise as they are growing up. In adulthood, corrected triscupid atresia requires regular monitoring by a cardiologist. It might be necessary to take medications to strengthen the HEARTBEAT and regulate the HEART RATE. There is an increased risk for developing CARDIOMYOPATHY and HEART FAILURE.

Risk Factors and Preventive Measures

Factors that appear to increase risk for tricuspid atresia include prenatal exposure to rubella (German measles), excessive alcohol, the acne medication Accutane, and the mood regulator lithium.

See also ARTERIAL SWITCH PROCEDURE; CARDIOVASCULAR SYSTEM; CYANOTIC CONGENITAL HEART DISEASE; HEART DISEASE; HEART DISEASE IN CHILDREN; BIDIRECTIONAL GLENN PROCEDURE; FONTAN PROCEDURE; NORWOOD PROCEDURE.

tricuspid valve See HEART AND CARDIOVASCULAR SYSTEM.

triglycerides, blood Lipids, or fatty acids, manufactured by the liver and stored in adipose (fatty)

FASTING BLOOD TRIGLYCERIDES LEVELS

Blood Level	Category	Cardiovascular Risk
150 mg/dL or lower	Normal	Not increased
150 to 199 mg/dL	Borderline	Moderately increased
200 to 499 mg/dL	High	Significantly increased
500 mg/dL or higher	Very high	Independent risk factor

tissue throughout the body and also in circulation in the bloodstream. Most dietary fat is in the form of triglycerides, which are digested into their component structures after ingestion and then reassembled within the body. The body uses triglycerides to transport fat-soluble substances such as vitamins and also as an energy source. Whatever triglycerides the body cannot immediately use become stored as body fat. Elevated levels of triglycerides in the blood present an increased risk for ATHEROSCLEROSIS, CORONARY ARTERY DISEASE (CAD), HEART ATTACK, and STROKE. Triglycerides may become elevated secondary to other health conditions such as DIABETES, METABOLIC, and OBESITY. Lowering blood triglycerides levels reduces their role in creating risk for HEART DISEASE.

Lifestyle modifications such as eating a low-fat diet and getting daily physical EXERCISE limit the body's ability to manufacture triglycerides and help the body to more efficiently use triglycerides for energy. Doctors typically attempt lifestyle modifications for several months when blood triglycerides levels are borderline, adding LIPID-LOWERING MEDICATIONS to the therapeutic approach when such modifications fail to produce the desired results or when blood triglycerides levels are high or very high.

See also CHOLESTEROL, BLOOD; HYPERLIPIDEMIA; LIFESTYLE AND HEART HEALTH.

truncus arteriosus A congenital malformation of the HEART in which the aorta and the pulmonary artery, instead of being separate structures, arise from the same site to form a single, oversized artery. As well, a VENTRICULAR SEPTAL DEFECT (VSD), in which there is an abnormal opening in the wall that separates the two ventricles, nearly always accompanies truncus arteriosus. This anomalous configuration allows unoxygenated blood the right ventricle pumps to the lungs to mix with oxygenated blood the left ventricle pumps out to the body, resulting in reduced oxygen in the blood the heart pumps to the body and increased oxygen in the blood the heart pumps to the lungs. The truncus allows a large volume of blood to enter the lungs, causing temporary congestive HEART FAILURE that further diminishes the heart's capacity.

Symptoms and Diagnostic Path

The infant develops a bluish hue to the skin (CYANOSIS) that signals the body is not receiving adequate oxygenation. Imaging technologies such as ECHOCARDIOGRAM, COMPUTED TOMOGRAPHY (CT) SCAN, and MAGNETIC RESONANCE IMAGING (MRI) allow doctors to diagnose truncus arteriosus. CARDIAC CATHETERIZATION, though invasive, allows conclusive diagnosis when there are any questions.

Treatment Options and Outlook

Treatment is OPEN-HEART SURGERY to divide the truncus into two arteries. This involves using a graft and prosthetic valve to construct a channel between the pulmonary artery and the right ventricle. Because the graft's size is fixed, the child will need two or three surgeries to replace this graft as he or she grows; cardiologists monitor heart function to time the operations so they take place before the heart experiences any distress from the graft being too small. In adulthood, the graft needs regular monitoring as well. As this operation is now seeing the first generation of recipients reach adulthood, cardiologists are unsure of the long-term consequences though expect there to be no more problems than with heart valve replacement.

Risk Factors and Preventive Measures

Truncus arteriosus is more common in children who have DOWN SYNDROME. Family history of congenital heart defect also increases the risk.

See also COARCTATION OF THE AORTA; CYANOTIC CONGENITAL HEART DISEASE; HEART DISEASE IN CHILDREN; SURGERY TO TREAT CARDIOVASCULAR DISEASE; TRANSPOSITION OF THE GREAT ARTERIES (TGA); VALVE REPAIR AND REPLACEMENT.

T-wave See ELECTROCARDIOGRAM (ECG).

twiddler's syndrome A malfunction of an implanted PACEMAKER in which the leads (wires that carry electrical impulses) become dislodged, often because the person "twiddles" with the area over the pacemaker pocket. The person is usually not aware that he or she is manipulating the pacemaker through the skin. Occasionally the same effect results from the pocket in the muscle not holding the pacemaker tightly in place. The movement of the pacemaker pulls and twists the leads, sometimes wrapping them around the pacemaker unit. They lose their positions in the HEART, and although they continue to deliver electrical impulses, the impulses do not properly activate the heart.

Symptoms and Diagnostic Path

Symptoms often are those of the original ARRHYTHMIA, or of HEART BLOCK or HEART FAILURE, because the heart's rhythm becomes seriously impaired. The person also might experience twitching of other muscles, such as in the arm or abdomen, depending on where the leads are. Diagnosis is by X-ray, which shows the displaced leads.

Treatment Options and Outlook

Treatment is removal and replacement of the pacemaker, at which time the surgeon attempts to make the new pocket as snug as possible or sutures the pacemaker unit into the pocket such that it cannot turn or move.

Risk Factors and Preventive Measures

Elderly people who have dementia are at greatest risk for twiddler's syndrome. Many surgeons attempt to minimize this risk by fitting the original pacemaker as tightly as possible.

See also PACEMAKER SYNDROME.

type A personality See PERSONALITY TYPES.

type B personality See PERSONALITY TYPES.

type D personality See PERSONALITY TYPES.

ultrafast CT scan See ELECTRON BEAM COMPUTED TOMOGRAPHY (EBCT) SCAN.

ultrasound An imaging technology in which high-frequency sound waves bounce, or "echo," from body tissues at varying rates to present visualization of internal organs and structures. An ultrasound of the HEART is called an ECHOCARDIOGRAM. An ultrasound transducer emits and focuses high frequency sound waves that, when aimed through the skin at targeted internal organs and structures, generate echoes that produce detailed images. The transducer collects and conveys the returning, or echoing, sound signals to the computerized ultrasound machine, which converts them into two-dimensional moving images that also can be enhanced with color. There is no radiation or other discharge from ultrasound; ultrasound has no known risks.

An ultrasound requires no preparation and generally causes no discomfort. The ultrasonographer spreads a conductive gel on the skin surface of the area to be scanned and then moves the transducer along the skin. The gel improves the quality of the contact for optimal quality of the signals being sent and accepted. An ultrasound scan may take 20 to 40 minutes, depending on the area of the scan. During the procedure the ultrasonographer may ask the person to lie in certain positions to facilitate clear images or to cause internal structures to shift position. A radiologist or cardiologist generally views the ultrasound once it is under way, then provides a comprehensive reading of the images at a later time. Results typically are back to the cardiologist within two days. The ultrasound may provide the diagnostic information the cardiologist seeks or result in further tests being ordered.

See also COMPUTED TOMOGRAPHY (CT) SCAN; DOPPLER ULTRASOUND; FLUOROSCOPY; MAGNETIC RESONANCE IMAGING (MRI).

urokinase An enzyme-based biopharmaceutical agent administered by intravenous or intra-arterial injection to dissolve BLOOD clots that have formed in the blood vessels. Doctors administer urokinase as thrombolytic treatment for ischemic STROKE and HEART ATTACK (MYOCARDIAL INFARCTION). Urokinase causes plasminogen to convert from its inert form to the active enzyme plasmin, which dissolves (a process called lysis) the fibrin in newly formed blood clots. Urokinase is a recombinant preparation derived from human protein sources and synthesized in the laboratory. As such, it has the potential to carry infectious agents and is handled in much the same way as are blood products. The primary risk of urokinase is excessive or easy bleeding (such as nosebleeds and bleeding gums) or hemorrhage (rapid and profuse loss of blood). Because urokinase is nondiscriminatory in its action, it dissolves the fibrin from any newly formed blood clot including clots that are therapeutic, such as ones that have formed at surgical or wound sites. People who recently have had surgery or serious injuries, or who may have experienced hemorrhagic stroke, should not receive urokinase. Generally urokinase is not administered to people over age 70 as there appears to be an increased risk of bleeding.

See also COAGULATION; STREPTOKINASE; THROMBOLYTIC MEDICATIONS; TISSUE PLASMINOGEN ACTIVATOR (TPA).

vagus nerve The tenth cranial nerve. With the widest distribution among the 12 pairs of cranial nerves, the vagus nerve serves as a conduit for both sensory and motor nerve signals. The word *vagus* means "wandering," an apt descriptor for the extensive reach of this nerve that emerges from the medulla oblongata in the BRAIN STEM and runs through the neck to the upper torso, where it branches to the pharynx (back of the throat), esophagus, trachea, lungs, HEART, stomach, liver, small intestine, and upper colon. The vagus nerve carries nerve signals that affect breathing, HEART RATE, BLOOD PRESSURE, and digestion, and that also transmit perceptions of pain. STROKE involving the lower regions of the brain or the brain stem can damage the vagus nerve near its point of origin, affecting swallowing, speech, breathing, and heart rate.

See also CARDIOVASCULAR SYSTEM; PULMONARY SYSTEM; SYNCOPE.

Valsalva maneuver A diagnostic procedure, generally done during ECHOCARDIOGRAM, that measures changes in BLOOD PRESSURE and HEART RATE in response to breathing against pressure. Breathing against pressure shuts down the return of venous BLOOD to the HEART, creating a sudden drop in the volume of blood entering the heart. This activates a cardiovascular response in which the heart compensate, when the breathing pressure is released, by accelerating the rate and force of its contractions. Within 15 to 30 seconds the heart rate jumps to tachycardia (rapid though regular heartbeat), which causes blood pressure to rise, then compensatorily drops to bradycardia (slow though regular heartbeat). The doctor may have the person breathe into a manometer, a device that measures

the pressure of resistance, to hold a pressure of 40 millimeters of mercury (mm Hg) for 30 seconds. A more informal method is to have the person bear down as though having a bowel movement. Sometimes doctors use the Valsalva maneuver therapeutically to correct minor arrhythmias such as might occur during CARDIAC CATHETERIZATION, as the changes in heart rate require the heart to alter its rhythm.

Inadvertent Valsalva maneuver can take place when bearing down for bowel movements, holding the breath while lifting heavy objects, or holding the nose and breathing out to relieve pressure against the eardrums such as when flying. The resulting cardiovascular changes can be significant enough to trigger HEART ATTACK or STROKE in someone who has moderate to severe CORONARY ARTERY DISEASE (CAD) by dislodging a blood clot or fragment of arterial plaque. People who have HYPERTENSION (high blood pressure) or CAD should avoid inadvertent Valsalva maneuvers.

See also ARRHYTHMIA; CONSTIPATION; PLAQUE, ARTERIAL.

valsartan A medication taken to treat HYPERTENSION (high BLOOD PRESSURE). Valsartan, marketed in the United States as the brand-name product Diovan, belongs to the family of ANGIOTENSIN II, RECEPTOR ANTAGONIST MEDICATIONS. It lowers BLOOD pressure by preventing angiotensin II, a powerful vasoconstrictor the body converts as part of the RENIN-ANGIOTENSIN-ALDOSTERONE (RAA) HORMONAL SYSTEM for regulating blood pressure, from binding with receptors in the smooth muscle cells of the arterioles, the body's tiniest arteries. This relaxes the arterioles, lowering the resistance blood encounters as it flows through them and inhibiting signals through the RAA system that would cause blood pressure to rise. Doctors often prescribe valsartan in combination with a DIURETIC MEDICATION for optimal blood pressure control. Because valsartan's inhibitory effect on the RAA system can affect the blood pressure regulatory mechanisms of a developing unborn child and cause its death, women who are pregnant should not take valsartan or other angiotensin II antagonists. Side effects are uncommon but when they do occur may include DIZZINESS, nausea, and headache.

See also ANGIOTENSIN-CONVERTING ENZYME (ACE) INHIBITOR MEDICATIONS; ANTIHYPERTENSIVE MEDICATIONS; MEDICATIONS TO TREAT HEART DISEASE.

valve, heart   See HEART.

valve disease   Damage to or deterioration of the valves in the HEART. BLOOD flows through the heart in only one direction; the heart's four valves maintain this directional flow. There is a valve between each atrium and ventricle, and at the root of the artery that arises from each ventricle. These valves open and close in synchronization, like doors, through a blend of mechanical and electrical stimuli to allow blood to flow from one part of the heart to another.

- The tricuspid valve separates the right atrium and right ventricle. It opens when the right atrium contracts, allowing unoxygenated blood returning from the body to flow into the right ventricle, and closes when the right atrium's contraction ends.
- The pulmonary valve separates the right ventricle and the pulmonary artery. It opens when the right ventricle contracts, allowing the ventricle to pump unoxygenated blood to the lungs, and closes when the right ventricle's contraction ends.
- The mitral valve separates the left atrium and left ventricle. It opens when the left atrium contracts to send oxygenated blood to the left ventricle, and closes when the left atrium's contraction ends.

- The aortic valve separates the left ventricle and the aorta. It opens when the left ventricle pumps oxygenated blood to the body, and closes when the left ventricle's contraction ends.

In the 1950s valve damage resulting from RHEUMATIC HEART DISEASE, associated with a streptococcal bacterial infection, was the leading cause of death due to heart disease among adults in the United States. With antibiotics that treat bacterial infections to prevent heart valve damage and operations to replace heart valves that are damaged, valve disease no longer is so deadly and now accounts for only about 3,500 deaths each year in the United States. Valve disease can affect the leaflets of the valve, the myocardial tissue that gives rise to the valve, or the fibrous cords that support the valve's functioning.

Valve disease can be acquired, as in the case of rheumatic heart disease and other infections, or congenital, and can affect any valve or multiple valves. HEART ATTACK (MYOCARDIAL INFARCTION) is another significant cause of valve damage, especially to the mitral valve. Acquired valve disease most commonly affects the aortic valve and the mitral valve; damage to the tricuspid and pulmonary valves is often congenital. Valve disease may not show symptoms until the valve's function becomes significantly compromised, and even then may manifest as HEART FAILURE or CARDIOMYOPATHY with symptoms such as shortness of breath (DYSPNEA) and CHEST PAIN (ANGINA) with exertion. ARRHYTHMIAS also are common with valve disorders.

Stenosis   STENOSIS of a valve exists when there is a narrowing or constricture of the valve's structure that restricts the amount of blood that can flow through the valve when it is open. The leaflets may be irregularly shaped (congenital stenosis) or contain calcifications, scar tissue from infection, or fibrous deposits that causes them to become stiff or partially fused (acquired stenosis). Though the valve opens incompletely, it usually closes properly. Tricuspid valve stenosis is generally a consequence of rheumatic heart disease and often occurs in combination with mitral valve stenosis, which also generally is acquired. Aortic valve stenosis and pulmonary valve stenosis are nearly always congenital malformations that may involve fused or malformed leaflets (the flaps of the valve that separate to allow blood to pass).

Regurgitation In valvular regurgitation, also called valve insufficiency, damage to the valve's structure prevents the valve from closing properly. This allows blood to leak back into the heart chamber from which it has come. The greater the insufficiency, the smaller the volume of blood that moves forward with each CARDIAC CYCLE. The heart pumps harder and faster to try to circulate an adequate supply of blood through the body, resulting in enlargement of the affected heart chamber and paving the way for heart failure and, especially when right-sided, PULMONARY HYPERTENSION. Regurgitation most commonly affects the mitral valve.

Prolapse Prolapse occurs when one of a valve's leaflets, or flaps, is elongated or becomes stretched or distended and bulges back into the atrium or the ventricle after shutting. A prolapsed valve often opens and closes properly, so it functions to the extent that it prevents blood from backflowing. MITRAL VALVE PROLAPSE (MVP) is the most common manifestation of valvular prolapse. MVP often runs in families, suggesting that there is a genetic component that allows weakness or a mild malformation to exist. MVP also is more common in people who have scoliosis, a deformity of the spine, and MARFAN SYNDROME, a disorder of connective tissue. In many people who have MVP the condition remains mild and requires no treatment; in some people it can progress to mitral valve regurgitation in which surgical intervention becomes necessary.

Symptoms and Diagnostic Path

A HEART MURMUR that the doctor can hear when listening to the heart through a STETHOSCOPE often is the first clue that valve disease or damage may be present. Each type of valve disorder (stenosis, regurgitation, prolapse) has a characteristic sound. An ECHOCARDIOGRAM, which uses ULTRASOUND (high-frequency sound waves) to generate images of the structure and function of the heart, can detect most valve disease and damage. When necessary the cardiologist can perform CARDIAC CATHETERIZATION to more accurately visualize the flow of blood through the chambers and vessels of the heart as well as through the CORONARY ARTER-

IES. ELECTROCARDIOGRAM (ECG) can highlight electrical irregularities in the cardiac cycle that point to valve problems as the source of arrhythmias, and MAGNETIC RESONANCE IMAGING (MRI) can present three-dimensional images of the heart in action, providing additional information to confirm the diagnosis and extent of the valve disorder.

Treatment Options and Outlook

Mild heart valve disorders often do not require treatment beyond careful monitoring. When treatment is necessary, there are three therapeutic paths available.

- **Medication** In some situations medications can support more efficient functioning of the heart, though drugs cannot remedy valve disease or damage. Medication might be the cardiologist's treatment of choice when the valve problem is minor or when surgery is not a viable option.

- **Valve repair** A cardiologist often can repair minor valve problems, particularly stenosis, through cardiac catheterization (also called percutaneous valvuloplasty), which is less invasive than OPEN-HEART SURGERY. Balloon valvuloplasty is one technique that allows the cardiologist to thread a tiny balloon through a blood vessel and into the heart. Using FLUOROSCOPY (real-time moving X-ray) for guidance, the cardiologist places the balloon in the opening of the stenotic valve and gently inflates it with liquid, pressing the valve open. Surgical repairs that can be done via open-heart surgery include suturing (sewing) together the edges of leaflets that have become distorted or that have minor structural anomalies and removal of calcifications and deposits.

- **Valve replacement** Replacing the defective or damaged valve is the only way to correct most valve disorders, and it requires open-heart surgery in which the surgeon stops the heart to open it and expose the damaged valve or valves. Replacement valves can be mechanical prostheses, ALLOGRAFTS (human donor), XENOGRAFTS (porcine or bovine tissue valves), and occasionally AUTOGRAFTS (one's own tissue) when reconstructing certain congenital malformations.

Medications to strengthen the heart and improve pumping efficiency can compensate for an inefficient valve for a period of time though cannot correct the valve's damage. However, correction of most valve disease requires surgery; cardiovascular surgeons perform 96,000 operations each year in the United States to repair (valvuloplasty) or replace damaged valves. Untreated valve disease can result in cardiomyopathy and heart failure as the heart progressively loses pumping efficiency and the affected ventricle thickens and enlarges to compensate.

Generally, people who have valve disease or have had valve operations need to take antibiotics before dental and surgical procedures to reduce the risk of infection. Some people also may need to take ANTICOAGULANT MEDICATIONS ("blood thinners") to prevent blood clots from forming on or around the valves; mechanical valves are particularly vulnerable to clot formation. It also is prudent to make appropriate lifestyle modifications to reduce as much as possible the risk factors for heart disease, to minimize stress on the valves and the heart.

Risk Factors and Preventive Measures

Most valve disease occurs in people over the age of 60; a small percentage of valve disease is congenital. Valve disease may also develop as a result of infection (bacterial or viral) that affects the heart valves, such as rheumatic fever and ENDOCARDITIS. Prompt diagnosis and treatment of strep throat is a crucial preventive measure for acquired valve disease. Cigarette smoking, hyperlipidemia (elevated blood lipids), untreated or poorly controlled hypertension, INSULIN RESISTANCE, and family history of heart disease are additional risk factors.

See also ANTIBIOTIC PROPHYLAXIS; AUSCULTATION; COAGULATION; ENDOCARDITIS; FIBROELASTOMA; LIVING WITH HEART DISEASE; RHEUMATIC HEART DISEASE; SURGERY TO TREAT CARDIOVASCULAR DISEASE; VALVE REPAIR AND REPLACEMENT.

valve repair and replacement Operations to correct damage, either acquired or congenital, to the HEART valves. The first mechanical valve replacement operations were performed in 1960, establishing a new avenue of treatment for VALVE DISEASE. Today valve repair and replacement operations have relegated valve damage and disease to the venue of routine cardiovascular problems; with treatment, valve conditions seldom cause health problems or interfere with the activities a person enjoys.

Valve Repair

Surgeons began trying to repair faulty heart valves in the 1920s, using hooklike cutting tools called valvotomes to release adhesions, scarring, and calcifications. The surgeon inserted the valvotome through an incision in the chest and into the aorta or the pulmonary artery, depending on the valve affected. The method, called commissurotomy or valvotomy, opened stenotic valves by cutting through fused or calcified valve leaflets, improving the flow of blood through the valve. However, the procedure often had a less than ideal outcome as the surgeon could not see the valve and sometimes created other valve problems, such as regurgitation, in which the valve allowed significant backflow of BLOOD. As well, infection was a serious consequence as antibiotics had not yet been discovered. Surgeons were not yet able to stop the heart for operations as the HEART-LUNG BYPASS MACHINE was only in its preliminary design stages, so surgery was typically a treatment of last resort before the 1960s.

When the heart-lung bypass machine and antibiotics made extended operations on the heart possible, surgeons could repair not only stenotic valves but also prolapsed and regurgitating valves. It became practical to patch tears in the valve leaflets, shorten or fortify the fibrous tendrils (the chordae tendinae) that tense and relax to facilitate valve function, reconstruct malformed leaflets, remove calcium and atherosclerotic deposits from valve leaflets, and reinforce the anchoring myocardial tissue bed where the valve attaches to the heart. The operations pioneered in the early 20th century have become refined and remain among the surgeon's repertoire today.

Valve Replacement

Valve repair has its limitations, however, and following World War II researchers turned their efforts to designing mechanical valves that could replace damaged heart valves. Many new materials such as Teflon, Dacron, Lucite, and Silicon—strong, lightweight composites—emerged from the military-oriented research of the war period. Doctors and engineers collaborated to bring a different dimension of usefulness to military technology. Among them were two Americans, cardiovascular surgeon Albert Starr and engineer Lowell Edwards, whose inventions were in widespread use in various industries including aerospace and forestry. The two met in Portland, Oregon, in 1958, and two years later debuted the Starr-Edwards ball valve for treating MITRAL STENOSIS. The design looked nothing like a natural heart valve but instead featured a steel ball that moved back and forth on a limited travel within a four-strut Lucite cage. The second person to receive a Starr-Edwards prototype prosthetic valve lived for 15 years with the replacement mitral valve (the first died shortly after surgery from an air embolism, a risk of heart-lung bypass).

A number of other researchers explored the viability of the ball-and-cage design, but it was Starr and Edwards who created a functional prototype. A modified version of their design remains the most commonly used ball valve today. Two other designs present surgeons with options: the double leaflet prosthetic valve, which looks and functions more like a natural heart valve, developed by cardiovascular pioneer Clarence Lillehei, M.D. (the St. Jude Medical heart valve remains in widespread use today); and the disc valve, which features a small disc that tilts forward to allow blood to flow past and then returns to an upright or "closed" position to stop blood flow. Each has its advantages and disadvantages; choice depends on what valve is diseased or damaged and the nature and extent of that damage.

Other sources for prosthetic valves include human donor valves (harvested from DONOR HEARTS that cannot be used for HEART TRANSPLANT) and valves crafted from a blend of synthetic materials and heart valves harvested from pig (porcine) or cow (bovine) hearts that are specially treated and prepared to reduce the likelihood of recipient rejection. These are called biological or bioprosthetic valves. Mechanical prosthetic valves are incredibly durable though are prone to blood clot formations on their structures; people who receive mechanical

valves generally take ANTICOAGULANT MEDICATIONS for the rest of their lives. Bioprosthetic valves are not as likely to develop clots though are not as durable; people who receive bioprosthetic valves typically need to have them replaced after 10 or 15 years. For this reason, age becomes a factor when determining which kind of replacement valve is most appropriate for an individual.

People who have valve disease or have had heart valves replaced need to take antibiotics before dental and medical procedures in which there is a chance of bleeding, as heart valves are particularly vulnerable to infection from bacteria that enter the bloodstream in such ways. This originally consisted of taking antibiotics for a few days before and up to two weeks after the procedure, though the current practice is to administer one dose of antibiotics one hour before the procedure.

See also ANTIBIOTIC PROPHYLAXIS; CARDIOVASCULAR SYSTEM; LIVING WITH HEART DISEASE; QUALITY OF LIFE; SURGERY TO TREAT CARDIOVASCULAR DISEASE.

valvuloplasty See VALVE REPAIR AND REPLACEMENT.

variant angina See ANGINA.

vasoconstriction Contraction of the smooth muscle cells in the walls of the arteries, causing the channel through which BLOOD flows to become narrower. Vasoconstriction is a normal physiological action that is part of the body's mechanisms for regulating BLOOD PRESSURE and blood flow. When blood volume, HEART RATE, or blood pressure itself falls, the body releases hormones, primarily EPINEPHRINE and NOREPINEPHRINE, that cause the smooth muscle cells to contract. In health this is a transient effect; the cells return to a normal state when there no longer is a need for the artery to be constricted.

The body also initiates peripheral vasoconstriction to help regulate body temperature during exposure to cold by drawing more blood into the body's core. The mechanisms that regulate vasoconstriction, including smooth muscle cell response to stimulation, can become dysfunctional, in which case HYPERTENSION (high blood pressure) results. Many ANTIHYPERTENSIVE MEDICATIONS work by inhibiting the ability of smooth muscle cells in the arterial walls to contract to cause the arteries to relax and dilate (VASODILATION).

Doctors may administer VASOCONSTRICTOR MEDICATIONS during cardiovascular crisis or SHOCK to stimulate the body to raise blood pressure and heart rate. Some over-the-counter medications, notably those taken to relieve viral and allergy symptoms such as pseudoephedrine, as well as CAFFEINE and NICOTINE, have vasoconstrictive effects. Though temporary, such medication-induced vasoconstriction can have a deleterious effect on control of hypertension.

See also CIRCULATION; COLD/FLU MEDICATION AND HYPERTENSION; CARDIOVASCULAR SYSTEM; MEDICATIONS TO TREAT HEART DISEASE.

vasoconstrictor medications Drugs that cause the BLOOD vessels to tighten, usually by initiating contractions of the smooth muscle cells that line the vessel walls. Doctors administer vasoconstrictor medications, also called vasopressor drugs in reference to their effect of raising BLOOD PRESSURE, to treat CARDIOGENIC SHOCK and HYPOTENSION (low BLOOD PRESSURE). Midodrine (ProAmitine) is a vasoconstrictor medication commonly prescribed to treat orthostatic hypotension (a sudden drop in blood pressure upon rising from a lying position) that causes troublesome symptoms and does not respond to other measures. Because hypotension is secondary (results as a consequence of other health conditions) or a MEDICATION SIDE EFFECT, doctors do not usually prescribe vasoconstrictor medications to treat it unless other efforts to maintain adequate blood pressure are not effective.

Vasoconstrictor medications also might be administered to people with significant respiratory impairment such as asthma or CHRONIC OBSTRUCTIVE PULMONARY DISEASE (COPD), as many of these drugs (such as ALPHA AGONIST MEDICATIONS) have a bronchodilating effect even as they constrict peripheral blood vessels. Vasoconstriction is a concern in people who receive such medications for pulmonary distress who also have HYPERTENSION (high blood pressure), as the vasoconstrictive effect causes blood pressure to rise.

Over-the-counter medications taken to relieve the symptoms of congestion and cough, such as with colds and flu, often contain ingredients that act as vasoconstrictors in the body. These include the decongestant PSEUDOEPHEDRINE, the cough suppressant dextromethorphan, and the expectorant guiaifenesin. Products with topical decongestants such as nasal sprays that act to locally constrict the blood vessels in the nose and nasal passages also can have systemic effects. CAFFEINE in beverages such as coffee, tea, and colas is a vasoconstrictor, as is NICOTINE, the addictive primary chemical ingredient in tobacco (cigarette smoke). Consuming these substances can cause blood pressure and HEART RATE to rise.

See also ANTIHYPERTENSIVE MEDICATIONS; COLD/FLU MEDICATION AND HYPERTENSION; MEDICATIONS TO TREAT HEART DISEASE; VASOCONSTRICTION; VASODILATION; VASODILATOR MEDICATIONS.

vasodilation Relaxation of the smooth muscle cells in the walls of the arteries, widening the channel through which BLOOD flows. Vasodilation causes BLOOD PRESSURE to drop, a normal physiological response within the body's blood pressure regulatory mechanisms and a counterbalance to VASOCONSTRICTION (narrowing of the arteries) as well as a desired therapeutic effect of VASODILATOR MEDICATIONS. Vasodilation is also part of the body's temperature regulation mechanisms, bringing blood closer to the surface of the skin for cooling.

Vasodilation occurs when the body's regulatory mechanisms—functions within the brain stem as well as the RENIN-ANGIOTENSIN-ALDOSTERONE (RAA) HORMONAL SYSTEM—cause a reduction in the release of endogenous (natural to the body) vasoconstrictors such as EPINEPHRINE, NOREPINEPHRINE, and ANGIOTENSIN II. Many ANTIHYPERTENSIVE MEDICATIONS work by inhibiting the release of these substances or blocking their actions on the blood vessels.

See also CIRCULATION; CARDIOVASCULAR SYSTEM; VASOCONSTRICTOR MEDICATIONS; VASODILATOR MEDICATIONS.

vasodilator medications Medications taken to relax and widen the BLOOD vessels, which increases

VASODILATOR MEDICATIONS PRESCRIBED TO TREAT HEART DISEASE

Type of Medication	Common Medications	Conditions Prescribed to Treat
Alpha antagonist (blocker) medications	Doxazosin, prazosin, terazosin, clonidine, guanfacine, methyldopa	Hypertension
Angiotensin-converting enzyme (ACE) inhibitor medications	Benazepril, captopril, enalapril, fosinopril, lisinopril, moexipril, ramipril, trandolapril	Hypertension, heart failure
Angiotensin II receptor antagonist (blocker) medications	Candesartan, eprosartan, irbesartan, losartan, telmisartan, valsartan	Hypertension
Calcium channel antagonist (blocker) medications	Amlodipine, diltiazem, nifedepine, verapamil	Hypertension
Nitrate medications	Nitroglyerin, amyl nitrate, isosorbide	Angina

the volume of blood the arteries can carry and decreases the resistance blood encounters as it flows through them. Doctors typically prescribe vasodilator medications to treat HYPERTENSION (high BLOOD PRESSURE), ANGINA (CHEST PAIN resulting from ISCHEMIC HEART DISEASE [IHD] or CORONARY ARTERY DISEASE [CAD]), and PERIPHERAL VASCULAR DISEASE (PVD). There are several classifications of drugs that have vasodilator actions; each classification has benefits and risks relative to the conditions being treated. In general one risk of taking vasodilator medications is orthostatic HYPOTENSION, a sudden drop in blood pressure when changing position from lying down to sitting or standing.

See also ALPHA ANTAGONIST MEDICATIONS; ANGIOTENSIN-CONVERTING ENZYME (ACE) INHIBITOR MEDICATIONS; ANGIOTENSIN II RECEPTOR ANTAGONIST MEDICATIONS; CALCIUM CHANNEL ANTAGONIST MEDICATIONS; MEDICATION SIDE EFFECTS; MEDICATIONS TO TREAT HEART DISEASE; NITRATE MEDICATIONS.

vasovagal syncope See SYNCOPE.

vein See CARDIOVASCULAR SYSTEM.

vena cava See CARDIOVASCULAR SYSTEM.

venogram A procedure in which a contrast medium (dye) is injected into a vein to make the vein's structure visible on X-ray or FLUOROSCOPY (real-time moving X-ray). Doctors may use venogram to explore structural anomalies and dysfunctions of the veins as well as to diagnose DEEP VEIN THROMBOSIS (DVT) when noninvasive imaging technologies such as DOPPLER ULTRASOUND fail to produce conclusive results.

Procedure

For a venogram, the radiologist injects dye into the vein being investigated and then takes X-ray images of the dye as it flows through the vein. The resulting visualization can show areas of STENOSIS (narrowing), ATHEROSCLEROSIS (accumulations of fatty acids and other debris along the inside walls of the veins), varicosities and other malformations of vein structure, and incompetent valves. Though atherosclerosis is more commonly a condition affecting the arteries, it can involve all blood vessels including veins. A venogram takes 20 to 60 minutes, depending on the location and number of veins being examined.

Risks and Complications

Some people experience mild discomfort when the dye is injected; side effects and complications are rare.

Outlook and Lifestyle Modifications

Most people return to usual activities the following day.

See also ANGIOGRAPHY; CIRCULATION; COMPUTED TOMOGRAPHY (CT) SCAN; MAGNETIC RESONANCE IMAGING (MRI); ULTRASOUND.

ventricle See HEART.

ventricular bigeminy See PREMATURE VENTRICU-LAR CONTRACTIONS (PVCs).

ventricular fibrillation See ARRHYTHMIA.

ventricular septal defect (VSD) A congenital malformation of the HEART in which there is an abnormal opening in the wall, or septum, separating the right ventricle from the left ventricle. This allows unoxygenated BLOOD and oxygenated blood to mingle in both ventricles, reducing the oxygen content of the blood the left ventricle pumps out to the body and increasing the volume of blood the right ventricle contains. Blood migrates from the left to the right ventricle because the pressure is higher in the left ventricle; when the volume of blood becomes equalized the heart sends a greater amount of blood flowing to the lungs and increases the pressure in the arteries of the lungs. This is called PULMONARY HYPERTENSION, and when undetected and untreated it can cause permanent damage to the heart and the lungs.

Symptoms and Diagnostic Path

Large VSDs are detectable at birth because they have a very characteristic sound heard during AUSCULTATION (listening to the heart with a STETHO-SCOPE). Minor VSDs may escape detection until a later routine examination when the doctor hears the abnormal movement of blood. Diagnostic procedures to confirm the diagnosis may include chest X-ray, ELECTROCARDIOGRAM (ECG), and ECHOCARDIOGRAM.

Treatment Options and Outlook

Many VSDs require OPEN-HEART SURGERY to close or patch the opening, though minor VSDs may close on their own by the time the child is two or three years old. A cardiologist is likely to adopt an approach of watchful waiting for a VSD that causes no symptoms and appears to be getting smaller as the child gets older. VSD is one of the most common

congenital heart defects, accounting for as many as 30 percent of heart problems in newborns.

Adults who have detectable but untreated VSDs may have symptoms that cause them to seek a cardiologist's evaluation, with a diagnosis of pulmonary hypertension as well as right-sided HEART FAILURE. An untreated VSD that does not cause symptoms generally does not cause further heart disease, either, though many cardiologists recommend ANTIBIOTIC PROPHYLAXIS for any dental or surgical procedures (including invasive diagnostic testing such as CARDIAC CATHETERIZATION). Such procedures can permit bacteria to enter the bloodstream. Normally the body's immune system neutralizes the bacteria before they can cause infection; however, the heart valves are particularly vulnerable to infection when there are any abnormalities of structure affecting the heart.

Risk Factors and Preventive Measures

VSD is often associated with other heart malformations such as TETRALOGY OF FALLOT that are far more significant and require immediate treatment. VSD also is more common in children who have DOWN SYNDROME. VSD is a congenital heart defect for which there are no known preventive measures.

See also ATRIOVENTRICULAR CANAL DEFECT; CYANOTIC CONGENITAL HEART DISEASE; HEART DISEASE; HEART DISEASE IN CHILDREN; SEPTAL DEFECT.

ventricular tachycardia An ARRHYTHMIA in which the HEART's ventricles (lower chambers) beat excessively fast (more than 100 beats per minute) due to abnormal electrical activation. Underlying HEART DISEASE is the most common cause of ventricular tachycardia. Other causes include ELECTROLYTE imbalance, over-the-counter decongestants and cold preparations, CAFFEINE, energy drinks and products, illicit drugs such as COCAINE, and MEDICATIONS TO TREAT HEART DISEASE such as ANTIARRHYTHMIA MEDICATIONS taken for irregularities in the HEARTBEAT other than ventricular tachycardia. Ventricular tachycardia may also occur following HEART ATTACK or heart surgery (including ANGIOPLASTY). No matter what its cause, ventricular tachycardia is hazardous because the heart can only sustain it for a short time. Although often the heart restores itself to a normal rhythm, if it cannot then the tachycardia disintegrates into ventricular fibrillation, a pattern of chaotic, dysrhythmic electrical activity and contractions that is life-threatening.

Symptoms and Diagnostic Path

Symptoms of ventricular tachycardia typically include PALPITATIONS, LIGHT-HEADEDNESS, and shortness of breath (DYSPNEA). Some people also experience CHEST PAIN (ANGINA pectoris) and SYNCOPE (fainting). ELECTROCARDIOGRAM (ECG) during an episode of tachycardia confirms the diagnosis. When symptoms are intermittent, a HOLTER MONITOR that records heart activity over a period of time (typically 48 to seven hours) can capture the episodes and provide diagnostic information. Other diagnostic procedures may be necessary to find the underlying cause of the tachycardia and may include EXERCISE STRESS TEST (or pharmacological stress test for those who cannot tolerate exercise stress testing), ECHOCARDIOGRAM, and ELECTROPHYSIOLOGY STUDIES.

Treatment Options and Outlook

Sustained ventricular tachycardia is life-threatening and requires immediate treatment, which might include IV administration of antiarrhythmia medications or CARDIOVERSION (administration of electrical shock) to interrupt the dysfunctional electrical activity in the heart and restore a normal rhythm. Treatment for intermittent ventricular tachycardia may be with antiarrhythmia medications or, because of the high risk for serious side effects with these drugs, an IMPLANTABLE CARDIOVERTER DEFIBRILLATOR (ICD). An ICD is similar to a PACEMAKER, with very thin wires (leads) going into the heart to automatically detect the tachycardia and administer an electrical shock to stop it. Other treatments may be necessary for underlying heart conditions.

Risk Factors and Preventive Measures

CORONARY ARTERY DISEASE (CAD), ISCHEMIC HEART DISEASE (IHD), CARDIOMYOPATHY, and HEART FAILURE are among the underlying heart conditions associated with ventricular tachycardia. Other risk factors include illicit drug use, excessive caffeine consumption, and chronic use of stimulants such as appetite suppressants and decongestants. Stopping the use of substances that cause the tachycardia also stops the tachycardia in most people. Preventive measures to lower the risk for heart disease overall are important.

See also AUTOMATED EXTERNAL DEFIBRILLATOR (AED); CARDIOVASCULAR EVENT; DRUG ABUSE AND HEART DISEASE; LIFESTYLE AND HEART HEALTH; MEDICATION SIDE EFFECTS; MEDICATIONS TO TREAT HEART DISEASE; SUDDEN CARDIAC ARREST; SURGERY TO TREAT CARDIOVASCULAR DISEASE.

ventricular trigeminy See PREMATURE VENTRICULAR CONTRACTIONS (PVCs).

verapamil A medication taken to treat HYPERTENSION (high BLOOD PRESSURE), ANGINA, and certain ARRHYTHMIAS. Verapamil belongs to the family of drugs called CALCIUM CHANNEL ANTAGONIST MEDICATIONS. It works by slowing the exchange of calcium during the CARDIAC CYCLE, which in turn slows the HEART RATE. By regulating the flow of ions (electrically charged particles), verapamil also stabilizes the heart's electrical activity and rhythm. Brand-name products available in the United States include Isoptin, Isoptin SR, Calan, Calan SR, Covera, Covera SR, Verelan, Verelan HS, Verelan PM; generic versions also are available. "SR" denotes sustained release formulations that dissolve in the gastrointestinal system over a period of time at a steady and predictable rate; "PM" and "HS" are delayed release formulations intended to be taken once daily at bedtime as treatment for hypertension.

Most people need to build up to, or titrate to, the dose that provides relief from symptoms. It is important to follow the dosages schedule, and to titrate back down when stopping verapamil. Verapamil interacts with certain chemotherapy (anticancer) drugs as well as some ANTIARRHYTHMIA MEDICATIONS, some ANTIHYPERTENSIVE MEDICATIONS, and DIGOXIN (taken to treat HEART FAILURE and arrhythmias). Side effects may include nausea, CONSTIPATION, headache, and SLEEP DISTURBANCES. It is important to let the doctor and the pharmacist know of all other medications being taken, prescription and over-the-counter (including herbal remedies), to check for potential interactions before beginning verapamil therapy.

See also MEDICATIONS TO TREAT HEART DISEASE.

very low-density lipoprotein (VLDL) See CHOLESTEROL, BLOOD.

Viagra See PDE5 INHIBITOR MEDICATIONS.

vital signs The term for key measurements of bodily function that help to ascertain relative health status. Typically vital signs include HEART RATE (PULSE rate), body temperature, BLOOD PRESSURE, breathing rate, and body height and weight. Body weight is particularly important for people who have HEART FAILURE as weight gain is one of the earliest indicators of fluid retention (EDEMA), a key factor in assessing the heart's pumping effectiveness because fluid accumulates in body tissues when the heart's pumping efficiency is diminished. Though doctors do not perform ELECTROCARDIOGRAM (ECG) as a routine procedure, people who have diagnosed HEART DISEASE often receive an ECG with routine visits to the cardiologist. Vital signs generally are taken at each visit to the doctor, regardless of the reason for the visit. This establishes a process for routine assessment of basic health.

Vital signs also help to provide monitoring of status and improvement following invasive diagnostic procedures (such as ANGIOGRAPHY), surgical procedures, and cardiovascular crises such as HEART ATTACK and STROKE. Within the range of normal readings for vital signs, each individual has his or her baseline. Doctors use both to determine general health status; deviations help to identify potential health concerns and to direct diagnostic efforts. A rapid, weak pulse with increased breathing rate and an elevated temperature suggests an infection, for example, while a rapid, weak pulse with no other deviations in vital signs may indicate a cardiovascular concern. Blood pressure that is elevated independent of changes in other vital signs may suggest HYPERTENSION (high blood pres-

sure). Inconsistent or erratic pulse may point to ARRHYTHMIAS.

See also CARDIOVASCULAR SYSTEM; HEART.

vitamin and mineral supplements Products containing natural or synthesized vitamins and minerals taken to bolster the nutrients provided through diet. Most healthy adults receive the vitamins and minerals their bodies need through the foods they eat. People who have HEART DISEASE, and especially those who are taking medications to treat their cardiovascular conditions, may not receive adequate nutrition through diet alone. Some medications deplete vitamin and mineral stores in the body or interfere with the absorption of nutrients. The reverse can also occur, with vitamins and minerals taken as dietary supplements interfering with the absorption of certain MEDICATIONS TO TREAT HEART DISEASE. People taking WARFARIN or other ANTICOAGULANT MEDICATIONS should not take supplements containing vitamin K, for example, as vitamin K affects the blood's clotting capability.

There is much speculation, though not an equitable level of objective evidence, that ANTIOXIDANT vitamins—notably vitamins C and E—reduce the risk for heart disease by decreasing the presence of FREE RADICALS in the body. Many health researchers believe free radicals (molecular debris remaining after METABOLISM) are responsible for most disease processes including those that result in nearly all forms of acquired heart disease. Antioxidants, which are metabolic components of many vitamins, attach to free radicals to allow them to be eliminated from the body as waste. Numerous clinical research studies have failed to provide conclusive evidence that such action helps to slow or prevent the development of heart disease. Recent research suggests vitamin B and folic acid supplements may actually increase the risk of heart disease.

Because mineral supplements are in salt forms, it is important to discuss their possible interference with medications being taken to treat conditions such as HYPERTENSION (high BLOOD PRESSURE) and HEART FAILURE for which doctors often prescribe diuretic medications ("water pills"). Diuretics alter the body's balance of electrolytes; it is important to know the amounts of minerals such as MAGNESIUM and POTASSIUM, which function as electrolytes in the body, that nutritional supplements contain. Generally, it is best to forgo vitamin and mineral supplement products (including HERBAL REMEDIES containing them) unless the doctor recommends or at least approves them. The American Heart Asso-ciation, along with other experts in heart health, recommends that people instead emphasize eating foods that are high in nutritional value to provide the body with needed vitamins and minerals.

See also COENZYME Q-10; DASH DIET; LIFESTYLE AND HEART HEALTH; NUTRITION AND DIET; ORNISH PROGRAM.

waist circumference The distance around the midsection, measured between the crests of the hip bones and the umbilicus (belly button). Waist circumference is a key indicator of abdominal adiposity, a pattern of fat distribution within the torso that is strongly linked with HEART DISEASE and increased risk for HEART ATTACK. A waist circumference of 35 inches or more for women and 40 inches or more for men is considered a risk factor for heart disease. To measure waist circumference:

- Remove clothing from around the waist area.
- Stand in a relaxed position.
- Locate the crest of the hip bones on the sides of the waist.
- Place a cloth measuring tape around the waist between the hip bones and the umbilicus (belly button).
- Pull the tape snug but not tight, and note the point where the end recontacts the measure. This is the distance around the waist or waist circumference.

If a cloth tape measure is not available, use a thick length of nonstretching string or cord to wrap around the waist. Note the point where the end recontacts the string. Measure the distance between the start of the string and the contact point using a ruler, yardstick, or conventional tape measure. This is the waist circumference. A large waist circumference often is associated with OBESITY, another risk factor for heart disease. Weight loss typically reduces waist circumference, lowering cardiovascular risk.

See also BODY MASS INDEX (BMI); BODY SHAPE AND HEART DISEASE; EXERCISE; LIFESTYLE AND HEART HEALTH; NUTRITION AND DIET; WAIST-TO-HIP RATIO; WEIGHT MANAGEMENT.

waist-to-hip ratio The relationship between the distance around the waist (waist circumference) and the distance around the hips at their broadest point. Waist-to-hip ratio is an important indicator of the risk for HEART DISEASE and HEART ATTACK; it can identify abdominal adiposity (a fat distribution pattern associated with HEART disease) in people who may not be overweight or obese yet have excessive body fat in the torso. A waist-to-hip ratio greater than 1.0 in men or greater than 0.8 in women is considered a risk factor for heart disease. To determine waist-to-hip ratio:

- Remove clothing from the waist and hips.
- Stand in a relaxed position.
- Measure the distance around the waist (see WAIST CIRCUMFERENCE entry for instructions on how to measure the waist).
- Use a cloth measuring tape to measure the distance around the hips at their widest point. Pull the tape snug but not tight and note the measurement at which the end recontacts the tape.
- Divide the waist measurement by the hip measurement.

For example, a waist measurement of 37 inches and a hip measurement of 41 inches gives a waist-to-hip ratio of 0.9. This example measurement is within the range of healthy for a man though suggests an increased risk of heart disease for a woman. There is some evidence that waist-to-hip ratio is more indicative of increased risk for stroke and waist circumference more indicative of increased risk for heart attack; both clearly correlate to an increased risk for cardiovascular disease.

See also BODY MASS INDEX (BMI); BODY SHAPE AND HEART DISEASE; EXERCISE; LIFESTYLE AND HEART HEALTH; NUTRITION AND DIET; WEIGHT MANAGEMENT.

walking   One of the most effective forms of aerobic EXERCISE. Health experts say that walking at a moderate pace for 30 to 45 minutes at a time at least five days a week is adequate physical EXERCISE for most people to maintain the health of the HEART and CARDIOVASCULAR SYSTEM. Walking has many advantages that make it an easy and manageable choice for physical exercise, key among them being that it can be integrated into most routine daily activities and requires no special equipment, gear, or preparation beyond comfortable clothing and supportive shoes. Walking at any pace benefits the cardiovascular system and health overall; walking at a rapid pace for 20 minutes at a time or longer results in an aerobic workout that provides even greater benefit.

Health experts encourage people to engage in whatever physical activities they enjoy, the point being to get the body in motion. People whose lifestyles are sedentary (without physical activity) or who have diagnosed HEART DISEASE should check with their doctors or have a health examination before initiating a new routine of physical exercise, including walking at a more strenuous level than that to which they are accustomed. As fitness level improves, it will be possible to walk longer distances or to walk at a faster pace if desired. Regular physical activity can affect the way the body metabolizes certain medications, as can weight loss that results. It is important to have the doctor review medications after six months of regular exercise or a significant weight loss (10 percent or greater). Some people find that they can reduce and sometimes eliminate medications taken to treat mild to moderate HYPERTENSION and non-insulin-dependent type 2 diabetes. This should be done only under the close supervision of a doctor.

See also AEROBIC CAPACITY; HEART RATE; LIFESTYLE AND HEART HEALTH.

warfarin   An ANTICOAGULANT MEDICATION taken to prevent BLOOD clots (thromboemboli) from forming. The most common brand-name product available in the United States is Coumadin. Doctors prescribe warfarin for people who have, have had, or are predisposed to having atrial fibrillation, DEEP VEIN THROMBOSIS (DVT), thromboembolism (sometimes called thrombophlebitis), ischemic STROKE, TRANSIENT ISCHEMIC ATTACK (TIA), HEART ATTACK, or pulmonary EMBOLISM. People who have mechanical heart valves may also take warfarin to reduce the risk for clots from forming on the synthetic components of these prosthetic replacement devices. Warfarin interferes with vitamin K's activation of certain clotting factors (clotting factors II, VII, IX, and X) in the blood, slowing the formation of blood clots. However warfarin, like other anticoagulant medications, cannot dissolve blood clots that have already formed.

It takes about three days after initiation of warfarin therapy to reach therapeutic blood levels for anticoagulation, and each dose of warfarin remains active in the body for three to five days. Doctors may begin anticoagulation therapy with HEPARIN injections to establish an immediate environment of reduced clotting ability, then follow with oral warfarin for extended anticoagulant effect. Regular blood tests to monitor blood clotting times are important as warfarin has a narrow therapeutic index (the margin of toxicity is narrow). The primary risk of warfarin therapy is bleeding and hemorrhage. Easy bruising, nosebleeds, cuts that take a long time to stop bleeding, persistent cough without signs of viral infection, and unexplained pain can by symptoms of excessive anticoagulation and should be reported to the doctor immediately.

Numerous lifestyle factors influence warfarin blood levels. Changes in the amounts of foods consumed that are high in vitamin K, such as spinach and broccoli, alters the effectiveness of warfarin; eating more such foods diminishes warfarin's effectiveness and eating fewer such foods allows warfarin levels in the blood to rise. Conditions that decrease the body's ability to produce vitamin K, such as extended diarrhea or liver disease, conversely increase warfarin's actions. The list of other medications that alter warfarin levels is extensive; people taking warfarin should not take other medications, prescription or over-the-counter, without first checking with their doctors or pharmacists. It is essential to identify all products being taken when initiating warfarin therapy, including prescription and over-the-counter medications as well as herbal remedies and vitamin and mineral supplements.

Side effects in general are uncommon with warfarin. A rare though serious side effect of warfarin therapy is called "purple toes syndrome"; the walking surfaces of the toes develop a mottled purple appearance that blanches with pressure. This sign signals significant interference with coagulation beyond that intended for therapeutic purposes and requires immediate medical attention. Warfarin therapy is an effective means of maintaining anticoagulation status to prevent the formation of blood clots and is one of the most commonly used therapeutic approaches for prophylactic anticoagulation. However, it requires close monitoring and careful attention to dosing for the duration of therapy.

See also COAGULATION; MEDICATIONS TO TREAT HEART DISEASE; NUTRITION AND DIET; VALVE REPAIR AND REPLACEMENT; VITAMIN AND MINERAL SUPPLEMENTS.

Washkansky, Louis   Recipient of the first HEART TRANSPLANT. Washkansky was a 53-year-old South African dentist whose diabetes had resulted in severe HEART FAILURE. A patient of pioneering heart surgeon CHRISTIAAN BARNARD in Capetown, South Africa, and dying from his HEART condition, Washkansky agreed to let Barnard try the radical treatment. The heart of 25-year-old DENISE DARVALL became available when the young woman suffered extensive brain injuries in an automobile accident, and on December 3, 1967, Barnard and a team of surgeons removed Washkansky's badly damaged heart and replaced it with Darvall's healthy heart. Washkansky lived only 18 days with the transplanted heart before pneumonia overwhelmed his immune system and he died. The operation opened the door to a new approach for treating otherwise untreatable HEART DISEASE, and by the 1980s heart transplant had become an accepted therapeutic approach.

See also ALLOGRAFT; COOLEY, DENTON; DEVRIES, WILLIAM C.; DONOR HEART; HEART-LUNG TRANSPLANT; JARVIK, ROBERT; LEFT VENTRICULAR ASSIST DEVICE (LVAD); SURGERY TO TREAT CARDIOVASCULAR DISEASE.

water pill   See DIURETIC MEDICATIONS.

weight management   Maintaining a body weight that supports cardiovascular and overall health. Current health statistics indicate that nearly two-thirds of the adult population in the United States is overweight (BMI between 25 and 29) and a third is obese (BMI greater than 29). Excess body weight (excess body fat) is a known contributor to numerous health conditions including type 2 diabetes and many forms of HEART DISEASE including HYPERTENSION (high BLOOD PRESSURE), ATHEROSCLEROSIS, CORONARY ARTERY DISEASE (CAD), and PERIPHERAL VASCULAR DISEASE (PVD). OBESITY now is considered an independent risk factor for heart disease and particularly for HEART ATTACK and STROKE.

Weight Loss

A small weight loss of 10 to 20 pounds can result in a decrease in blood pressure of 10 mm Hg or more; for people with mild to moderate hypertension, this can be enough to reduce or eliminate ANTIHYPERTENSIVE MEDICATIONS (which should be done only with the doctor's approval and supervision). Such a level of weight loss also dramatically improves insulin sensitivity among cells throughout the body, lowering the risk for diabetes. The most effective way to lose weight and keep it off is through lifestyle changes that incorporate nutritious eating habits with daily physical exercise.

Methods that often do *not* achieve the desired results include:

- **Fad and very low calorie diets**   Though restrictive diets may result in short-term weight loss, they are difficult as well as unhealthy to maintain and fail to establish nutritious eating habits.
- **Appetite suppressant medications**   Drugs that suppress the urge to eat can provide a short-term boost to efforts to reduce the amount of food consumed. However, those that are effective act on neurotransmitters in the brain and produce other, less desired consequences such as mood swings and dependence on the drug.

Appetite suppressant medications generally are stimulants, which can affect the HEART AND CARDIOVASCULAR SYSTEM. None of the prescription appetite suppressants currently on the market can be taken for longer than 12 months because of the risk for potentially harmful side effects. Over-the-counter appetite suppressant products typically contain CAFFEINE and other stimulant-type substances. These products are harmful to people who have hypertension, HEART FAILURE, ARRHYTHMIAS, and other forms of heart disease.

- **Gastric reduction surgery**   Generally reserved for people who need to lose 100 pounds or more, gastric reduction surgery reduces the volume of food the stomach can hold. Some procedures, such as gastric banding, are intended to be temporary. Others are permanent. Though initial results can be significant, such methods are fraught with potential health hazards including the risk of infection from surgery and various gastrointestinal and nutritional disturbances. As well the stomach can eventually distend (stretch) to accommodate nearly the normal volume of food in just a few years.

Methods that *do* work for weight loss and sustained weight management include:

- nutritious eating habits that emphasize fruits, vegetables, and whole grains and whole grain products; appropriate portion sizes; and low-fat foods.
- daily physical EXERCISE (30 to 45 minutes).

Weight Gain

In people who have heart disease, unexplained weight gain is an important symptom that can signal the development or worsening of heart failure. Weight gain is one of the early indications of edema, the abnormal accumulation of fluid in the tissues of the body. People with New York Heart Association (NYHA) category II and III heart failure often are instructed to weigh themselves several times daily to help monitor fluid accumulation. EDEMA also occurs as a side effect of some medications. Unexplained weight gain should be reported to the doctor.

See also BODY MASS INDEX (BMI); DIABETES AND HEART DISEASE; LIFESTYLE AND HEART HEALTH; MEDICATION SIDE EFFECTS.

Welchol   See COLESEVELAM.

Wenckebach phenomenon   A type of HEART BLOCK, also called ATRIOVENTRICULAR (AV) NODE block or Mobitz I block, with a characteristic set of symptoms and ELECTROCARDIOGRAM (ECG) findings. Heart block is a disorder of conduction, or the way in which electrical impulses move through the HEART. The AV node is a cluster of specialized cells in the heart that functions as a circuit breaker between the atria (heart's upper chambers) and the ventricles (heart's lower chambers). With each CARDIAC CYCLE, the AV node gathers and momentarily holds the wave of electrical impulses that causes the atria to contract. This momentary delay allows the ventricles to completely fill with BLOOD and also refocuses the heart's electrical energy. When the AV node discharges, the wave of electrical impulses activates the ventricles in a synchronized pattern for maximum efficiency in contraction. With Wenckebach phenomenon, there is a progressive increased delay, called a lengthening PR interval, before the AV node discharges the electrical impulse to contract the ventricles, until the heart misses an entire beat (called a dropped QRS complex).

Symptoms and Diagnostic Path

Wenckebach phenomenon is a second-degree block, which means it causes symptoms and they are intermittent. Symptoms usually begin suddenly and may include episodes of LIGHT-HEADEDNESS, DIZZINESS, nausea, or SYNCOPE (fainting). Diagnosis is primarily by ECG, which shows the characteristic progressive increase in the PR interval. The cardiologist may request other diagnostic procedures if underlying HEART DISEASE is suspected.

Treatment Options and Outlook

Treatment depends on symptoms and may include no treatment other than regular follow-up visits, medications to help regulate the heart rate such as ADENOSINE or DILTIAZEM, or the implantation of a PACEMAKER. When other heart disease, such as CORONARY ARTERY DISEASE (CAD) or VALVE DISEASE, is the cause of the ARRHYTHMIA, treatment for those conditions may eliminate the heart block. With appropriate treatment, most people are able to enjoy regular activities and a normal lifestyle.

Risk Factors and Preventive Measures

In about half of people with Wenckebach phenomenon, underlying heart disease, and especially MYOCARDIAL INFARCTION (MI), is the cause. In the rest, the CONDUCTION PATHWAY dysfunction may be congenital (present from birth), may result from the formation of fibrous tissue in the area of the AV node (such as following OPEN-HEART SURGERY), or may be an undesired MEDICATION SIDE EFFECT from medications such as DIGITOXIN, ADENOSINE, DILTIAZEM, and BETA ANTAGONIST MEDICATIONS.

See also LENERGE-LEV DISEASE; MEDICATIONS TO TREAT HEART DISEASE.

wine See ALCOHOL CONSUMPTION AND HEART DISEASE.

Wolff-Parkinson-White (WPW) syndrome A disorder of HEART rhythm in which there is an extra, or accessory, conduction path from the atrium to the ventricle. This causes a loop of electrical activation to form, called atrioventricular REENTRY, where electricity travels from the atrium through the Kent bundle to the ventricle, then traveling the wrong way (antidromic) through the atrioventricular (AV) node back to the atrium. This rhythm can be mistaken for VENTRICULAR TACHYCARDIA on an ELECTROCARDIOGRAM (ECG).

Symptoms and Diagnostic Path

Symptoms, when they occur, include PALPITATIONS and DIZZINESS; many people who have Wolff-Parkinson-White syndrome do not have symptoms. Rather, the doctor discovers the condition during evaluation for other health problems or routine health examination. Wolff-Parkinson-White syndrome produces characteristic ECG patterns that reveal the accessory pathway. The condition generally manifests in people under age 50 and can affect those in their teens. Researchers do not know what causes the congenital accessory pathway that characterizes this ARRHYTHMIA disorder to become active, and there is no known way to prevent Wolff-Parkinson-White syndrome from developing.

Treatment Options and Outlook

Treatment targets disrupting the accessory conduction path so that electrical activation must take the normal path from the atrium to the ventricles. It may consist of taking ANTIARRHYTHMIA MEDICATIONS or undergoing RADIOFREQUENCY CATHETER ABLATION. The antiarrhythmics ADENOSINE (Adenocard) and procainamide (Procan) are the medications of choice when cardiologists choose the medication route. However, these medications can cause serious side effects including life-threatening arrhythmias different from those being treated. With radiofrequency ablation, an invasive procedure conducted via cardiac catheterization, the cardiologist uses bursts of radiofrequency energy to ablate, or kill, cells along the accessory conduction pathway. This results in scar tissue that usually forms a permanent barrier across the accessory conduction pathway to prevent it from conveying electrical impulses. For most people in whom Wolff-Parkinson-White syndrome causes symptoms or serious ECG anomalies, radiofrequency ablation is the treatment of choice as it eliminates the need for medications.

Risk Factors and Preventive Measures

Because the accessory pathway responsible for Wolff-Parkinson-White syndrome is congenital, it is important for people with a family history of the syndrome to receive regular cardiology evaluations to determine whether they, too, have it and if so to receive appropriate treatment. However, there are no known measures to prevent Wolff-Parkinson-White syndrome from developing.

See also BRUGADA SYNDROME; LIVING WITH HEART DISEASE; MEDICATIONS TO TREAT HEART DISEASE; REENTRY; SUDDEN CARDIAC ARREST (SCA).

women and heart disease For decades HEART DISEASE has been thought of as a man's disease. Though men are more likely than women to develop HEART disease in their 40s and 50s, overall more women than men are diagnosed with and die from heart disease. Though deaths due to CARDIOVASCULAR DISEASE (CVD) among men have steadily declined since 1979, deaths due to CVD among women surpassed those of men in 1983 and have continued to rise. Women who have HEART ATTACKS seem to suffer more extensive damage and are more likely to die from their heart attacks or to experience subsequent heart attacks within the five years following the first heart attack. HEART FAILURE causes full disability in nearly half the women who have it. Researchers are not certain of the reasons for this though believe several key factors are contributing to this trend. Among them are:

- **Delayed recognition of heart attack symptoms**   Though doctors have known for some time that women often experience heart attack differently than men, the classic heart attack symptoms of crushing CHEST PAIN and rapid collapse continue to dominate perceptions even among health-care providers. Women are more likely than men to experience heart attack with less specific symptoms, even when the resulting damage to the heart is significant.

- **Delays in seeking medical attention**   Women are less likely than men to suspect they are having heart attacks, partly because their symptoms may not fit the classic perceptions and partly because women, too, tend to believe that heart disease is more of a "man's problem." Women may be more willing to dismiss their symptoms as gastrointestinal or viral, or to wait to see whether they improve. Such delays allow the heart damage to become more extensive and reduce the likelihood of mitigating damage through the use of THROMBOLYTIC MEDICATIONS.

- **Increased obesity**   Though OBESITY is a health concern affecting men and women alike, more women have high BODY MASS INDEX (BMI) and women have higher BMI values. Health experts classify obesity as an independent RISK FACTOR for heart disease. Obesity directly contributes to HYPERTENSION (high blood pressure), ATHEROSCLEROSIS, CORONARY ARTERY DISEASE (CAD), CARDIOMYOPATHY, and HEART FAILURE as the additional weight pressures body structures and their functions and also requires the heart to increase its workload.

- **Increased sedentary lifestyle habits**   Women are increasingly less active physically, which has significant health consequences for cardiovascular disease as well as health overall. Physical inactivity contributes to hypertension, HYPERCHOLESTEROLEMIA (high blood cholesterol), diabetes, DEEP VEIN THROMBOSIS (DVT), PERIPHERAL VASCULAR DISEASE (PVD), and increased risk for heart attack and STROKE.

The Estrogen Effect

Researchers have long believed that ESTROGEN, the primary female HORMONE, provides a protective effect for a woman's CARDIOVASCULAR SYSTEM, though are unable to explain why this is. It is in part an extrapolation based on comparing the rates of heart disease in women before and after MENOPAUSE (when the woman's estrogen levels significantly decline). Until about age 60, a woman's risk of heart disease is three to four times less the risk of a man of comparable age and health status. In the first five years following menopause a woman's risk for heart disease and especially heart attack skyrockets past that of a man's, then returns to remain slightly less until she is in her mid-80s when the risk between men and women is again the same. Among the questions researchers have yet to answer adequately is whether there is a protective effect from estrogen or a detrimental effect from testosterone, the primary male hormone.

After Menopause

Until 1998 health experts recommended long-term HORMONE REPLACEMENT THERAPY (HRT) for women past menopause as a means of extending what was perceived to be estrogen's protective effect. The HEART AND ESTROGEN/PROGESTIN REPLACEMENT STUDY (HERS), completed in 1998, provided the first major body of objective clinical evidence that this effect was not what doctors assumed it to be and raised significant concerns about the relationship between HRT and heart disease in postmenopausal women. Four years later the HRT study of the WOMEN'S HEALTH INITIATIVE (WHI) was cut short when researchers realized the evidence was overwhelming that HRT not only did not provide protection against heart disease in women past menopause but that it in fact contributed to the accelerated development of heart disease (as well as some cancers). Doctors now recommend that women take HRT only if necessary to mitigate the discomforts of the menopause transition, and for the shortest length of time necessary to obtain relief. After menopause, health experts recommend that women follow lifestyle guidelines similar to those long in place for men:

- Eat a nutritious, low-fat diet.
- Get daily physical EXERCISE.
- Maintain a healthy weight.
- Regularly monitor blood cholesterol levels, blood pressure, and blood glucose levels (for diabetes).
- Avoid TOBACCO USE.

Symptoms of Heart Attack in Women

The classic presentation of heart attack is crushing chest pain followed by rapid incapacitation. Though many people experience heart attack in just this way, many—and most women—do not. A woman's experience of heart attack might instead feature:

- general feeling of discomfort
- weakness or tiredness
- achy discomfort in the left shoulder and jaw
- sensations similar to gastrointestinal distress
- chills and breaking into cold sweats

Such symptoms that persist for longer than 20 minutes should be evaluated as to whether they represent a heart attack or cardiac event (less than a full-fledged heart attack but stress to the heart), especially in women who are beyond menopause.

See also CHOLESTEROL, BLOOD; DIABETES AND HEART DISEASE; NURSES' HEALTH STUDY.

Women's Health Initiative (WHI) A long-term research program, launched in 1991, to improve treatment for and prevention of the leading causes of disease and death among women in the United States between the ages of 50 and 79. Those causes are identified as HEART DISEASE, breast cancer, colorectal cancer, and osteoporosis. More than 160,000 women are enrolled in the WHI, which is a combination of clinical research trials, observational studies, and a five-year community prevention study. The National Heart, Lung, and Blood Institute (NHLBI) of the National Institutes of Health (NIH) sponsors the WHI; the Fred Hutchinson Cancer Research Center in Seattle, Washington, is the clinical coordination center for the trials and studies.

Contact information for the WHI is:

Women's Health Initiative Program Office
1 Rockledge Centre
Suite 300, MS 7966
6705 Rockledge Drive
Bethesda, MD 20892-7966
(301) 402-2900
http://www.nhlbi.nih.gov/whi

In 2002 the WHI ended early its study of HORMONE REPLACEMENT THERAPY (HRT) and heart disease as data conclusively demonstrated that not only did HRT fail to provide cardiovascular benefits as long assumed, but also it conveyed a significantly increased risk for accelerated onset and severity of heart disease in women past menopause who took HRT. The WHI study corroborated the findings of the HERS completed in 1998. The landmark findings resulted in a reversal of recommendation for HRT, with health experts now taking the position that women should take HRT only for short-term relief of the discomforts associated with the transition to menopause, and for the shortest amount of time possible. The WHI HRT study findings made it clear that the risk for heart disease increases, rather than decreases, with extended HRT. The WHI study also showed that taking HRT for longer than five years also increases a woman's risk for endometrial (uterine) cancer.

See also FRAMINGHAM HEART STUDY; LIFESTYLE AND HEART HEALTH; NURSES' HEALTH STUDY; WOMEN AND HEART DISEASE.

X

xanthoma A benign (noncancerous) skin lesion that is common in people who have high BLOOD lipid levels (TRIGLYCERIDES and cholesterol) as well as diabetes. Xanthomas contain deposits of fatty tissue and can appear anywhere on the body though are most common at joints, on the eyelids, and on the hands and feet. The presence of xanthoma is a key indication of HYPERCHOLESTEROLEMIA, often familial. Though xanthomas have a characteristic appearance—flat, soft, and yellowish in color with distinct, palpable edges—doctors may choose to biopsy them to be certain they are xanthomas. Once a xanthoma forms it can be removed surgically if its appearance is undesirable or it is in a troublesome location, although xanthoma does not cause pain or other discomfort. Xanthomas have a tendency to grow back, particularly when blood lipid levels remain elevated.

See also CHOLESTEROL, BLOOD; HYPERCHOLESTEROLEMIA; HYPERLIPIDEMIA; HYPERTRIGLYCERIDEMIA.

xenograft A tissue or an organ transplant that comes from a different species, also called a xenotransplant. These grafts sometimes are referred to as bioprosthetics. Bovine (cow) or porcine (pig) heart valves are among the most common xenografts used in treating HEART DISEASE. These tissues are sterilized and prepared to remove proteins that might initiate an immune response in a human recipient. Typically bovine and porcine heart valves contain synthetic parts as well, as the tissue is not itself strong enough to support the valve's function when implanted in the human heart. Xenograft heart valves have a limited life expectancy of eight to 10 years, after which they must be replaced.

Cross-species organ transplants have not been successful in humans and raise a number of ethical questions. The effort that received widespread public attention was the attempt to transplant the heart of a baboon into an infant, known as Baby Faye, at California's Loma Linda Medical Center in 1994. Baby Faye was born with severe HYPOPLASTIC LEFT HEART SYNDROME (HLHS) and was certain to die without a HEART TRANSPLANT. Researchers hoped the baboon heart would at minimum serve as a "bridge" until a human donor heart became available, but Baby Faye's body strongly rejected the xenograft despite IMMUNOSUPPRESSIVE MEDICATIONS.

See also ALLOGRAFT; SURGERY TO TREAT CARDIOVASCULAR DISEASE; VALVE REPAIR AND REPLACEMENT.

yoga A centuries-old practice that integrates physical postures with meditation. The word *yoga* means "to yoke," a reference to the union of body and mind that yoga aspires to achieve. Yoga emphasizes the breath; all yoga postures incorporate focused breathing techniques to open the lungs and airways and improve the flow of oxygen, via the bloodstream, throughout the body. Yoga's MEDITATION component helps to quiet the mind and focus the thoughts, replacing stress and anxiety with a sense of calm. Performing yoga postures in structured sequences can provide an invigorating aerobic workout, improving physical flexibility and balance as well. When practiced regularly yoga provides physical and emotional benefits. The best way to learn yoga is to take classes; it is important to perform the postures correctly for maximum benefit as well as to prevent injury. As with any change in physical activity, it is a good idea to check with the doctor before embarking on yoga. The following four yoga postures are particularly beneficial for cardiovascular health.

- **Corpse pose** *(shavasana)* This yoga posture relaxes the body and clears the mind. It is a prone posture, though is not intended as a prelude to sleep. In corpse pose the focus first is on relaxing all of the muscles, from head to toe, then on clearing the mind, and lastly on the breath.

- **Mountain pose** *(tadasana)* This standing pose stretches and opens the body, improving breath control, OXYGENATION, and CIRCULATION. It also enhances balance.

- **Downward Facing Dog** *(adho mukha shvanasana)* This pose stretches the body, as the feet and hands are both on the floor with the tailbone to the sky. It can be modified for comfort with the knees and hands down and takes pressure from the heart.

- **Sun Salutation** *(surya namaskura)* This series of poses is performed in sequence, with emphasis on smooth, steady movements that transition from one pose to the next. When performed with speed, Sun Salutation provides a vigorous aerobic workout.

Many community centers, health centers, and senior centers provide classes in yoga that can teach these and other yoga poses. Search for a qualified teacher who can adapt poses to accommodate physical limitations as well as improved strength and flexibility after yoga becomes part of the everyday routine.

See also EXERCISE; STRESS AND HEART DISEASE; STRESS REDUCTION TECHNIQUES.

APPENDIXES

APPENDIX I
ORGANIZATIONS AND RESOURCES

Heart Health Information

American Heart Association
1701 North Beauregard Street
Alexandria, VA 22311
(800) DIABETES (or [800] 342-2383)
http://www.diabetes.org

American Heart Association
National Center
7272 Greenville Avenue
Dallas, TX 75231
(800) AHA-USA-1 (or [800] 242-8721)
http://www.americanheart.org

American Lung Association
1301 Pennsylvania Avenue NW
Washington, DC 20004
(202) 785-3355
http://www.lungusa.org

American Stroke Association
7272 Greenville Avenue
Dallas, TX 75231
(888) 4-STROKE (or [888] 478-7653)
http://www.strokeassociation.org

Centers for Disease Control and Prevention
1600 Clifton Road
Atlanta, GA 30333
(800) CDC-INFO or
(800) 232-4636
http://www.cdc.gov

National Center for Complementary and Alternative Medicine (NCCAM)
National Institutes of Health
9000 Rockville Pike
Bethesda, MD 20892
(888) 644-6226 (toll-free voice)

(866) 464-3615 (toll-free TTY)
http://www.nccam.nih.gov

National Cholesterol Education Program (NCEP)
NHLBI Health Information Network
P.O. Box 30105
Bethesda, MD 20824-0105
(301) 592-8573
http://www.nhlbi.nih.gov

National Heart, Lung, and Blood Institute (NHLBI)
NHLBI Health Information Network
P.O. Box 30105
Bethesda, MD 20824-0105
(301) 592-8573 (voice)
(240) 629-3255 (TTY)
http://www.nhlbi.nih.gov

National Institute of Neurological Disorders and Stroke (NINDS)
P.O. Box 5801
Bethesda, MD 20824
(800) 352-9424 (toll-free) or (301) 496-5751
(301) 468-5981 (TTY)
http://www.ninds.nih.gov

National Institutes of Health (NIH)
9000 Rockville Pike
Bethesda, MD 20892
(301) 496-4000
http://www.nih.gov

National Library of Medicine
8600 Rockville Pike
Bethesda, MD 20894
(888) 346-3656 or (301) 594-5983
http://www.nlm.nih.gov

United Network for Organ Sharing (UNOS)
700 North Fourth Street
Richmond, Virginia 23219
(888) 894-6361 (toll-free)
http://www.unos.org

WomenHeart: The National Coalition for Women with Heart Disease
818 18th Street NW
Suite 1000
Washington, DC 20006
(202) 728-7199 or (877) 771-0030 (toll-free)
http://www.womenheart.org

PROFESSIONAL ORGANIZATIONS

American Board of Internal Medicine
510 Walnut Street
Suite 1700
Philadelphia, PA 19106
(800) 441-ABIM (2246) or (215) 446-3500
http://www.abim.org

American Board of Thoracic Surgery
633 St. Clair Street
Suite 232
Chicago, IL 60611
(312) 202-5900
http://www.abts.org

American College of Cardiology
Heart House
2400 N Street NW
Washington, DC 20037
(800) 253-4636
http://www.acc.org

American College of Physicians
190 North Independence Mall West
Philadelphia, PA 19106-1572
(800) 523-1546 or (215) 351-2600
http://www.acponline.org

American Medical Association
515 North State Street
Chicago, IL 60654
(800) 621-8335
http://www.ama-assn.org

Association of Black Cardiologists
5355 Hunter Road
Atlanta, GA 30349

(404) 201-6600
http://www.abcardio.org

Heart Rhythm Society
7400 K Street NW
Suite 500
Washington, DC 20005
(202) 464-3400
www.hrsonline.org

Society of Thoracic Surgeons
633 North St. Clair Street
Suite 2320
Chicago, IL 60611-3658
(312) 202-5800
http://www.sts.org

WEB-SITE-BASED INTERNET RESOURCES

Children's Heart Society
http://www.childrensheart.org

Congenital Heart Information Network
http://www.tchin.org

Healthfinder
http://www.healthfinder.gov/

MEDLINE Plus Health Information
http://www.nlm.nih.gov/medlineplus/

The Healthy Refrigerator: Open the Door to a Healthy Heart
http://www.healthyfridge.org

CLINICAL RESEARCH STUDY INFORMATION

National Institutes of Health
Clinical Trials Database
http://www.clinicaltrials.gov

Women's Health Initiative (WHI)
2 Rockledge Centre
Suite 1018, MS 7936
6701 Rockledge Drive
Bethesda, Maryland 20892-7936
(301) 402-2900
http://www.nhlbi.nih.gov/whi

WORKPLACE AND DISABILITY

Americans with Disabilities Act (ADA)
U.S. Department of Justice

950 Pennsylvania Avenue NW
Civil Rights Division, Disability Rights
    Section—NYA
Washington, DC 20530
(800) 514-0301 (voice)
(800) 514-0383 (TTY)
http://www.ada.gov

U.S. Department of Labor
Office of Disability Employment Policy
200 Constitution Avenue NW
Washington, DC 20210
(866) 4-USA-DOL
or (866) 487-2365
http://www.dol.gov/odep/

APPENDIX II
COMMON ABBREVIATIONS AND SYMBOLS

α alpha

AAA   abdominal aortic aneurysm

ACE   angiotensin-converting enzyme

ADL   activities of daily living

AIDS   acquired immunodeficiency syndrome

AED   automated external defibrillator

AHA   American Heart Association

ALLTHAT   Antihypertensive and Lipid-Lowering Treatment to Prevent Heart Attack Trial

AMA   American Medical Association

APLS   antiphospholipid syndrome

AV   atrioventricular

β beta

BMI   body mass index

BVAD   biventricular assist device

Ca   calcium

CABG   coronary artery bypass graft

CAD   coronary artery disease

CHD   coronary heart disease; congestive heart disease

CHF   congestive heart failure

CICU   cardiac intensive care unit

COPD   chronic obstructive pulmonary disease

CPR   cardiopulmonary resuscitation

CT   computed tomography

CVA   cerebrovascular accident

CVD   cardiovascular disease; cerebrovascular disease

DASH   Dietary Approaches to Stop Hypertension

DGA   digital cardiac angiography

DNR   do not resuscitate

DPHC   durable power of attorney for health care

DSA   digital subtraction angiography

DVT   deep vein thrombosis

EBCT   electron beam computed tomography

ECC   emergency cardiovascular care

ECG   electrocardiogram

ED   erectile dysfunction; emergency department

EECP   enhanced external counterpulsation

EEG   electroencephalogram

EPO   erythropoietin

ERT   estrogen replacement therapy

FDA   U.S. Food and Drug Administration

HCM   hypertrophic cardiomyopathy

HCTZ   hydrochlorothiazide

HDL   high-density lipoprotein

HERS   Heart and Estrogen/Progestin Replacement Study

HLHS   hyperplastic left heart syndrome

HIV   human immunodeficiency virus

HOCM   hypertrophic obstructive cardiomyopathy

HRT   hormone replacement therapy

IABP   intra-aortic balloon pump

ICD   implantable cardioverter defibrillator

IHD   ischemic heart disease

IHSS   idiopathic hypertrophic subaortic stenosis

IND   investigational new drug

K   potassium

LDL   low-density lipoprotein

LQTS   long QT syndrome

LVAD   left ventricular assist device

LVEF   left ventricular ejection fraction

MAOI   monoamine oxidase inhibitor

MCS   mechanical circulatory support

Mg   magnesium

MET   metabolic equivalent

MI   myocardial infarction

MRI   magnetic resonance imaging

MVP   mitral valve prolapse

MUGA   multi-unit gated acquisition

Na   sodium

NCCAM   National Center for Complementary and Alternative Medicine

NCEP   National Cholesterol Education Program

NHLBI   National Heart, Lung, and Blood Institute

NINDS National Institute of Neurological Disorders and Stroke

NSAID nonsteroidal anti-inflammatory drug

NTI narrow therapeutic index

NYHA New York Heart Association

PCTA percutaneous transluminal coronary angioplasty

PDA patent ductus arteriosus

PET positron emission tomography

PPH primary pulmonary hypertension

PVD peripheral vascular disease

PVC premature ventricular contraction

RAA renin-angiotensin-aldosterone

RVAD right ventricular assist device

SA sinoatrial

SASD sudden arrhythmia death syndrome

SAECG signal-averaged electrocardiogram

SCA sudden cardiac arrest

SNF skilled nursing facility

SPECT single photon emission computed tomography

SSRI selective serotonin reuptake inhibitor

SUDS sudden unexpected death syndrome

TdP Torsades de Pointes

TEE transesophageal echocardiography

TGA transposition of the great arteries

TIA transient ischemic attack

TMLR transmyocardial laser revascularization

tPA tissue plasminogen activator

VLDL very low-density lipoprotein

VSD ventricular septal defect

WHI Women's Health Initiative

APPENDIX III
DIAGRAMS

Location and structure of the heart

The heart is a muscular organ that pumps blood around the body. It is located between the lungs, and two-thirds of the heart lies to the left of the body's midline. It is shaped like a closed fist and sits in a loose-fitting membrane called the pericardium or pericardial sac.

Chambers of the heart

The heart has four chambers: two atria (upper chambers) and two ventricles (lower chambers).
The four chambers are the

a right atrium;
b right ventricle;
c left atrium; and
d left ventricle.

Blood vessels of the heart

These are the

e superior vena cava;
f inferior vena cava;
g aorta;
h pulmonary artery; and
i pulmonary vein.

Heart valves

These are the
j aortic valve;
k tricuspid valve;
l mitral valve; and
m pulmonary valve.

Heart wall

The heart wall consists of the
n epicardium;
o myocardium; and
p endocardium.

The myocardium is muscle tissue and makes up the bulk of the heart:
q pericardial cavity;
r serous pericardium; and
s fibrous pericardium.

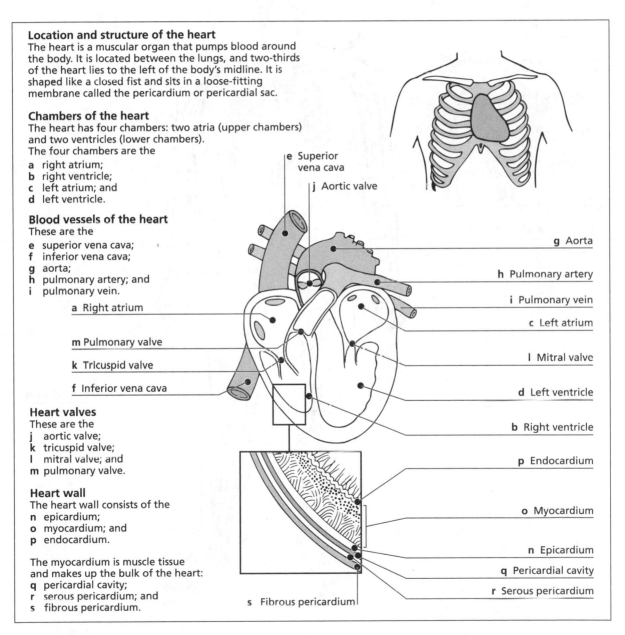

e Superior vena cava

j Aortic valve

g Aorta

h Pulmonary artery

i Pulmonary vein

c Left atrium

l Mitral valve

d Left ventricle

b Right ventricle

p Endocardium

o Myocardium

n Epicardium

q Pericardial cavity

r Serous pericardium

a Right atrium

m Pulmonary valve

k Tricuspid valve

f Inferior vena cava

s Fibrous pericardium

Anterior View Showing Major Arteries (white) and Veins (black)

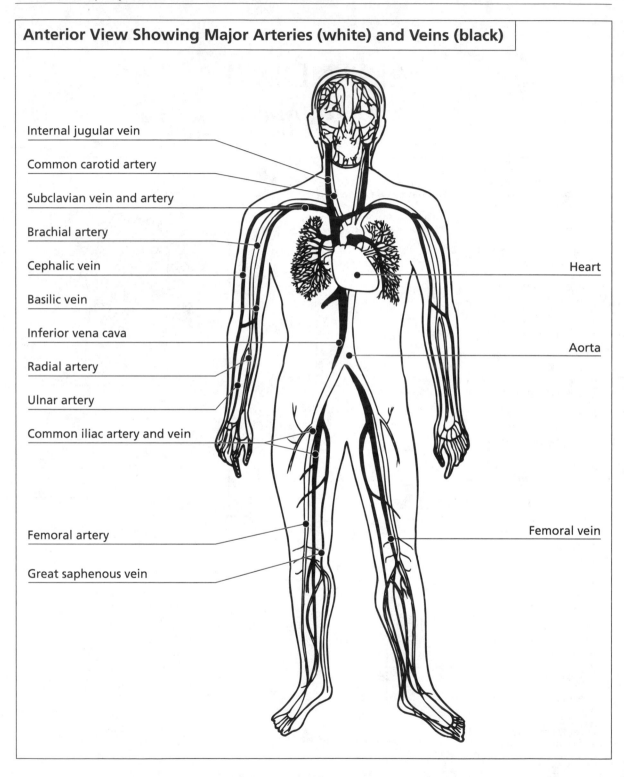

Internal jugular vein

Common carotid artery

Subclavian vein and artery

Brachial artery

Cephalic vein

Basilic vein

Inferior vena cava

Radial artery

Ulnar artery

Common iliac artery and vein

Femoral artery

Great saphenous vein

Heart

Aorta

Femoral vein

Anterior View

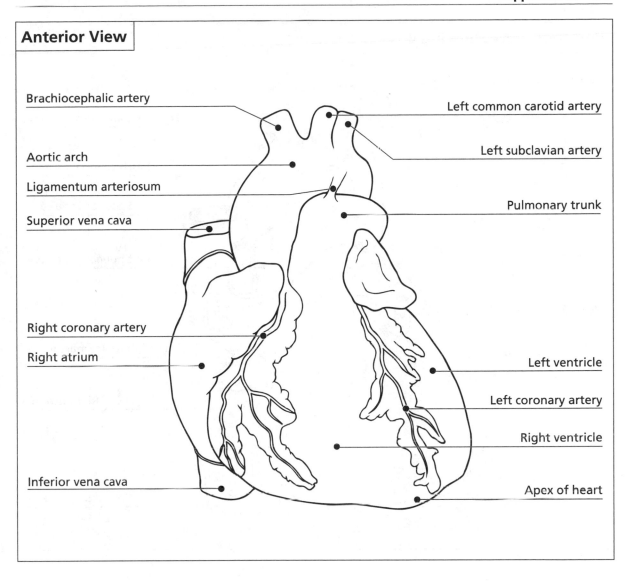

Brachiocephalic artery

Aortic arch

Ligamentum arteriosum

Superior vena cava

Right coronary artery

Right atrium

Inferior vena cava

Left common carotid artery

Left subclavian artery

Pulmonary trunk

Left ventricle

Left coronary artery

Right ventricle

Apex of heart

Posterior View Showing Base of the Heart

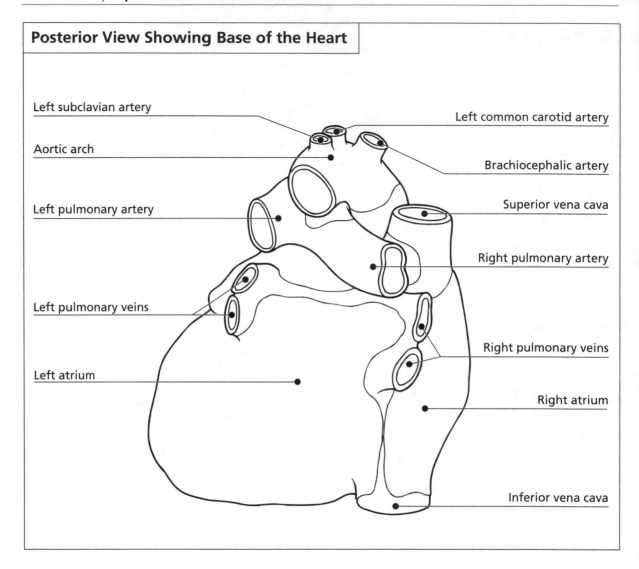

Left subclavian artery

Left common carotid artery

Aortic arch

Brachiocephalic artery

Left pulmonary artery

Superior vena cava

Right pulmonary artery

Left pulmonary veins

Left atrium

Right pulmonary veins

Right atrium

Inferior vena cava

Section Showing Blood Flow through Atria and Ventricles

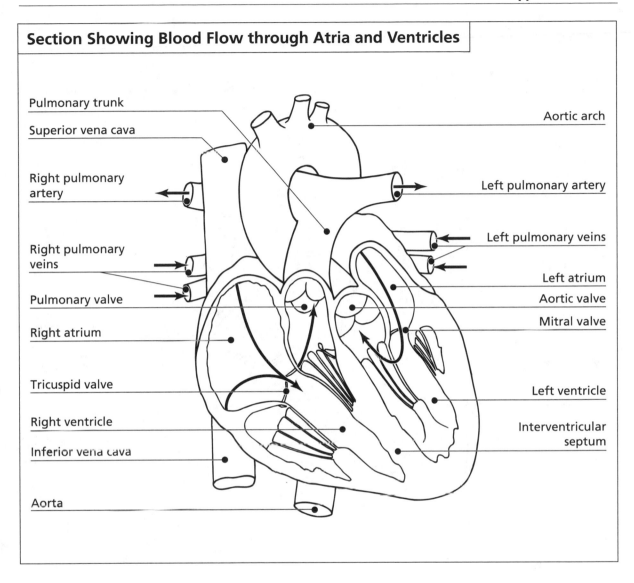

Pulmonary trunk

Superior vena cava

Right pulmonary artery

Right pulmonary veins

Pulmonary valve

Right atrium

Tricuspid valve

Right ventricle

Inferior vena cava

Aorta

Aortic arch

Left pulmonary artery

Left pulmonary veins

Left atrium

Aortic valve

Mitral valve

Left ventricle

Interventricular septum

Section Showing Impulse-Conducting System

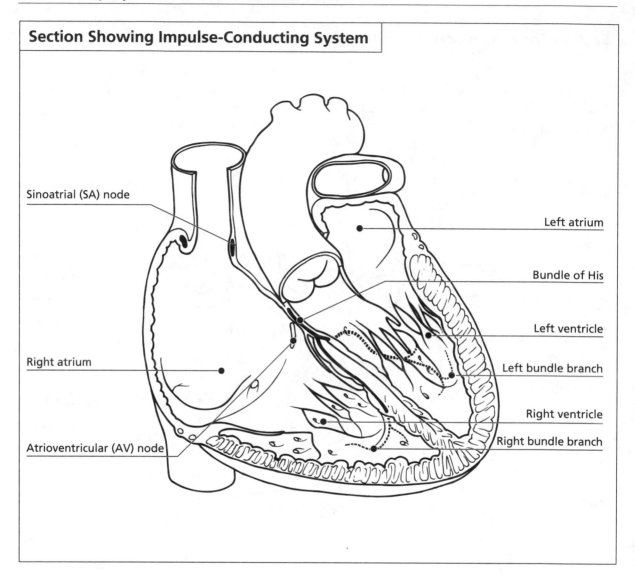

Sinoatrial (SA) node

Right atrium

Atrioventricular (AV) node

Left atrium

Bundle of His

Left ventricle

Left bundle branch

Right ventricle

Right bundle branch

Circulation in Pulmonary Veins and Left Heart

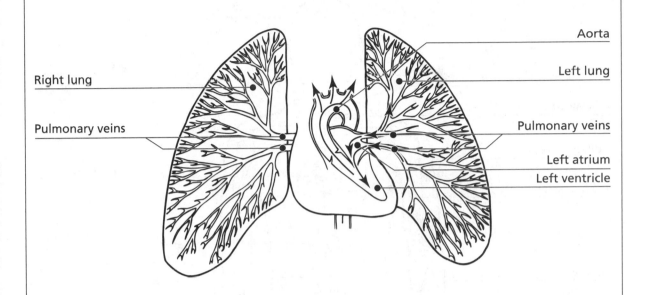

Right lung

Pulmonary veins

Aorta

Left lung

Pulmonary veins

Left atrium

Left ventricle

Circulation in right heart and pulmonary artery

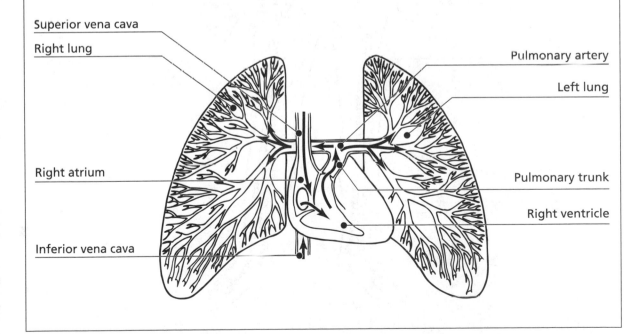

Superior vena cava

Right lung

Right atrium

Inferior vena cava

Pulmonary artery

Left lung

Pulmonary trunk

Right ventricle

Anterior View, Showing Arteries

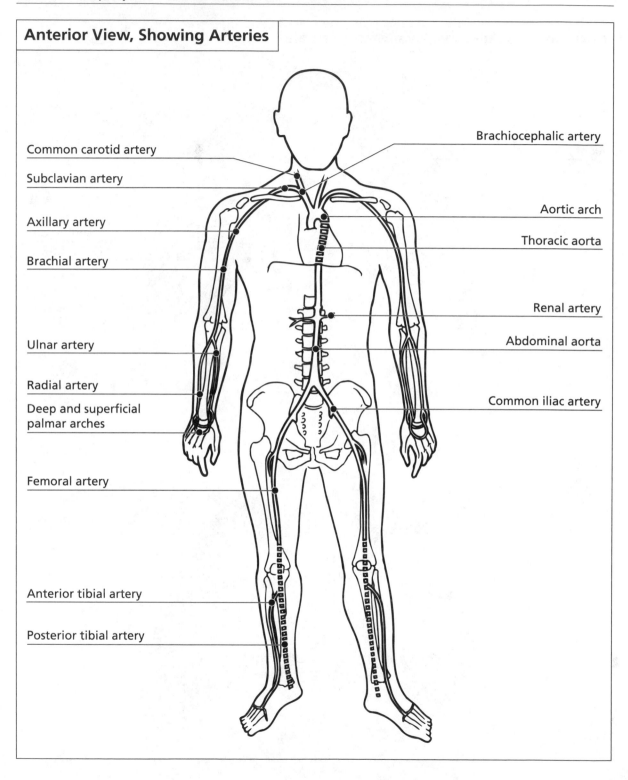

Common carotid artery

Subclavian artery

Axillary artery

Brachial artery

Ulnar artery

Radial artery

Deep and superficial
palmar arches

Femoral artery

Anterior tibial artery

Posterior tibial artery

Brachiocephalic artery

Aortic arch

Thoracic aorta

Renal artery

Abdominal aorta

Common iliac artery

Anterior View, Showing Veins

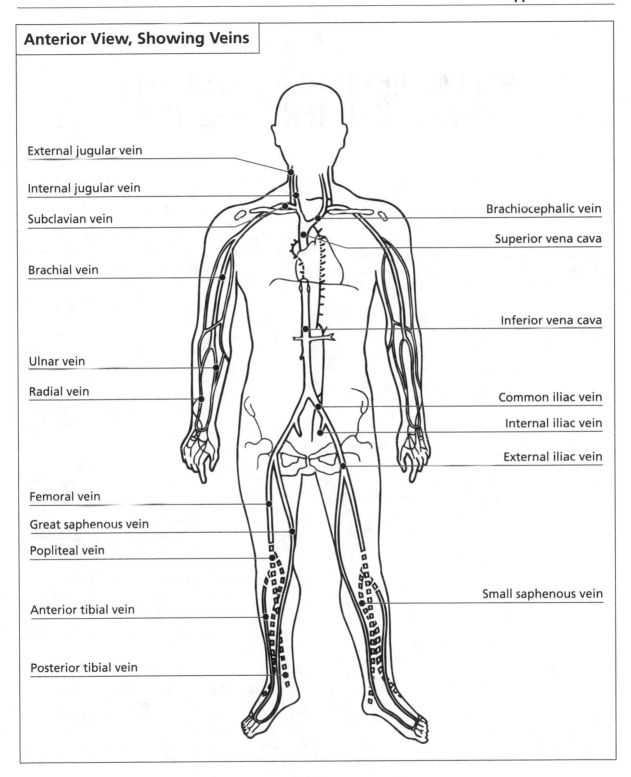

External jugular vein

Internal jugular vein

Subclavian vein

Brachial vein

Ulnar vein

Radial vein

Femoral vein

Great saphenous vein

Popliteal vein

Anterior tibial vein

Posterior tibial vein

Brachiocephalic vein

Superior vena cava

Inferior vena cava

Common iliac vein

Internal iliac vein

External iliac vein

Small saphenous vein

SELECTED BIBLIOGRAPHY
AND FURTHER READING

BOOKS: CLINICAL

Armstrong, William F., and Thomas Ryan. *Feigenbaum's Echocardiography*. 7th ed. *New York: Lippencott Williams & Wilkins*, 2009.

Artman, Michael, D. Woodrow Benson, Deepak Srivastava, and Makoto Nakazawa, eds. *Cardiovascular Development and Congenital Malformations: Molecular and Genetic Mechanisms*. Malden, Mass.: Blackwell Futura, 2005.

Ballantyne, Christie M. *Clinical Lipidology: A Companion to Braunwald's Heart Disease*. Philadelphia: Saunders Elsevier, 2008.

Cohn, Lawrence. *Cardiac Surgery in the Adult*. 3rd ed. New York: McGraw-Hill Professional, 2007.

Davidson, Michael H., Peter P. Toth, and Kevin C. Maki, eds. *Therapeutic Lipidology*. Totowa, N.J.: Humana Press, 2007.

Dzau, Victor J., and Choong-Chin Liew, eds. *Cardiovascular Genetics and Genomics for the Cardiologist*. Malden, Mass.: Blackwell Futura, 2007.

Fogoros, Richard N. *Electrophysiologic Testing*. 4th ed. Oxford, U.K.: Wiley-Blackwell, 2006.

Hoffman, Julien. *The Natural and Unnatural History of Congenital Heart Disease*. Oxford, U.K.: Wiley-Blackwell, 2009.

Houston, Mark. *Handbook of Hypertension*. Oxford, U.K.: Wiley-Blackwell, 2009.

Furster, Valentin, Robert O'Rourke, Richard Walsh, and Phillip Poole-Wilson. *Hurst's The Heart*. 12th ed. New York: McGraw-Hill Professional, 2007.

Klein, Allan L. W., and Mario J. Garcia. *Diastology: Clinical Approach to Diastolic Heart Failure*. Philadelphia: Saunders Elsevier, 2008.

Leri, Annarosa, Piero Anversa, and William H. Frishman, eds. *Cardiovascular Regeneration and Stem Cell Therapy*. Malden, Mass.: Blackwell Futura, 2007.

Libby, Peter, Robert O. Bonow, Douglas L. Mann, and Douglas P. Zipes, eds. *Braunwald's Heart Disease: A Textbook of Cardiovascular Medicine*. 8th ed. Philadelphia: Saunders Elsevier, 2007.

Nichols, David G. et al. *Critical Heart Disease in Infants and Children*. 2nd ed. Philadelphia: Mosby, 2006.

Otto, Catherine M. *Textbook of Clinical Echocardiography*. 4th ed. Philadelphia: Saunders Elsevier, 2009.

Otto, Catherine M., and Robert O. Bonow. *Valvular Heart Disease: A Companion to Braunwald's Heart Disease*. 3rd ed. Philadelphia: Saunders Elsevier, 2009.

Perloff, Joseph K., John S. Child, and Jamil Aboulhosn. *Congenital Heart Disease in Adults*. 3rd ed. Philadelphia: Saunders Elsevier, 2008.

Polak, Joseph F. *Peripheral Vascular Sonography: A Practical Guide*. 2nd ed. New York: Lippencott Williams & Wilkins, 2004.

Roden, Dan M., ed. *Cardiovascular Genetics and Genomics*. Oxford, U.K.: Wiley-Blackwell, 2009.

Rudolph, Abraham. *Congenital Diseases of the Heart: Clinical-Physiological Considerations*. 3rd ed. Oxford, U.K.: Wiley-Blackwell, 2009.

Surawicz, Borys, and Timothy Knilans. *Chou's Electrocardiography in Clinical Practice*. 6th ed. Philadelphia: Saunders Elsevier, 2008.

Toth, Peter P., and Kevin C. Maki. *Practical Lipid Management: Concepts and Controversies*. Oxford, U.K.: Wiley-Blackwell, 2008.

West, John B. *Respiratory Physiology: The Essentials*. New York: Lippencott Williams & Wilkins, 2008.

Wilber, David J., Douglas L. Packer, and William G. Stevenson, eds. *Catheter Ablation of Cardiac Arrhythmias: Basic Concepts and Clinical Applications*. 3rd ed. Oxford, U.K.: Wiley-Blackwell, 2008.

Wilcox, Benson R., Andrew C. Cook, and Robert H. Anderson. *Surgical Anatomy of the Heart*. Cambridge: Cambridge University Press, 2005.

Zipes, Douglas P., and Jose Jalif. *Cardiac Electrophysiology: From Cell to Bedside*. 5th ed. Philadelphia: Saunders Elsevier, 2009.

BOOKS: GENERAL

Cannon, Christopher P., and Elizabeth Vierck. *The New Heart Disease Handbook: Everything You Need to Know to Effectively Reverse and Manage Heart Disease*. Beverly, Mass.: Fair Winds Press, 2009.

Cutlip, M. Laurel with Sari Budgazad. *The Cardiac Recovery Cookbook: Heart Healty Recipes for Life after Heart*

Attack or Heart Surgery. New York: Hatherleigh Press, 2005.

Chilnick, Lawrence D. *The First Year: Heart Disease, An Essential Guide for the Newly Diagnosed.* Philadelphia: De Capo Press, 2008.

Fisher, Miles, ed. *Heart Disease and Diabetes.* New York: Oxford University Press, 2009.

Gerber, Max S. *My Heart vs. the Real World: Children with Heart Disease, in Photographs & Interviews.* Cold Spring Harbor, N.Y.: Cold Spring Harbor Laboratory Press, 2008.

Granato, Jerome E. *Living with Coronary Heart Disease: A Guide for Patients and Families.* Baltimore: The Johns Hopkins University Press, 2008.

Heller, Marla. *The DASH Diet Action Plan: Based on the National Institutes of Health Research: Dietary Approaches to Stop Hypertension.* Deerfield, Ill.: Amidon Press, 2007.

Kligfield, Paul. *The Cardiac Recovery Handbook: The Complete Guide to Life after Heart Attack or Heart Surgery.* 2nd ed. New York: Hatherleigh Press, 2006.

Lyle, Theresa A. *Balancing Your Life with Congenital Heart Disease.* Atlanta, Ga.: Pritchett & Hull Associates, 2009.

McRae, Donald. *Every Second Counts: The Race to Transplant the First Human Heart.* New York: Berkley Trade, 2007.

Monagan, David, with David O. Williams. *Journey into the Heart: A Tale of Pioneering Doctors and Their Race to Transform Cardiovascular Medicine.* New York: Gotham Books/Penguin, 2007.

Phibbs, Brendan. *The Human Heart: A Basic Guide to Heart Disease.* 2nd ed. New York: Lippencott Williams & Wilkins, 2007.

Piscatella, Joseph C. *The Healthy Heart Cookbook: Over 700 Recipes for Every Day and Every Occasion.* New York: Black Dog & Leventhal Publishers, 2004.

Stoney, William S. *Pioneers of Cardiac Surgery.* Nashville, Tenn.: Vanderbilt University Press, 2008.

JOURNALS

Alberti, K.G.M.M., et al. "Harmonizing the Metabolic Syndrome: A Joint Interim Statement of the International Diabetes Federation Task Force on Epidemiology and Prevention; National Heart, Lung, and Blood Institute; American Heart Association; World Heart Federation; International Atherosclerosis Society; and International Association for the Study of Obesity." *Circulation* 120 (2009): 1,640–1,645.

———. "Heart Disease and Stroke Statistics: Our Guide to Current Statistics and the Supplement to Our *Heart and Stroke Facts,* 2009 Update At-A-Glance."

Arnett, Donna K., et al. "AHA Scientific Statement: Relevance of Genetics and Genomics for Prevention and Treatment of Cardiovascular Disease." *Circulation* 115 (2007): 2,878–2,901.

Cambien, François, and Laurence Tiret. "Genetics of Cardiovascular Diseases: From Single Mutations to the Whole Genome." *Circulation* 116 (2007): 1,714–1,724.

Cassaburi, Richard, and Richard ZuWallack. "Pulmonary Rehabilitation for Management of Chronic Obstructive Pulmonary Disease." *The New England Journal of Medicine* 360 (2009): 1,329–1,335.

Chen, Huei-Sheng Vincent, Changsung Kim, and Mark Mercola. "Electrophysiological Challenges of Cell-Based Myocardial Repair." *Circulation* 120 (2009): 2,496–2,508.

Ding, Keyue, and Iftikhar J. Kullo. "Evolutionary Genetics of Coronary Heart Disease." *Circulation* 119 (2009): 459–467.

Fletcher, Barbara, et al. AHA Scientific Statement: Managing Abnormal Blood Lipids, A Collaborative Approach." *Circulation* 112 (2005): 3,184–3,209.

Gidding, Samuel S., et al. "Implementing American Heart Association Pediatric and Adult Nutrition Guidelines: A Scientific Statement from the American Heart Association Nutrition Committee of the Council on Nutrition, Physical Activity and Metabolism, Council on Cardiovascular Disease in the Young, Council on Arteriosclerosis, Thrombosis and Vascular Biology, Council on Cardiovascular Nursing, Council on Epidemiology and Prevention, and Council for High Blood Pressure Research." *Circulation* 119 (2009): 1,161–1,175.

Grundy, Scott M., et al. "Diagnosis and Management of the Metabolic Syndrome: An American Heart Association/National Heart, Lung, and Blood Institute Scientific Statement: Executive Summary." *Circulation* 112 (2005): e285–e290.

Haïssaguerre, Michel, et al. "Sudden Cardiac Arrest Associated with Early Repolarization." *The New England Journal of Medicine* 358 (2008): 2,016–2,023.

Lichtenstein, Alice H., et al. "Diet and Lifestyle Recommendations Revision 2006: A Scientific Statement from the American Heart Association Nutrition Committee." *Circulation* 114 (2006): 82–96.

Mosca, Lori, et al. "Evidence-Based Guidelines for Cardiovascular Disease Prevention in Women: 2007 Update." *Circulation* 115 (2007): 1,481–1,501.

Moss, Arthur, et al. "Cardiac Resynchronization Therapy for Prevention of Heart-Failure Events." *The New England Journal of Medicine* 361 (2009): 1,329–1,338.

Pelliccia, Antonio, et al. "Outcomes in Athletes with Marked ECG Repolarization Abnormalities." *The New England Journal of Medicine* 358 (2008): 152–161.

Poirier, Paul, et al. "AHA Scientific Statement: Obesity and Cardiovascular Disease: Pathophysiology, Evaluation and Effect of Weight Loss." *Circulation* 113 (2006): 898–918.

INDEX